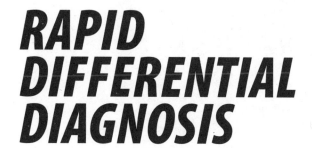

RAPID
DIFFERENTIAL
DIAGNOSIS

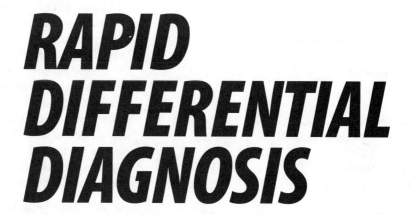

RAPID DIFFERENTIAL DIAGNOSIS

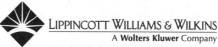

LIPPINCOTT WILLIAMS & WILKINS
A **Wolters Kluwer** Company

Philadelphia • Baltimore • New York • London
Buenos Aires • Hong Kong • Sydney • Tokyo

STAFF

Publisher
Judith A. Schilling McCann, RN, MSN

Editorial Director
David Moreau

Clinical Director
Joan M. Robinson, RN, MSN, CCRN

Senior Art Director
Arlene Putterman

Clinical Editors
Kate McGovern (project manager), RN, BSN, CCRN;
Laura Herm, RN; Colleen Fries, RN, MSN, CCRN, CRNP;
Jill Curry, RN, BSN; Deborah Becker, RN, MSN, CCRN, CRNP, CS

Editors
Jaime Stockslager (senior associate editor), Ty Eggenberger,
Kevin Haworth, Julie Munden

Copy Editors
Peggy Williams (supervisor), Kimberly Bilotta, Scotti Cohn,
Shana Harrington, Marcia Ryan

Designers
Susan Hopkins Rodzewich (book designer), Linda Franklin,
Donna S. Morris, Susan L. Sheridan

Editor (electronic products)
Liz Schaeffer

Electronic Production Services
Diane Paluba (manager), Joyce Rossi Biletz

Manufacturing
Patricia K. Dorshaw (senior manager), Beth Janae Orr

Editorial Assistants
Danielle J. Barsky, Beverly Lane, Linda Ruhf

Indexer
Barbara Hodgson

The clinical procedures described and recommended in this publication are based on research and consultation with medical and nursing authorities. To the best of our knowledge, these procedures reflect currently accepted clinical practice; nevertheless, they can't be considered absolute and universal recommendations. For individual application, treatment recommendations must be considered in light of the patient's clinical condition and, before administration of new or infrequently used drugs, in light of the latest package-insert information. The authors and the publisher disclaim responsibility for any adverse effects resulting directly or indirectly from the suggested procedures, from any undetected errors, or from the reader's misunderstanding of the text.

Printed in the United States of America.

RDD – D N O S A J J M A M F J

04 03 02   10 9 8 7 6 5 4 3 2 1

Library of Congress Cataloging-in-Publication Data

Rapid differential diagnosis.
    p. : cm.
    Includes index.
1. Diagnosis, Differential — Handbooks, manuals, etc. 2. Nurse practitioners — Handbooks, manual, etc. I. Lippincott Williams & Wilkins.
    [DNLM: 1. Diagnosis, Differential — Nurses' Instruction. 2. Nurse Practitioners — Nurses' Instruction. WB 141.5 R218 2002]
RC71.5 .R37 2002
616.07'5—dc21
ISBN 1-58255-174-X (alk. paper)   2001050825

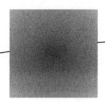

Contents

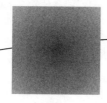

Contributors

W. Chad Barefoot, MSN, CRNP
Acute Care Nurse Practitioner
Abington (Pa.) Pulmonary and Critical Care Associates

Joseph L. DuFour, RN, MS, CS, FNP
Lecturer
Nurse Practitioner
State University of New York at New Paltz

M. Susan Emerson, RN, PhD, ACNP, ANP, CNS, CS
Clinical Assistant Professor
University of Missouri
Kansas City, Mo.

Eileen R. Giardino, RN, PhD, CRNP
Associate Professor
LaSalle University
Philadelphia

April Lewis, MS, NP
Acute Care Nurse
Adult Nurse Practitioner
Johns Hopkins Hospital — Urgent Care
Baltimore

Ellen Mangin, RN, MSN, CRNP, CS
Director of Resident Care
Rydal Park of Philadelphia Presbyterian Homes

Debi Murphy, MSN, CRNP
Stroke Program Research Coordinator
Abington (Pa.) Memorial Hospital

Maryellen Stahley-Brown, MSN, CRNP
Nurse Practitioner
Concentra Medical Center
Baltimore

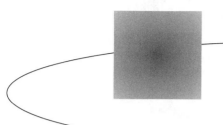

Foreword

Dramatic changes in health care over the last several decades have afforded nurse practitioners (NPs) unique opportunities as health care providers. With each opportunity, however, a challenge emerges. The greatest challenge for NPs throughout these changing times has been to render exceptional health care in an efficient, cost-effective manner — one of the most difficult aspects of which is the ability to arrive at a correct differential diagnosis in a timely fashion.

When a patient presents with a clear diagnosis, an NP can choose from many protocol references that adequately outline the appropriate treatment. However, when a patient presents with a symptom, as is more often the case, an NP needs a resource with well-organized, straightforward, and manageable information that will expedite her arrival at an appropriate differential diagnosis — without the overwhelmingly detailed information found in medical texts.

That resource is finally here! *Rapid Differential Diagnosis* is practical, concise, and current. Easy to use and loaded with useful information, this revolutionary reference is essential for every NP — from the anxious novice to the seasoned veteran.

As NPs, we follow the cues of our patients' chief complaints to guide our algorithms of health care. Using a primary sign or symptom as a starting point, we advance through the history of the present illness and the focused physical examination — all the time picking up clues that lead us to our diagnosis. What makes *Rapid Differential Diagnosis* so helpful is that its format is based on this familiar diagnostic process.

Both the student learner and the novice NP find the book an indispensable partner in their evolving professions. It provides easy access to the authoritative and invaluable information they can't do without.

The unique presentation of information in *Rapid Differential Diagnosis* appeals to all types of health care practitioners, including nurses, medical students, and physician assistants. It's also an excellent reference for health care professionals who are treating patients with specific symptoms but elusive diagnoses.

Each entry in the book follows a standard format that begins with an introduction to and description of the specific sign or symptom. It goes on to discuss specific information related to the history and physical examination, providing relevant questions that will help guide diagnosis. The more than 200 signs and symptoms covered in the book are presented alphabetically, making them easy to find and saving the NP even more time.

Each sign or symptom is accompanied by a chart that leads the NP through the diagnostic process. Beginning with a common symptom, each chart quickly and easily guides the practitioner to an accurate differential diagnosis. But the information doesn't end there. Each diagnosis is expanded by the addition of its corresponding diagnostic tests, treatments, and follow-up, ensuring that the NP considers all possibilities and makes sound and rational patient care decisions.

More so than other health care providers, NPs focus on preventive heath care rather than disease management. We never forget that a disease is a symptom long before it becomes a diagnosis and that preventive health care begins at the level of the symptom, not the diagnosis. *Rapid Differential Diagnosis* will help NPs deliver excellent health care one symptom and one correct diagnosis at a time.

Joyce E. Clement, MSN, ANP, CS, FNP
Clinical Instructor, Family Nurse Practitioner Program
University of Missouri-Kansas City School of Nursing
Family Practice and Gynecology
Joplin

Judy Willis Hileman, PhD, ARNP
Clinical Assistant Professor
University of Missouri-Kansas City School of Nursing
Parish and Hospice Nursing

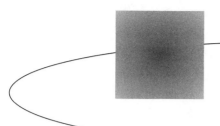

How to use this book

One of your most important roles as an NP is to arrive at an accurate diagnosis based on a patient's history, physical examination, and diagnostic test results — all in a timely manner. *Rapid Differential Diagnosis* will help you accomplish this difficult task by putting thousands of indispensable facts about more than 200 signs and symptoms, their possible causes, and the diagnostic tests that can confirm potential diagnoses at your fingertips.

In this book, you'll find several timesaving features designed to aid you in your quest for a quick diagnosis:
- practical organization — entries are alphabetically arranged by presenting sign or symptom
- unique layout — most entries take up a single two-page spread, with text on the left and a flowchart on the right
- bulleted lists — the flowcharts are easy to read, shaving valuable minutes off your diagnosis time.

The text

The left-hand page of each entry begins with a concise description of the sign or symptom. This information is enhanced by the "History and physical examination" section, which provides step-by-step guidance for exploring the patient's chief complaint.

Also included on the left-hand pages are easy-to-spot icons that highlight important details:
- *Pediatric pointers* and *Elder care cues* identify special findings, tests, causes, and follow-up care specific to each population. They also call attention to age-related circumstances or conditions that can influence the meaning or severity of a sign or symptom.
- *Women's health tips* distinguish differences that you may need to keep in mind when diagnosing and caring for a female patient.

The flowchart

Each sign or symptom discussed in the book contains at least one flowchart that will lead you through the process of diagnosis. Signs and symptoms that may present in more than one way, such as coughing (which can be barking, nonproductive, or productive), have three associated flowcharts.

Each flowchart begins at the top with the patient's presenting sign or symptom. It then guides you through the diagnostic process, beginning with the history of present illness (HPI) and the focused physical examination (PE), which lists areas that you should concentrate on while performing the assessment.

The flowchart then directs you to and provides valuable information about the most common differential diagnoses for each sign or symptom, helping you to reach an accurate diagnosis. Each differential diagnosis appears in a rectangular box and is introduced by a black arrow. Within each of these boxes is an easy-to-reference bulleted list of other signs and symptoms that you may see in a patient with that diagnosis. Several diagnoses share signs and symptoms. On the flowchart, these shared signs and symptoms appear in a white oval.

Each differential diagnosis is followed by diagnostic tests (DX) that help confirm the medical diagnosis, possible treatments (TX), and associated follow-up (F/U) care. Gray arrows within the flowchart point the NP to shared diagnostic tests, treatments, and follow-up for related disorders, which appear in gray rectangular boxes.

If applicable, other differential diagnoses and possible causes are listed in separate boxes at the bottom of the page. They help guide your consideration of other important factors if you're unable to confidently diagnose the patient.

Common medical abbreviations have been used throughout to make the charts easier to read. Appendix E, *Commonly used medical abbreviations,* on page 440, includes a list of abbreviations that you may find helpful when looking at a flowchart. Other valuable appendices in the book include *Normal laboratory test values, X-ray interpretation, Types of cardiac arrhythmias,* and *Resources for professionals, patients, and caregivers.*

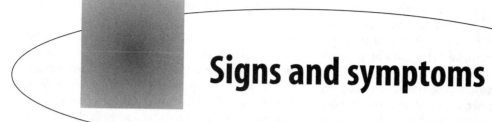

Signs and symptoms

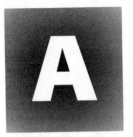

Abdominal distention

Abdominal distention refers to increased abdominal girth — the result of increased intra-abdominal pressure forcing the abdominal wall outward. Distention may be mild or severe, depending on the amount of pressure. It may be localized or diffuse and may occur gradually or suddenly. Acute abdominal distention may signal life-threatening peritonitis or acute bowel obstruction.

Abdominal distention may result from fat, flatus, intra-abdominal mass, or fluid. Fluid and gas are normally present in the GI tract but not in the peritoneal cavity. However, if fluid and gas can't pass freely through the GI tract, abdominal distention occurs. In the peritoneal cavity, distention may reflect acute bleeding, accumulation of ascitic fluid, or air from perforation of an abdominal organ.

History and physical examination

If the patient's abdominal distention isn't acute, ask about its onset and duration and associated signs. A patient with localized distention may report a sensation of pressure, fullness, or tenderness in the affected area. A patient with generalized distention may report a bloated feeling, a pounding heart, difficulty breathing deeply, or difficulty breathing when lying flat. The patient may also feel unable to bend at his waist. Be sure to ask about abdominal pain, fever, nausea, vomiting, anorexia, altered bowel habits, and weight gain or loss.

Obtain a medical history, noting GI or biliary disorders that may cause peritonitis or ascites, such as cirrhosis, hepatitis, or inflammatory bowel disease. Also note chronic constipation. Has the patient recently had abdominal surgery, which can lead to abdominal distention? Ask about recent accidents, even minor ones, such as a fall from a stepladder.

Perform a complete physical examination. Don't restrict the examination to the abdomen or you could miss important clues to the cause of abdominal symptoms. Next, stand at the foot of the bed and observe the recumbent patient for abdominal asymmetry to determine if distention is localized or generalized. Then assess abdominal contour by stooping at his side. Inspect for tense, glistening skin and bulging flanks, which may indicate ascites. Observe the umbilicus. An everted umbilicus may indicate ascites or umbilical hernia. An inverted umbilicus may indicate distention from gas; it's also common in obese patients. Inspect the abdomen for signs of inguinal or femoral hernia and for incisions that may point to adhesions. Both may lead to intestinal obstruction. Then auscultate for bowel sounds, abdominal friction rubs (indicating peritoneal inflammation), and bruits (indicating an aneurysm). Listen for succussion splash — a splashing sound normally heard in the stomach when the patient moves or when palpation disturbs the viscera. An abnormally loud splash indicates fluid accumulation, suggesting gastric dilatation or obstruction.

Next, percuss and palpate the abdomen to determine if distention results from air, fluid, or both. A tympanic note in the left lower quadrant suggests an air-filled descending or sigmoid colon. A tympanic note throughout a generally distended abdomen suggests an air-filled peritoneal cavity. A dull percussion note throughout a generally distended abdomen suggests a fluid-filled peritoneal cavity. Shifting of dullness laterally with the patient in the decubitus position also indicates a fluid-filled abdominal cavity. A pelvic or intra-abdominal mass should be palpable and causes local dullness on percussion. Obesity causes a large abdomen without shifting dullness, prominent tympany, or palpable bowel or other masses, with generalized rather then localized dullness.

Palpate the abdomen for tenderness, noting whether it's localized or generalized. Watch for peritoneal signs, such as rebound tenderness, guarding, rigidity, McBurney's sign, obturator sign, and psoas sign. Female patients should undergo a pelvic examination; male patients, a genital examination. All patients who report abdominal pain should undergo a digital rectal examination with fecal occult blood testing. Finally, measure abdominal girth for a baseline value. Mark the flanks with a felt-tipped pen; use this as a reference for subsequent measurements.

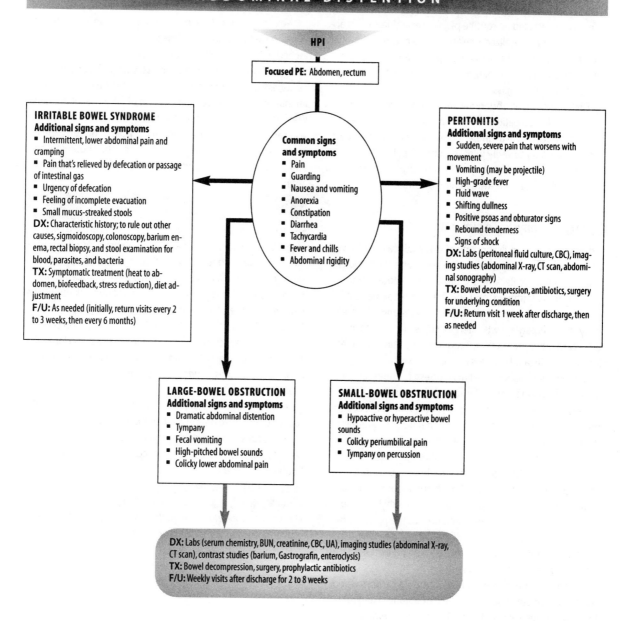

HPI

Focused PE: Abdomen, rectum

Common signs and symptoms
- Pain
- Guarding
- Nausea and vomiting
- Anorexia
- Constipation
- Diarrhea
- Tachycardia
- Fever and chills
- Abdominal rigidity

IRRITABLE BOWEL SYNDROME
Additional signs and symptoms
- Intermittent, lower abdominal pain and cramping
- Pain that's relieved by defecation or passage of intestinal gas
- Urgency of defecation
- Feeling of incomplete evacuation
- Small mucus-streaked stools

DX: Characteristic history; to rule out other causes, sigmoidoscopy, colonoscopy, barium enema, rectal biopsy, and stool examination for blood, parasites, and bacteria
TX: Symptomatic treatment (heat to abdomen, biofeedback, stress reduction), diet adjustment
F/U: As needed (initially, return visits every 2 to 3 weeks, then every 6 months)

PERITONITIS
Additional signs and symptoms
- Sudden, severe pain that worsens with movement
- Vomiting (may be projectile)
- High-grade fever
- Fluid wave
- Shifting dullness
- Positive psoas and obturator signs
- Rebound tenderness
- Signs of shock

DX: Labs (peritoneal fluid culture, CBC), imaging studies (abdominal X-ray, CT scan, abdominal sonography)
TX: Bowel decompression, antibiotics, surgery for underlying condition
F/U: Return visit 1 week after discharge, then as needed

LARGE-BOWEL OBSTRUCTION
Additional signs and symptoms
- Dramatic abdominal distention
- Tympany
- Fecal vomiting
- High-pitched bowel sounds
- Colicky lower abdominal pain

SMALL-BOWEL OBSTRUCTION
Additional signs and symptoms
- Hypoactive or hyperactive bowel sounds
- Colicky periumbilical pain
- Tympany on percussion

DX: Labs (serum chemistry, BUN, creatinine, CBC, UA), imaging studies (abdominal X-ray, CT scan), contrast studies (barium, Gastrografin, enteroclysis)
TX: Bowel decompression, surgery, prophylactic antibiotics
F/U: Weekly visits after discharge for 2 to 8 weeks

Additional differential diagnoses: abdominal cancer ▪ abdominal trauma ▪ abdominal tumor ▪ cirrhosis ▪ heart failure ▪ mesenteric artery occlusion ▪ nephrotic syndrome ▪ paralytic ileus ▪ toxic megacolon

Other causes: ascites ▪ bladder distention ▪ gastric dilation

Abdominal mass

Commonly detected on routine physical examination, an abdominal mass is a localized swelling in one of the abdominal quadrants. Typically, this sign develops insidiously and may represent an enlarged organ, a neoplasm, an abscess, a vascular defect, or a fecal mass.

Distinguishing an abdominal mass from normal structures requires skillful palpation. At times, palpation must be repeated with the patient in a different position or performed by a second examiner to verify initial findings. A palpable abdominal mass is an important clinical sign and usually represents a serious and, perhaps, life-threatening disorder.

History and physical examination

If the patient has a pulsating midabdominal mass and severe abdominal or back pain, suspect an aortic aneurysm. Quickly take his vital signs. Because the patient may require emergency surgery, withhold food and fluids until the patient is examined. Obtain routine preoperative tests, and prepare the patient for angiography. Be alert for signs of shock, such as tachycardia, hypotension, and cool, clammy skin, which may indicate significant blood loss.

If the patient's abdominal mass doesn't suggest an aortic aneurysm, obtain a detailed history. Ask the patient if the mass is painful. If so, ask if the pain is constant or if it occurs only on palpation. Is it localized or generalized? Determine if the patient was already aware of the mass. If he was, find out if the patient noticed any change in its size or location.

Next, review the patient's medical history, paying special attention to GI disorders. Ask the patient about GI signs and symptoms, such as constipation, diarrhea, rectal bleeding, abnormally colored stools, and vomiting. Has the patient noticed a change in his appetite? If the patient is female, ask whether her menstrual cycles are regular and ask when the first day of her last menses was.

A complete physical examination should be performed. Auscultate for bowel sounds in each quadrant. Listen for bruits or friction rubs, and check for enlarged veins. Lightly palpate, and then deeply palpate, the abdomen, assessing painful or suspicious areas last. Be sure to note the patient's position when you locate the mass. Some masses can be detected only with the patient in the supine position; others require the patient to be in a side-lying position.

Estimate the size of the mass in centimeters. Determine its shape. Is it round or sausage-shaped? Describe its contour as smooth, rough, sharply defined, nodular, or irregular. Further determine the consistency of the mass. Is it doughy, soft, solid,

or hard? Also, percuss the mass. A dull sound indicates a fluid-filled mass; a tympanic sound, an air-filled mass.

Next, determine if the mass moves when you palpate it or in response to respiration. Is the mass free-floating or attached to intra-abdominal structures? To determine whether the mass is located in the abdominal wall or the abdominal cavity, ask the patient to lift his head and shoulders off the examination table, thereby contracting his abdominal muscles. While these muscles are contracted, try to palpate the mass. If you can, the mass is in the abdominal wall; if you can't, the mass is within the abdominal cavity. After the abdominal examination is complete, perform pelvic, genital, and rectal examinations.

HPI

Focused PE: Abdomen, rectum

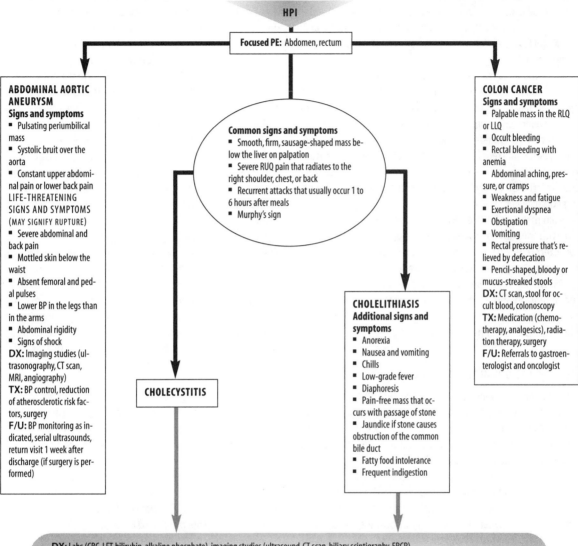

Common signs and symptoms
- Smooth, firm, sausage-shaped mass below the liver on palpation
- Severe RUQ pain that radiates to the right shoulder, chest, or back
- Recurrent attacks that usually occur 1 to 6 hours after meals
- Murphy's sign

ABDOMINAL AORTIC ANEURYSM
Signs and symptoms
- Pulsating periumbilical mass
- Systolic bruit over the aorta
- Constant upper abdominal pain or lower back pain

LIFE-THREATENING SIGNS AND SYMPTOMS (MAY SIGNIFY RUPTURE)
- Severe abdominal and back pain
- Mottled skin below the waist
- Absent femoral and pedal pulses
- Lower BP in the legs than in the arms
- Abdominal rigidity
- Signs of shock

DX: Imaging studies (ultrasonography, CT scan, MRI, angiography)
TX: BP control, reduction of atherosclerotic risk factors, surgery
F/U: BP monitoring as indicated, serial ultrasounds, return visit 1 week after discharge (if surgery is performed)

CHOLECYSTITIS

CHOLELITHIASIS
Additional signs and symptoms
- Anorexia
- Nausea and vomiting
- Chills
- Low-grade fever
- Diaphoresis
- Pain-free mass that occurs with passage of stone
- Jaundice if stone causes obstruction of the common bile duct
- Fatty food intolerance
- Frequent indigestion

COLON CANCER
Signs and symptoms
- Palpable mass in the RLQ or LLQ
- Occult bleeding
- Rectal bleeding with anemia
- Abdominal aching, pressure, or cramps
- Weakness and fatigue
- Exertional dyspnea
- Obstipation
- Vomiting
- Rectal pressure that's relieved by defecation
- Pencil-shaped, bloody or mucus-streaked stools

DX: CT scan, stool for occult blood, colonoscopy
TX: Medication (chemotherapy, analgesics), radiation therapy, surgery
F/U: Referrals to gastroenterologist and oncologist

DX: Labs (CBC, LFT, bilirubin, alkaline phosphate), imaging studies (ultrasound, CT scan, biliary scintigraphy, ERCP)
TX: Low-fat diet, gallstone solubilizing agent, surgery
F/U: Liver enzyme tests, serum cholesterol, imaging studies (if on medication), return visit 1 week after procedure or discharge (if surgery is performed)

Additional differential diagnoses: Crohn's disease ▪ diverticulitis ▪ gallbladder cancer ▪ gastric cancer ▪ hepatic cancer ▪ hernia (inguinal or ventral) ▪ hydronephrosis ▪ ovarian cyst ▪ pancreatic abscess ▪ pancreatic pseudocysts ▪ renal cell carcinoma ▪ splenomegaly ▪ uterine leiomyoma

Other causes: hepatomegaly

Abdominal pain

Abdominal pain usually results from GI disorders; however, it can also be caused by reproductive, genitourinary (GU), musculoskeletal, and vascular disorders as well as drug use and ingestion of toxins. At times, this symptom signals life-threatening complications.

Abdominal pain arises from the abdominopelvic viscera, the parietal peritoneum, or the capsules of the liver, kidney, or spleen. It may be acute or chronic, diffuse or localized. Visceral pain develops slowly into a deep, dull, aching pain that's poorly localized in the epigastric, periumbilical, or lower midabdominal (hypogastric) region. In contrast, somatic (parietal, peritoneal) pain produces a sharp, more intense, and well-localized discomfort that rapidly follows the insult. Movement or coughing aggravates this pain.

Pain may also be referred to the abdomen from another site with the same or a similar nerve supply. This sharp, well-localized, referred pain is felt in skin or deeper tissues and may coexist with skin hyperesthesia and muscle hyperalgesia.

Mechanisms that produce abdominal pain include stretching or tension of the gut wall, traction on the peritoneum or mesentery, vigorous intestinal contraction, inflammation, ischemia, and sensory nerve irritation.

History and physical examination

If the patient is experiencing sudden, severe abdominal pain, quickly take his vital signs and palpate the pulses below the waist. Be alert for signs of hypovolemic shock, such as tachycardia and hypotension. Emergency surgery may be required if the patient also has mottled skin below the waist and a pulsating epigastric mass or rebound tenderness and rigidity.

If the patient has no life-threatening signs or symptoms, take his history. Ask the patient if the pain is constant or intermittent, and ask when the pain began. Constant, steady abdominal pain suggests organ perforation, ischemia, or inflammation or blood in the peritoneal cavity. Intermittent, cramping abdominal pain suggests that the patient may have an obstruction of a hollow organ.

If pain is intermittent, determine the duration of a typical episode. In addition, ask the patient where the pain is located and whether it radiates to other areas. Find out if movement, coughing, exertion, vomiting, eating, elimination, and walking worsen or relieve the pain. The patient may report abdominal pain as indigestion or gas pain, so ask him to describe it in detail.

Ask the patient about drug and alcohol use and any history of vascular, GI, GU, or reproductive disorders. When appropriate, ask the female patient about the date of her last menses, changes in her menstrual pattern, or dyspareunia. Also ask the patient about appetite changes. In addition, ask about the onset and frequency of nausea or vomiting. Find out about changes in bowel habits, such as constipation, diarrhea, and changes in stool consistency. When was the patient's last bowel movement? Ask about urinary frequency, urgency, or pain. Is the urine cloudy or pink?

Perform a physical examination. Take the patient's vital signs, and assess skin turgor and mucous membranes. Inspect his abdomen for distention or visible peristaltic waves and, if indicated, measure his abdominal girth.

Auscultate for bowel sounds and characterize their motility. Percuss all quadrants, carefully noting the percussion sounds. Palpate the entire abdomen for masses, rigidity, and tenderness. Check specifically for costovertebral angle tenderness, abdominal tenderness with guarding, and rebound tenderness.

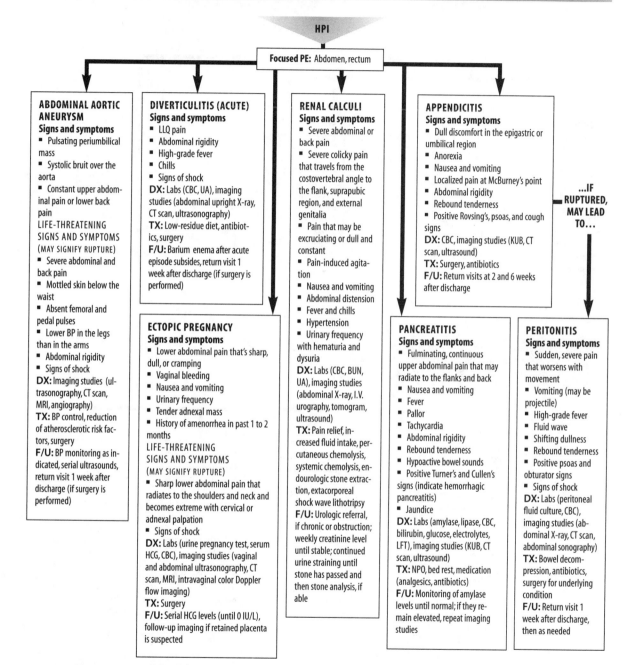

HPI

Focused PE: Abdomen, rectum

ABDOMINAL AORTIC ANEURYSM
Signs and symptoms
- Pulsating periumbilical mass
- Systolic bruit over the aorta
- Constant upper abdominal pain or lower back pain

LIFE-THREATENING SIGNS AND SYMPTOMS (MAY SIGNIFY RUPTURE)
- Severe abdominal and back pain
- Mottled skin below the waist
- Absent femoral and pedal pulses
- Lower BP in the legs than in the arms
- Abdominal rigidity
- Signs of shock

DX: Imaging studies (ultrasonography, CT scan, MRI, angiography)
TX: BP control, reduction of atherosclerotic risk factors, surgery
F/U: BP monitoring as indicated, serial ultrasounds, return visit 1 week after discharge (if surgery is performed)

DIVERTICULITIS (ACUTE)
Signs and symptoms
- LLQ pain
- Abdominal rigidity
- High-grade fever
- Chills
- Signs of shock

DX: Labs (CBC, UA), imaging studies (abdominal upright X-ray, CT scan, ultrasonography)
TX: Low-residue diet, antibiotics, surgery
F/U: Barium enema after acute episode subsides, return visit 1 week after discharge (if surgery is performed)

ECTOPIC PREGNANCY
Signs and symptoms
- Lower abdominal pain that's sharp, dull, or cramping
- Vaginal bleeding
- Nausea and vomiting
- Urinary frequency
- Tender adnexal mass
- History of amenorrhea in past 1 to 2 months

LIFE-THREATENING SIGNS AND SYMPTOMS (MAY SIGNIFY RUPTURE)
- Sharp lower abdominal pain that radiates to the shoulders and neck and becomes extreme with cervical or adnexal palpation
- Signs of shock

DX: Labs (urine pregnancy test, serum HCG, CBC), imaging studies (vaginal and abdominal ultrasonography, CT scan, MRI, intravaginal color Doppler flow imaging)
TX: Surgery
F/U: Serial HCG levels (until 0 IU/L), follow-up imaging if retained placenta is suspected

RENAL CALCULI
Signs and symptoms
- Severe abdominal or back pain
- Severe colicky pain that travels from the costovertebral angle to the flank, suprapubic region, and external genitalia
- Pain that may be excruciating or dull and constant
- Pain-induced agitation
- Nausea and vomiting
- Abdominal distension
- Fever and chills
- Hypertension
- Urinary frequency with hematuria and dysuria

DX: Labs (CBC, BUN, UA), imaging studies (abdominal X-ray, I.V. urography, tomogram, ultrasound)
TX: Pain relief, increased fluid intake, percutaneous chemolysis, systemic chemolysis, endourologic stone extraction, extracorporeal shock wave lithotripsy
F/U: Urologic referral, if chronic or obstruction; weekly creatinine level until stable; continued urine straining until stone has passed and then stone analysis, if able

APPENDICITIS
Signs and symptoms
- Dull discomfort in the epigastric or umbilical region
- Anorexia
- Nausea and vomiting
- Localized pain at McBurney's point
- Abdominal rigidity
- Rebound tenderness
- Positive Rovsing's, psoas, and cough signs

DX: CBC, imaging studies (KUB, CT scan, ultrasound)
TX: Surgery, antibiotics
F/U: Return visits at 2 and 6 weeks after discharge

PANCREATITIS
Signs and symptoms
- Fulminating, continuous upper abdominal pain that may radiate to the flanks and back
- Nausea and vomiting
- Fever
- Pallor
- Tachycardia
- Abdominal rigidity
- Rebound tenderness
- Hypoactive bowel sounds
- Positive Turner's and Cullen's signs (indicate hemorrhagic pancreatitis)
- Jaundice

DX: Labs (amylase, lipase, CBC, bilirubin, glucose, electrolytes, LFT), imaging studies (KUB, CT scan, ultrasound)
TX: NPO, bed rest, medication (analgesics, antibiotics)
F/U: Monitoring of amylase levels until normal; if they remain elevated, repeat imaging studies

...IF RUPTURED, MAY LEAD TO...

PERITONITIS
Signs and symptoms
- Sudden, severe pain that worsens with movement
- Vomiting (may be projectile)
- High-grade fever
- Fluid wave
- Shifting dullness
- Rebound tenderness
- Positive psoas and obturator signs
- Signs of shock

DX: Labs (peritoneal fluid culture, CBC), imaging studies (abdominal X-ray, CT scan, abdominal sonography)
TX: Bowel decompression, antibiotics, surgery for underlying condition
F/U: Return visit 1 week after discharge, then as needed

Additional differential diagnoses: abdominal cancer ▪ abdominal trauma ▪ acute cholecystitis ▪ acute cholelithiasis ▪ acute hepatitis ▪ adrenal crisis ▪ cholangitis ▪ diabetic ketoacidosis ▪ gastroenteritis ▪ heart failure ▪ hepatic abscess ▪ hepatic amebiasis ▪ hernia (inguinal or ventral) ▪ herpes zoster ▪ intestinal obstruction ▪ intestinal perforation ▪ Meckel's diverticulitis ▪ mesenteric artery ischemia ▪ MI ▪ perforated ulcer ▪ pneumonia ▪ pyelonephritis ▪ retroperitoneal bleed ▪ ruptured ovarian cyst ▪ ruptured spleen ▪ sickle cell crisis ▪ SLE

Other causes: insect toxins

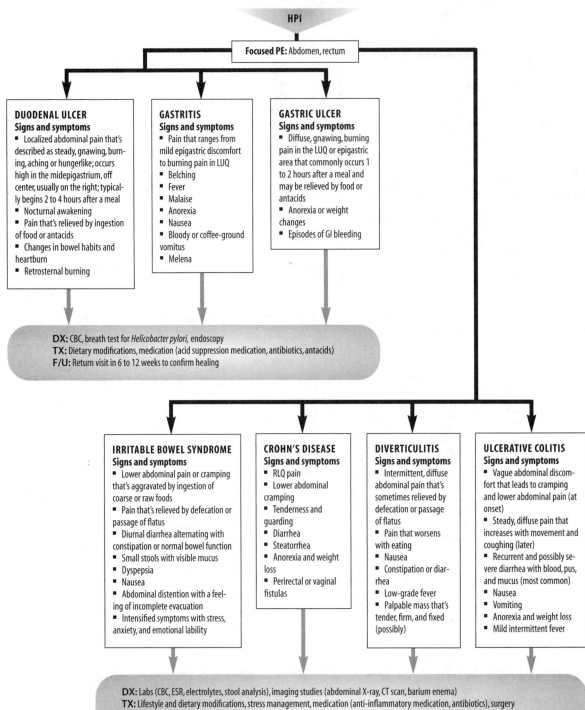

HPI

Focused PE: Abdomen, rectum

DUODENAL ULCER
Signs and symptoms
- Localized abdominal pain that's described as steady, gnawing, burning, aching or hungerlike; occurs high in the midepigastrium, off center, usually on the right; typically begins 2 to 4 hours after a meal
- Nocturnal awakening
- Pain that's relieved by ingestion of food or antacids
- Changes in bowel habits and heartburn
- Retrosternal burning

GASTRITIS
Signs and symptoms
- Pain that ranges from mild epigastric discomfort to burning pain in LUQ
- Belching
- Fever
- Malaise
- Anorexia
- Nausea
- Bloody or coffee-ground vomitus
- Melena

GASTRIC ULCER
Signs and symptoms
- Diffuse, gnawing, burning pain in the LUQ or epigastric area that commonly occurs 1 to 2 hours after a meal and may be relieved by food or antacids
- Anorexia or weight changes
- Episodes of GI bleeding

DX: CBC, breath test for *Helicobacter pylori,* endoscopy
TX: Dietary modifications, medication (acid suppression medication, antibiotics, antacids)
F/U: Return visit in 6 to 12 weeks to confirm healing

IRRITABLE BOWEL SYNDROME
Signs and symptoms
- Lower abdominal pain or cramping that's aggravated by ingestion of coarse or raw foods
- Pain that's relieved by defecation or passage of flatus
- Diurnal diarrhea alternating with constipation or normal bowel function
- Small stools with visible mucus
- Dyspepsia
- Nausea
- Abdominal distention with a feeling of incomplete evacuation
- Intensified symptoms with stress, anxiety, and emotional lability

CROHN'S DISEASE
Signs and symptoms
- RLQ pain
- Lower abdominal cramping
- Tenderness and guarding
- Diarrhea
- Steatorrhea
- Anorexia and weight loss
- Perirectal or vaginal fistulas

DIVERTICULITIS
Signs and symptoms
- Intermittent, diffuse abdominal pain that's sometimes relieved by defecation or passage of flatus
- Pain that worsens with eating
- Nausea
- Constipation or diarrhea
- Low-grade fever
- Palpable mass that's tender, firm, and fixed (possibly)

ULCERATIVE COLITIS
Signs and symptoms
- Vague abdominal discomfort that leads to cramping and lower abdominal pain (at onset)
- Steady, diffuse pain that increases with movement and coughing (later)
- Recurrent and possibly severe diarrhea with blood, pus, and mucus (most common)
- Nausea
- Vomiting
- Anorexia and weight loss
- Mild intermittent fever

DX: Labs (CBC, ESR, electrolytes, stool analysis), imaging studies (abdominal X-ray, CT scan, barium enema)
TX: Lifestyle and dietary modifications, stress management, medication (anti-inflammatory medication, antibiotics), surgery
F/U: Regular appointments (every 3 to 6 months) to evaluate weight, bowel activity, and complications

HPI

Focused PE: Abdomen, rectum, pelvis

CYSTITIS
Signs and symptoms
- Suprapubic abdominal pain
- Flank pain
- Lower back pain
- Malaise
- Nausea and vomiting
- Urinary frequency
- Nocturia
- Dysuria
- Fever and chills

DX: Labs (UA, urine culture), ultrasound
TX: Antibiotic, increased fluid intake
F/U: Reculture, if symptoms persist or recur

HEPATITIS
Signs and symptoms
- Dull pain in the RUQ
- Dark urine
- Clay-colored stools
- Nausea and vomiting
- Anorexia and weight loss
- Jaundice
- Pruritus
- Malaise

DX: Labs (serologic markers for virus, LFT, coagulation studies), possible liver biopsy to confirm type and extent of liver damage
TX: Medication (interferon alpha therapy, corticosteroids), liver transplant, lifestyle modifications
F/U: Monitoring for complications while on medication

...MAY LEAD TO...

CIRRHOSIS
Signs and symptoms
- Dull abdominal aching
- RUQ pain that worsens when the patient sits up or leans forward
- Fever
- Ascites
- Leg edema
- Weight gain
- Hepatomegaly
- Jaundice
- Severe pruritus
- Bleeding tendencies and bruising
- Palmar erythema
- Spider angiomas
- Gynecomastia and testicular atrophy

DX: LFT, imaging studies (CT scan, ultrasound), laparoscopic liver biopsy
TX: Lifestyle modifications, dietary modifications (for underlying cause)
F/U: Annual checkups with LFT

PROSTATITIS
Signs and symptoms
- Vague lower abdominal pain
- Pain in the groin, perineum, or rectum
- Scrotal pain, penile pain, and pain on ejaculation (in chronic cases)
- Dysuria
- Urinary frequency and urgency
- Nocturia
- Fever and chills
- Lower back pain
- Myalgia
- Arthralgia

DX: Labs (fractional urine examination, urine culture), imaging studies (CT scan, transrectal ultrasound)
TX: Medication (analgesics, antibiotics, stool softener), surgery
F/U: UA and urine culture every 30 days until infection resolves

PID
Signs and symptoms
- Pain in the RLQ or LLQ that ranges from vague discomfort to deep, severe and progressive pain
- Metrorrhagia that sometimes precedes or accompanies pain
- Cervical or adnexal palpation that causes extreme pain
- Pelvic mass (possibly)
- Fever and chills
- Nausea and vomiting
- Urinary discomfort
- Abnormal vaginal bleeding or discharge

OVARIAN CYST
Signs and symptoms
- Torsion or hemorrhage causes RLQ or LLQ pain
- Sharp and severe pain when suddenly standing or stooping
- Fever
- Anorexia
- Vomiting
- Palpable abdominal mass (possibly)
- Rupture (may cause peritonitis)

ENDOMETRIOSIS
Signs and symptoms
- Constant, severe pain in the lower abdomen that usually occurs 5 to 7 days before menstruation
- Pain that may be aggravated by defecation
- Dysmenorrhea
- Dyspareunia
- Deep sacral pain

DX: Labs (pregnancy test, CBC, ESR, serum tumor markers), imaging studies (transabdominal or transvaginal ultrasound, CT scan, MRI), laparoscopy
TX: Medication (for PID, antibiotics; for ovarian cyst, monophasic contraceptive pill; for endometriosis, gonadotropin-releasing hormone agonist), laparoscopy, or surgery
F/U: Yearly ultrasound to monitor adnexal mass (if present), varies according to symptoms

Abdominal rigidity

Detected by palpation, abdominal rigidity refers to abdominal muscle tension or inflexibility of the abdomen. Rigidity may be voluntary or involuntary. Voluntary rigidity reflects the patient's fear of or nervousness about palpation; involuntary rigidity reflects potentially life-threatening peritoneal irritation or inflammation.

Involuntary rigidity most commonly results from GI disorders but may also result from pulmonary and vascular disorders and from the effects of insect toxins. Usually, it's accompanied by fever, nausea, vomiting, abdominal tenderness, distention, and pain. (See *Recognizing voluntary rigidity*.)

History and physical examination

After palpating abdominal rigidity, quickly take the patient's vital signs. Even though the patient may not appear gravely ill or have markedly abnormal vital signs, abdominal rigidity calls for emergency interventions. Because emergency surgery may be necessary, the patient should be prepared for laboratory tests and X-rays.

If the patient's condition allows further assessment, take a brief history. Find out when the abdominal rigidity began. Is it associated with abdominal pain? If so, did the pain begin at the same time? Determine whether abdominal rigidity is localized or generalized. Is it always present? Has its site changed or remained constant? Next, ask about aggravating or alleviating factors, such as position changes, coughing, vomiting, elimination, and walking.

Then explore other signs and symptoms. Inspect the abdomen for peristaltic waves, which may be visible in very thin patients. Also, check for a visible distended bowel loop. Next, auscultate bowel sounds. Perform light palpation to locate the rigidity and determine its severity. Avoid deep palpation, which may exacerbate abdominal pain. Finally, check for poor skin turgor and dry mucous membranes, which indicate dehydration.

PEDIATRIC POINTERS

- *Voluntary rigidity may be difficult to distinguish from involuntary rigidity if associated pain makes the child restless, tense, or apprehensive. However, in any child with suspected involuntary rigidity, your priority is early detection of dehydration and shock, which can rapidly become life-threatening.*
- *Abdominal rigidity in the child can stem from gastric perforations, hypertrophic pyloric stenosis, duodenal obstruction, meconium ileus, intussusception, cystic fibrosis, celiac disease, and appendicitis.*

ELDER CARE CUE

Advanced age and impaired cognition decrease pain perception and intensity. Weakening of abdominal muscles may decrease muscle spasms and rigidity.

Recognizing voluntary rigidity

Distinguishing voluntary rigidity from involuntary rigidity is essential for accurate assessment.

Voluntary rigidity is:
- usually symmetrical
- more rigid on inspiration (expiration causes muscle relaxation)
- eased by relaxation techniques, such as positioning the patient comfortably and talking to him in a calm, soothing manner
- painless when the patient sits up using his abdominal muscles alone.

Involuntary rigidity is:
- usually asymmetrical
- equally rigid on inspiration and expiration
- unaffected by relaxation techniques
- painful when the patient sits up using his abdominal muscles.

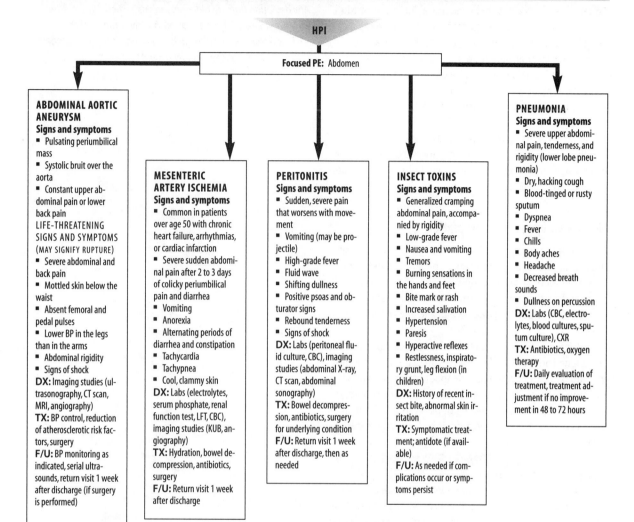

HPI

Focused PE: Abdomen

ABDOMINAL AORTIC ANEURYSM
Signs and symptoms
- Pulsating periumbilical mass
- Systolic bruit over the aorta
- Constant upper abdominal pain or lower back pain

LIFE-THREATENING SIGNS AND SYMPTOMS (MAY SIGNIFY RUPTURE)
- Severe abdominal and back pain
- Mottled skin below the waist
- Absent femoral and pedal pulses
- Lower BP in the legs than in the arms
- Abdominal rigidity
- Signs of shock

DX: Imaging studies (ultrasonography, CT scan, MRI, angiography)
TX: BP control, reduction of atherosclerotic risk factors, surgery
F/U: BP monitoring as indicated, serial ultrasounds, return visit 1 week after discharge (if surgery is performed)

MESENTERIC ARTERY ISCHEMIA
Signs and symptoms
- Common in patients over age 50 with chronic heart failure, arrhythmias, or cardiac infarction
- Severe sudden abdominal pain after 2 to 3 days of colicky periumbilical pain and diarrhea
- Vomiting
- Anorexia
- Alternating periods of diarrhea and constipation
- Tachycardia
- Tachypnea
- Cool, clammy skin

DX: Labs (electrolytes, serum phosphate, renal function test, LFT, CBC), imaging studies (KUB, angiography)
TX: Hydration, bowel decompression, antibiotics, surgery
F/U: Return visit 1 week after discharge

PERITONITIS
Signs and symptoms
- Sudden, severe pain that worsens with movement
- Vomiting (may be projectile)
- High-grade fever
- Fluid wave
- Shifting dullness
- Positive psoas and obturator signs
- Rebound tenderness
- Signs of shock

DX: Labs (peritoneal fluid culture, CBC), imaging studies (abdominal X-ray, CT scan, abdominal sonography)
TX: Bowel decompression, antibiotics, surgery for underlying condition
F/U: Return visit 1 week after discharge, then as needed

INSECT TOXINS
Signs and symptoms
- Generalized cramping abdominal pain, accompanied by rigidity
- Low-grade fever
- Nausea and vomiting
- Tremors
- Burning sensations in the hands and feet
- Bite mark or rash
- Increased salivation
- Hypertension
- Paresis
- Hyperactive reflexes
- Restlessness, inspiratory grunt, leg flexion (in children)

DX: History of recent insect bite, abnormal skin irritation
TX: Symptomatic treatment; antidote (if available)
F/U: As needed if complications occur or symptoms persist

PNEUMONIA
Signs and symptoms
- Severe upper abdominal pain, tenderness, and rigidity (lower lobe pneumonia)
- Dry, hacking cough
- Blood-tinged or rusty sputum
- Dyspnea
- Fever
- Chills
- Body aches
- Headache
- Decreased breath sounds
- Dullness on percussion

DX: Labs (CBC, electrolytes, blood cultures, sputum culture), CXR
TX: Antibiotics, oxygen therapy
F/U: Daily evaluation of treatment, treatment adjustment if no improvement in 48 to 72 hours

Agitation

Agitation refers to a state of hyperarousal, increased tension, and irritability that can lead to confusion, hyperactivity, and overt hostility. This common sign can result from various disorders, pain, fever, anxiety, drug use and withdrawal, and hypersensitivity reactions. It can arise gradually or suddenly and can last for minutes or months. Whether it's mild or severe, agitation worsens with increased fever, pain, stress, or external stimuli.

Agitation alone merely signals a change in the patient's condition. However, it's a useful indicator of a developing disorder when considered with the patient's history, current status, and other findings.

History and physical examination

Determine the severity of the patient's agitation by examining the number and quality of agitation-induced behaviors, such as emotional lability, confusion, memory loss, hyperactivity, and hostility. Obtain a history from the patient or a family member; include the patient's diet and any known allergies.

Ask if the patient is being treated for any illnesses. Has the patient had any recent infections, trauma, stress, or changes in sleep patterns? Ask the patient about prescription and over-the-counter drug use. Check for signs of drug abuse, such as needle tracks and dilated pupils. Also ask about alcohol intake. Obtain baseline vital signs and neurologic status for future comparison.

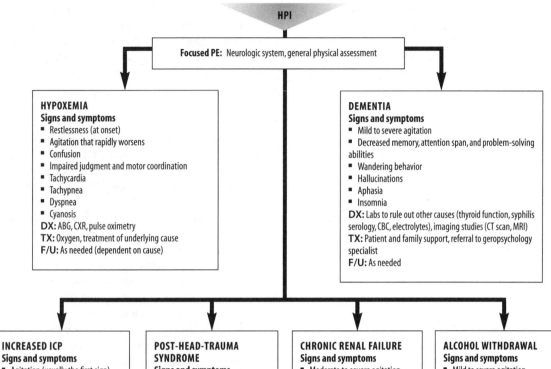

HPI

Focused PE: Neurologic system, general physical assessment

HYPOXEMIA
Signs and symptoms
- Restlessness (at onset)
- Agitation that rapidly worsens
- Confusion
- Impaired judgment and motor coordination
- Tachycardia
- Tachypnea
- Dyspnea
- Cyanosis

DX: ABG, CXR, pulse oximetry
TX: Oxygen, treatment of underlying cause
F/U: As needed (dependent on cause)

DEMENTIA
Signs and symptoms
- Mild to severe agitation
- Decreased memory, attention span, and problem-solving abilities
- Wandering behavior
- Hallucinations
- Aphasia
- Insomnia

DX: Labs to rule out other causes (thyroid function, syphilis serology, CBC, electrolytes), imaging studies (CT scan, MRI)
TX: Patient and family support, referral to geropsychology specialist
F/U: As needed

INCREASED ICP
Signs and symptoms
- Agitation (usually the first sign)
- Headache
- Nausea and vomiting
- Cheyne-Stokes respirations
- Ataxia
- Sluggish, nonreactive pupils
- Widened pulse pressure
- Tachycardia
- Decreased LOC
- Abnormal posturing

DX: Intracranial CT scan, intracranial MRI
TX: Treatment of underlying cause, osmotic diuretics, surgery
F/U: As needed (dependent on cause)

POST-HEAD-TRAUMA SYNDROME
Signs and symptoms
- Disorientation
- Loss of concentration
- Emotional lability
- Fatigue
- Wandering behavior
- Poor judgment

DX: History of head trauma
TX: Safety precautions
F/U: Daily visits until behavior returns to baseline or stabilizes

CHRONIC RENAL FAILURE
Signs and symptoms
- Moderate to severe agitation
- Decreased urine output
- Increased BP
- Nausea and vomiting
- Anorexia
- Ammonia breath odor
- GI bleeding
- Pallor
- Dry skin
- Uremic frost
- Edema

DX: Labs (renal function studies, electrolytes, ABG), imaging studies (renal ultrasound, CT scan, MRI)
TX: Control of associated cause, diet modification, dialysis, kidney transplant
F/U: Weekly to monthly visits, depending on response to treatment

ALCOHOL WITHDRAWAL
Signs and symptoms
- Mild to severe agitation
- Hyperactivity
- Tremors
- Anxiety

LIFE-THREATENING SIGNS AND SYMPTOMS (DELIRIUM TREMENS)
- Severe agitation
- Visual hallucinations
- Insomnia
- Diaphoresis
- Tachycardia
- Depression
- Seizures
- Cardiac arrest
- Shock

DX: History of ETOH use, labs (LFT, electrolytes)
TX: Medication (benzodiazepines, barbiturates, beta-adrenergic blocker, anticonvulsant)
F/U: Referral to addiction program

Additional differential diagnoses: affective disturbance ▪ anxiety ▪ drug withdrawal syndrome ▪ endocrine disorder ▪ hepatic encephalopathy ▪ hypersensitivity reaction ▪ intracranial bleed ▪ organic brain syndrome ▪ vitamin B_6 deficiency ▪ vitamin B_{12} deficiency

---

Other causes: medication (famotidine, lorazepam, haloperidol) ▪ radiographic contrast media

Alopecia

Occurring most commonly on the scalp, alopecia typically develops gradually and may be diffuse or patchy. It can be classified as scarring or nonscarring. Scarring alopecia, or permanent hair loss, results from hair follicle destruction, which smoothes the skin surface, erasing follicular openings. Nonscarring alopecia, or temporary hair loss, results from hair follicle damage that spares follicular openings, allowing future hair growth. (See *Recognizing patterns of alopecia*.)

One of the most common causes of alopecia is the use of certain chemotherapeutic drugs. Alopecia may also result from the use of other drugs; radiation therapy; skin, connective tissue, endocrine, nutritional, and psychological disorders; neoplasms; infections; burns; and the effects of toxins.

Normally, a person loses about 50 hairs per day, and these hairs are replaced by new ones. However, aging, genetic predisposition, and hormonal changes may contribute to gradual hair thinning and hairline recession. This type of alopecia occurs in about 40% of adult men and may also occur in postmenopausal women.

History and physical examination

If the patient isn't receiving chemotherapeutic drugs or radiation therapy, begin by asking when he first noticed the hair loss or thinning. Does it affect only the scalp or does it occur elsewhere on the body? Do itching or rashes accompany it? Then carefully explore other signs and symptoms to help distinguish between normal and pathologic hair loss. Ask about recent weight change, anorexia, nausea, vomiting, and altered bowel habits. Also ask about changes in urination habits, such as hematuria or oliguria. Has the patient been especially tired or irritable? Does he have a cough or difficulty breathing? Ask about joint pain or stiffness and about heat or cold intolerance. Inquire about exposure to insecticides. If the patient is female, find out if she has had menstrual irregularities and note her pregnancy history. If the patient is male, ask about sexual dysfunction, such as decreased libido or impotence.

Next, ask about hair care. Does the patient frequently use a hot blow-dryer or electric curlers? Does he periodically dye or bleach his hair or receive a permanent? Ask the black patient if he uses a hot comb to straighten his hair or a long-toothed comb to achieve an Afro. Does he ever braid his hair in cornrows? Check for a family history of alopecia. Ask what age relatives were when they started experiencing hair loss, if appropriate. Also ask about nervous habits, such as pulling the hair or twirling it around a finger.

Begin the physical examination by taking vital signs and then assessing the extent and pattern of scalp hair loss. Is it patchy or symmetrical? Is the hair surrounding a bald area brittle or lusterless? Is it a different color than other scalp hair? Does it fall out easily? Inspect the underlying skin for follicular openings, erythema, loss of pigment, scaling, induration, broken hair shafts, and hair regrowth.

Then examine the rest of the skin. Note the size, color, texture, and location of any lesions. Check for jaundice, edema, hyperpigmentation, pallor, or duskiness. Examine nails for vertical or horizontal pitting, thickening, brittleness, or whitening. As you do so, watch for fine tremors in the hands. Observe for muscle weakness and ptosis. Palpate for lymphadenopathy, enlarged thyroid or salivary glands, and masses in the abdomen or chest.

PEDIATRIC POINTERS

- *Alopecia normally occurs during the first 6 months of life, as either a sudden, diffuse hair loss or a gradual thinning that's hardly noticeable. Reassure the infant's parents that this hair loss is normal and temporary.*

- *Common causes of alopecia in children include use of chemotherapy, seborrheic dermatitis (cradle cap in infancy), alopecia mucinosa, tinea capitis, and hypopituitarism. Tinea capitis may produce a kerion lesion — a boggy, raised, tender, and hairless lesion. Trichotillomania, a psychological disorder that's more common in children than adults, may produce patchy baldness with stubby hair growth due to habitual hair pulling. Other causes include progeria and congenital hair shaft defects such as trichorrhexis nodosa.*

Recognizing patterns of alopecia

Distinctive patterns of alopecia result from different causes.

Alopecia areata causes expanding patches of nonscarring hair loss bordered by "exclamation point" hairs.

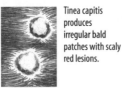

Tinea capitis produces irregular bald patches with scaly red lesions.

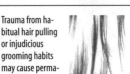

Trauma from habitual hair pulling or injudicious grooming habits may cause permanent peripheral alopecia.

Chemotherapeutic medication produces diffuse temporary hair loss.

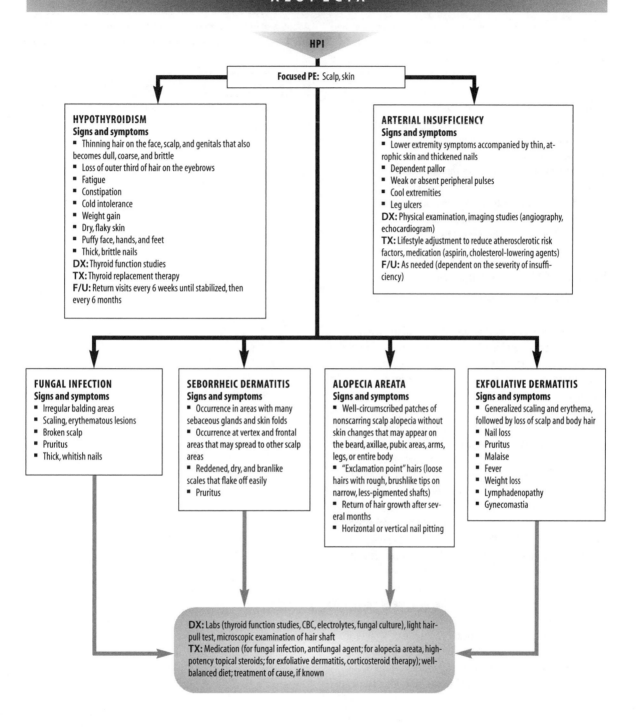

HPI

Focused PE: Scalp, skin

HYPOTHYROIDISM
Signs and symptoms
- Thinning hair on the face, scalp, and genitals that also becomes dull, coarse, and brittle
- Loss of outer third of hair on the eyebrows
- Fatigue
- Constipation
- Cold intolerance
- Weight gain
- Dry, flaky skin
- Puffy face, hands, and feet
- Thick, brittle nails

DX: Thyroid function studies
TX: Thyroid replacement therapy
F/U: Return visits every 6 weeks until stabilized, then every 6 months

ARTERIAL INSUFFICIENCY
Signs and symptoms
- Lower extremity symptoms accompanied by thin, atrophic skin and thickened nails
- Dependent pallor
- Weak or absent peripheral pulses
- Cool extremities
- Leg ulcers

DX: Physical examination, imaging studies (angiography, echocardiogram)
TX: Lifestyle adjustment to reduce atherosclerotic risk factors, medication (aspirin, cholesterol-lowering agents)
F/U: As needed (dependent on the severity of insufficiency)

FUNGAL INFECTION
Signs and symptoms
- Irregular balding areas
- Scaling, erythematous lesions
- Broken scalp
- Pruritus
- Thick, whitish nails

SEBORRHEIC DERMATITIS
Signs and symptoms
- Occurrence in areas with many sebaceous glands and skin folds
- Occurrence at vertex and frontal areas that may spread to other scalp areas
- Reddened, dry, and branlike scales that flake off easily
- Pruritus

ALOPECIA AREATA
Signs and symptoms
- Well-circumscribed patches of nonscarring scalp alopecia without skin changes that may appear on the beard, axillae, pubic areas, arms, legs, or entire body
- "Exclamation point" hairs (loose hairs with rough, brushlike tips on narrow, less-pigmented shafts)
- Return of hair growth after several months
- Horizontal or vertical nail pitting

EXFOLIATIVE DERMATITIS
Signs and symptoms
- Generalized scaling and erythema, followed by loss of scalp and body hair
- Nail loss
- Pruritus
- Malaise
- Fever
- Weight loss
- Lymphadenopathy
- Gynecomastia

DX: Labs (thyroid function studies, CBC, electrolytes, fungal culture), light hair-pull test, microscopic examination of hair shaft
TX: Medication (for fungal infection, antifungal agent; for alopecia areata, high-potency topical steroids; for exfoliative dermatitis, corticosteroid therapy); well-balanced diet; treatment of cause, if known

Additional differential diagnoses: arsenic poisoning ▪ burns ▪ cutaneous T-cell lymphoma ▪ dissecting cellulitis of the scalp ▪ Hodgkin's disease ▪ hypopituitarism ▪ lichen planus ▪ myotonic dystrophy ▪ protein deficiency ▪ sarcoidosis ▪ scleroderma ▪ secondary syphilis ▪ skin metastases ▪ thallium poisoning ▪ thyrotoxicosis

Amenorrhea

Amenorrhea, the absence of menstrual flow, can be classified as primary or secondary. In primary amenorrhea, menstruation fails to begin before age 16. In secondary amenorrhea, it begins at an appropriate age but later ceases for 3 or more months in the absence of normal physiologic causes, such as pregnancy, lactation, and menopause.

Pathologic amenorrhea results from anovulation or physical obstruction to menstrual outflow, such as from an imperforate hymen, cervical stenosis, or intrauterine adhesions. Anovulation may result from hormonal imbalance, debilitating disease, stress or emotional disturbances, strenuous exercise, malnutrition, obesity, or anatomic abnormalities, such as congenital absence of the ovaries or uterus. Amenorrhea may also result from drug or hormonal treatments.

History and physical examination

Begin by determining whether the amenorrhea is primary or secondary. If it's primary, ask the patient at what age her mother first menstruated, because the age of menarche is fairly consistent in families. Form an overall impression of the patient's physical, mental, and emotional development because these factors, as well as heredity and climate, may delay menarche until after age 16.

If menstruation began at an appropriate age but has since ceased, determine the frequency and duration of the patient's previous menstrual cycles. Ask her about the onset and nature of any changes in her normal menstrual pattern, and determine the date of her last menstruation. Find out if she has noticed related signs, such as breast swelling or weight changes.

Determine when the patient last had a physical examination. Review her health history, especially noting long-term illnesses, such as anemia, or use of oral contraceptives. Ask about exercise habits, especially running, and ask whether she experiences stress on the job or at home. Probe the patient's eating habits, including number and size of daily meals and snacks, and ask if she has recently gained weight.

Observe her appearance for secondary sex characteristics or signs of virilization. If you're responsible for performing a pelvic examination, check for anatomic aberrations of the outflow tract, such as cervical adhesions, fibroids, or an imperforate hymen.

PEDIATRIC POINTER

Adolescent girls are especially prone to amenorrhea caused by emotional upsets, typically stemming from school, social, or family problems.

ELDER CARE CUE

In women older than age 50, amenorrhea usually represents the onset of menopause.

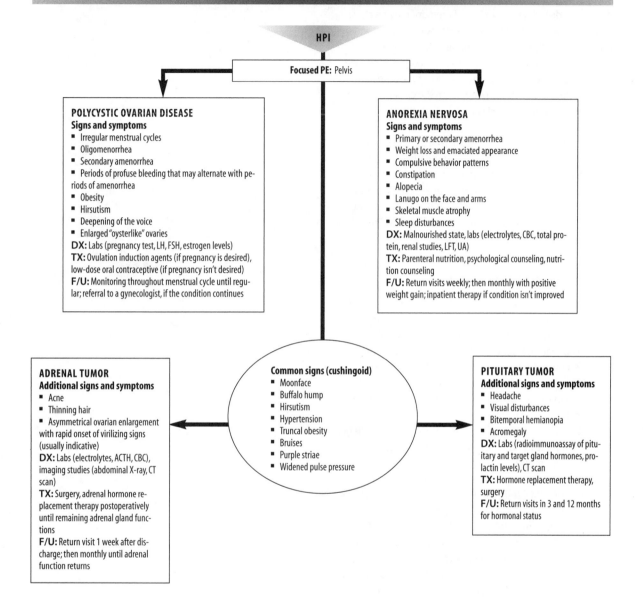

HPI

Focused PE: Pelvis

POLYCYSTIC OVARIAN DISEASE
Signs and symptoms
- Irregular menstrual cycles
- Oligomenorrhea
- Secondary amenorrhea
- Periods of profuse bleeding that may alternate with periods of amenorrhea
- Obesity
- Hirsutism
- Deepening of the voice
- Enlarged "oysterlike" ovaries

DX: Labs (pregnancy test, LH, FSH, estrogen levels)
TX: Ovulation induction agents (if pregnancy is desired), low-dose oral contraceptive (if pregnancy isn't desired)
F/U: Monitoring throughout menstrual cycle until regular; referral to a gynecologist, if the condition continues

ANOREXIA NERVOSA
Signs and symptoms
- Primary or secondary amenorrhea
- Weight loss and emaciated appearance
- Compulsive behavior patterns
- Constipation
- Alopecia
- Lanugo on the face and arms
- Skeletal muscle atrophy
- Sleep disturbances

DX: Malnourished state, labs (electrolytes, CBC, total protein, renal studies, LFT, UA)
TX: Parenteral nutrition, psychological counseling, nutrition counseling
F/U: Return visits weekly; then monthly with positive weight gain; inpatient therapy if condition isn't improved

ADRENAL TUMOR
Additional signs and symptoms
- Acne
- Thinning hair
- Asymmetrical ovarian enlargement with rapid onset of virilizing signs (usually indicative)

DX: Labs (electrolytes, ACTH, CBC), imaging studies (abdominal X-ray, CT scan)
TX: Surgery, adrenal hormone replacement therapy postoperatively until remaining adrenal gland functions
F/U: Return visit 1 week after discharge; then monthly until adrenal function returns

Common signs (cushingoid)
- Moonface
- Buffalo hump
- Hirsutism
- Hypertension
- Truncal obesity
- Bruises
- Purple striae
- Widened pulse pressure

PITUITARY TUMOR
Additional signs and symptoms
- Headache
- Visual disturbances
- Bitemporal hemianopia
- Acromegaly

DX: Labs (radioimmunoassay of pituitary and target gland hormones, prolactin levels), CT scan
TX: Hormone replacement therapy, surgery
F/U: Return visits in 3 and 12 months for hormonal status

Additional differential diagnoses: adrenocortical hyperplasia ▪ adrenocortical hypofunction ▪ amenorrhea-lactation disorders ▪ chronic renal failure ▪ congenital absence of the ovaries ▪ congenital absence of the uterus ▪ corpus luteum cysts ▪ hypothalamic tumor ▪ hypothyroidism ▪ mosaicism ▪ ovarian insensitivity to gonadotropins ▪ ovarian tumor ▪ PID ▪ physiologic delay of puberty ▪ pituitary infarction ▪ pregnancy ▪ pseudoamenorrhea ▪ pseudocyesis ▪ Sertoli-Leydig cell tumor ▪ testicular feminization ▪ thyrotoxicosis ▪ uterine hypoplasia

Amnesia

Amnesia, a disturbance in or loss of memory, may be classi-fied as partial or complete and as anterograde or retrograde. Anterograde amnesia denotes memory loss for events that occurred after the onset of the causative trauma or disease; retrograde amnesia denotes memory loss for events that oc-curred before the onset. Depending on the cause, amnesia may arise suddenly or slowly and may be temporary or per-manent.

Organic, or true, amnesia results from temporal lobe dys-function, and it characteristically spares patches of memory. A common symptom among patients with seizures or head trauma, organic amnesia can also be an early indicator of Alzheimer's disease. Hysterical amnesia has a psychogenic origin and typically causes complete memory loss. Treatment-induced amnesia is usually transient.

History and physical examination

Because the patient often isn't aware of his amnesia, you'll usually need to obtain information from his family and friends. Throughout your assessment, notice the patient's general appearance, behavior, mood, and train of thought. Ask when the amnesia first appeared and what types of things the patient can't remember. Can he learn new informa-tion? How long does he remember it? Does the amnesia en-compass a recent or remote period?

Test the patient's recent memory by asking him to identify and repeat three items. Retest him after 3 minutes. Test his in-termediate memory by asking, "Who was president before the person who is currently in office?" or "What was the last type of car you bought?" Test remote memory with such questions as "How old are you?" and "Where were you born?"

Take the patient's vital signs and assess his level of con-sciousness. Check his pupils: They should be equal in size and should constrict quickly when exposed to direct light. Also as-sess his extraocular movements. Test motor function by hav-ing the patient move his arms and legs through their range of motion. Evaluate sensory function with pinpricks on the pa-tient's skin.

PEDIATRIC POINTER

A child who suffers amnesia during seizures may mistakenly be labeled as "learning disabled." To prevent this mislabeling, stress the importance of adherence to the prescribed medication schedule, and discuss ways that the child, his parents, and his teachers can cope with the amnesia.

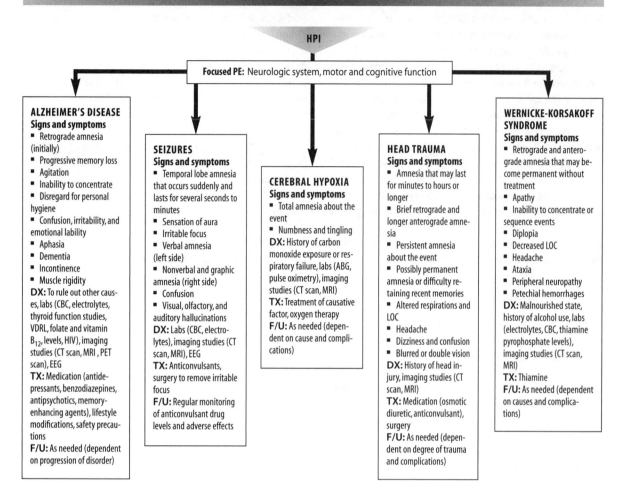

HPI

Focused PE: Neurologic system, motor and cognitive function

ALZHEIMER'S DISEASE
Signs and symptoms
- Retrograde amnesia (initially)
- Progressive memory loss
- Agitation
- Inability to concentrate
- Disregard for personal hygiene
- Confusion, irritability, and emotional lability
- Aphasia
- Dementia
- Incontinence
- Muscle rigidity

DX: To rule out other causes, labs (CBC, electrolytes, thyroid function studies, VDRL, folate and vitamin B_{12}, levels, HIV), imaging studies (CT scan, MRI, PET scan), EEG

TX: Medication (antidepressants, benzodiazepines, antipsychotics, memory-enhancing agents), lifestyle modifications, safety precautions

F/U: As needed (dependent on progression of disorder)

SEIZURES
Signs and symptoms
- Temporal lobe amnesia that occurs suddenly and lasts for several seconds to minutes
- Sensation of aura
- Irritable focus
- Verbal amnesia (left side)
- Nonverbal and graphic amnesia (right side)
- Confusion
- Visual, olfactory, and auditory hallucinations

DX: Labs (CBC, electrolytes), imaging studies (CT scan, MRI), EEG

TX: Anticonvulsants, surgery to remove irritable focus

F/U: Regular monitoring of anticonvulsant drug levels and adverse effects

CEREBRAL HYPOXIA
Signs and symptoms
- Total amnesia about the event
- Numbness and tingling

DX: History of carbon monoxide exposure or respiratory failure, labs (ABG, pulse oximetry), imaging studies (CT scan, MRI)

TX: Treatment of causative factor, oxygen therapy

F/U: As needed (dependent on cause and complications)

HEAD TRAUMA
Signs and symptoms
- Amnesia that may last for minutes to hours or longer
- Brief retrograde and longer anterograde amnesia
- Persistent amnesia about the event
- Possibly permanent amnesia or difficulty retaining recent memories
- Altered respirations and LOC
- Headache
- Dizziness and confusion
- Blurred or double vision

DX: History of head injury, imaging studies (CT scan, MRI)

TX: Medication (osmotic diuretic, anticonvulsant), surgery

F/U: As needed (dependent on degree of trauma and complications)

WERNICKE-KORSAKOFF SYNDROME
Signs and symptoms
- Retrograde and anterograde amnesia that may become permanent without treatment
- Apathy
- Inability to concentrate or sequence events
- Diplopia
- Decreased LOC
- Headache
- Ataxia
- Peripheral neuropathy
- Petechial hemorrhages

DX: Malnourished state, history of alcohol use, labs (electrolytes, CBC, thiamine pyrophosphate levels), imaging studies (CT scan, MRI)

TX: Thiamine

F/U: As needed (dependent on causes and complications)

Additional differential diagnoses: anoxia ▪ cerebral lesion ▪ cerebral mass ▪ dissociative disorder ▪ herpes simplex encephalitis ▪ stroke

Other causes: medication (general anesthetics, barbiturates, certain benzodiazepines) ▪ ECT ▪ temporal lobe surgery

Analgesia

Analgesia, the absence of sensitivity to pain, is an important sign of central nervous system disease that commonly indicates a specific type and location of spinal cord lesion. It always occurs with loss of temperature sensation (thermanesthesia) because these two sensory nerve impulses travel together in the spinal cord. It can also occur with other sensory deficits (such as paresthesia, loss of proprioception and vibratory sense, and tactile anesthesia) that are common in disorders involving the peripheral nerves, spinal cord, and brain. However, when accompanied only by thermanesthesia, analgesia points to an incomplete lesion of the spinal cord.

Analgesia can be classified as partial or total below the level of the lesion and as unilateral or bilateral, depending on the cause and level of the lesion. Its onset may be slow and progressive (such as with a tumor) or abrupt (such as with trauma). Often transient, analgesia may resolve spontaneously.

History and physical examination

Suspect spinal cord injury if the patient complains of unilateral or bilateral analgesia over a large body area that's accompanied by paralysis. Immobilize his spine in proper alignment, using a cervical collar and a long backboard, if possible. If a collar or backboard isn't available, position the patient supine on a flat surface and place sandbags around his head, neck, and torso. Use correct technique and extreme caution when moving him to prevent exacerbating spinal injury. Continuously monitor respiratory rate and rhythm, and observe for accessory muscle use because a complete lesion above the T6 level may cause diaphragmatic and intercostal muscle paralysis. Have an artificial airway and handheld resuscitation bag on hand, and be prepared to initiate emergency resuscitation measures in case of respiratory failure.

When you're satisfied that the patient's spine and respiratory status are stabilized — or if the analgesia isn't severe and isn't accompanied by signs of spinal cord injury — perform a physical examination and baseline neurologic evaluation. First, take the patient's vital signs and assess his level of consciousness. Then test pupillary, corneal, cough, and gag reflexes to rule out brain stem and cranial nerve involvement. If the patient is conscious, evaluate his speech and ability to swallow.

If possible, observe the patient's gait and posture and assess his balance and coordination. Evaluate muscle tone and strength in all extremities. Test for other sensory deficits over all dermatomes (individual skin segments innervated by a specific spinal nerve) by applying light tactile stimulation with a tongue depressor or cotton swab. Perform a more thorough check of pain sensitivity, if necessary, using a pin.

Also, test temperature sensation over all dermatomes, using two test tubes — one filled with hot water, the other with cold water. In each arm and leg, test vibration sense (using a tuning fork), proprioception, and superficial and deep tendon reflexes. Check for increased muscle tone by extending and flexing the patient's elbows and knees as he tries to relax.

Focus your history taking on the onset of analgesia (sudden or gradual) and on any recent trauma. Obtain a complete medical history, especially noting any incidence of cancer in the patient or his family.

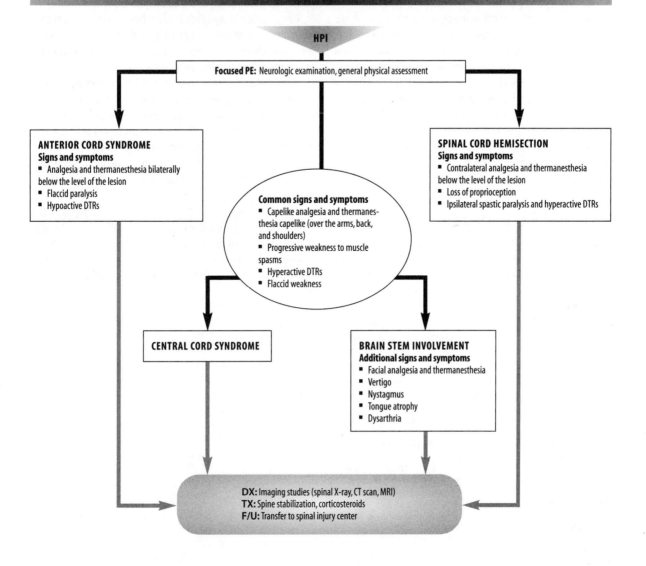

HPI

Focused PE: Neurologic examination, general physical assessment

ANTERIOR CORD SYNDROME
Signs and symptoms
- Analgesia and thermanesthesia bilaterally below the level of the lesion
- Flaccid paralysis
- Hypoactive DTRs

Common signs and symptoms
- Capelike analgesia and thermanes-thesia capelike (over the arms, back, and shoulders)
- Progressive weakness to muscle spasms
- Hyperactive DTRs
- Flaccid weakness

SPINAL CORD HEMISECTION
Signs and symptoms
- Contralateral analgesia and thermanesthesia below the level of the lesion
- Loss of proprioception
- Ipsilateral spastic paralysis and hyperactive DTRs

CENTRAL CORD SYNDROME

BRAIN STEM INVOLVEMENT
Additional signs and symptoms
- Facial analgesia and thermanesthesia
- Vertigo
- Nystagmus
- Tongue atrophy
- Dysarthria

DX: Imaging studies (spinal X-ray, CT scan, MRI)
TX: Spine stabilization, corticosteroids
F/U: Transfer to spinal injury center

Other causes: medication, such as topical and local anesthetics

Anorexia

Anorexia is a lack of appetite in the presence of a physiologic need for food. This symptom is common of GI and endocrine disorders and is characteristic of certain severe psychological disturbances such as anorexia nervosa. It can also result from such factors as anxiety, chronic pain, poor oral hygiene, increased blood temperature due to hot weather or fever, and changes in taste or smell that normally accompany aging. Anorexia can also result from drug therapy or abuse. Short-term anorexia rarely jeopardizes health, but chronic anorexia can lead to life-threatening malnutrition. (See *Common signs of malnutrition*.)

History and physical examination

Take the patient's vital signs and weight. Ask about previous minimum and maximum weights. Explore dietary habits, such as when and what the patient eats. Ask what foods he likes and dislikes, and why. The patient may identify tastes and smells that nauseate him and cause loss of appetite. Ask about dental problems that interfere with chewing, including poorly fitting dentures. Ask if he has difficulty or pain when swallowing or if he vomits or has diarrhea after meals. Ask the patient how frequently and intensely he exercises.

Check for a history of stomach or bowel disorders, which can interfere with the ability to digest, absorb, or metabolize nutrients. Ask about changes in bowel habits. Also ask about alcohol and drug use, including dosages.

If the medical history doesn't reveal an organic basis for anorexia, consider psychological factors. Ask the patient if he knows what's causing his decreased appetite. Situational factors — such as a death in the family or problems at school or at work — can lead to depression and subsequent loss of appetite. Be alert for signs of malnutrition, consistent refusal of food, and a 7% to 10% loss of body weight in the preceding month.

PEDIATRIC POINTER

In children, anorexia commonly accompanies many illnesses but usually resolves promptly. However, in preadolescent and adolescent girls, be alert for the commonly subtle signs of anorexia nervosa.

Common signs of malnutrition

When assessing a patient with anorexia, be sure to check for these common signs of malnutrition:
- **hair** — dull, dry, thin, fine, and straight; easily plucked; areas of lighter or darker spots; hair loss
- **face** — generalized swelling, dark areas on the cheeks and under the eyes, lumpy or flaky skin around the nose and mouth, enlarged parotid glands
- **eyes** — dull appearance; dry and pale or red membranes; triangular, shiny gray spots on the conjunctivae; red, fissured eyelid corners; bloodshot ring around the cornea
- **lips** — red and swollen, especially at the corners
- **tongue** — swollen, purple, raw-looking; sores or abnormal papillae
- **teeth** — missing or emerging abnormally; visible cavities or dark spots; spongy, bleeding gums
- **neck** — swollen thyroid gland
- **skin** — dry, flaky, and swollen; dark with lighter or darker spots, some resembling bruises; tight and drawn with poor turgor
- **nails** — spoon-shaped, brittle and ridged
- **musculoskeletal system** — muscle wasting, knock-knee or bowlegs, bumps on the ribs, swollen joints, musculoskeletal hemorrhages
- **cardiovascular system** — heart rate greater than 100 beats/minute, arrhythmias, elevated blood pressure
- **abdomen** — enlarged liver and spleen
- **reproductive system** — decreased libido, amenorrhea
- **nervous system** — irritability, confusion, paresthesia in the hands and feet, loss of proprioception, decreased ankle and knee reflexes.

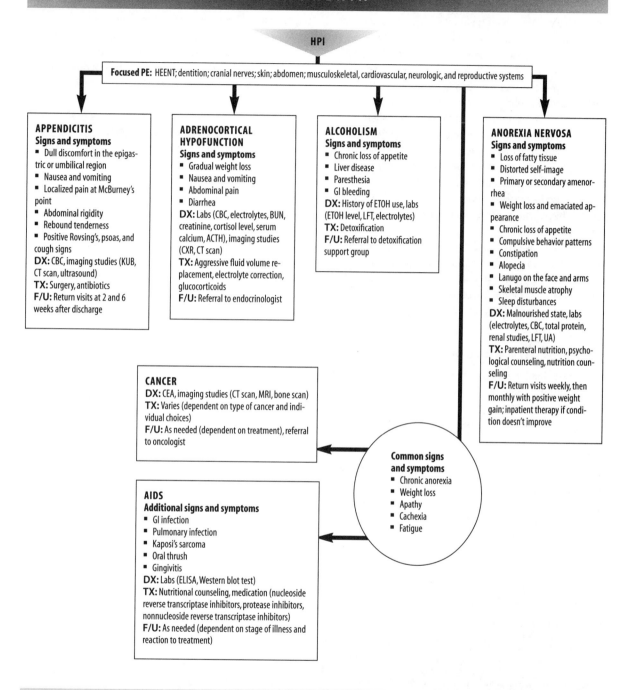

HPI

Focused PE: HEENT; dentition; cranial nerves; skin; abdomen; musculoskeletal, cardiovascular, neurologic, and reproductive systems

APPENDICITIS
Signs and symptoms
- Dull discomfort in the epigastric or umbilical region
- Nausea and vomiting
- Localized pain at McBurney's point
- Abdominal rigidity
- Rebound tenderness
- Positive Rovsing's, psoas, and cough signs

DX: CBC, imaging studies (KUB, CT scan, ultrasound)
TX: Surgery, antibiotics
F/U: Return visits at 2 and 6 weeks after discharge

ADRENOCORTICAL HYPOFUNCTION
Signs and symptoms
- Gradual weight loss
- Nausea and vomiting
- Abdominal pain
- Diarrhea

DX: Labs (CBC, electrolytes, BUN, creatinine, cortisol level, serum calcium, ACTH), imaging studies (CXR, CT scan)
TX: Aggressive fluid volume replacement, electrolyte correction, glucocorticoids
F/U: Referral to endocrinologist

ALCOHOLISM
Signs and symptoms
- Chronic loss of appetite
- Liver disease
- Paresthesia
- GI bleeding

DX: History of ETOH use, labs (ETOH level, LFT, electrolytes)
TX: Detoxification
F/U: Referral to detoxification support group

ANOREXIA NERVOSA
Signs and symptoms
- Loss of fatty tissue
- Distorted self-image
- Primary or secondary amenorrhea
- Weight loss and emaciated appearance
- Chronic loss of appetite
- Compulsive behavior patterns
- Constipation
- Alopecia
- Lanugo on the face and arms
- Skeletal muscle atrophy
- Sleep disturbances

DX: Malnourished state, labs (electrolytes, CBC, total protein, renal studies, LFT, UA)
TX: Parenteral nutrition, psychological counseling, nutrition counseling
F/U: Return visits weekly, then monthly with positive weight gain; inpatient therapy if condition doesn't improve

CANCER
DX: CEA, imaging studies (CT scan, MRI, bone scan)
TX: Varies (dependent on type of cancer and individual choices)
F/U: As needed (dependent on treatment), referral to oncologist

Common signs and symptoms
- Chronic anorexia
- Weight loss
- Apathy
- Cachexia
- Fatigue

AIDS
Additional signs and symptoms
- GI infection
- Pulmonary infection
- Kaposi's sarcoma
- Oral thrush
- Gingivitis

DX: Labs (ELISA, Western blot test)
TX: Nutritional counseling, medication (nucleoside reverse transcriptase inhibitors, protease inhibitors, nonnucleoside reverse transcriptase inhibitors)
F/U: As needed (dependent on stage of illness and reaction to treatment)

Additional differential diagnoses: chronic renal failure ▪ cirrhosis ▪ Crohn's disease ▪ decreased gastric emptying ▪ depressive syndrome ▪ electrolyte imbalance ▪ esophagitis ▪ gastritis ▪ hepatitis ▪ hypopituitarism ▪ hypothyroidism ▪ ketoacidosis ▪ osteoporosis ▪ pernicious anemia

Other causes: cardiomegaly ▪ constipation ▪ digitalis toxicity ▪ medication (amphetamines, chemotherapeutic agents, sympathomimetics such as ephedrine, and some antibiotics) ▪ radiation therapy ▪ TPN

Anosmia

Although it's usually an insignificant consequence of nasal congestion or obstruction, anosmia — absence of the sense of smell — occasionally heralds a serious defect. (See *Understanding the sense of smell.*) Temporary anosmia can result from any condition that irritates and causes swelling of the nasal mucosa and obstructs the olfactory area in the nose, such as heavy smoking, rhinitis, or sinusitis. Permanent anosmia usually results when the olfactory neuroepithelium, or any part of the olfactory nerve, is destroyed. Permanent or temporary anosmia can also result from inhaling irritants, such as cocaine or acid fumes, that paralyze nasal cilia. Anosmia may also be reported — without an identifiable organic cause — by patients suffering from hysteria, depression, or schizophrenia.

Anosmia is invariably perceived as bilateral; unilateral anosmia can also occur but is seldom recognized by the patient. Because combined stimulation of taste buds and olfactory cells produces the sense of taste, anosmia is usually accompanied by ageusia, loss of the sense of taste.

History and physical examination

Begin the patient history by asking about the onset and duration of anosmia and its related symptoms — stuffy nose, nasal discharge or bleeding, postnasal drip, sneezing, dry or sore mouth and throat, ageusia, loss of appetite, excessive tearing, and facial or eye pain. Pinpoint any history of nasal disease, allergies, or head trauma. Ask about heavy smoking and the use of prescribed or over-the-counter nasal drops or sprays. Be sure to rule out cocaine use.

Inspect and palpate nasal structures for obvious injury, inflammation, deformities, and septal deviation or perforation. Observe the contour and color of the nasal mucosa and the size and color of the turbinates. Check for polyps, which appear as translucent, white masses around the middle meatus. Note the source and character of any nasal discharge. Palpate the sinus areas for tenderness and contour.

Assess for nasal obstruction by occluding one nostril at a time with your thumb as the patient breathes quietly; listen for breath sounds and for sounds of moisture or mucus. Test olfactory nerve (first cranial nerve) function by having the patient identify common odors.

PEDIATRIC POINTER

Anosmia in children usually results from nasal obstruction by a foreign body or enlarged adenoids.

Understanding the sense of smell

Our noses can distinguish the odors of thousands of chemicals, thanks to a highly developed complex of sensory cells. The olfactory epithelium contains olfactory receptor cells, along with olfactory glands and sustentacular cells — both of which secrete mucus to keep the epithelial surface moist. The mucus covering the olfactory cells probably traps airborne odorous molecules, which then fit into the appropriate receptors on the cell surface. In response to this stimulus, the receptor cell transmits an impulse along the olfactory nerve (cranial nerve I) to the olfactory area of the cortex, where it's interpreted. Any disruption along this transmission pathway, or any obstruction of the epithelial surface due to dryness or congestion, can cause anosmia.

ANOSMIA

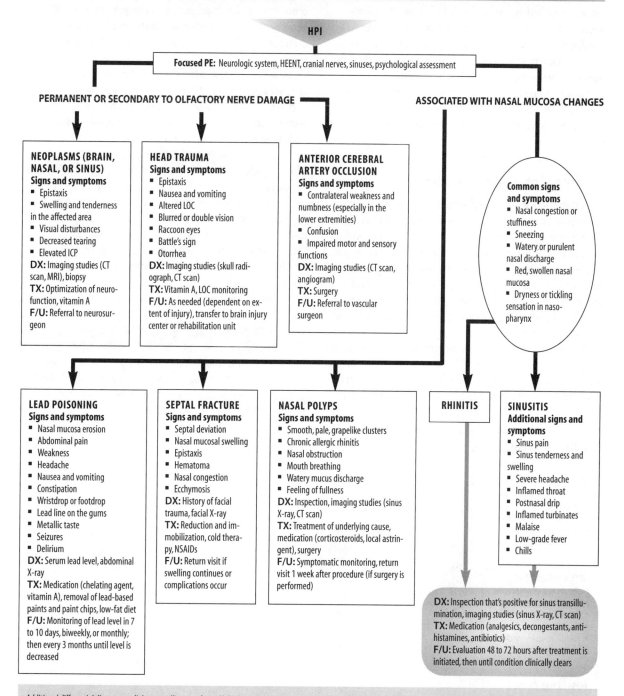

HPI

Focused PE: Neurologic system, HEENT, cranial nerves, sinuses, psychological assessment

PERMANENT OR SECONDARY TO OLFACTORY NERVE DAMAGE

NEOPLASMS (BRAIN, NASAL, OR SINUS)
Signs and symptoms
- Epistaxis
- Swelling and tenderness in the affected area
- Visual disturbances
- Decreased tearing
- Elevated ICP

DX: Imaging studies (CT scan, MRI), biopsy
TX: Optimization of neurofunction, vitamin A
F/U: Referral to neurosurgeon

HEAD TRAUMA
Signs and symptoms
- Epistaxis
- Nausea and vomiting
- Altered LOC
- Blurred or double vision
- Raccoon eyes
- Battle's sign
- Otorrhea

DX: Imaging studies (skull radiograph, CT scan)
TX: Vitamin A, LOC monitoring
F/U: As needed (dependent on extent of injury), transfer to brain injury center or rehabilitation unit

ANTERIOR CEREBRAL ARTERY OCCLUSION
Signs and symptoms
- Contralateral weakness and numbness (especially in the lower extremities)
- Confusion
- Impaired motor and sensory functions

DX: Imaging studies (CT scan, angiogram)
TX: Surgery
F/U: Referral to vascular surgeon

ASSOCIATED WITH NASAL MUCOSA CHANGES

Common signs and symptoms
- Nasal congestion or stuffiness
- Sneezing
- Watery or purulent nasal discharge
- Red, swollen nasal mucosa
- Dryness or tickling sensation in nasopharynx

LEAD POISONING
Signs and symptoms
- Nasal mucosa erosion
- Abdominal pain
- Weakness
- Headache
- Nausea and vomiting
- Constipation
- Wristdrop or footdrop
- Lead line on the gums
- Metallic taste
- Seizures
- Delirium

DX: Serum lead level, abdominal X-ray
TX: Medication (chelating agent, vitamin A), removal of lead-based paints and paint chips, low-fat diet
F/U: Monitoring of lead level in 7 to 10 days, biweekly, or monthly; then every 3 months until level is decreased

SEPTAL FRACTURE
Signs and symptoms
- Septal deviation
- Nasal mucosal swelling
- Epistaxis
- Hematoma
- Nasal congestion
- Ecchymosis

DX: History of facial trauma, facial X-ray
TX: Reduction and immobilization, cold therapy, NSAIDs
F/U: Return visit if swelling continues or complications occur

NASAL POLYPS
Signs and symptoms
- Smooth, pale, grapelike clusters
- Chronic allergic rhinitis
- Nasal obstruction
- Mouth breathing
- Watery mucus discharge
- Feeling of fullness

DX: Inspection, imaging studies (sinus X-ray, CT scan)
TX: Treatment of underlying cause, medication (corticosteroids, local astringent), surgery
F/U: Symptomatic monitoring, return visit 1 week after procedure (if surgery is performed)

RHINITIS

SINUSITIS
Additional signs and symptoms
- Sinus pain
- Sinus tenderness and swelling
- Severe headache
- Inflamed throat
- Postnasal drip
- Inflamed turbinates
- Malaise
- Low-grade fever
- Chills

DX: Inspection that's positive for sinus transillumination, imaging studies (sinus X-ray, CT scan)
TX: Medication (analgesics, decongestants, antihistamines, antibiotics)
F/U: Evaluation 48 to 72 hours after treatment is initiated, then until condition clinically clears

---

Additional differential diagnoses: diabetes mellitus ▪ frontal lobe brain tumor ▪ lethal midline granulomas ▪ nasal polyps ▪ optic chiasm ▪ pernicious anemia ▪ septal hematoma

---

Other causes: medication (prolonged use of nasal decongestants, naphazoline, reserpine and, less commonly, amphetamines, phenothiazines, and estrogen) ▪ radiation therapy ▪ surgery

Anuria

Clinically defined as urine output of less than 75 ml daily, anuria indicates either urinary tract obstruction or renal failure due to various mechanisms. (See *Major causes of renal failure.*) Fortunately, anuria is rare; even in renal failure, the kidneys usually produce at least 75 ml of urine daily.

Because urine output is easily measured, anuria rarely goes undetected. However, without immediate treatment, it can rapidly cause uremia and other complications of urine retention.

History and physical examination

After detecting anuria, your priorities are to determine if urine formation is occurring and to intervene appropriately. The patient may require catheterization to relieve a lower urinary tract obstruction and to check for residual urine. You may find that an obstruction hinders catheter insertion and that urine return is cloudy and foul smelling. If more than 75 ml of urine are collected, suspect lower urinary tract obstruction; less than 75 ml, suspect renal dysfunction or obstruction higher in the urinary tract.

Take the patient's vital signs and obtain a complete history. First ask about changes in voiding patterns. Determine the amount of fluid normally ingested each day, the amount of fluid ingested in the last 24 to 48 hours, and the time and amount of the patient's last urination. Review his medical history, especially noting previous kidney disease, urinary tract obstruction or infection, prostate enlargement, renal calculi, neurogenic bladder, or congenital abnormalities. Ask about drug use as well as previous abdominal, renal, or urinary tract surgery.

Inspect and palpate the abdomen for asymmetry, distention, or bulging. Inspect the flank area for edema or erythema, and percuss and palpate the bladder. Palpate the kidneys anteriorly and posteriorly, and percuss them at the costovertebral angle. Auscultate for bruits over the renal arteries.

Major causes of acute renal failure

PRERENAL CAUSES
- Decreased cardiac output
- Hypovolemia
- Peripheral vasodilation
- Renovascular obstruction
- Severe vasoconstriction

INTRARENAL CAUSES
- Acute tubular necrosis
- Cortical necrosis
- Glomerulonephritis
- Papillary necrosis
- Renal vascular occlusion
- Vasculitis

POSTRENAL CAUSES
- Bladder obstruction
- Ureteral obstruction
- Urethral obstruction

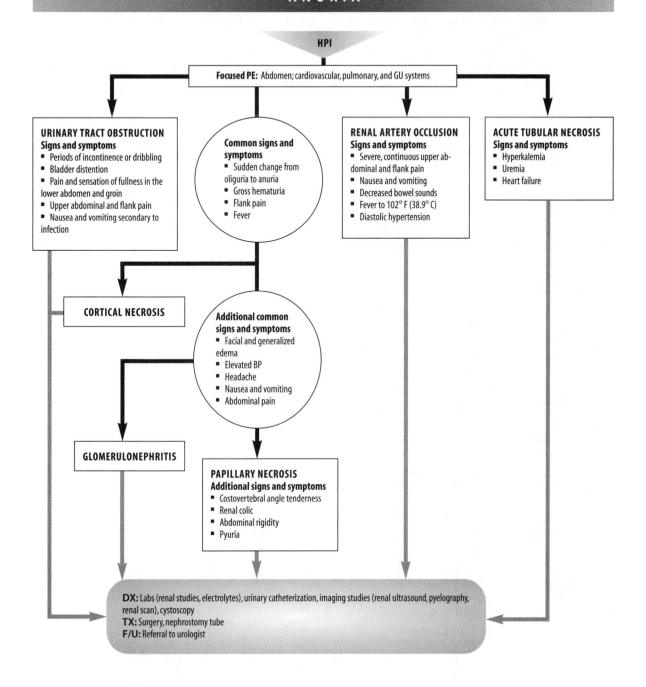

HPI

Focused PE: Abdomen; cardiovascular, pulmonary, and GU systems

URINARY TRACT OBSTRUCTION
Signs and symptoms
- Periods of incontinence or dribbling
- Bladder distention
- Pain and sensation of fullness in the lower abdomen and groin
- Upper abdominal and flank pain
- Nausea and vomiting secondary to infection

Common signs and symptoms
- Sudden change from oliguria to anuria
- Gross hematuria
- Flank pain
- Fever

RENAL ARTERY OCCLUSION
Signs and symptoms
- Severe, continuous upper abdominal and flank pain
- Nausea and vomiting
- Decreased bowel sounds
- Fever to 102° F (38.9° C)
- Diastolic hypertension

ACUTE TUBULAR NECROSIS
Signs and symptoms
- Hyperkalemia
- Uremia
- Heart failure

CORTICAL NECROSIS

Additional common signs and symptoms
- Facial and generalized edema
- Elevated BP
- Headache
- Nausea and vomiting
- Abdominal pain

GLOMERULONEPHRITIS

PAPILLARY NECROSIS
Additional signs and symptoms
- Costovertebral angle tenderness
- Renal colic
- Abdominal rigidity
- Pyuria

DX: Labs (renal studies, electrolytes), urinary catheterization, imaging studies (renal ultrasound, pyelography, renal scan), cystoscopy
TX: Surgery, nephrostomy tube
F/U: Referral to urologist

Additional differential diagnoses: burns ▪ crush injury ▪ hemolytic-uremic syndrome ▪ hepatic renal syndrome ▪ renal artery or vein occlusion ▪ vasculitis

Other causes: medication (antibiotics, especially aminoglycosides; anesthetics; heavy metals; ethyl alcohol; adrenergics; anticholinergics; NSAIDs; ACE inhibitors; amphotericin B; ASA; methotrexate) ▪ contrast dye for imaging studies

Anxiety

A subjective reaction to a real or imagined threat, anxiety is a nonspecific feeling of uneasiness or dread. It may be mild, moderate, or severe. Mild anxiety may cause slight physical or psychological discomfort. Severe anxiety may be incapacitating or even life-threatening.

Everyone experiences anxiety from time to time — it's a normal response to actual danger, prompting the body (through stimulation of the sympathetic and parasympathetic nervous systems) to purposeful action. It's also a normal response to physical and emotional stress, which can be produced by virtually any illness. In addition, anxiety can be precipitated or exacerbated by many nonpathologic factors, including lack of sleep, poor diet, and excessive intake of caffeine or other stimulants. However, excessive, unwarranted anxiety may indicate an underlying psychological problem.

History and physical examination

If the patient displays acute, severe anxiety, quickly take his vital signs and determine his chief complaint; this will serve as a guide for how to proceed. For example, if the patient's anxiety occurs with chest pain and shortness of breath, you might suspect myocardial infarction and act accordingly. While examining the patient, try to keep him as calm as possible. Suggest relaxation techniques and talk in a reassuring, soothing voice. Uncontrolled anxiety can alter vital signs and exacerbate the causative disorder.

If the patient displays mild or moderate anxiety, ask about its duration. Is the anxiety constant or sporadic? Did he notice any precipitating factors? Find out if the anxiety is exacerbated by stress, lack of sleep, or excessive caffeine intake. Does rest, tranquilizers, or exercise alleviate it?

Obtain a complete medical history, especially noting drug use. Then perform a physical examination, focusing on any complaints that may trigger or be aggravated by anxiety.

If significant physical signs don't accompany the patient's anxiety, suspect a psychological basis. Determine the patient's level of consciousness and observe his behavior. If appropriate, refer the patient for psychiatric evaluation.

PEDIATRIC POINTER

Anxiety in children usually results from painful physical illness or inadequate oxygenation. Its autonomic signs tend to be more common and dramatic than in adults.

ELDER CARE CUE

In elderly patients, distractions from the patient's ritual activity may provoke anxiety or agitation.

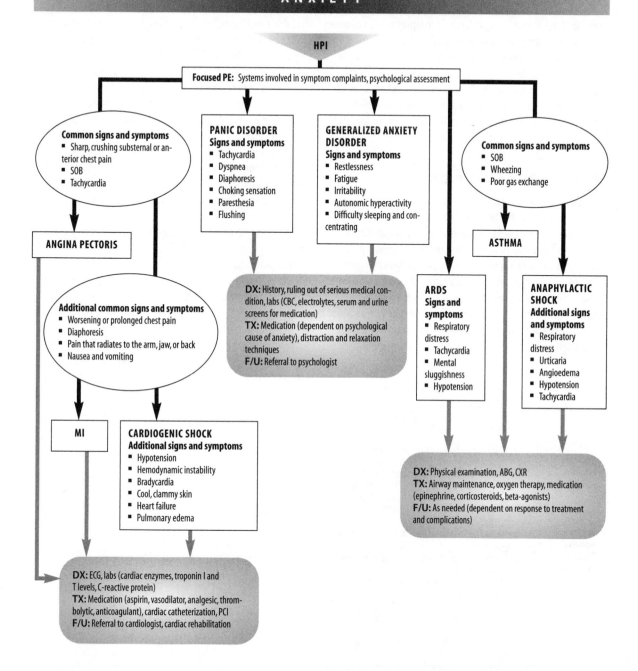

HPI

Focused PE: Systems involved in symptom complaints, psychological assessment

Common signs and symptoms
- Sharp, crushing substernal or anterior chest pain
- SOB
- Tachycardia

ANGINA PECTORIS

Additional common signs and symptoms
- Worsening or prolonged chest pain
- Diaphoresis
- Pain that radiates to the arm, jaw, or back
- Nausea and vomiting

MI

CARDIOGENIC SHOCK
Additional signs and symptoms
- Hypotension
- Hemodynamic instability
- Bradycardia
- Cool, clammy skin
- Heart failure
- Pulmonary edema

DX: ECG, labs (cardiac enzymes, troponin I and T levels, C-reactive protein)
TX: Medication (aspirin, vasodilator, analgesic, thrombolytic, anticoagulant), cardiac catheterization, PCI
F/U: Referral to cardiologist, cardiac rehabilitation

PANIC DISORDER
Signs and symptoms
- Tachycardia
- Dyspnea
- Diaphoresis
- Choking sensation
- Paresthesia
- Flushing

DX: History, ruling out of serious medical condition, labs (CBC, electrolytes, serum and urine screens for medication)
TX: Medication (dependent on psychological cause of anxiety), distraction and relaxation techniques
F/U: Referral to psychologist

GENERALIZED ANXIETY DISORDER
Signs and symptoms
- Restlessness
- Fatigue
- Irritability
- Autonomic hyperactivity
- Difficulty sleeping and concentrating

ARDS
Signs and symptoms
- Respiratory distress
- Tachycardia
- Mental sluggishness
- Hypotension

Common signs and symptoms
- SOB
- Wheezing
- Poor gas exchange

ASTHMA

ANAPHYLACTIC SHOCK
Additional signs and symptoms
- Respiratory distress
- Urticaria
- Angioedema
- Hypotension
- Tachycardia

DX: Physical examination, ABG, CXR
TX: Airway maintenance, oxygen therapy, medication (epinephrine, corticosteroids, beta-agonists)
F/U: As needed (dependent on response to treatment and complications)

Additional differential diagnoses: autonomic hyperreflexia ▪ COPD ▪ hyperthyroidism ▪ hyperventilation syndrome ▪ hypoglycemia ▪ mitral valve prolapse ▪ obsessive-compulsive disorder ▪ pheochromocytoma ▪ phobias ▪ pneumonia ▪ pneumothorax ▪ postconcussion syndrome ▪ posttraumatic stress disorder ▪ pulmonary embolism ▪ rabies ▪ somatoform disorder

Other causes: sympathomimetics ▪ CNS stimulants ▪ antidepressants

Aphasia

Aphasia is the impaired expression or comprehension of written or spoken language and reflects disease or injury of the brain's language centers. Depending on its severity, aphasia may slightly impede communication or it may make speech impossible. It can be classified as Broca's, Wernicke's, anomic, or global aphasia. Anomic aphasia eventually resolves in more than 50% of patients, but global aphasia is commonly irreversible. (See *Identifying types of aphasia*.)

History and physical examination

If the patient doesn't display signs of increased intracranial pressure (such as a change in his level of consciousness [LOC], headaches, or increased blood pressure) or if his aphasia has developed gradually, perform a thorough neurologic examination, starting with his history. You'll probably need to obtain information from the patient's family or companion because of the patient's impairment. Ask about a history of headaches, hypertension, or seizure disorders as well as drug use. Also ask about the patient's ability to communicate and to perform routine activities before the aphasia began.

Check for obvious signs of neurologic deficit, such as ptosis or fluid leakage from the nose and ears. Take the patient's vital signs and assess his LOC. Be aware, however, that assessing LOC is difficult in many cases because the patient's verbal responses may be unreliable. Also, recognize that dysarthria (impaired articulation due to weakness or paralysis of the muscles necessary for speech) or speech apraxia (inability to voluntarily control the muscles of speech) may accompany aphasia. Speak slowly and distinctly, and allow the patient ample time to respond. Assess the patient's pupillary response, eye movements, and motor function, especially his mouth and tongue movement, swallowing ability, and spontaneous movements and gestures. To best assess motor function, first demonstrate the motions and then have the patient imitate them.

PEDIATRIC POINTERS

- *Recognize that the term* childhood aphasia *is sometimes mistakenly applied to children who fail to develop normal language skills but who aren't considered mentally retarded or developmentally delayed. Aphasia refers solely to loss of previously developed communication skills.*
- *Brain damage associated with aphasia in children most commonly follows anoxia — the result of near-drowning or airway obstruction.*

Identifying types of aphasia

TYPE	CLINICAL FINDINGS
Broca's aphasia (expressive aphasia)	- Ability to understand written and spoken language intact - Nonfluent speech, evidenced by word-finding difficulty, jargon, paraphasia, limited vocabulary, and simple sentence construction - Inability to repeat words or phrases
Wernicke's aphasia (receptive aphasia)	- Difficulty understanding written and spoken language - Inability to repeat words or phrases or follow directions - Fluent speech but may be rapid and rambling with paraphasia - Difficulty naming objects (anomia) - Lack of awareness of speech errors
Anomic aphasia	- Ability to understand written and spoken language intact - Fluent speech but lacks meaningful content - Difficulty finding words and circumlocution - Paraphasia (rarely)
Global aphasia	- Profoundly impaired receptive and expressive aphasia ability - Inability to repeat words or phrases or follow directions - Speech marked by paraphasia or jargon

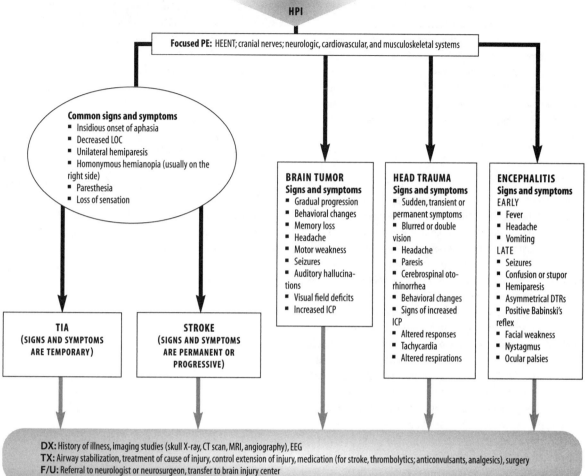

HPI

Focused PE: HEENT; cranial nerves; neurologic, cardiovascular, and musculoskeletal systems

Common signs and symptoms
- Insidious onset of aphasia
- Decreased LOC
- Unilateral hemiparesis
- Homonymous hemianopia (usually on the right side)
- Paresthesia
- Loss of sensation

TIA
(SIGNS AND SYMPTOMS ARE TEMPORARY)

STROKE
(SIGNS AND SYMPTOMS ARE PERMANENT OR PROGRESSIVE)

BRAIN TUMOR
Signs and symptoms
- Gradual progression
- Behavioral changes
- Memory loss
- Headache
- Motor weakness
- Seizures
- Auditory hallucinations
- Visual field deficits
- Increased ICP

HEAD TRAUMA
Signs and symptoms
- Sudden, transient or permanent symptoms
- Blurred or double vision
- Headache
- Paresis
- Cerebrospinal otorhinorrhea
- Behavioral changes
- Signs of increased ICP
- Altered responses
- Tachycardia
- Altered respirations

ENCEPHALITIS
Signs and symptoms
EARLY
- Fever
- Headache
- Vomiting
LATE
- Seizures
- Confusion or stupor
- Hemiparesis
- Asymmetrical DTRs
- Positive Babinski's reflex
- Facial weakness
- Nystagmus
- Ocular palsies

DX: History of illness, imaging studies (skull X-ray, CT scan, MRI, angiography), EEG
TX: Airway stabilization, treatment of cause of injury, control extension of injury, medication (for stroke, thrombolytics; anticonvulsants, analgesics), surgery
F/U: Referral to neurologist or neurosurgeon, transfer to brain injury center

Additional differential diagnoses: Alzheimer's disease ▪ brain abscess ▪ Creutzfeldt-Jakob disease

Apnea

Apnea, the cessation of spontaneous respiration, is occasionally temporary and self-limiting, as occurs during Cheyne-Stokes and Biot's respirations. More commonly, however, it's a life-threatening emergency that requires immediate intervention to prevent death.

Apnea usually results from one or more of six pathophysiologic mechanisms, each of which has numerous causes. Its most common causes include trauma, cardiac arrest, neurologic disease, aspiration of foreign objects, bronchospasm, and drug overdose.

History and physical examination

If you detect apnea, first establish and maintain a patent airway. Place the patient in the supine position and open his airway using the head-tilt or chin-lift maneuver. (*Caution:* Use the jaw-thrust technique on a patient with an obvious or suspected head or neck injury to prevent hyperextension of the neck.) Next, quickly look, listen, and feel for spontaneous respiration; if it's absent, begin artificial ventilation until it occurs or until mechanical ventilation can be initiated.

Because apnea may result from cardiac arrest (or it may cause it), be sure to assess the patient's carotid pulse immediately after you've established a patent airway. If the patient is an infant or a small child, assess the brachial pulse instead. If you can't palpate a pulse, begin cardiac compression.

When the patient's respiratory and cardiac status is stable, investigate the underlying cause of apnea. Ask him about the onset of apnea and the events immediately preceding it. If the patient is unable to answer, ask someone who witnessed the episode. The cause may become readily apparent, as in trauma.

Take a patient history, especially noting reports of headache, chest pain, muscle weakness, sore throat, or dyspnea. Ask about a history of respiratory, cardiac, or neurologic disease and about allergies and drug use.

Inspect the head, face, neck, and trunk for soft-tissue injury, hemorrhage, or skeletal deformity. Don't overlook obvious clues, such as oral and nasal secretions, reflecting fluid-filled airways and alveoli, or facial soot and singed nasal hair, suggesting thermal injury to the tracheobronchial tree.

Auscultate over all lung lobes for adventitious breath sounds, particularly crackles and rhonchi, and percuss the lung fields for increased dullness or hyperresonance. Move on to the heart, auscultating for murmurs, pericardial friction rub, and arrhythmias. Check for cyanosis, pallor, jugular vein distention, and edema. If appropriate, perform a neurologic assessment. Evaluate level of consciousness, orientation, and mental status; test cranial nerve and motor function, sensation, and reflexes in all extremities.

PEDIATRIC POINTERS

- *Premature infants are especially susceptible to periodic apneic episodes because of central nervous system immaturity.*
- *Other common causes of apnea in infants include sepsis, intraventricular and subarachnoid hemorrhage, seizures, bronchiolitis, and sudden infant death syndrome.*
- *In toddlers and older children, the primary cause of apnea is acute airway obstruction from aspiration of foreign objects. Other causes include acute epiglottiditis, croup, asthma, and such systemic disorders as muscular dystrophy and cystic fibrosis.*

ELDER CARE CUE

In elderly patients, increased sensitivity to analgesics, sedative-hypnotics, or any combination of these drugs may produce apnea, even within normal dosage ranges.

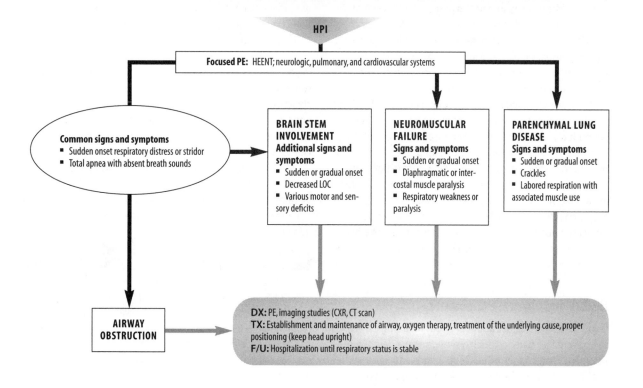

HPI

Focused PE: HEENT; neurologic, pulmonary, and cardiovascular systems

Common signs and symptoms
- Sudden onset respiratory distress or stridor
- Total apnea with absent breath sounds

BRAIN STEM INVOLVEMENT
Additional signs and symptoms
- Sudden or gradual onset
- Decreased LOC
- Various motor and sensory deficits

NEUROMUSCULAR FAILURE
Signs and symptoms
- Sudden or gradual onset
- Diaphragmatic or intercostal muscle paralysis
- Respiratory weakness or paralysis

PARENCHYMAL LUNG DISEASE
Signs and symptoms
- Sudden or gradual onset
- Crackles
- Labored respiration with associated muscle use

AIRWAY OBSTRUCTION

DX: PE, imaging studies (CXR, CT scan)
TX: Establishment and maintenance of airway, oxygen therapy, treatment of the underlying cause, proper positioning (keep head upright)
F/U: Hospitalization until respiratory status is stable

Additional differential diagnoses: pleural pressure gradient disruption ■ pulmonary capillary perfusion decrease

Apraxia

Apraxia is the inability to perform purposeful movements in the absence of significant weakness, sensory loss, poor coordination, or lack of comprehension or motivation. This neurologic sign usually indicates a lesion in the cerebral hemisphere. Its onset, severity, and duration vary, depending on the location and extent of the lesion.

Apraxia is classified as ideational, ideomotor, or kinetic, depending on the stage at which voluntary movement is impaired. It can also be classified by type of motor or skill impairment. For example, facial and gait apraxia involve specific motor groups and are easily perceived. Constructional apraxia refers to inability to copy simple drawings or patterns. Dressing apraxia refers to inability to dress oneself correctly. Callosal apraxia refers to normal motor function on one side of the body accompanied by an inability to reproduce movements on the other side. (See *How apraxia interferes with purposeful movement*.)

History and physical examination

If you detect apraxia, ask about previous neurologic disease. If the patient fails to report such disease, begin a neurologic assessment. First, take the patient's vital signs and assess his level of consciousness. Be alert for evidence of aphasia or dysarthria. Ask the patient if he has recently experienced headaches or dizziness. Then test the patient's motor function, observing for weakness and tremors. Next, use a small pin or other pointed object to test sensory function. Check deep tendon reflexes for quality and symmetry. Finally, test the patient for visual field deficits.

During your assessment, be alert for signs of increased intracranial pressure, such as headache and vomiting. If you detect these signs, elevate the head of the bed 30 degrees and monitor the patient closely for altered pupil size and reactivity, bradycardia, widened pulse pressure, and irregular respirations. Have emergency resuscitation equipment nearby.

If the patient is having seizures, maintain his airway patency and safety. Avoid restraining the patient. Help him to a lying position, loosen tight clothing, and place a pillow or other soft object beneath his head. If the patient's teeth are clenched, don't force anything into his mouth. If his mouth is open, protect the tongue by placing a soft object, such as a washcloth, between his teeth. Turn the patient's head to provide an open airway.

After completing the examination and ensuring the patient's safety, take a history. Ask about previous cerebrovascular disease, atherosclerosis, neoplastic disease, infection, or hepatic disease. Then further assess the apraxia to help determine its type.

How apraxia interferes with purposeful movement

TYPE OF APRAXIA	DESCRIPTION
Ideational apraxia	The patient can physically perform the steps required to complete a task but fails to remember the sequence in which they're performed.
Ideomotor apraxia	The patient understands and can physically perform the steps required to complete the task but can't formulate a plan to carry them out.
Kinetic apraxia	The patient understands the task and formulates a plan but fails to set the proper muscles in motion.

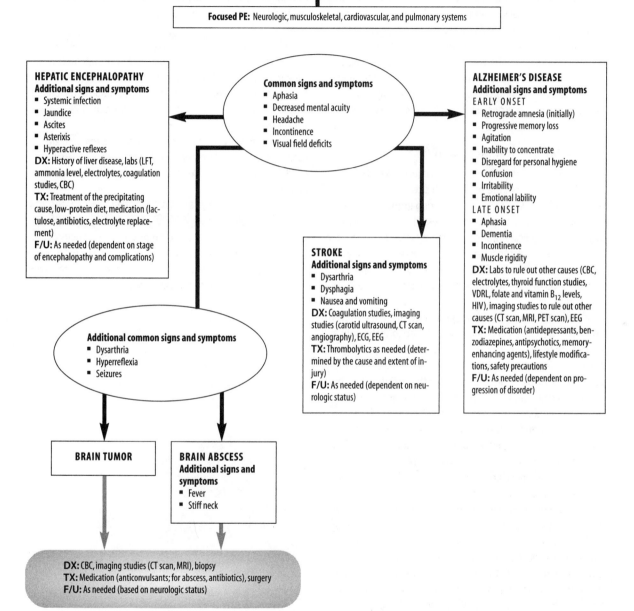

HPI

Focused PE: Neurologic, musculoskeletal, cardiovascular, and pulmonary systems

Common signs and symptoms
- Aphasia
- Decreased mental acuity
- Headache
- Incontinence
- Visual field deficits

HEPATIC ENCEPHALOPATHY
Additional signs and symptoms
- Systemic infection
- Jaundice
- Ascites
- Asterixis
- Hyperactive reflexes

DX: History of liver disease, labs (LFT, ammonia level, electrolytes, coagulation studies, CBC)
TX: Treatment of the precipitating cause, low-protein diet, medication (lactulose, antibiotics, electrolyte replacement)
F/U: As needed (dependent on stage of encephalopathy and complications)

ALZHEIMER'S DISEASE
Additional signs and symptoms
EARLY ONSET
- Retrograde amnesia (initially)
- Progressive memory loss
- Agitation
- Inability to concentrate
- Disregard for personal hygiene
- Confusion
- Irritability
- Emotional lability
LATE ONSET
- Aphasia
- Dementia
- Incontinence
- Muscle rigidity

DX: Labs to rule out other causes (CBC, electrolytes, thyroid function studies, VDRL, folate and vitamin B_{12} levels, HIV), imaging studies to rule out other causes (CT scan, MRI, PET scan), EEG
TX: Medication (antidepressants, benzodiazepines, antipsychotics, memory-enhancing agents), lifestyle modifications, safety precautions
F/U: As needed (dependent on progression of disorder)

STROKE
Additional signs and symptoms
- Dysarthria
- Dysphagia
- Nausea and vomiting

DX: Coagulation studies, imaging studies (carotid ultrasound, CT scan, angiography), ECG, EEG
TX: Thrombolytics as needed (determined by the cause and extent of injury)
F/U: As needed (dependent on neurologic status)

Additional common signs and symptoms
- Dysarthria
- Hyperreflexia
- Seizures

BRAIN TUMOR

BRAIN ABSCESS
Additional signs and symptoms
- Fever
- Stiff neck

DX: CBC, imaging studies (CT scan, MRI), biopsy
TX: Medication (anticonvulsants; for abscess, antibiotics), surgery
F/U: As needed (based on neurologic status)

Arm pain

Arm pain usually results from musculoskeletal disorders, but it can also stem from neurovascular or cardiovascular disorders. In some cases, it may be referred pain from another area, such as the chest, neck, or abdomen. Its location, onset, and character provide clues to its cause. The pain may affect the entire arm or only the upper arm or forearm. It may arise suddenly or gradually and be constant or intermittent. Arm pain can be described as sharp or dull, burning or numbing, and shooting or penetrating. Diffuse arm pain, however, may be difficult to describe, especially if it isn't associated with injury.

History and physical examination

If the patient reports arm pain after an injury, take a brief history of the injury from the patient or his companion. Then quickly assess for severe injuries requiring immediate treatment. If you've ruled out severe injuries, check pulses, capillary refill time, sensation, and movement distal to the affected area because circulatory impairment or nerve injury may require immediate surgery. Inspect the arm for deformities, assess the level of pain, and immobilize the arm to prevent further injury.

If the patient reports continuous or intermittent arm pain, ask him to describe it and relate when it began. Is the pain associated with repetitive or specific movements or positions? Ask the patient about activities that he performs during the day at work. Also ask him to point out other painful areas because arm pain may be referred. For example, arm pain commonly accompanies the characteristic chest pain of myocardial infarction, and right shoulder pain may be referred from the right-upper-quadrant abdominal pain of cholecystitis. Ask the patient if the pain worsens in the morning or in the evening, if it prevents him from performing his job, and if it restricts any movements. Also ask if the pain is relieved by heat, rest, or drugs. Finally, ask about any preexisting illnesses, a family history of gout or arthritis, and current drug therapy.

Next, perform a focused examination. Observe the way the patient walks, sits, and holds his arm. Inspect the entire arm, comparing it with the opposite arm for symmetry, movement, and muscle atrophy. (It's important to know if the patient is right- or left-handed.) Palpate the entire arm for swelling, nodules, and tender areas. In both arms, compare active range of motion, muscle strength, and reflexes.

If the patient reports numbness or tingling, check his sensation to vibration, temperature, and pinprick. Compare bilateral hand grasps and shoulder strength to detect weakness.

If a patient has a cast, splint, or restrictive dressing, check for circulation, sensation, and mobility distal to the dressing.

Ask the patient about edema and if the pain has worsened within the last 24 hours. Also ask what activities he has been performing.

Examine the neck for pain on motion, point tenderness, muscle spasms, or arm pain when the neck is extended with the head toward the involved side.

PEDIATRIC POINTERS

- *In children, arm pain commonly results from fractures, muscle sprain, muscular dystrophy, or rheumatoid arthritis.*
- *In young children especially, the exact location of the pain may be difficult to establish. Watch for nonverbal clues, such as wincing or guarding.*
- *If the child has a fracture or sprain, obtain a complete account of the injury. Closely observe interactions between the child and his family, and don't rule out the possibility of child abuse.*

ELDER CARE CUE

Elderly patients with osteoporosis may experience fractures from simple trauma or even from heavy lifting or unexpected movements. They're also prone to degenerative joint disease that can involve several joints in the arm or neck.

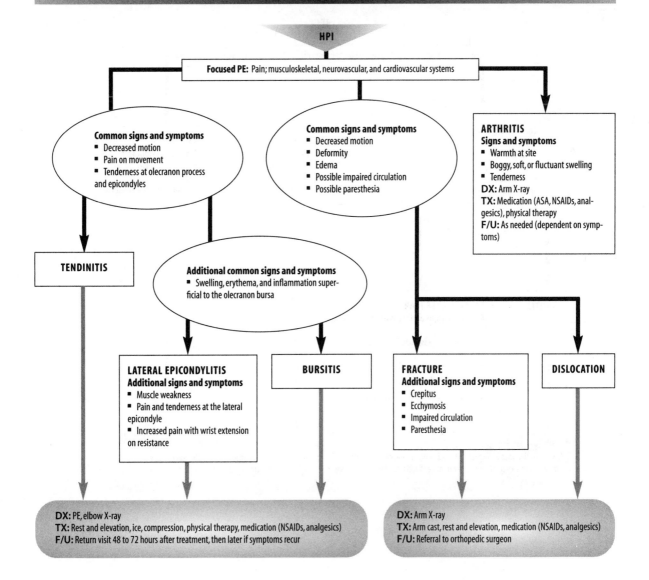

HPI

Focused PE: Pain; musculoskeletal, neurovascular, and cardiovascular systems

Common signs and symptoms
- Decreased motion
- Pain on movement
- Tenderness at olecranon process and epicondyles

Common signs and symptoms
- Decreased motion
- Deformity
- Edema
- Possible impaired circulation
- Possible paresthesia

ARTHRITIS
Signs and symptoms
- Warmth at site
- Boggy, soft, or fluctuant swelling
- Tenderness
DX: Arm X-ray
TX: Medication (ASA, NSAIDs, analgesics), physical therapy
F/U: As needed (dependent on symptoms)

TENDINITIS

Additional common signs and symptoms
- Swelling, erythema, and inflammation superficial to the olecranon bursa

LATERAL EPICONDYLITIS
Additional signs and symptoms
- Muscle weakness
- Pain and tenderness at the lateral epicondyle
- Increased pain with wrist extension on resistance

BURSITIS

FRACTURE
Additional signs and symptoms
- Crepitus
- Ecchymosis
- Impaired circulation
- Paresthesia

DISLOCATION

DX: PE, elbow X-ray
TX: Rest and elevation, ice, compression, physical therapy, medication (NSAIDs, analgesics)
F/U: Return visit 48 to 72 hours after treatment, then later if symptoms recur

DX: Arm X-ray
TX: Arm cast, rest and elevation, medication (NSAIDs, analgesics)
F/U: Referral to orthopedic surgeon

Additional differential diagnoses: angina ▪ ankylosis ▪ biceps rupture ▪ cellulitis ▪ compartment syndrome ▪ medical epicondylitis ▪ MI ▪ muscle contusion ▪ neoplasm of the arm ▪ osteomyelitis

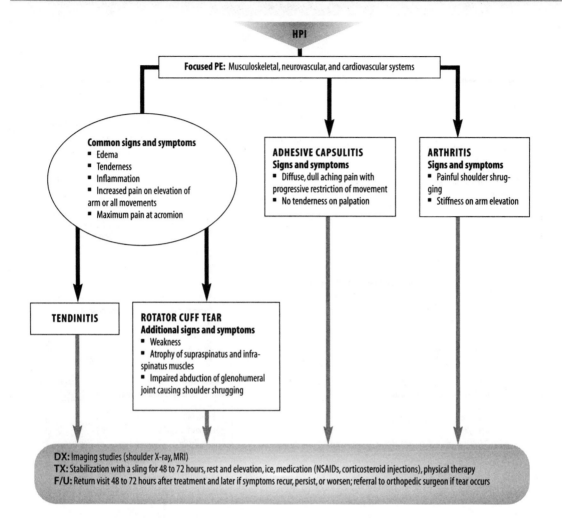

HPI

Focused PE: Musculoskeletal, neurovascular, and cardiovascular systems

Common signs and symptoms
- Edema
- Tenderness
- Inflammation
- Increased pain on elevation of arm or all movements
- Maximum pain at acromion

ADHESIVE CAPSULITIS
Signs and symptoms
- Diffuse, dull aching pain with progressive restriction of movement
- No tenderness on palpation

ARTHRITIS
Signs and symptoms
- Painful shoulder shrugging
- Stiffness on arm elevation

TENDINITIS

ROTATOR CUFF TEAR
Additional signs and symptoms
- Weakness
- Atrophy of supraspinatus and infra-spinatus muscles
- Impaired abduction of glenohumeral joint causing shoulder shrugging

DX: Imaging studies (shoulder X-ray, MRI)
TX: Stabilization with a sling for 48 to 72 hours, rest and elevation, ice, medication (NSAIDs, corticosteroid injections), physical therapy
F/U: Return visit 48 to 72 hours after treatment and later if symptoms recur, persist, or worsen; referral to orthopedic surgeon if tear occurs

Additional differential diagnoses: acromioclavicular separation ▪ acute pancreatitis ▪ angina pectoris ▪ bursitis ▪ cellulitis ▪ cervical nerve root compression ▪ cholecystitis ▪ cholelithiasis ▪ clavicle fracture ▪ diaphragmatic pleurisy ▪ dislocation ▪ dissecting aortic aneurysm ▪ gastritis ▪ humeral neck fracture ▪ infection ▪ MI ▪ muscle contusion ▪ neoplasm of the arm ▪ osteomyelitis ▪ Pancoast's syndrome ▪ pneumothorax ▪ ruptured spleen ▪ shoulder-hand syndrome ▪ subphrenic abscess

Other causes: laparoscopy

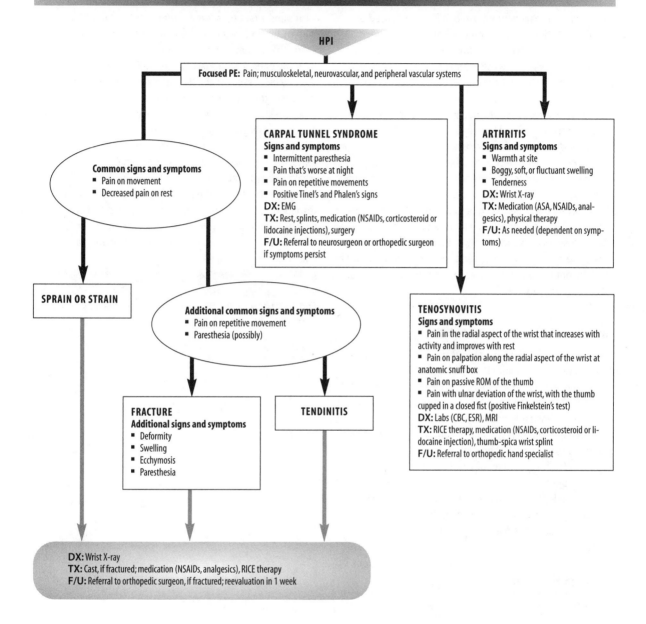

HPI

Focused PE: Pain; musculoskeletal, neurovascular, and peripheral vascular systems

Common signs and symptoms
- Pain on movement
- Decreased pain on rest

CARPAL TUNNEL SYNDROME
Signs and symptoms
- Intermittent paresthesia
- Pain that's worse at night
- Pain on repetitive movements
- Positive Tinel's and Phalen's signs
DX: EMG
TX: Rest, splints, medication (NSAIDs, corticosteroid or lidocaine injections), surgery
F/U: Referral to neurosurgeon or orthopedic surgeon if symptoms persist

ARTHRITIS
Signs and symptoms
- Warmth at site
- Boggy, soft, or fluctuant swelling
- Tenderness
DX: Wrist X-ray
TX: Medication (ASA, NSAIDs, analgesics), physical therapy
F/U: As needed (dependent on symptoms)

SPRAIN OR STRAIN

Additional common signs and symptoms
- Pain on repetitive movement
- Paresthesia (possibly)

TENOSYNOVITIS
Signs and symptoms
- Pain in the radial aspect of the wrist that increases with activity and improves with rest
- Pain on palpation along the radial aspect of the wrist at anatomic snuff box
- Pain on passive ROM of the thumb
- Pain with ulnar deviation of the wrist, with the thumb cupped in a closed fist (positive Finkelstein's test)
DX: Labs (CBC, ESR), MRI
TX: RICE therapy, medication (NSAIDs, corticosteroid or lidocaine injection), thumb-spica wrist splint
F/U: Referral to orthopedic hand specialist

FRACTURE
Additional signs and symptoms
- Deformity
- Swelling
- Ecchymosis
- Paresthesia

TENDINITIS

DX: Wrist X-ray
TX: Cast, if fractured; medication (NSAIDs, analgesics), RICE therapy
F/U: Referral to orthopedic surgeon, if fractured; reevaluation in 1 week

Additional differential diagnoses: biceps rupture ▪ cellulitis ▪ compartment syndrome ▪ muscle contusion ▪ neoplasm of the arm ▪ osteomyelitis

Asterixis

A bilateral, coarse movement, asterixis is characterized by sudden relaxation of muscle groups holding a sustained posture. This elicited sign is most commonly observed in the wrists and fingers but may also appear during sustained voluntary action. Typically, it signals hepatic, renal, or pulmonary disease.

To elicit asterixis, have the patient extend his arms, dorsiflex his wrists, and spread his fingers (or do this for him, if necessary). Briefly observe for asterixis. Alternately, if the patient has a decreased level of consciousness but can follow verbal commands, ask him to squeeze two of your fingers. Consider rapid clutching and unclutching positive for asterixis. Alternatively, elevate the patient's leg off the bed and dorsiflex the foot. Briefly observe for asterixis in the ankle. If the patient can tightly close his eyes and mouth, observe for irregular tremulous movements of the eyelids and corners of the mouth. If he can stick out his tongue, observe for continuous quivering. (See *Recognizing asterixis*.)

History and physical examination

Because asterixis may signal serious metabolic deterioration, quickly evaluate the patient's neurologic status and vital signs. Compare these data to his baseline, and watch carefully for acute changes. Continue to closely monitor neurologic status, vital signs, and urine output.

Watch for signs of respiratory insufficiency, and be prepared to provide endotracheal intubation and ventilatory support. Also, be alert for complications of end-stage hepatic, renal, or pulmonary disease.

If the patient has hepatic disease, assess for early signs of hemorrhage, including restlessness, tachypnea, and cool, moist, pale skin. (If the patient is jaundiced, check for pallor in the conjunctivae and mucous membranes of the mouth.) Perform an abdominal examination.

It's important to recognize that hypotension, oliguria, hematemesis, and melena are late signs of hemorrhage. Be aware that emergency measures may need to be instituted.

If the patient has renal disease, briefly review what type of therapy he has received. If he's on dialysis, ask about the frequency of treatments to help gauge the severity of the disease. Question a family member if the patient's level of consciousness is significantly decreased.

Then assess for hyperkalemia and metabolic acidosis. Look for tachycardia, nausea, diarrhea, abdominal cramps, muscle weakness, hyperreflexia, and Kussmaul's respirations.

If the patient has pulmonary disease, assess for labored respirations, tachypnea, accessory muscle use, and cyanosis, which are critical signs. Prepare to provide ventilatory support through a nasal cannula, a mask, or intubation and mechanical ventilation, if necessary.

PEDIATRIC POINTER

End-stage hepatic, renal, and pulmonary disease may also cause asterixis in children.

Recognizing asterixis

In asterixis, the patient's wrists and fingers appear to "flap" because there's a brief, rapid relaxation of dorsiflexion of the wrist.

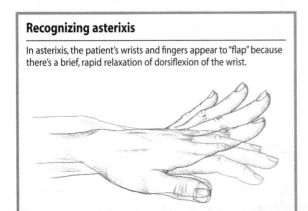

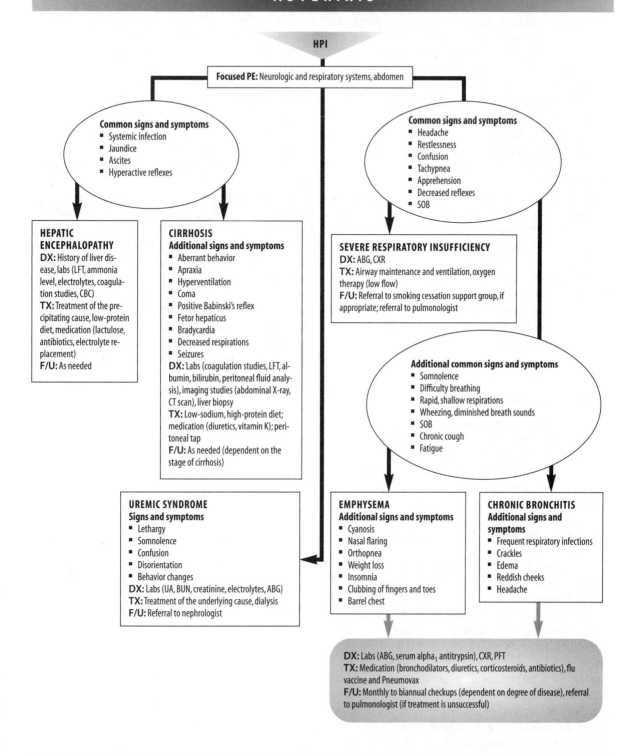

HPI

Focused PE: Neurologic and respiratory systems, abdomen

Common signs and symptoms
- Systemic infection
- Jaundice
- Ascites
- Hyperactive reflexes

Common signs and symptoms
- Headache
- Restlessness
- Confusion
- Tachypnea
- Apprehension
- Decreased reflexes
- SOB

HEPATIC ENCEPHALOPATHY
DX: History of liver disease, labs (LFT, ammonia level, electrolytes, coagulation studies, CBC)
TX: Treatment of the precipitating cause, low-protein diet, medication (lactulose, antibiotics, electrolyte replacement)
F/U: As needed

CIRRHOSIS
Additional signs and symptoms
- Aberrant behavior
- Apraxia
- Hyperventilation
- Coma
- Positive Babinski's reflex
- Fetor hepaticus
- Bradycardia
- Decreased respirations
- Seizures

DX: Labs (coagulation studies, LFT, albumin, bilirubin, peritoneal fluid analysis), imaging studies (abdominal X-ray, CT scan), liver biopsy
TX: Low-sodium, high-protein diet; medication (diuretics, vitamin K); peritoneal tap
F/U: As needed (dependent on the stage of cirrhosis)

SEVERE RESPIRATORY INSUFFICIENCY
DX: ABG, CXR
TX: Airway maintenance and ventilation, oxygen therapy (low flow)
F/U: Referral to smoking cessation support group, if appropriate; referral to pulmonologist

Additional common signs and symptoms
- Somnolence
- Difficulty breathing
- Rapid, shallow respirations
- Wheezing, diminished breath sounds
- SOB
- Chronic cough
- Fatigue

UREMIC SYNDROME
Signs and symptoms
- Lethargy
- Somnolence
- Confusion
- Disorientation
- Behavior changes

DX: Labs (UA, BUN, creatinine, electrolytes, ABG)
TX: Treatment of the underlying cause, dialysis
F/U: Referral to nephrologist

EMPHYSEMA
Additional signs and symptoms
- Cyanosis
- Nasal flaring
- Orthopnea
- Weight loss
- Insomnia
- Clubbing of fingers and toes
- Barrel chest

CHRONIC BRONCHITIS
Additional signs and symptoms
- Frequent respiratory infections
- Crackles
- Edema
- Reddish cheeks
- Headache

DX: Labs (ABG, serum alpha$_1$ antitrypsin), CXR, PFT
TX: Medication (bronchodilators, diuretics, corticosteroids, antibiotics), flu vaccine and Pneumovax
F/U: Monthly to biannual checkups (dependent on degree of disease), referral to pulmonologist (if treatment is unsuccessful)

Other causes: medication such as phenytoin

Ataxia

Classified as cerebellar or sensory, ataxia refers to incoordination and irregularity of voluntary, purposeful movements. *Cerebellar ataxia* results from disease of the cerebellum and its pathways to and from the cerebral cortex, brain stem, and spinal cord. It causes gait, trunk, limb and, possibly, speech disorders. *Sensory ataxia,* which can cause gait disorders, typically results from impaired position sense (proprioception) due to interruption of afferent nerve fibers in the peripheral nerves, posterior roots, posterior columns of the spinal cord, or medial lemnisci. It may also be caused by a lesion in either parietal lobe.

Ataxia occurs in acute and chronic forms. *Acute ataxia* may result from cerebrovascular accident, hemorrhage, or a large tumor in the posterior fossa. In this life-threatening condition, the cerebellum may herniate downward through the foramen magnum behind the cervical spinal cord or upward through the tentorium on the cerebral hemispheres. Herniation may also compress the brain stem. Acute ataxia may also result from drug toxicity or poisoning. *Chronic ataxia* can be progressive and, at times, can result from acute disease. It can also occur in metabolic and chronic degenerative neurologic disease.

History and physical examination

If ataxic movements develop suddenly, examine the patient for signs of increased intracranial pressure and impending herniation. Determine his level of consciousness, and be alert for pupillary changes, motor weakness or paralysis, neck stiffness or pain, and vomiting. Check his vital signs, especially respirations; abnormal respiratory patterns may quickly lead to respiratory arrest. Have emergency resuscitation equipment readily available. Prepare the patient for computed tomography scanning or surgery.

If the patient isn't in distress, review his history. Ask about multiple sclerosis, diabetes, central nervous system infection, neoplastic disease, previous cerebrovascular accident, and a family history of ataxia. Also ask about chronic alcohol abuse or prolonged exposure to industrial toxins such as mercury. Find out if the patient's ataxia developed suddenly or gradually.

If necessary, perform Romberg's test to help distinguish between cerebellar and sensory ataxia. Instruct the patient to stand with his feet together and his arms at his side. Note his posture and balance, first with his eyes open and then with them closed. Test results may indicate normal posture and balance (minimal swaying), cerebellar ataxia (swaying and inability to maintain balance with eyes open or closed), or sensory ataxia (increased swaying and inability to maintain balance with eyes closed). Stand close to the patient during this test to prevent him from falling.

If you test for gait and limb ataxia, be aware that motor weakness may mimic ataxic movements, so also check motor strength. Gait ataxia may be severe, even when there's minimal limb ataxia. In gait ataxia, ask the patient if he tends to fall to one side or if falling occurs more often at night. In truncal ataxia, remember that the patient's inability to walk or stand, combined with the absence of other signs while he's lying down, may give the impression of hysteria or drug or alcohol intoxication.

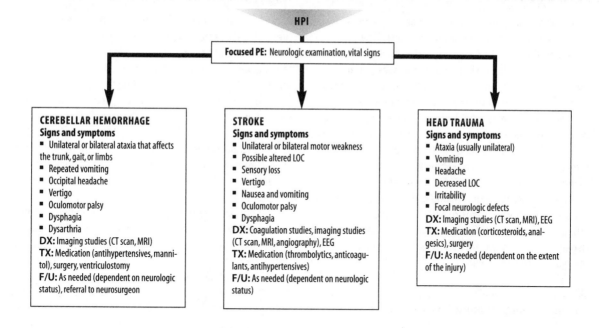

HPI

Focused PE: Neurologic examination, vital signs

CEREBELLAR HEMORRHAGE
Signs and symptoms
- Unilateral or bilateral ataxia that affects the trunk, gait, or limbs
- Repeated vomiting
- Occipital headache
- Vertigo
- Oculomotor palsy
- Dysphagia
- Dysarthria

DX: Imaging studies (CT scan, MRI)
TX: Medication (antihypertensives, mannitol), surgery, ventriculostomy
F/U: As needed (dependent on neurologic status), referral to neurosurgeon

STROKE
Signs and symptoms
- Unilateral or bilateral motor weakness
- Possible altered LOC
- Sensory loss
- Vertigo
- Nausea and vomiting
- Oculomotor palsy
- Dysphagia

DX: Coagulation studies, imaging studies (CT scan, MRI, angiography), EEG
TX: Medication (thrombolytics, anticoagulants, antihypertensives)
F/U: As needed (dependent on neurologic status)

HEAD TRAUMA
Signs and symptoms
- Ataxia (usually unilateral)
- Vomiting
- Headache
- Decreased LOC
- Irritability
- Focal neurologic defects

DX: Imaging studies (CT scan, MRI), EEG
TX: Medication (corticosteroids, analgesics), surgery
F/U: As needed (dependent on the extent of the injury)

Additional differential diagnoses: cerebellar abscess ▪ Creutzfeldt-Jakob disease ▪ diabetic neuropathy ▪ diphtheria ▪ encephalomyelitis ▪ Friedreich's ataxia ▪ Guillain-Barré syndrome ▪ hepatocerebral degeneration ▪ hyperthermia ▪ metastatic cancer ▪ multiple sclerosis ▪ olivopontocerebellar atrophy ▪ poisoning ▪ polyarteritis nodosa ▪ polyneuropathy ▪ porphyria ▪ posterior fossa tumor ▪ spinocerebellar ataxia ▪ syringomyelia ▪ Wernicke's disease

Other causes: anticonvulsants (phenytoin) ▪ anticholinergics ▪ tricyclic antidepressants ▪ aminoglutethimide

Athetosis

Athetosis, an extrapyramidal sign, is characterized by slow, continuous, twisting involuntary movements. Typically, these movements involve the face, neck, and distal extremities, such as the forearm, wrist, and hand. Facial grimaces, jaw and tongue movements, and occasional phonation are associated with neck movements. Athetosis worsens during stress and voluntary activity, may subside during relaxation, and disappears during sleep. Commonly a lifelong affliction, athetosis is sometimes difficult to distinguish from chorea (hence the term *choreoathetosis*). Typically, however, athetoid movements are slower than choreiform movements.

Athetosis usually begins during childhood, resulting from hypoxia at birth, kernicterus, or a genetic disorder. In adults, athetosis usually results from vascular or neoplastic lesions, degenerative disease, drug toxicity, or hypoxia. (See *Distinguishing athetosis from chorea*.)

Distinguishing athetosis from chorea

In *athetosis*, movements are typically slow, twisting, and writhing. They're associated with spasticity and most commonly involve the face, neck, and distal extremities.

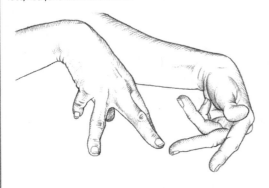

In *chorea*, movements are brief, rapid, jerky, and unpredictable. They can occur at rest or during normal movement. Typically, they involve the hands, lower arm, face, and head.

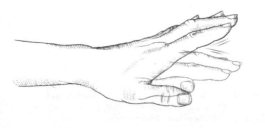

History and physical examination

Begin your neurologic evaluation by taking a comprehensive prenatal and postnatal history, covering maternal and child health, labor and delivery, and possible trauma. Obtain a family health history because many genetic disorders can cause athetosis. Also, ask about current drug therapy.

Continue your evaluation by asking about the decline in the patient's functional abilities: When was he last able to roll over, sit up, or carry out daily activities? Find out what problem — uncontrollable movements, mental deterioration, or a speech impediment — prompted him to seek medical help. Ask about the effects of rest, stress, and routine activity on his symptoms.

Test the patient's muscle strength and tone, range of motion, fine muscle movements, and ability to perform rapidly alternating movements. Observe the limb muscles during voluntary movements, noting the rhythm and duration of contraction and relaxation.

PEDIATRIC POINTERS

- *Childhood athetosis may be acquired or inherited. It can result from hypoxia at birth, which causes an athetoid cerebral palsy, kernicterus, Sydenham's chorea (in school-age children), and paroxysmal choreoathetosis. Inherited causes of athetosis include Lesch-Nyhan syndrome, Tay-Sachs disease, and phenylketonuria.*
- *Help the child develop self-esteem and a positive self-image. Encourage the child and his family to set realistic goals, tailoring educational plans to the child's level of intelligence. Refer the child to special education services, rehabilitation centers, and support groups. Provide him with emotional support during the frequent medical evaluations he'll be required to undergo.*

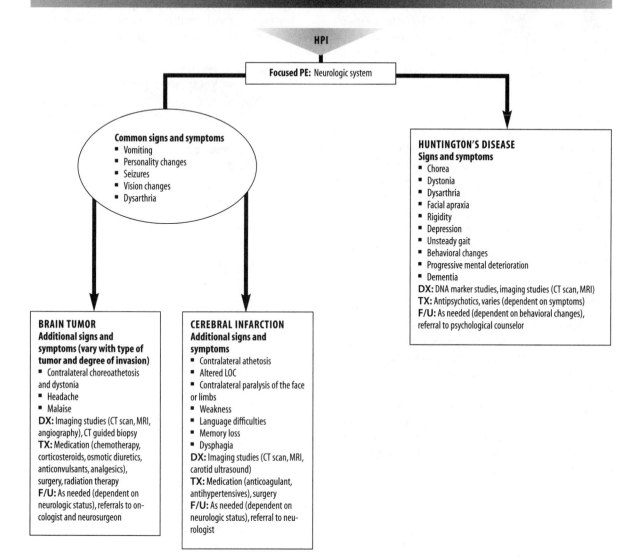

HPI

Focused PE: Neurologic system

Common signs and symptoms
- Vomiting
- Personality changes
- Seizures
- Vision changes
- Dysarthria

BRAIN TUMOR
Additional signs and symptoms (vary with type of tumor and degree of invasion)
- Contralateral choreoathetosis and dystonia
- Headache
- Malaise

DX: Imaging studies (CT scan, MRI, angiography), CT guided biopsy
TX: Medication (chemotherapy, corticosteroids, osmotic diuretics, anticonvulsants, analgesics), surgery, radiation therapy
F/U: As needed (dependent on neurologic status), referrals to on-cologist and neurosurgeon

CEREBRAL INFARCTION
Additional signs and symptoms
- Contralateral athetosis
- Altered LOC
- Contralateral paralysis of the face or limbs
- Weakness
- Language difficulties
- Memory loss
- Dysphagia

DX: Imaging studies (CT scan, MRI, carotid ultrasound)
TX: Medication (anticoagulant, antihypertensives), surgery
F/U: As needed (dependent on neurologic status), referral to neu-rologist

HUNTINGTON'S DISEASE
Signs and symptoms
- Chorea
- Dystonia
- Dysarthria
- Facial apraxia
- Rigidity
- Depression
- Unsteady gait
- Behavioral changes
- Progressive mental deterioration
- Dementia

DX: DNA marker studies, imaging studies (CT scan, MRI)
TX: Antipsychotics, varies (dependent on symptoms)
F/U: As needed (dependent on behavioral changes), referral to psychological counselor

Additional differential diagnoses: calcification of the basal ganglia ▪ hepatic encephalopathy ▪ Wilson's disease

Other causes: levodopa ▪ phenothiazines and other antipsychotics ▪ phenytoin

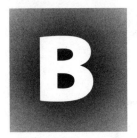

Babinski's reflex

Babinski's reflex (extensor plantar reflex) involves dorsiflexion of the great toe with extension and fanning of the other toes. It's an abnormal reflex elicited by firmly stroking the lateral aspect of the sole of the foot with a blunt object. In some patients, this reflex can be triggered by noxious stimuli, such as pain, noise, or even bumping of the bed. An indicator of corticospinal damage, Babinski's reflex may occur unilaterally or bilaterally. It may also be temporary or permanent. A temporary Babinski's reflex commonly occurs during the postictal phase of a seizure, whereas a permanent Babinski's reflex occurs with corticospinal damage. A positive Babinski's reflex is normal in neonates and in infants up to age 24 months. (See *Positive Babinski's reflex.*)

History and physical examination

After eliciting a positive Babinski's reflex, evaluate the patient for other neurologic signs. Evaluate muscle strength in each extremity by asking the patient to push or pull against your resistance. Passively flex and extend the extremity to assess muscle tone. Intermittent resistance to flexion and extension indicates spasticity, and a lack of resistance indicates flaccidity.

Next, check for evidence of incoordination by asking the patient to perform a repetitive activity. Test deep tendon reflexes (DTRs) in the patient's elbow, antecubital area, wrist, knee, and ankle by striking the tendon with a reflex hammer.

An exaggerated muscle response indicates hyperactive DTRs; little or no muscle response indicates hypoactivity.

Then evaluate pain sensation and proprioception in the feet. As you move the patient's toes up and down, ask the patient to identify (without looking at his feet) the direction in which the toes have been moved.

Positive Babinski's reflex

In a positive Babinski's reflex, the great toe dorsiflexes and the other toes fan out, as shown below right.

NORMAL TOE FLEXION

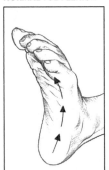

POSITIVE BABINSKI'S REFLEX

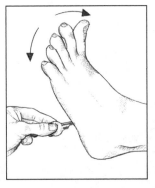

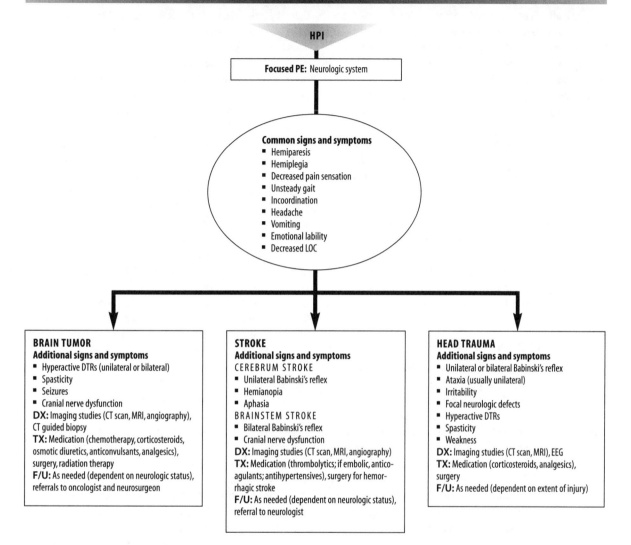

HPI

Focused PE: Neurologic system

Common signs and symptoms
- Hemiparesis
- Hemiplegia
- Decreased pain sensation
- Unsteady gait
- Incoordination
- Headache
- Vomiting
- Emotional lability
- Decreased LOC

BRAIN TUMOR
Additional signs and symptoms
- Hyperactive DTRs (unilateral or bilateral)
- Spasticity
- Seizures
- Cranial nerve dysfunction

DX: Imaging studies (CT scan, MRI, angiography), CT guided biopsy
TX: Medication (chemotherapy, corticosteroids, osmotic diuretics, anticonvulsants, analgesics), surgery, radiation therapy
F/U: As needed (dependent on neurologic status), referrals to oncologist and neurosurgeon

STROKE
Additional signs and symptoms
CEREBRUM STROKE
- Unilateral Babinski's reflex
- Hemianopia
- Aphasia
BRAINSTEM STROKE
- Bilateral Babinski's reflex
- Cranial nerve dysfunction

DX: Imaging studies (CT scan, MRI, angiography)
TX: Medication (thrombolytics; if embolic, anticoagulants; antihypertensives), surgery for hemorrhagic stroke
F/U: As needed (dependent on neurologic status), referral to neurologist

HEAD TRAUMA
Additional signs and symptoms
- Unilateral or bilateral Babinski's reflex
- Ataxia (usually unilateral)
- Irritability
- Focal neurologic defects
- Hyperactive DTRs
- Spasticity
- Weakness

DX: Imaging studies (CT scan, MRI), EEG
TX: Medication (corticosteroids, analgesics), surgery
F/U: As needed (dependent on extent of injury)

Additional differential diagnoses: ALS ▪ familial spastic paraparesis ▪ Friedreich's ataxia ▪ hepatic encephalopathy ▪ meningitis ▪ multiple sclerosis ▪ pernicious anemia ▪ rabies ▪ spinal cord injury ▪ spinal cord tumor ▪ spinal paralytic poliomyelitis ▪ spinal tuberculosis ▪ syringomyelia

Back pain

Back pain affects an estimated 80% of the population; in fact, it's the second leading reason — after the common cold — for lost time from work. Although this symptom may herald a spondylogenic disorder, it may also result from genitourinary, GI, cardiovascular, and neoplastic disorders. Postural imbalance associated with pregnancy may also cause back pain.

The onset, location, and distribution of pain and its response to activity and rest provide important clues about the causative disorder. Pain may be acute or chronic, constant or intermittent. It may remain localized in the back or radiate along the spine or down one or both legs. Pain may be exacerbated by activity — usually, bending, stooping, or lifting — and alleviated by rest, or it may be unaffected by both.

Intrinsic back pain results from muscle spasm, nerve root irritation, fracture, or a combination of these mechanisms. It usually occurs in the lower back, or lumbosacral area. Back pain may also be referred from the abdomen or flank, possibly signaling a life-threatening perforated ulcer, acute pancreatitis, or dissecting abdominal aortic aneurysm.

History and physical examination

If the patient reports acute, severe back pain, quickly take his vital signs. Then perform a rapid evaluation to rule out life-threatening causes. Ask him when the pain began. Can he relate it to a cause? For example, did the pain occur after eating? After falling on ice? Have the patient describe the pain. Is it burning, stabbing, throbbing, or aching? Is it constant or intermittent? Does it radiate to the buttocks or legs? Does he have any leg weakness? Or, does the pain seem to originate in the abdomen and radiate to the back? Has he had a pain like this before? What makes it better or worse? Is it affected by activity or rest? Is it worse in the morning or evening? Does it wake him up?

Typically, visceral referred back pain is unaffected by activity and rest. In contrast, pain of spondylogenic origin worsens with activity and improves with rest. Pain of neoplastic origin is usually relieved by walking and worsens at night.

If the patient describes deep lumbar pain unaffected by activity, palpate for a pulsating epigastric mass. If this sign is present, suspect dissecting abdominal aortic aneurysm.

If the patient describes severe epigastric pain that radiates through the abdomen to the back, assess for absent bowel sounds and for abdominal rigidity and tenderness. If these occur, suspect a perforated ulcer or acute pancreatitis.

If life-threatening causes of back pain are ruled out, continue with a more complete history and physical examination. Be aware of the patient's expressions of pain as you do so. Obtain a medical history, including past injuries and illnesses, and a family history. Ask about occupational activities that may affect the back. Also ask about diet and alcohol intake. Take a drug history, including past and present prescriptions as well as over-the-counter drugs.

Next, perform a thorough physical examination. Observe skin color, especially in the patient's legs, and palpate skin temperature. Palpate femoral, popliteal, posterior tibial, and pedal pulses. Ask about unusual sensations in the legs, such as numbness and tingling. Observe the patient's posture if the pain doesn't prohibit standing. Does he stand erect or tend to lean toward one side? Observe the level of the shoulders and pelvis and the curvature of the back. Ask the patient to bend forward, backward, and from side to side while you palpate for paravertebral muscle spasms. Note rotation of the spine on the trunk. Palpate the dorsolumbar spine for point tenderness. Then ask the patient to walk — first on his heels, then on his toes; protect him from falling as he does so. Weakness may reflect a muscular disorder or spinal nerve root irritation. Place the patient in a sitting position to evaluate and compare patellar tendon, Achilles tendon, and Babinski's reflexes. Evaluate the strength of the extensor hallucis longus by asking the patient to hold up his big toe against resistance. Measure leg length and hamstring and quadriceps muscles bilaterally. Note a difference of more than 1 cm in muscle size, especially in the calf.

To reproduce leg and back pain, place the patient in the supine position on the examination table. Grasp his heel and slowly lift his leg. If he feels pain, note its exact location and the angle between the table and his leg when it occurs. Repeat this maneuver with the opposite leg. Pain along the sciatic nerve may indicate disk herniation or sciatica. Also, note the range of motion of the hip and knee. Palpate the flanks and percuss with the fingertips or perform fist percussion to elicit costovertebral angle tenderness.

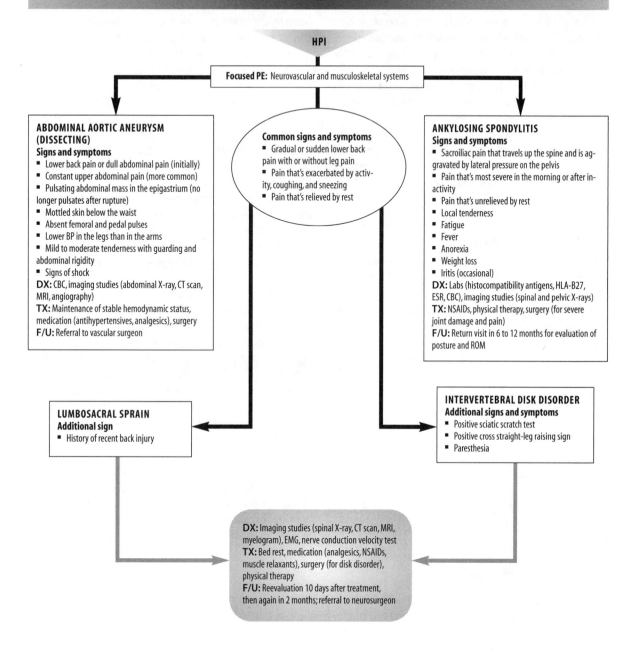

HPI

Focused PE: Neurovascular and musculoskeletal systems

ABDOMINAL AORTIC ANEURYSM (DISSECTING)
Signs and symptoms
- Lower back pain or dull abdominal pain (initially)
- Constant upper abdominal pain (more common)
- Pulsating abdominal mass in the epigastrium (no longer pulsates after rupture)
- Mottled skin below the waist
- Absent femoral and pedal pulses
- Lower BP in the legs than in the arms
- Mild to moderate tenderness with guarding and abdominal rigidity
- Signs of shock

DX: CBC, imaging studies (abdominal X-ray, CT scan, MRI, angiography)
TX: Maintenance of stable hemodynamic status, medication (antihypertensives, analgesics), surgery
F/U: Referral to vascular surgeon

Common signs and symptoms
- Gradual or sudden lower back pain with or without leg pain
- Pain that's exacerbated by activity, coughing, and sneezing
- Pain that's relieved by rest

ANKYLOSING SPONDYLITIS
Signs and symptoms
- Sacroiliac pain that travels up the spine and is aggravated by lateral pressure on the pelvis
- Pain that's most severe in the morning or after inactivity
- Pain that's unrelieved by rest
- Local tenderness
- Fatigue
- Fever
- Anorexia
- Weight loss
- Iritis (occasional)

DX: Labs (histocompatibility antigens, HLA-B27, ESR, CBC), imaging studies (spinal and pelvic X-rays)
TX: NSAIDs, physical therapy, surgery (for severe joint damage and pain)
F/U: Return visit in 6 to 12 months for evaluation of posture and ROM

LUMBOSACRAL SPRAIN
Additional sign
- History of recent back injury

INTERVERTEBRAL DISK DISORDER
Additional signs and symptoms
- Positive sciatic scratch test
- Positive cross straight-leg raising sign
- Paresthesia

DX: Imaging studies (spinal X-ray, CT scan, MRI, myelogram), EMG, nerve conduction velocity test
TX: Bed rest, medication (analgesics, NSAIDs, muscle relaxants), surgery (for disk disorder), physical therapy
F/U: Reevaluation 10 days after treatment, then again in 2 months; referral to neurosurgeon

Additional differential diagnoses: acute cauda equina ▪ appendicitis ▪ cholecystitis ▪ chordoma ▪ endometriosis ▪ metastatic tumors ▪ myeloma ▪ pancreatitis (acute) ▪ perforated ulcer ▪ prostate cancer ▪ pyelonephritis (acute) ▪ Reiter's syndrome ▪ renal calculi ▪ sacroiliac strain ▪ spinal neoplasm (benign) ▪ spinal stenosis ▪ spondylolisthesis ▪ transverse process fracture ▪ vertebral compression fracture ▪ vertebral osteomyelitis ▪ vertebral osteoporosis

Other causes: neurologic tests, such as lumbar puncture and myelography

Barrel chest

In barrel chest, the normal elliptical configuration of the chest is replaced by a rounded one in which the anteroposterior diameter enlarges to approximate the transverse diameter. The diaphragm is depressed and the sternum is pushed forward with the ribs attached in a horizontal, not angular, fashion. As a result, the chest appears continuously in the inspiratory position. (See *Recognizing barrel chest.*)

Typically a late sign of chronic obstructive pulmonary disease (COPD), barrel chest results from augmented lung volumes due to chronic airflow obstruction. The patient may not notice it because it develops gradually.

Recognizing barrel chest

In the normal adult chest, the ratio of anteroposterior to transverse (or lateral) diameter is 1:2. In barrel chest, the ratio approaches 1:1 as the anteroposterior diameter enlarges.

NORMAL CHEST

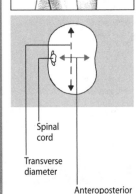

BARREL CHEST

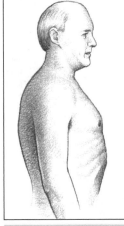
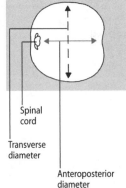

Spinal cord

Transverse diameter

Anteroposterior diameter

Spinal cord

Transverse diameter

Anteroposterior diameter

History and physical examination

Begin by asking about a history of pulmonary disease. Note chronic exposure to environmental irritants such as asbestos. Also ask about the patient's smoking habits.

Then explore other symptoms of pulmonary disease. Does the patient have a cough? Is it productive or nonproductive? If it's productive, have him describe the sputum color and consistency. Does the patient experience shortness of breath? Is it related to activity? Although dyspnea is common in COPD, many patients fail to associate it with the disease. Instead, they blame "old age" or "getting out of shape" for causing dyspnea.

Auscultate for abnormal breath sounds, such as crackles and wheezes. Then percuss the chest; hyperresonant sounds indicate trapped air, whereas dull or flat sounds indicate mucus buildup. Be alert for accessory muscle use, intercostal retractions, and tachypnea, which may signal respiratory distress.

Finally, you should observe the patient's general appearance. Look for central cyanosis in the cheeks, nose, and mucosa inside the lips. In addition, look for peripheral cyanosis in the nail beds. Also note clubbing, a late sign of COPD.

PEDIATRIC POINTERS

- In infants, the ratio of anteroposterior to transverse diameter normally approximates 1:1. As the child grows, this ratio gradually changes, reaching 1:2 by age 5 or 6.
- Cystic fibrosis and chronic asthma may cause barrel chest in the child.

ELDER CARE CUE

In elderly patients, senile kyphosis of the thoracic spine may be mistaken for barrel chest. However, unlike barrel chest, patients with senile kyphosis lack signs of pulmonary disease.

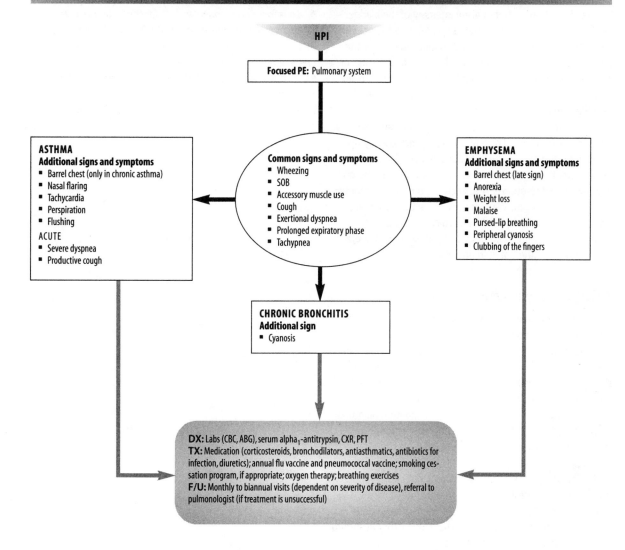

HPI

Focused PE: Pulmonary system

ASTHMA
Additional signs and symptoms
- Barrel chest (only in chronic asthma)
- Nasal flaring
- Tachycardia
- Perspiration
- Flushing

ACUTE
- Severe dyspnea
- Productive cough

Common signs and symptoms
- Wheezing
- SOB
- Accessory muscle use
- Cough
- Exertional dyspnea
- Prolonged expiratory phase
- Tachypnea

EMPHYSEMA
Additional signs and symptoms
- Barrel chest (late sign)
- Anorexia
- Weight loss
- Malaise
- Pursed-lip breathing
- Peripheral cyanosis
- Clubbing of the fingers

CHRONIC BRONCHITIS
Additional sign
- Cyanosis

DX: Labs (CBC, ABG), serum alpha$_1$-antitrypsin, CXR, PFT
TX: Medication (corticosteroids, bronchodilators, antiasthmatics, antibiotics for infection, diuretics); annual flu vaccine and pneumococcal vaccine; smoking cessation program, if appropriate; oxygen therapy; breathing exercises
F/U: Monthly to biannual visits (dependent on severity of disease), referral to pulmonologist (if treatment is unsuccessful)

Bladder distention

Bladder distention — abnormal enlargement of the bladder — results from an inability to excrete urine, leading to its accumulation. Distention can be caused by mechanical and anatomic obstructions, neuromuscular disorders, and the use of certain drugs. Relatively common in all ages and in both sexes, it occurs most frequently in older men with prostate disorders that cause urine retention.

Distention usually develops gradually but occasionally has a sudden onset. Gradual distention usually remains asymptomatic until stretching of the bladder produces discomfort. Acute distention produces suprapubic fullness, pressure, and pain. If severe distention isn't corrected promptly by catheterization or massage, the bladder rises within the abdomen, its walls become thin, and renal function can be impaired.

Bladder distention is aggravated by intake of caffeine, alcohol, large quantities of fluid, and diuretics.

History and physical examination

If distention is severe, immediately arrange for bladder catheterization. If distention isn't severe, begin by reviewing the patient's voiding patterns. Find out the time and amount of the patient's last voiding and the amount of fluid consumed since then. Ask if he has difficulty urinating. Does he use Valsalva's or Credé's maneuver to initiate urination? Does he urinate with urgency or without warning? Is urination painful or irritating? Ask about the force and continuity of his urine stream and whether he feels that his bladder is empty after voiding.

Explore the patient's history for urinary tract obstruction or infections; venereal disease; neurologic, intestinal, or pelvic surgery; lower abdominal or urinary tract trauma; and systemic or neurologic disorders. Note his drug history, including use of over-the-counter preparations.

Take the patient's vital signs, and percuss and palpate the bladder. (Remember that if the bladder is empty, it can't be palpated through the abdominal wall.) Inspect the urethral meatus. Describe the appearance and amount of any discharge. Finally, test for perineal sensation and anal sphincter tone and, in male patients, examine the prostate gland.

PEDIATRIC POINTERS

- Look for urine retention and bladder distention in any infant who fails to void normal amounts. (In the first 48 hours of life, an infant excretes about 60 ml of urine; during the next week, he excretes about 300 ml of urine daily.)
- In males, posterior urethral valves, meatal stenosis, phimosis, spinal cord anomalies, bladder diverticula, and other congenital defects may cause urinary obstruction and resultant bladder distention.

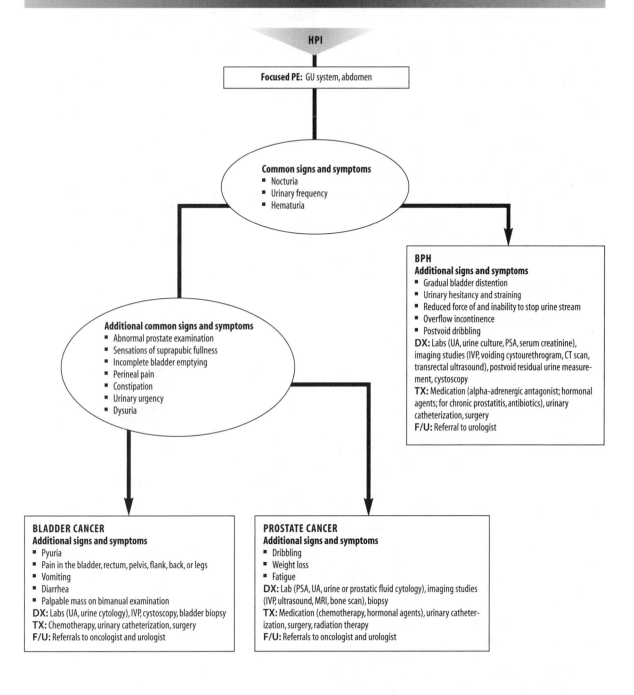

HPI

Focused PE: GU system, abdomen

Common signs and symptoms
- Nocturia
- Urinary frequency
- Hematuria

BPH
Additional signs and symptoms
- Gradual bladder distention
- Urinary hesitancy and straining
- Reduced force of and inability to stop urine stream
- Overflow incontinence
- Postvoid dribbling

DX: Labs (UA, urine culture, PSA, serum creatinine), imaging studies (IVP, voiding cystourethrogram, CT scan, transrectal ultrasound), postvoid residual urine measurement, cystoscopy
TX: Medication (alpha-adrenergic antagonist; hormonal agents; for chronic prostatitis, antibiotics), urinary catheterization, surgery
F/U: Referral to urologist

Additional common signs and symptoms
- Abnormal prostate examination
- Sensations of suprapubic fullness
- Incomplete bladder emptying
- Perineal pain
- Constipation
- Urinary urgency
- Dysuria

BLADDER CANCER
Additional signs and symptoms
- Pyuria
- Pain in the bladder, rectum, pelvis, flank, back, or legs
- Vomiting
- Diarrhea
- Palpable mass on bimanual examination

DX: Labs (UA, urine cytology), IVP, cystoscopy, bladder biopsy
TX: Chemotherapy, urinary catheterization, surgery
F/U: Referrals to oncologist and urologist

PROSTATE CANCER
Additional signs and symptoms
- Dribbling
- Weight loss
- Fatigue

DX: Lab (PSA, UA, urine or prostatic fluid cytology), imaging studies (IVP, ultrasound, MRI, bone scan), biopsy
TX: Medication (chemotherapy, hormonal agents), urinary catheterization, surgery, radiation therapy
F/U: Referrals to oncologist and urologist

Additional differential diagnoses: bladder calculi ▪ multiple sclerosis ▪ prostatitis ▪ spinal neoplasms ▪ urethral calculi ▪ urethral stricture

Other causes: catheterization ▪ parasympatholytics ▪ anticholinergics ▪ ganglionic blockers ▪ sedatives ▪ anesthetics ▪ opiates

Blood pressure decrease

Low blood pressure (hypotension) refers to inadequate intravascular pressure to maintain the oxygen requirements of the body's tissues. Although commonly linked to shock, this sign may also result from cardiovascular, respiratory, neurologic, and metabolic disorders. Low blood pressure may be drug-induced or may accompany diagnostic tests — usually, those using contrast media. It may stem from stress or change of position — specifically, rising abruptly from a supine or sitting position to a standing position (orthostatic hypotension).

Normal blood pressure varies considerably; what qualifies as low blood pressure for one person may be perfectly normal for another. Consequently, every blood pressure reading must be compared with the patient's baseline. Typically, a reading below 90/60 mm Hg or a drop of 30 mm Hg from the baseline is considered low blood pressure.

Low blood pressure can reflect an expanded intravascular space (as in severe infections, allergic reactions, or adrenal insufficiency), reduced intravascular volume (as in dehydration and hemorrhage), or decreased cardiac output (as in impaired cardiac muscle contractility). Because the body's pressure-regulating mechanisms are complex and interrelated, a combination of these factors usually contributes to low blood pressure.

History and physical examination

If the patient's systolic pressure is less than 80 mm Hg, or is 30 mm Hg below his baseline, suspect shock immediately. Quickly evaluate for a decreased level of consciousness. Check the apical pulse for tachycardia and check respirations for tachypnea. Also, inspect for cool, clammy skin. Elevate the patient's legs above the level of his heart or place him in Trendelenburg's position. Institute emergency measures. Throughout emergency interventions, keep the patient's spinal column immobile until spinal cord trauma is ruled out.

If the patient is conscious, ask him about associated symptoms. For example, does he feel unusually weak or fatigued? Is his vision blurred? Gait unsteady? Does he have chest or abdominal pain or difficulty breathing? Has he had episodes of dizziness or fainting? Do these episodes occur when he stands up suddenly? If so, take the blood pressure with the patient lying down, sitting, and then standing; compare readings. A drop in systolic or diastolic pressure of 10 to 20 mm Hg or more and an increase in heart rate of more than 15 beats/minute between position changes suggest orthostatic hypotension.

Next, continue with a physical examination. Inspect the skin for pallor, diaphoresis, and clamminess. Palpate the peripheral pulses. Note paradoxical pulse — an accentuated fall in systolic pressure during inspiration, which suggests pericardial tamponade. Then auscultate for abnormal heart sounds (gallops, murmurs), rate (bradycardia, tachycardia), or rhythm. Auscultate the lungs for abnormal breath sounds (diminished sounds, crackles, wheezing), rate (bradypnea, tachypnea), or rhythm (agonal or Cheyne-Stokes respirations). Look for signs of hemorrhage, including visible bleeding and palpable masses, bruising, and tenderness. Assess for abdominal rigidity and rebound tenderness; auscultate for abnormal bowel sounds. Also carefully assess for possible sources of infection such as open wounds.

PEDIATRIC POINTERS

■ *Normal blood pressure in children is lower than that in adults. Because accidents occur frequently with children, suspect trauma or shock first as a possible cause of low blood pressure.*

■ *Remember that low blood pressure typically doesn't accompany head injury in adults because intracranial hemorrhage is insufficient to cause hypovolemia. However, it does accompany head injury in infants and young children; their expandable cranial vaults allow significant blood loss into the cranial space, resulting in hypovolemia.*

■ *Another common cause of low blood pressure in children is dehydration, which results from failure to thrive or from persistent diarrhea and vomiting for as little as 24 hours.*

ELDER CARE CUES

■ *In elderly patients, low blood pressure commonly results from using multiple drugs that have low blood pressure as a potential adverse reaction.*

■ *Orthostatic hypotension due to autonomic dysfunction is another common cause of low blood pressure in elderly patients.*

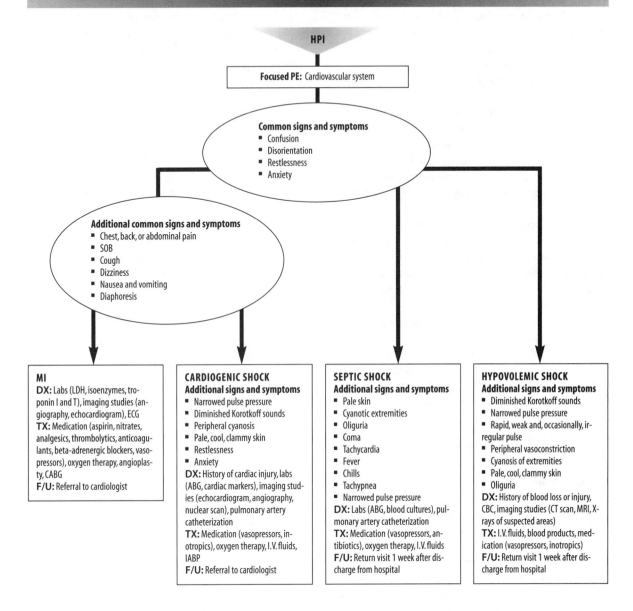

HPI

Focused PE: Cardiovascular system

Common signs and symptoms
- Confusion
- Disorientation
- Restlessness
- Anxiety

Additional common signs and symptoms
- Chest, back, or abdominal pain
- SOB
- Cough
- Dizziness
- Nausea and vomiting
- Diaphoresis

MI
DX: Labs (LDH, isoenzymes, troponin I and T), imaging studies (angiography, echocardiogram), ECG
TX: Medication (aspirin, nitrates, analgesics, thrombolytics, anticoagulants, beta-adrenergic blockers, vasopressors), oxygen therapy, angioplasty, CABG
F/U: Referral to cardiologist

CARDIOGENIC SHOCK
Additional signs and symptoms
- Narrowed pulse pressure
- Diminished Korotkoff sounds
- Peripheral cyanosis
- Pale, cool, clammy skin
- Restlessness
- Anxiety
DX: History of cardiac injury, labs (ABG, cardiac markers), imaging studies (echocardiogram, angiography, nuclear scan), pulmonary artery catheterization
TX: Medication (vasopressors, inotropics), oxygen therapy, I.V. fluids, IABP
F/U: Referral to cardiologist

SEPTIC SHOCK
Additional signs and symptoms
- Pale skin
- Cyanotic extremities
- Oliguria
- Coma
- Tachycardia
- Fever
- Chills
- Tachypnea
- Narrowed pulse pressure
DX: Labs (ABG, blood cultures), pulmonary artery catheterization
TX: Medication (vasopressors, antibiotics), oxygen therapy, I.V. fluids
F/U: Return visit 1 week after discharge from hospital

HYPOVOLEMIC SHOCK
Additional signs and symptoms
- Diminished Korotkoff sounds
- Narrowed pulse pressure
- Rapid, weak and, occasionally, irregular pulse
- Peripheral vasoconstriction
- Cyanosis of extremities
- Pale, cool, clammy skin
- Oliguria
DX: History of blood loss or injury, CBC, imaging studies (CT scan, MRI, X-rays of suspected areas)
TX: I.V. fluids, blood products, medication (vasopressors, inotropics)
F/U: Return visit 1 week after discharge from hospital

Additional differential diagnoses: acute adrenal insufficiency ▪ alcohol toxicity ▪ anaphylactic shock ▪ cardiac arrhythmias ▪ cardiac contusion ▪ cardiac tamponade ▪ cardiomyopathy ▪ diabetic ketoacidosis ▪ heart failure ▪ hyperosmolar hyperglycemic nonketotic coma ▪ hypoxemia ▪ MI ▪ neurogenic shock ▪ pulmonary embolism ▪ vasovagal syncope

Other causes: gastric acid stimulation test with histamine ▪ X-ray studies with contrast media ▪ calcium channel blockers ▪ diuretics ▪ vasodilators ▪ alpha- and beta-adrenergic blockers ▪ general anesthetics ▪ narcotic analgesic ▪ MAO inhibitors ▪ antianxiety agents such as benzodiazepines ▪ tranquilizers ▪ most I.V. antiarrhythmics

Blood pressure increase

Elevated blood pressure (hypertension) — an intermittent or sustained increase in blood pressure to 140/90 mm Hg — strikes more men than women and twice as many blacks as whites. By itself, this common sign is easily ignored by the patient; after all, he can't see or feel it. However, its causes can be life-threatening.

Elevated blood pressure may develop suddenly or gradually. A sudden, severe rise in blood pressure (to more than 200/120 mm Hg) indicates life-threatening hypertensive crisis. However, even a less dramatic rise may be equally significant if it heralds dissecting aortic aneurysm, increased intracranial pressure, myocardial infarction, eclampsia, or thyrotoxicosis.

Usually associated with essential hypertension, elevated blood pressure may also result from renal and endocrine disorders; treatments that affect fluid status, such as dialysis; and drug adverse effects. Ingestion of large amounts of certain foods, such as black licorice and cheddar cheese, may temporarily elevate blood pressure.

Sometimes, elevated blood pressure may simply reflect an inaccurate blood pressure measurement. However, careful measurement alone doesn't ensure a clinically useful reading. To be useful, each blood pressure reading must be compared with the patient's baseline. Also, serial readings may be necessary to establish elevated blood pressure.

History and physical examination

If you detect sharply elevated blood pressure, quickly rule out possible life-threatening causes. If blood pressure exceeds 200/120 mm Hg, the patient is experiencing hypertensive crisis and emergency measures should be taken. In a female patient who is pregnant, suspect pregnancy-induced hypertension.

After ruling out life-threatening causes, complete a more leisurely history and physical examination. Ask about a family history of high blood pressure — a likely finding in essential hypertension — pheochromocytoma, and polycystic kidney disease. Then ask about its onset. Did high blood pressure appear abruptly? Ask the patient's age. Sudden onset of high blood pressure in middle-aged or elderly patients suggests renovascular stenosis. Although essential hypertension may begin in childhood, it typically isn't diagnosed until age 35. Pheochromocytoma and primary aldosteronism usually occur between ages 40 and 60. If you suspect either, check for orthostatic hypotension. Take the patient's blood pressure while he's lying in a supine position, sitting, and standing. Nor-

mally, systolic pressure falls and diastolic pressure rises on standing. In orthostatic hypotension, both pressures fall.

Note headache, palpitations, blurred vision, and sweating. Ask about wine-colored urine and decreased urine output; these signs suggest glomerulonephritis, which can cause elevated blood pressure.

Obtain a drug history, including past and present prescriptions and over-the-counter drugs (especially decongestants). If the patient is already taking an antihypertensive, determine how well he complies with the regimen. Ask about his perception of elevated blood pressure. How serious does he believe it is? Does he expect drug therapy to help?

Follow up the history with a well-directed physical examination. Using a funduscope, check for intraocular hemorrhage, exudate, and papilledema, which characterize severe hypertension. Perform a thorough cardiovascular assessment. Check for carotid bruits and neck vein distention. Assess skin color, temperature, and turgor. Palpate peripheral pulses. Auscultate for abnormal heart sounds (gallops, louder second sound, murmurs), rate (bradycardia, tachycardia), or rhythm. Then auscultate for abnormal breath sounds (crackles, wheezing), rate (bradypnea, tachypnea), or rhythm.

Palpate the abdomen for tenderness, masses, or liver enlargement. Auscultate for abdominal bruits. Renal artery stenosis produces bruits over the upper abdomen or in the costovertebral angles. Easily palpable, enlarged kidneys and a large, tender liver suggest polycystic kidney disease. Obtain a urine sample to check for microscopic hematuria.

PEDIATRIC POINTERS

- *Normally, blood pressure in children is lower than that in adults.*
- *Elevated blood pressure in children may result from lead or mercury poisoning, essential hypertension, renovascular stenosis, chronic pyelonephritis, coarctation of the aorta, patent ductus arteriosus, glomerulonephritis, adrenogenital syndrome, and neuroblastoma.*
- *Treatment typically begins with drug therapy. Surgery may follow for a patient with patent ductus arteriosus, coarctation of the aorta, or neuroblastoma and for some cases of renovascular stenosis.*
- *Diuretics and antibiotics are used to treat glomerulonephritis and chronic pyelonephritis; hormonal therapy, to treat adrenogenital syndrome.*

ELDER CARE CUE

Atherosclerosis commonly produces isolated systolic hypertension in elderly patients. Treatment is warranted to prevent long-term complications.

HPI

Focused PE: Cardiovascular and neurologic systems

HYPERTENSION
Signs and symptoms
- Systolic BP >140 mm Hg; diastolic > 90 mm Hg
- Headache
- Retinopathy
- Signs and symptoms of underlying disorder, if present

DX: History of risk factors, sustained elevated BP, test for suspected underlying disorder, labs (CBC, electrolytes, cholesterol)

TX: Treatment of underlying cause, if present; reduction of controllable risk factors; low-fat, low-salt diet; medication (diuretics, alpha-adrenergic blockers, ACE inhibitors, angiotension II receptor blocker, calcium channel blockers, beta-adrenergic blockers)

F/U: Return visits every 3 to 6 months (when condition is stable)

RENOVASCULAR STENOSIS
Signs and symptoms
- Abruptly elevated systolic and diastolic BP
- Bruits over the upper abdomen or in the costovertebral angles
- Hematuria
- Headache (occasionally)
- Acute flank pain

DX: Imaging studies (renal scan, angiography, IVP)

TX: Medication (diuretics, beta-adrenergic blockers, calcium channel blockers, ACE inhibitors), balloon angioplasty of renal artery, surgery

F/U: Referral to nephrologist

ATHEROSCLEROSIS
Signs and symptoms
- Increased systolic BP
- Normal or slightly elevated diastolic BP
- Weak pulse
- Flushed skin
- Tachycardia
- Anginal pain
- Claudication of extremities

DX: Labs (cholesterol level, LDL, HDL), imaging studies (ultrasound of affected area, arteriography of affected area)

TX: Treatment of affected area; medication (aspirin, antilipemic agents); low-fat, low-cholesterol, low-salt diet; exercise program

F/U: As needed (dependent on symptoms)

PHEOCHROMOCYTOMA
Signs and symptoms
- Paroxysmal or sustained elevated BP
- Orthostatic hypotension
- Anxiety
- Tremors
- Diaphoresis
- Palpitations
- Pallor
- Nausea
- Weight loss
- Headache

DX: Labs (urine metanephrine, urine catecholamines), imaging studies (MRI, MIBG scintiscan), adrenal biopsy

TX: Combined alpha- and beta-adrenergic blockers (preoperatively), surgery

F/U: Daily BP monitoring preoperatively, urine catecholamine level 2 weeks postoperatively

---

Additional differential diagnoses: aldosteronism (primary) ▪ anemia ▪ aortic aneurysm (dissecting) ▪ Cushing's syndrome ▪ eclampsia ▪ essential hypertension ▪ increased ICP ▪ malignant hypertension ▪ MI ▪ polycystic kidney disease ▪ preeclampsia ▪ thyrotoxicosis

---

Other causes: medication (CNS stimulants [such as amphetamines], sympathomimetics, corticosteroids, oral contraceptives, MAO inhibitors, cocaine) ▪ ephedra ▪ ginseng ▪ licorice ▪ St. John's wort ▪ treatments (kidney dialysis and transplantation)

Bowel sounds, abnormal

Absent bowel sounds refers to an inability to hear bowel sounds through a stethoscope after listening for at least 5 minutes in each abdominal quadrant. Bowel sounds cease when mechanical or vascular obstruction or neurogenic inhibition halts peristalsis. When peristalsis stops, gas from bowel contents and fluid secreted from the intestinal walls accumulate and distend the lumen, leading to life-threatening complications, such as perforation, peritonitis and sepsis, or hypovolemic shock.

Simple mechanical obstruction, resulting from adhesions, hernia, or tumor, causes loss of fluids and electrolytes and induces dehydration. Vascular obstruction cuts off circulation to the intestinal walls, leading to ischemia, necrosis, and shock. Neurogenic inhibition, affecting innervation of the intestinal wall, may result from infection, bowel distention, or trauma.

Abrupt cessation of bowel sounds, when accompanied by abdominal pain, rigidity, and distention, signals a life-threatening crisis requiring immediate intervention. Absent bowel sounds following a period of hyperactive sounds are equally ominous and may indicate strangulation of a mechanically obstructed bowel.

Sometimes audible without a stethoscope, *hyperactive bowel sounds* reflect increased intestinal motility (peristalsis). They're commonly characterized as rapid, rushing, gurgling waves of sounds. They may stem from life-threatening bowel obstruction or GI hemorrhage as well as from GI infection, inflammatory bowel disease, food allergies, and stress.

Hypoactive bowel sounds, detected by auscultation, are diminished in regularity, tone, and loudness from normal bowel sounds. By themselves, hypoactive bowel sounds don't herald an emergency; in fact, they're considered normal during sleep. However, they may lead to absent bowel sounds, which can indicate a life-threatening disorder.

Hypoactive bowel sounds result from decreased peristalsis which, in turn, can result from a developing bowel obstruction. The obstruction may be mechanical (as from hernia, tumor, or twisting), vascular (as from embolism or thrombosis), or neurogenic (as from mechanical, ischemic, or toxic impairment of bowel innervation).

History and physical examination

If you fail to detect bowel sounds and the patient reports sudden, severe abdominal pain and cramping or exhibits severe abdominal distention, decompression of the bowel may be needed, as well as abdominal surgery. If you detect hyperactive bowel sounds, quickly check vital signs and ask the patient about associated symptoms, such as abdominal pain, vomiting, and diarrhea. If he reports cramping abdominal

pain or vomiting, continue to auscultate for bowel sounds. If bowel sounds stop abruptly, suspect complete bowel obstruction.

If the patient's condition permits, proceed with a brief history. Start with abdominal pain. When did it begin? Has it gotten worse? Where does he feel it? Ask about a sensation of bloating and about flatulence. Find out if the patient has had diarrhea or has passed pencil-thin stools — possible signs of a developing luminal obstruction. The patient may have had no bowel movements at all — a possible sign of complete obstruction or paralytic ileus.

Ask about conditions that commonly lead to mechanical obstruction, such as abdominal tumors, hernias, and adhesions from past surgery. Determine if the patient was involved in an accident — even a seemingly minor one such as falling off a stepladder — that may have caused vascular clots. Check for a history of acute pancreatitis, diverticulitis, or gynecologic infection, which may have led to intra-abdominal infection and bowel dysfunction. Be sure to ask about previous toxic conditions, such as uremia, and about spinal cord injury, which can lead to paralytic ileus.

If the patient's pain isn't severe or accompanied by other life-threatening signs, obtain a detailed medical and surgical history and perform a complete physical examination followed by an abdominal assessment and pelvic examination.

Start your assessment by inspecting abdominal contour. Stoop at the recumbent patient's side and then at the foot of his bed to detect localized or generalized distention. Listen for dullness over fluid-filled areas and tympany over pockets of gas. Percuss and palpate the abdomen gently. Palpate for abdominal rigidity and guarding, which suggest peritoneal irritation that can lead to paralytic ileus.

In addition, determine whether stress may have contributed to the patient's problem. Ask about food allergies and recent ingestion of unusual foods or fluids. Check for fever, which suggests infection.

PEDIATRIC POINTERS

- *Absent bowel sounds in children may result from Hirschsprung's disease or intussusception, both of which can lead to life-threatening obstructions.*
- *Hyperactive bowel sounds in children usually result from gastroenteritis, erratic eating habits, excessive ingestion of certain foods (such as unripened fruit), or food allergy.*
- *Hypoactive bowel sounds in a child may simply be due to bowel distention from excessive swallowing of air while the child was eating or crying. However, be sure to observe the child for further signs of illness.*
- *As with an adult, sluggish bowel sounds in a child may signal the onset of paralytic ileus or peritonitis.*

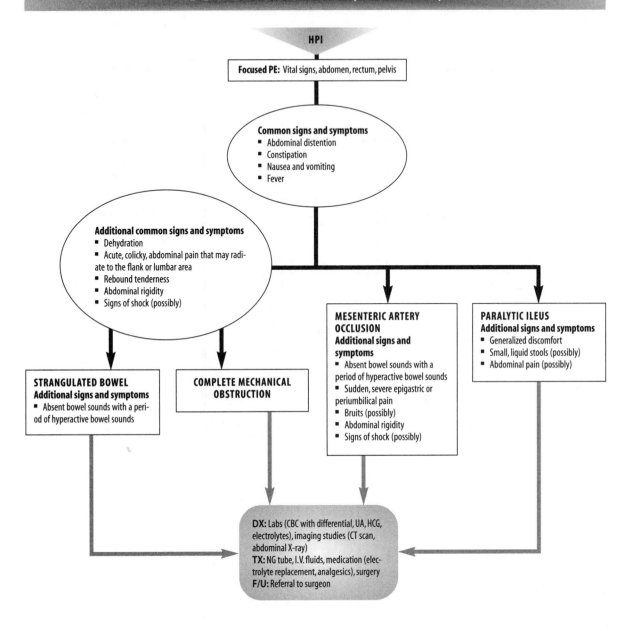

HPI

Focused PE: Vital signs, abdomen, rectum, pelvis

Common signs and symptoms
- Abdominal distention
- Constipation
- Nausea and vomiting
- Fever

Additional common signs and symptoms
- Dehydration
- Acute, colicky, abdominal pain that may radiate to the flank or lumbar area
- Rebound tenderness
- Abdominal rigidity
- Signs of shock (possibly)

MESENTERIC ARTERY OCCLUSION
Additional signs and symptoms
- Absent bowel sounds with a period of hyperactive bowel sounds
- Sudden, severe epigastric or periumbilical pain
- Bruits (possibly)
- Abdominal rigidity
- Signs of shock (possibly)

PARALYTIC ILEUS
Additional signs and symptoms
- Generalized discomfort
- Small, liquid stools (possibly)
- Abdominal pain (possibly)

STRANGULATED BOWEL
Additional signs and symptoms
- Absent bowel sounds with a period of hyperactive bowel sounds

COMPLETE MECHANICAL OBSTRUCTION

DX: Labs (CBC with differential, UA, HCG, electrolytes), imaging studies (CT scan, abdominal X-ray)
TX: NG tube, I.V. fluids, medication (electrolyte replacement, analgesics), surgery
F/U: Referral to surgeon

Other causes: abdominal surgery

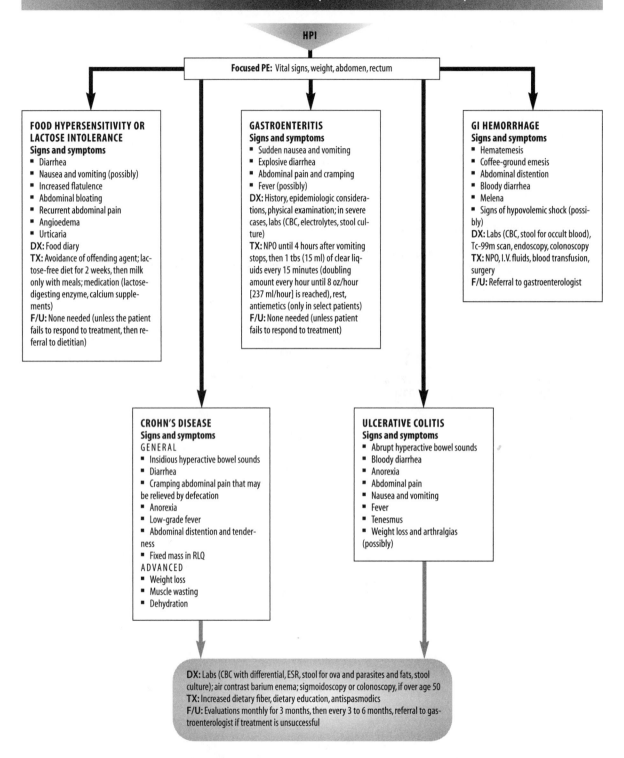

HPI

Focused PE: Vital signs, weight, abdomen, rectum

FOOD HYPERSENSITIVITY OR LACTOSE INTOLERANCE
Signs and symptoms
- Diarrhea
- Nausea and vomiting (possibly)
- Increased flatulence
- Abdominal bloating
- Recurrent abdominal pain
- Angioedema
- Urticaria

DX: Food diary
TX: Avoidance of offending agent; lactose-free diet for 2 weeks, then milk only with meals; medication (lactose-digesting enzyme, calcium supplements)
F/U: None needed (unless the patient fails to respond to treatment, then referral to dietitian)

GASTROENTERITIS
Signs and symptoms
- Sudden nausea and vomiting
- Explosive diarrhea
- Abdominal pain and cramping
- Fever (possibly)

DX: History, epidemiologic considerations, physical examination; in severe cases, labs (CBC, electrolytes, stool culture)
TX: NPO until 4 hours after vomiting stops, then 1 tbs (15 ml) of clear liquids every 15 minutes (doubling amount every hour until 8 oz/hour [237 ml/hour] is reached), rest, antiemetics (only in select patients)
F/U: None needed (unless patient fails to respond to treatment)

GI HEMORRHAGE
Signs and symptoms
- Hematemesis
- Coffee-ground emesis
- Abdominal distention
- Bloody diarrhea
- Melena
- Signs of hypovolemic shock (possibly)

DX: Labs (CBC, stool for occult blood), Tc-99m scan, endoscopy, colonoscopy
TX: NPO, I.V. fluids, blood transfusion, surgery
F/U: Referral to gastroenterologist

CROHN'S DISEASE
Signs and symptoms
GENERAL
- Insidious hyperactive bowel sounds
- Diarrhea
- Cramping abdominal pain that may be relieved by defecation
- Anorexia
- Low-grade fever
- Abdominal distention and tenderness
- Fixed mass in RLQ
ADVANCED
- Weight loss
- Muscle wasting
- Dehydration

ULCERATIVE COLITIS
Signs and symptoms
- Abrupt hyperactive bowel sounds
- Bloody diarrhea
- Anorexia
- Abdominal pain
- Nausea and vomiting
- Fever
- Tenesmus
- Weight loss and arthralgias (possibly)

DX: Labs (CBC with differential, ESR, stool for ova and parasites and fats, stool culture); air contrast barium enema; sigmoidoscopy or colonoscopy, if over age 50
TX: Increased dietary fiber, dietary education, antispasmodics
F/U: Evaluations monthly for 3 months, then every 3 to 6 months, referral to gastroenterologist if treatment is unsuccessful

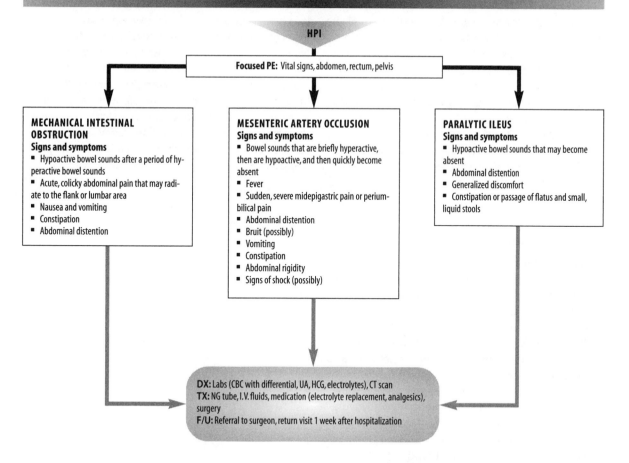

HPI

Focused PE: Vital signs, abdomen, rectum, pelvis

MECHANICAL INTESTINAL OBSTRUCTION
Signs and symptoms
- Hypoactive bowel sounds after a period of hyperactive bowel sounds
- Acute, colicky abdominal pain that may radiate to the flank or lumbar area
- Nausea and vomiting
- Constipation
- Abdominal distention

MESENTERIC ARTERY OCCLUSION
Signs and symptoms
- Bowel sounds that are briefly hyperactive, then are hypoactive, and then quickly become absent
- Fever
- Sudden, severe midepigastric pain or periumbilical pain
- Abdominal distention
- Bruit (possibly)
- Vomiting
- Constipation
- Abdominal rigidity
- Signs of shock (possibly)

PARALYTIC ILEUS
Signs and symptoms
- Hypoactive bowel sounds that may become absent
- Abdominal distention
- Generalized discomfort
- Constipation or passage of flatus and small, liquid stools

DX: Labs (CBC with differential, UA, HCG, electrolytes), CT scan
TX: NG tube, I.V. fluids, medication (electrolyte replacement, analgesics), surgery
F/U: Referral to surgeon, return visit 1 week after hospitalization

Other causes: opiates such as codeine ▪ anticholinergics such as propantheline bromide ▪ phenothiazines such as chlorpromazine ▪ vinca alkaloids such as vincristine ▪ radiation therapy ▪ surgery

Bradycardia

Bradycardia refers to a heart rate of less than 60 beats/minute. It occurs normally in young adults, trained athletes, and elderly people and during sleep. It's also a normal response to vagal stimulation caused by coughing, vomiting, or straining during defecation. When bradycardia results from these causes, the heart rate rarely drops below 40 beats/minute. However, when it results from pathologic causes (such as cardiovascular disorders), the heart rate may be slower.

By itself, bradycardia is a nonspecific sign. However, in conjunction with such symptoms as chest pain, dizziness, syncope, and shortness of breath, it can signal a life-threatening disorder.

History and physical examination

After detecting bradycardia, check for related signs of life-threatening disorders. Bradycardia can signal a life-threatening disorder when accompanied by such other symptoms as pain, shortness of breath, dizziness, syncope, prolonged exposure to cold, or head or neck trauma.

If the patient's bradycardia isn't accompanied by untoward signs, ask the patient if he or a family member has a history of a slow pulse rate because bradycardia may be inherited. Also, find out if he has an underlying metabolic disorder, such as hypothyroidism, which can precipitate bradycardia. Ask which medications he's taking and if he's complying with the prescribed schedule and dosage.

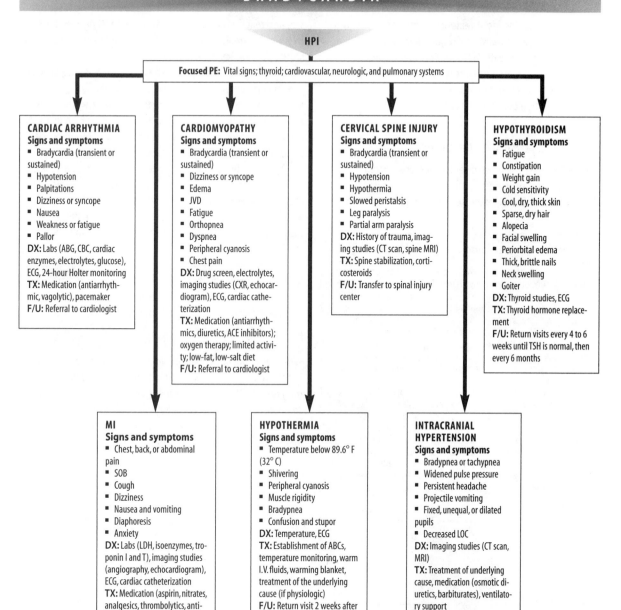

HPI

Focused PE: Vital signs; thyroid; cardiovascular, neurologic, and pulmonary systems

CARDIAC ARRHYTHMIA
Signs and symptoms
- Bradycardia (transient or sustained)
- Hypotension
- Palpitations
- Dizziness or syncope
- Nausea
- Weakness or fatigue
- Pallor

DX: Labs (ABG, CBC, cardiac enzymes, electrolytes, glucose), ECG, 24-hour Holter monitoring
TX: Medication (antiarrhythmic, vagolytic), pacemaker
F/U: Referral to cardiologist

CARDIOMYOPATHY
Signs and symptoms
- Bradycardia (transient or sustained)
- Dizziness or syncope
- Edema
- JVD
- Fatigue
- Orthopnea
- Dyspnea
- Peripheral cyanosis
- Chest pain

DX: Drug screen, electrolytes, imaging studies (CXR, echocardiogram), ECG, cardiac catheterization
TX: Medication (antiarrhythmics, diuretics, ACE inhibitors); oxygen therapy; limited activity; low-fat, low-salt diet
F/U: Referral to cardiologist

CERVICAL SPINE INJURY
Signs and symptoms
- Bradycardia (transient or sustained)
- Hypotension
- Hypothermia
- Slowed peristalsis
- Leg paralysis
- Partial arm paralysis

DX: History of trauma, imaging studies (CT scan, spine MRI)
TX: Spine stabilization, corticosteroids
F/U: Transfer to spinal injury center

HYPOTHYROIDISM
Signs and symptoms
- Fatigue
- Constipation
- Weight gain
- Cold sensitivity
- Cool, dry, thick skin
- Sparse, dry hair
- Alopecia
- Facial swelling
- Periorbital edema
- Thick, brittle nails
- Neck swelling
- Goiter

DX: Thyroid studies, ECG
TX: Thyroid hormone replacement
F/U: Return visits every 4 to 6 weeks until TSH is normal, then every 6 months

MI
Signs and symptoms
- Chest, back, or abdominal pain
- SOB
- Cough
- Dizziness
- Nausea and vomiting
- Diaphoresis
- Anxiety

DX: Labs (LDH, isoenzymes, troponin I and T), imaging studies (angiography, echocardiogram), ECG, cardiac catheterization
TX: Medication (aspirin, nitrates, analgesics, thrombolytics, anticoagulants, beta-adrenergic blockers, vasopressors), oxygen therapy, angioplasty, CABG
F/U: Referral to cardiologist; return visit 3 to 6 weeks after hospitalization, then every 3 months

HYPOTHERMIA
Signs and symptoms
- Temperature below 89.6° F (32° C)
- Shivering
- Peripheral cyanosis
- Muscle rigidity
- Bradypnea
- Confusion and stupor

DX: Temperature, ECG
TX: Establishment of ABCs, temperature monitoring, warm I.V. fluids, warming blanket, treatment of the underlying cause (if physiologic)
F/U: Return visit 2 weeks after hospitalization

INTRACRANIAL HYPERTENSION
Signs and symptoms
- Bradypnea or tachypnea
- Widened pulse pressure
- Persistent headache
- Projectile vomiting
- Fixed, unequal, or dilated pupils
- Decreased LOC

DX: Imaging studies (CT scan, MRI)
TX: Treatment of underlying cause, medication (osmotic diuretics, barbiturates), ventilatory support
F/U: Referral to neurologist or neurosurgeon

Other causes: diagnostic tests (cardiac catheterization, electrophysiologic studies) ▪ beta-adrenergic blockers ▪ some calcium channel blockers ▪ cardiac glycosides ▪ topical miotics ▪ protamine sulfate ▪ quinidine and other antiarrhythmics ▪ sympatholytics ▪ failure to take thyroid replacements ▪ suctioning ▪ cardiac surgery

Bradypnea

Commonly preceding life-threatening apnea or respiratory arrest, bradypnea is a pattern of regular respirations with a rate of less than 12 breaths/minute. This sign results from neurologic and metabolic disorders or drug overdose, which depress the brain's respiratory control centers. (See *Understanding neurologic control of breathing*.)

History and physical examination

Depending on the degree of central nervous system depression, the patient may require constant stimulation to breathe. If the patient seems excessively sleepy, try to arouse him by shaking and instructing him to breathe. Quickly take his vital signs and assess his neurologic status by checking his pupil size and reactions and by evaluating his level of consciousness and his ability to move his extremities. Be prepared to institute emergency measures.

Obtain a brief history from the patient, if possible, or whoever accompanied him to the hospital. Ask if he may be having a drug overdose and, if so, try to determine what drugs he took, how much, when, and by what route. Check his arms for needle marks, indicating possible drug abuse. You may need to administer I.V. naloxone, a narcotic antagonist.

If you rule out a drug overdose, ask about chronic illnesses, such as diabetes and renal failure. Check for a medical identification bracelet or an identification card that identifies an underlying condition. Also, ask whether the patient has a history of head trauma, brain tumor, neurologic infection, or stroke.

PEDIATRIC POINTER

Because respiratory rates are higher in children than adults, bradypnea in children is defined according to age.

ELDER CARE CUE

When drugs are prescribed for older patients, keep in mind that they have a higher risk of developing bradypnea secondary to drug toxicity. That's because they often take several drugs that can potentiate this effect and they typically have other conditions that predispose them to it. Warn older patients about this potentially life-threatening complication.

Understanding neurologic control of breathing

The mechanical aspects of breathing are regulated by respiratory centers, groups of discrete neurons in the medulla and pons that function as a unit. In the medullary respiratory center, neurons associated with inspiration and neurons associated with expiration interact to control respiratory rate and depth. In the pons, two additional centers interact with the medullary center to regulate rhythm: the apneustic center stimulates inspiratory neurons in the medulla to precipitate inspiration; these, in turn, stimulate the pneumotaxic center to inhibit inspiration, allowing passive expiration to occur.

Normally, the breathing mechanism is stimulated by increased carbon dioxide levels and decreased oxygen levels in the blood. Chemoreceptors in the medulla and in the carotid and aortic bodies respond to changes in $PaCO_2$, pH, and PaO_2, signaling respiratory centers to adjust respiratory rate and depth. Respiratory depression occurs when decreased cerebral perfusion inactivates respiratory center neurons, when changes in $PaCO_2$ and arterial blood pH affect chemoreceptor responsiveness, or when neuron responsiveness to $PaCO_2$ changes is reduced — for example, in narcotic overdose.

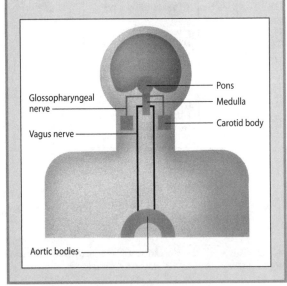

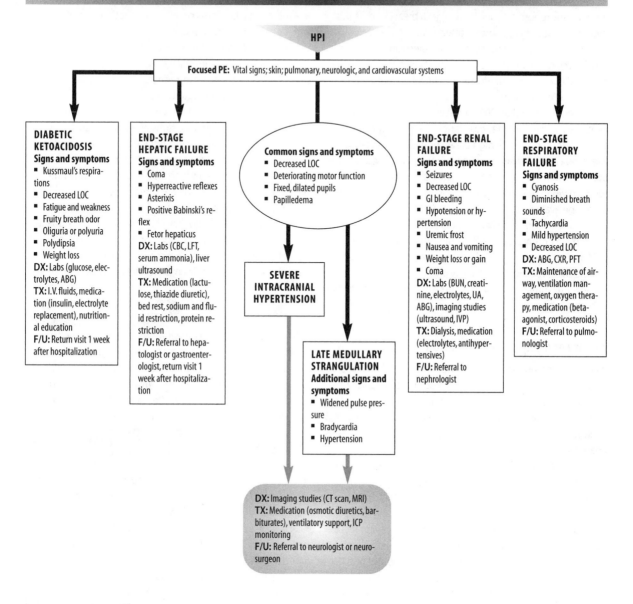

HPI

Focused PE: Vital signs; skin; pulmonary, neurologic, and cardiovascular systems

DIABETIC KETOACIDOSIS
Signs and symptoms
- Kussmaul's respirations
- Decreased LOC
- Fatigue and weakness
- Fruity breath odor
- Oliguria or polyuria
- Polydipsia
- Weight loss
DX: Labs (glucose, electrolytes, ABG)
TX: I.V. fluids, medication (insulin, electrolyte replacement), nutritional education
F/U: Return visit 1 week after hospitalization

END-STAGE HEPATIC FAILURE
Signs and symptoms
- Coma
- Hyperreactive reflexes
- Asterixis
- Positive Babinski's reflex
- Fetor hepaticus
DX: Labs (CBC, LFT, serum ammonia), liver ultrasound
TX: Medication (lactulose, thiazide diuretic), bed rest, sodium and fluid restriction, protein restriction
F/U: Referral to hepatologist or gastroenterologist, return visit 1 week after hospitalization

Common signs and symptoms
- Decreased LOC
- Deteriorating motor function
- Fixed, dilated pupils
- Papilledema

SEVERE INTRACRANIAL HYPERTENSION

LATE MEDULLARY STRANGULATION
Additional signs and symptoms
- Widened pulse pressure
- Bradycardia
- Hypertension

DX: Imaging studies (CT scan, MRI)
TX: Medication (osmotic diuretics, barbiturates), ventilatory support, ICP monitoring
F/U: Referral to neurologist or neurosurgeon

END-STAGE RENAL FAILURE
Signs and symptoms
- Seizures
- Decreased LOC
- GI bleeding
- Hypotension or hypertension
- Uremic frost
- Nausea and vomiting
- Weight loss or gain
- Coma
DX: Labs (BUN, creatinine, electrolytes, UA, ABG), imaging studies (ultrasound, IVP)
TX: Dialysis, medication (electrolytes, antihypertensives)
F/U: Referral to nephrologist

END-STAGE RESPIRATORY FAILURE
Signs and symptoms
- Cyanosis
- Diminished breath sounds
- Tachycardia
- Mild hypertension
- Decreased LOC
DX: ABG, CXR, PFT
TX: Maintenance of airway, ventilation management, oxygen therapy, medication (beta-agonist, corticosteroids)
F/U: Referral to pulmonologist

Other causes: overdose of narcotic analgesics or, less commonly, sedatives, barbiturates, phenothiazines, or other CNS depressants (use of any of these medications with alcohol can also cause bradypnea)

Breast nodule

A frequently reported gynecologic sign, a breast nodule has two chief causes: benign breast disease and cancer. Benign breast disease, the leading cause of nodules, can stem from cyst formation in obstructed and dilated lactiferous ducts, hypertrophy or tumor formation in the ductal system, and inflammation or infection.

Although fewer than 20% of breast nodules are malignant, the clinical signs of breast cancer aren't easily distinguished from those of benign breast disease. Breast cancer is a leading cause of death among women but also occasionally occurs in men, with signs and symptoms mimicking those found in women. Thus, breast nodules in both sexes should always be evaluated.

A woman who is familiar with the feel of her breasts and performs monthly breast self-examinations can detect a nodule 5 mm or less in size, considerably smaller than the 1-cm nodule that's readily detectable by an experienced examiner. However, a woman may fail to report a nodule because of fear of breast cancer.

History and physical examination

If your patient reports a lump, ask her how and when she discovered it. Does the size and tenderness of the lump vary with her menstrual cycle? Has the lump changed since she first noticed it? Has she noticed other breast signs, such as a change in breast shape, size, or contour; a discharge; or nipple changes?

Is she lactating? Does she have fever, chills, fatigue, or other flulike symptoms? Ask her to describe pain or tenderness associated with the lump. Is the pain in one breast only? Has she sustained recent trauma to the breast?

Explore the patient's medical and family history for factors that increase her risk of breast cancer. These include a high-fat diet, high caffeine consumption, having a mother or sister with breast cancer, or having a history of cancer, especially cancer in the other breast. Other risk factors include nulliparity and a first pregnancy after age 30.

Next, perform a thorough breast examination. Pay special attention to the upper outer quadrant of each breast, where half the ductal tissue is located. This is the most common site of malignant breast tumors.

Carefully palpate a suspected breast nodule, noting its location, shape, size, consistency, mobility, and delineation. Does the nodule feel soft, rubbery, and elastic or hard? Is it mobile, slipping away from your fingers as you palpate it, or firmly fixed to adjacent tissue? Does the nodule seem to limit the mobility of the entire breast? Note the nodule's delineation. Are the borders clearly defined or indefinite? Or does the area feel more like a hardness or diffuse induration than a nodule with definite borders? Is it painful?

Do you feel one nodule or several small ones? Is the shape round, oval, lobular, or irregular? Inspect and palpate the skin over the nodule for warmth, redness, and edema. Palpate the lymph nodes of the breast and axilla for enlargement.

Observe the contour of the breasts, looking for asymmetry and irregularities. Be alert for signs of retraction, such as skin dimpling and nipple deviation, retraction, or flattening. (To exaggerate dimpling, have your patient raise her arms over her head or press her hands against her hips.) Gently pull the breast skin toward the clavicle. Is dimpling evident? Mold the breast skin and again observe for dimpling.

Be alert for a nipple discharge that's spontaneous, unilateral, and nonmilky (serous, bloody, or purulent). Be careful not to confuse it with the grayish discharge that can commonly be elicited from the nipples of a woman who has been pregnant.

WOMEN'S HEALTH TIP

A Breast Cancer Risk Assessment Tool has been developed by the National Cancer Institute and the National Surgical Adjuvant Breast and Bowel Project. This tool is to be used by the health professional to estimate the risk for invasive breast cancer over a 5-year period and over a lifetime (to age 90). It's available at the following Web site: www.bcra.nci.nih.gov/brc.

PEDIATRIC POINTERS

- *Most nodules in children and adolescents reflect the normal response of breast tissue to hormonal fluctuations. For instance, the breasts of young teenage girls may normally contain cord-like nodules that become tender just before menstruation.*
- *A transient breast nodule in young boys (as well as women between ages 20 and 30) may result from juvenile mastitis, which usually affects one breast. Signs of inflammation are present in a firm mass beneath the nipple.*

ELDER CARE CUE

In women age 70 and older, three-quarters of all breast lumps are malignant.

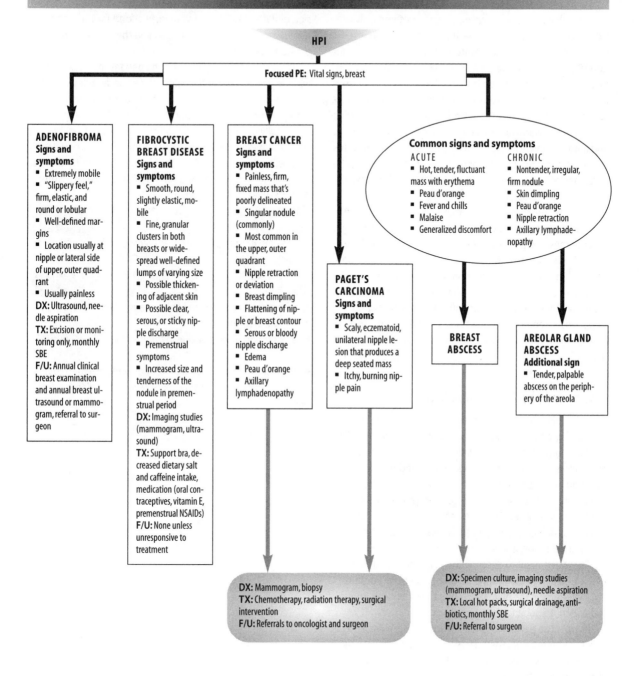

HPI

Focused PE: Vital signs, breast

ADENOFIBROMA
Signs and symptoms
- Extremely mobile
- "Slippery feel," firm, elastic, and round or lobular
- Well-defined margins
- Location usually at nipple or lateral side of upper, outer quadrant
- Usually painless

DX: Ultrasound, needle aspiration
TX: Excision or monitoring only, monthly SBE
F/U: Annual clinical breast examination and annual breast ultrasound or mammogram, referral to surgeon

FIBROCYSTIC BREAST DISEASE
Signs and symptoms
- Smooth, round, slightly elastic, mobile
- Fine, granular clusters in both breasts or widespread well-defined lumps of varying size
- Possible thickening of adjacent skin
- Possible clear, serous, or sticky nipple discharge
- Premenstrual symptoms
- Increased size and tenderness of the nodule in premenstrual period

DX: Imaging studies (mammogram, ultrasound)
TX: Support bra, decreased dietary salt and caffeine intake, medication (oral contraceptives, vitamin E, premenstrual NSAIDs)
F/U: None unless unresponsive to treatment

BREAST CANCER
Signs and symptoms
- Painless, firm, fixed mass that's poorly delineated
- Singular nodule (commonly)
- Most common in the upper, outer quadrant
- Nipple retraction or deviation
- Breast dimpling
- Flattening of nipple or breast contour
- Serous or bloody nipple discharge
- Edema
- Peau d'orange
- Axillary lymphadenopathy

PAGET'S CARCINOMA
Signs and symptoms
- Scaly, eczematoid, unilateral nipple lesion that produces a deep seated mass
- Itchy, burning nipple pain

Common signs and symptoms
ACUTE
- Hot, tender, fluctuant mass with erythema
- Peau d'orange
- Fever and chills
- Malaise
- Generalized discomfort

CHRONIC
- Nontender, irregular, firm nodule
- Skin dimpling
- Peau d'orange
- Nipple retraction
- Axillary lymphadenopathy

BREAST ABSCESS

AREOLAR GLAND ABSCESS
Additional sign
- Tender, palpable abscess on the periphery of the areola

DX: Mammogram, biopsy
TX: Chemotherapy, radiation therapy, surgical intervention
F/U: Referrals to oncologist and surgeon

DX: Specimen culture, imaging studies (mammogram, ultrasound), needle aspiration
TX: Local hot packs, surgical drainage, antibiotics, monthly SBE
F/U: Referral to surgeon

Additional differential diagnoses: actinomycosis ▪ hydatid cyst ▪ intraductal papilloma ▪ mastitis ▪ sebaceous cyst

Breast pain

An unreliable indicator of cancer, breast pain commonly results from benign breast disease. It may occur during rest or movement and may be aggravated by manipulation or palpation. (*Breast tenderness* refers to pain elicited by physical contact.) Breast pain may be unilateral or bilateral; cyclic, intermittent, or constant; and dull or sharp. It may result from surface cuts, furuncles, contusions, and similar lesions (superficial pain); nipple fissures and inflammation in the papillary ducts and areolae (severe localized pain); stromal distention in the breast parenchyma; or a tumor that affects nerve endings (severe, constant pain). Breast pain may radiate to the back, the arms and, sometimes, the neck.

Breast tenderness in women may occur before menstruation and during pregnancy. Before menstruation, breast pain or tenderness stems from increased mammary blood flow due to hormonal changes. During pregnancy, breast tenderness and throbbing, tingling, or pricking sensations may occur, also from hormonal changes. In men, breast pain may stem from gynecomastia (especially during puberty and senescence), reproductive tract anomalies, and organic disease of the liver or pituitary, adrenal cortex, and thyroid glands.

History and physical examination

Begin by asking the patient if breast pain is constant or intermittent. For either type, ask about onset and character. If it's intermittent, determine the relationship of pain to the phase of the menstrual cycle. Is the patient a nursing mother? If not, ask about any nipple discharge and have her describe it. Is she pregnant? Does she use oral contraceptives? Has she reached menopause? Has she recently experienced flulike symptoms or sustained injury to the breast? Has she noticed any change in breast shape or contour?

Ask your patient to describe the pain. She may describe it as sticking, stinging, shooting, stabbing, throbbing, or burning. Determine if the pain affects one breast or both, and ask the patient to point to the painful area.

Instruct the patient to place her arms at her sides, and inspect the breast. Note their size, symmetry, and contour as well as the appearance of the skin. Remember that breast shape and size vary widely and that breasts normally change during the menstrual cycle, pregnancy, and lactation and with aging. Are the breasts red or edematous? Are the veins prominent?

Note the size, shape, and symmetry of the nipples and areolae. Do you detect ecchymosis, a rash, ulceration, or a discharge? Do the nipples point in the same direction? Do you see signs of retraction, such as skin dimpling or nipple inversion or flattening? Repeat your inspection, first with the patient's arms raised above her head and then with her hands pressed against her hips.

Palpate the breasts, first with the patient seated and then with her lying down and a pillow placed under her shoulder on the side being examined. Use the pads of your fingers to compress breast tissue against the chest wall. Proceed systematically from the sternum to the midline and from the axilla to the midline, noting any warmth, tenderness, nodules, masses, or irregularities. Palpate the nipple, noting tenderness and nodules, and check for discharge. Palpate axillary lymph nodes, noting any enlargement.

PEDIATRIC POINTER

Transient gynecomastia can cause breast pain in males during puberty.

ELDER CARE CUES

- *Breast pain secondary to benign breast disease is rare in postmenopausal women.*
- *Breast pain can also be due to trauma from falls or physical abuse.*
- *Because of decreased pain perception and decreased cognitive function, breast pain may not be reported by elderly patients.*

BREAST PAIN

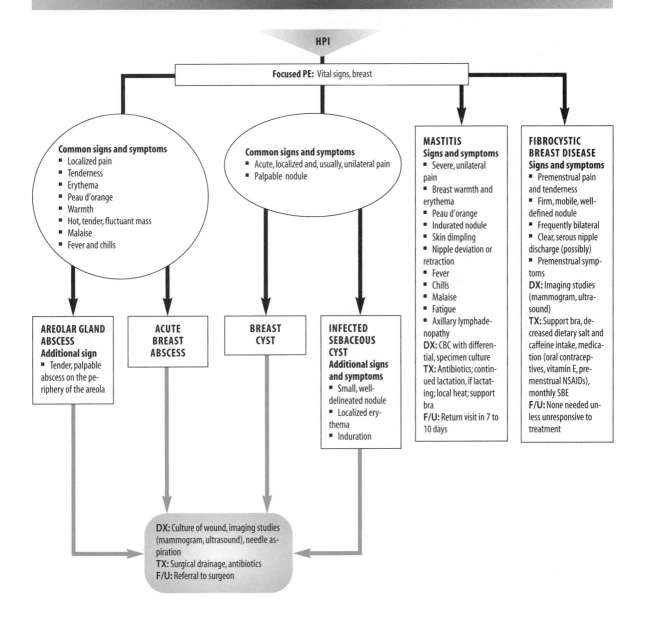

HPI

Focused PE: Vital signs, breast

Common signs and symptoms
- Localized pain
- Tenderness
- Erythema
- Peau d'orange
- Warmth
- Hot, tender, fluctuant mass
- Malaise
- Fever and chills

Common signs and symptoms
- Acute, localized and, usually, unilateral pain
- Palpable nodule

MASTITIS
Signs and symptoms
- Severe, unilateral pain
- Breast warmth and erythema
- Peau d'orange
- Indurated nodule
- Skin dimpling
- Nipple deviation or retraction
- Fever
- Chills
- Malaise
- Fatigue
- Axillary lymphadenopathy

DX: CBC with differential, specimen culture
TX: Antibiotics; continued lactation, if lactating; local heat; support bra
F/U: Return visit in 7 to 10 days

FIBROCYSTIC BREAST DISEASE
Signs and symptoms
- Premenstrual pain and tenderness
- Firm, mobile, well-defined nodule
- Frequently bilateral
- Clear, serous nipple discharge (possibly)
- Premenstrual symptoms

DX: Imaging studies (mammogram, ultrasound)
TX: Support bra, decreased dietary salt and caffeine intake, medication (oral contraceptives, vitamin E, premenstrual NSAIDs), monthly SBE
F/U: None needed unless unresponsive to treatment

AREOLAR GLAND ABSCESS
Additional sign
- Tender, palpable abscess on the periphery of the areola

ACUTE BREAST ABSCESS

BREAST CYST

INFECTED SEBACEOUS CYST
Additional signs and symptoms
- Small, well-delineated nodule
- Localized erythema
- Induration

DX: Culture of wound, imaging studies (mammogram, ultrasound), needle aspiration
TX: Surgical drainage, antibiotics
F/U: Referral to surgeon

Breast ulcer

Appearing on the nipple or areola or on the breast itself, an ulcer indicates destruction of the skin and subcutaneous tissue. A breast ulcer is usually a late sign of cancer, appearing well after the confirming diagnosis. However, it may be the presenting sign of breast cancer in men, who are more apt to dismiss earlier breast changes. Breast ulcers can also result from trauma, infection, or radiation.

History and physical examination

Begin the history by asking when the patient first noticed the ulcer and if it was preceded by other breast changes, such as nodules, edema, and nipple discharge, deviation, or retraction. Does the ulcer seem to be getting better or worse? Does it cause pain or produce drainage? Has the patient noticed any change in breast shape? Has she had a skin rash? If she has been treating the ulcer at home, find out how.

Review the patient's personal and family history for factors that increase the risk of breast cancer. Ask, for example, about previous cancer, especially of the breast, and mastectomy. Ask whether the patient's mother or sister has had breast cancer. Also ask the patient's age at menarche and menopause because more than 30 years of menstrual activity increases the risk of breast cancer. Also ask about pregnancy because nulliparity and birth of a first child after age 30 also increase the risk of breast cancer.

If the patient recently gave birth, ask if she breast-feeds her infant or has recently weaned him. Ask if she's currently taking oral antibiotics and if she's diabetic. All these factors predispose the patient to *Candida albicans* infections.

Inspect the patient's breast, noting any asymmetry or flattening. Look for a rash, scaling, cracking, or red excoriation on the nipples, areola, and inframammary fold. Check especially for skin changes such as warmth, erythema, or peau d'orange. Palpate the breast for masses, noting any induration beneath the ulcer. Then carefully palpate for tenderness or nodules around the areola and the axillary lymph nodes.

ELDER CARE CUES

- *Because of increased breast cancer risk in this population, breast ulcers should be considered cancerous until proved otherwise.*
- *Ulcers can result from normal skin changes in elderly patients, such as thinning, decreased vascularity, and loss of elasticity as well as from poor skin hygiene.*
- *Pressure ulcers may also result from tight brassieres; traumatic ulcers may result from falls or abuse.*

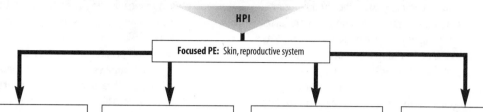

HPI

Focused PE: Skin, reproductive system

BREAST CANCER
Signs and symptoms
- Painless, firm, fixed mass that's poorly delineated
- Singular nodule (commonly)
- Most common in the upper, outer quadrant
- Nipple retraction or deviation
- Breast dimpling
- Flattening of nipple or breast contour
- Serous or bloody nipple discharge
- Edema
- Peau d'orange
- Axillary lymphadenopathy

DX: Mammogram, biopsy
TX: Chemotherapy, radiation therapy, surgery
F/U: Referrals to oncologist and surgeon

CANDIDA ALBICANS INFECTION
Signs and symptoms
- Well-defined, bright red papular patches with scaly borders
- Location in breast folds (usually)
- Occurrence in breast feeding women with dry, cracked nipples
- Burning pain that penetrates the chest wall

DX: Inspection of site, labs (wound culture, blood cultures, ELISA test, analgesics)
TX: Antifungals, wound care
F/U: Return visit 1 week after treatment

PAGET'S DISEASE
Signs and symptoms
- Bright red nipple excoriation that may extend to the areola
- Serous or bloody discharge
- Symptoms (usually unilateral)
- Local hyperemia
- Local edema

DX: Mammography, biopsy
TX: Chemotherapy, surgery
F/U: Referrals to oncologist and surgeon

BREAST TRAUMA
Signs and symptoms
- Pain at the affected site
- Ecchymosis
- Laceration
- Abrasions
- Swelling
- Hematoma

DX: History of injury or surgery, inspection of site
TX: Varies (based on extent of injury), medication (NSAIDs; analgesics; if infection present, antibiotics), surgery
F/U: As needed (dependent on extent of injury, 7 to 10 days after treatment), referral to surgeon (if injury is extensive or isn't responding to treatment)

Other causes: radiation therapy

Breath, abnormal

Ammonia breath odor — commonly described as urinous or "fishy" breath — typically occurs in end-stage chronic renal failure. This sign improves slightly after hemodialysis and persists throughout the course of the disorder but isn't of great concern.

Ammonia breath odor reflects the long-term metabolic disturbances and biochemical abnormalities associated with uremia and end-stage chronic renal failure. It's produced by metabolic end products blown off by the lungs and the breakdown of urea in the saliva to ammonia. A specific uremic toxin hasn't yet been identified.

Fecal breath odor typically accompanies fecal vomiting associated with a long-standing intestinal obstruction or gastrojejunocolic fistula. It represents an important late diagnostic clue to a potentially life-threatening GI disorder because complete obstruction of any part of the bowel, if untreated, can cause death within hours from vascular collapse and shock.

When the obstructed or adynamic intestine attempts self-decompression by regurgitating its contents, vigorous peristaltic waves propel bowel contents backward into the stomach. When the stomach fills with intestinal fluid, further reverse peristalsis results in vomiting. The odor of feculent vomitus lingers in the mouth.

Fruity breath odor results from respiratory elimination of excess acetone. This sign characteristically occurs in ketoacidosis — a potentially life-threatening condition that requires immediate treatment to prevent severe dehydration, irreversible coma, and death.

Ketoacidosis results from the excessive catabolism of fats for cellular energy in the absence of usable carbohydrates. This process begins when insulin levels are insufficient to transport glucose into the cells, as in diabetes mellitus, or when glucose is unavailable and hepatic glycogen stores are depleted, as in low-carbohydrate diets and malnutrition. Lacking glucose, the cells burn fat faster than enzymes can handle the ketones, the acidic end products. As a result, the ketones accumulate in the blood and urine. To compensate for increased acidity, Kussmaul's respirations expel carbon dioxide with enough acetone to flavor the breath. Eventually, this compensatory mechanism fails, producing ketoacidosis.

History and physical examination

When you detect ammonia breath odor, the diagnosis of chronic renal failure will probably already be well established. However, look for associated GI symptoms so that palliative care and support can be individualized.

Inspect the patient's oral cavity for bleeding, swollen gums or tongue, and ulceration with drainage. Ask the patient if he has experienced a metallic taste, loss of smell, increased thirst, heartburn, difficulty swallowing, loss of appetite at the sight of food, and early morning vomiting. Ask about bowel habits, noting especially melenic stools or constipation. Take the patient's vital signs. Watch for indications of hypertension or hypotension. Be alert for other signs of shock (such as tachycardia, tachypnea, and cool, clammy skin) and altered mental status.

When you detect fecal breath odor, if the patient's condition permits, ask about previous abdominal surgery because adhesions can cause an obstruction. Also ask about loss of appetite. Is the patient experiencing abdominal pain? If so, have him describe its onset, duration, and location. Ask if the pain is intense, persistent, or spasmodic. Have the patient describe his normal bowel habits, especially noting constipation, diarrhea, or leakage of stool. Ask when the patient's last bowel movement occurred, and have him describe the stool's color and consistency.

Auscultate for bowel sounds — hyperactive, high-pitched sounds may indicate impending bowel obstruction, whereas hypoactive or absent sounds occur late in obstruction and paralytic ileus. Inspect the abdomen, noting contour and any surgical scars. Measure abdominal girth to provide baseline data for subsequent assessment of distention. Palpate for tenderness, distention, and rigidity. Percuss for tympany, indicating a gas-filled bowel, and dullness, indicating fluid.

When you detect fruity breath odor, check for Kussmaul's respirations and examine the patient's level of consciousness. Ask about the onset and duration of fruity breath odor. Find out about changes in breathing pattern. Ask about increased thirst, frequent urination, weight loss, fatigue, and abdominal pain. Ask the female patient if she has had monilial vaginitis or vaginal secretions with itching. If the patient has a history of diabetes mellitus, ask about stress, infections, and noncompliance with therapy — the most common causes of ketoacidosis in known diabetics. If the patient is suspected of having anorexia nervosa, obtain a dietary and weight history.

PEDIATRIC POINTERS

- *Carefully monitor the child with fecal breath odor for fluid and electrolyte imbalance because dehydration can occur rapidly from persistent vomiting.*
- *Fruity breath odor in an infant or a child usually stems from uncontrolled diabetes mellitus. Ketoacidosis develops rapidly in this age-group because of low glycogen reserves.*

ELDER CARE CUE

Elderly patients may have poor oral hygiene, increased dental caries, decreased salivary function with dryness, and poor dietary intake. In addition, they're commonly taking multiple medications. Consider all of these factors when evaluating an elderly patient with mouth odor.

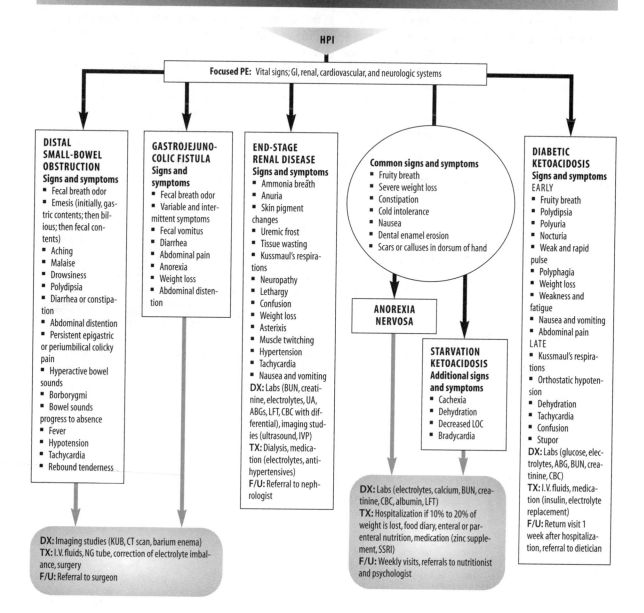

HPI

Focused PE: Vital signs; GI, renal, cardiovascular, and neurologic systems

DISTAL SMALL-BOWEL OBSTRUCTION
Signs and symptoms
- Fecal breath odor
- Emesis (initially, gastric contents; then bilious; then fecal contents)
- Aching
- Malaise
- Drowsiness
- Polydipsia
- Diarrhea or constipation
- Abdominal distention
- Persistent epigastric or periumbilical colicky pain
- Hyperactive bowel sounds
- Borborygmi
- Bowel sounds progress to absence
- Fever
- Hypotension
- Tachycardia
- Rebound tenderness

GASTROJEJUNO-COLIC FISTULA
Signs and symptoms
- Fecal breath odor
- Variable and intermittent symptoms
- Fecal vomitus
- Diarrhea
- Abdominal pain
- Anorexia
- Weight loss
- Abdominal distention

END-STAGE RENAL DISEASE
Signs and symptoms
- Ammonia breath
- Anuria
- Skin pigment changes
- Uremic frost
- Tissue wasting
- Kussmaul's respirations
- Neuropathy
- Lethargy
- Confusion
- Weight loss
- Asterixis
- Muscle twitching
- Hypertension
- Tachycardia
- Nausea and vomiting

DX: Labs (BUN, creatinine, electrolytes, UA, ABGs, LFT, CBC with differential), imaging studies (ultrasound, IVP)
TX: Dialysis, medication (electrolytes, antihypertensives)
F/U: Referral to nephrologist

Common signs and symptoms
- Fruity breath
- Severe weight loss
- Constipation
- Cold intolerance
- Nausea
- Dental enamel erosion
- Scars or calluses in dorsum of hand

ANOREXIA NERVOSA

STARVATION KETOACIDOSIS
Additional signs and symptoms
- Cachexia
- Dehydration
- Decreased LOC
- Bradycardia

DIABETIC KETOACIDOSIS
Signs and symptoms
EARLY
- Fruity breath
- Polydipsia
- Polyuria
- Nocturia
- Weak and rapid pulse
- Polyphagia
- Weight loss
- Weakness and fatigue
- Nausea and vomiting
- Abdominal pain
LATE
- Kussmaul's respirations
- Orthostatic hypotension
- Dehydration
- Tachycardia
- Confusion
- Stupor

DX: Labs (glucose, electrolytes, ABG, BUN, creatinine, CBC)
TX: I.V. fluids, medication (insulin, electrolyte replacement)
F/U: Return visit 1 week after hospitalization, referral to dietician

DX: Imaging studies (KUB, CT scan, barium enema)
TX: I.V. fluids, NG tube, correction of electrolyte imbalance, surgery
F/U: Referral to surgeon

DX: Labs (electrolytes, calcium, BUN, creatinine, CBC, albumin, LFT)
TX: Hospitalization if 10% to 20% of weight is lost, food diary, enteral or parenteral nutrition, medication (zinc supplement, SSRI)
F/U: Weekly visits, referrals to nutritionist and psychologist

Other causes: medication (any drug known to cause metabolic acidosis) ▪ fad diets (especially those encouraging little or no carbohydrate intake)

Brudzinski's sign

A positive Brudzinski's sign (flexion of the hips and knees in response to passive flexion of the neck) signals meningeal irritation. Passive flexion of the neck stretches the nerve roots, causing pain and involuntary flexion of the knees and hips.

Brudzinski's sign is a common and important early indicator of life-threatening meningitis and subarachnoid hemorrhage. It can be elicited in children as well as adults, although more reliable indicators of meningeal irritation exist for infants.

Testing for Brudzinski's sign isn't part of the routine examination, unless meningeal irritation is suspected. (See *Testing for Brudzinski's sign*.)

History and physical examination

If the patient is alert, ask him about headache, neck pain, nausea, and visual disturbances (blurred or double vision and photophobia) — all symptoms of increased intracranial pressure (ICP). Next, observe for signs of increased ICP, such as altered level of consciousness (restlessness, irritability, confusion, lethargy, personality changes, and coma), pupillary changes, bradycardia, widened pulse pressure, irregular respiratory patterns (Cheyne-Stokes or Kussmaul's respirations), vomiting, and moderate fever. Institute emergency measures if your patient's condition deteriorates suddenly.

Continue your neurologic examination by evaluating the patient's cranial nerve function and noting motor or sensory deficits. Also, be sure to look for Kernig's sign (resistance to knee extension after flexion of the hip), which is a further indication of meningeal irritation. In addition, you should look for signs of central nervous system infection, such as fever and nuchal rigidity.

Ask the patient or his family, if necessary, about a history of hypertension, spinal arthritis, or recent head trauma. Also ask about dental work and abscessed teeth (a possible cause of meningitis), open head injury, endocarditis, and I.V. drug abuse. Ask about sudden onset of headaches, which may be associated with subarachnoid hemorrhage.

Brudzinski's sign may not be the most useful indicator of meningeal irritation in infants; more reliable signs, such as bulging fontanels, weak cry, fretfulness, vomiting, and poor feeding, will commonly signal meningeal irritation before you assess for Brudzinski's sign.

Testing for Brudzinski's sign

Here's how to test for Brudzinski's sign, which will help to confirm meningeal irritation.

With the patient in the supine position, place your hands behind her head and lift her head toward her chest.

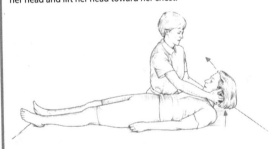

If your patient has meningeal irritation, you'll observe a positive Brudzinski's sign — the patient's hips and knees will flex in response to the passive neck flexion.

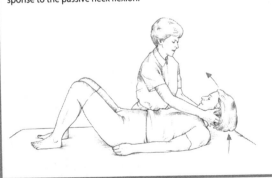

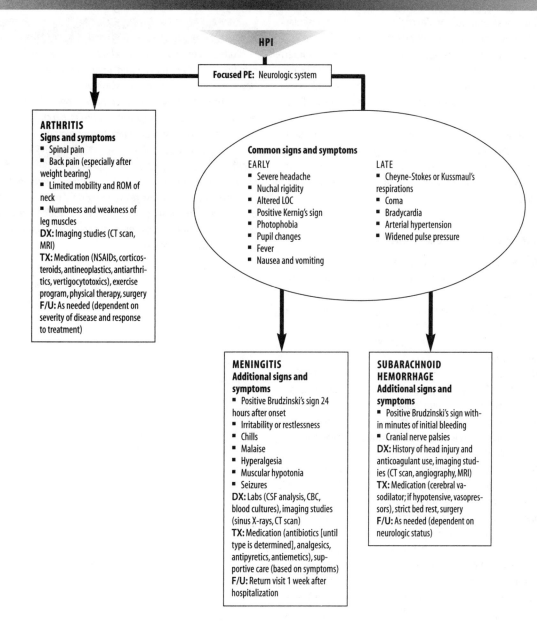

HPI

Focused PE: Neurologic system

ARTHRITIS
Signs and symptoms
- Spinal pain
- Back pain (especially after weight bearing)
- Limited mobility and ROM of neck
- Numbness and weakness of leg muscles

DX: Imaging studies (CT scan, MRI)
TX: Medication (NSAIDs, corticosteroids, antineoplastics, antiarthritics, vertigocytotoxics), exercise program, physical therapy, surgery
F/U: As needed (dependent on severity of disease and response to treatment)

Common signs and symptoms
EARLY
- Severe headache
- Nuchal rigidity
- Altered LOC
- Positive Kernig's sign
- Photophobia
- Pupil changes
- Fever
- Nausea and vomiting

LATE
- Cheyne-Stokes or Kussmaul's respirations
- Coma
- Bradycardia
- Arterial hypertension
- Widened pulse pressure

MENINGITIS
Additional signs and symptoms
- Positive Brudzinski's sign 24 hours after onset
- Irritability or restlessness
- Chills
- Malaise
- Hyperalgesia
- Muscular hypotonia
- Seizures

DX: Labs (CSF analysis, CBC, blood cultures), imaging studies (sinus X-rays, CT scan)
TX: Medication (antibiotics [until type is determined], analgesics, antipyretics, antiemetics), supportive care (based on symptoms)
F/U: Return visit 1 week after hospitalization

SUBARACHNOID HEMORRHAGE
Additional signs and symptoms
- Positive Brudzinski's sign within minutes of initial bleeding
- Cranial nerve palsies

DX: History of head injury and anticoagulant use, imaging studies (CT scan, angiography, MRI)
TX: Medication (cerebral vasodilator; if hypotensive, vasopressors), strict bed rest, surgery
F/U: As needed (dependent on neurologic status)

Bruits

Commonly an indicator of life- or limb-threatening vascular disease, bruits are swishing sounds caused by turbulent blood flow. They're characterized by location, duration, intensity, pitch, and time of onset in the cardiac cycle. Loud bruits produce intense vibration and a palpable thrill. A thrill, however, doesn't provide any further clue to the causative disorder or to its severity.

Bruits are most significant when heard over the abdominal aorta; the renal, carotid, femoral, popliteal, and subclavian arteries; and the thyroid gland. They're also significant when heard consistently despite changes in patient position and when heard during diastole.

History and physical examination

If you detect bruits over the abdominal aorta, check for a pulsating mass or a bluish discoloration around the umbilicus (Cullen's sign). Either of these signs — or severe, tearing pain in the abdomen, flank, or lower back — may signal life-threatening dissection of an aortic aneurysm. Also check peripheral pulses, comparing intensity in the upper extremities versus the lower extremities.

If you suspect dissection, monitor the patient's vital signs, and withhold food and fluids until a definitive diagnosis is made. Watch for signs of hypovolemic shock, such as thirst; hypotension; tachycardia; weak, thready pulse; tachypnea; altered level of consciousness (LOC); mottled knees and elbows; and cool, clammy skin.

If you detect bruits over the thyroid gland, ask the patient if he has a history of hyperthyroidism or signs that suggest it, such as nervousness, tremors, weight loss, palpitations, heat intolerance and, in female patients, amenorrhea. Watch for symptoms of life-threatening thyroid storm, such as tremor, restlessness, diarrhea, abdominal pain, and hepatomegaly.

If you detect carotid artery bruits, be alert for signs and symptoms of a transient ischemic attack, including dizziness, diplopia, slurred speech, flashing lights, and syncope. These findings may indicate an impending stroke. Be sure to evaluate the patient frequently for changes in LOC and muscle function.

If you detect bruits over the femoral, popliteal, or subclavian arteries, watch for signs of decreased or absent peripheral circulation — edema, weakness, and paresthesia. Ask the patient if he has a history of intermittent claudication. Watch for sudden absence of pulse, pallor, or coolness, which may indicate a threat to the affected limb.

If you detect a bruit, be sure to check for further vascular damage and perform a thorough cardiac assessment.

PEDIATRIC POINTERS

- *Bruits are common in young children but are usually of little significance; for example, cranial bruits are normal until age 4. However, certain bruits may be significant.*
- *Because birthmarks often accompany congenital arteriovenous fistulas, carefully auscultate for bruits in a child with port-wine spots or cavernous or diffuse hemangiomas.*

ELDER CARE CUE

Elderly people with atherosclerosis can present with bruits heard over several arteries. Those related to carotid artery stenosis are particularly important because of the high incidence of associated stroke. Close follow-up is mandatory as well as prompt surgical referral when indicated.

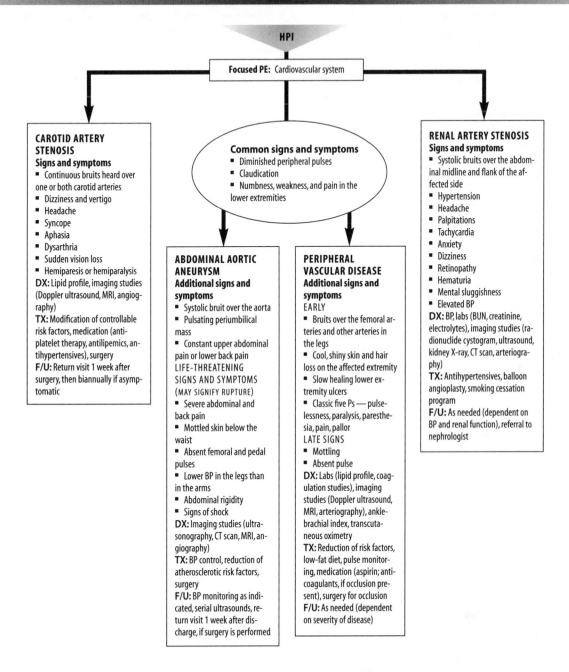

HPI

Focused PE: Cardiovascular system

CAROTID ARTERY STENOSIS
Signs and symptoms
- Continuous bruits heard over one or both carotid arteries
- Dizziness and vertigo
- Headache
- Syncope
- Aphasia
- Dysarthria
- Sudden vision loss
- Hemiparesis or hemiparalysis

DX: Lipid profile, imaging studies (Doppler ultrasound, MRI, angiography)

TX: Modification of controllable risk factors, medication (antiplatelet therapy, antilipemics, antihypertensives), surgery

F/U: Return visit 1 week after surgery, then biannually if asymptomatic

Common signs and symptoms
- Diminished peripheral pulses
- Claudication
- Numbness, weakness, and pain in the lower extremities

ABDOMINAL AORTIC ANEURYSM
Additional signs and symptoms
- Systolic bruit over the aorta
- Pulsating periumbilical mass
- Constant upper abdominal pain or lower back pain

LIFE-THREATENING SIGNS AND SYMPTOMS (MAY SIGNIFY RUPTURE)
- Severe abdominal and back pain
- Mottled skin below the waist
- Absent femoral and pedal pulses
- Lower BP in the legs than in the arms
- Abdominal rigidity
- Signs of shock

DX: Imaging studies (ultrasonography, CT scan, MRI, angiography)

TX: BP control, reduction of atherosclerotic risk factors, surgery

F/U: BP monitoring as indicated, serial ultrasounds, return visit 1 week after discharge, if surgery is performed

PERIPHERAL VASCULAR DISEASE
Additional signs and symptoms
EARLY
- Bruits over the femoral arteries and other arteries in the legs
- Cool, shiny skin and hair loss on the affected extremity
- Slow healing lower extremity ulcers
- Classic five Ps — pulselessness, paralysis, paresthesia, pain, pallor

LATE SIGNS
- Mottling
- Absent pulse

DX: Labs (lipid profile, coagulation studies), imaging studies (Doppler ultrasound, MRI, arteriography), ankle-brachial index, transcutaneous oximetry

TX: Reduction of risk factors, low-fat diet, pulse monitoring, medication (aspirin; anticoagulants, if occlusion present), surgery for occlusion

F/U: As needed (dependent on severity of disease)

RENAL ARTERY STENOSIS
Signs and symptoms
- Systolic bruits over the abdominal midline and flank of the affected side
- Hypertension
- Headache
- Palpitations
- Tachycardia
- Anxiety
- Dizziness
- Retinopathy
- Hematuria
- Mental sluggishness
- Elevated BP

DX: BP, labs (BUN, creatinine, electrolytes), imaging studies (radionuclide cystogram, ultrasound, kidney X-ray, CT scan, arteriography)

TX: Antihypertensives, balloon angioplasty, smoking cessation program

F/U: As needed (dependent on BP and renal function), referral to nephrologist

---

Additional differential diagnoses: abdominal aortic atherosclerosis ▪ anemia ▪ carotid cavernous fistula ▪ peripheral arteriovenous fistula ▪ subclavian steal syndrome ▪ thyrotoxicosis

Butterfly rash

The presence of a butterfly rash is commonly a sign of systemic lupus erythematosus; however, it can also signal dermatologic disorders. Typically, butterfly rash appears in a malar distribution across the nose and cheeks. (See *Recognizing butterfly rash*.) Similar rashes may appear on the neck, scalp, and other areas. Butterfly rash is sometimes mistaken for sunburn because it can be provoked or aggravated by ultraviolet rays, but it has more substance, is more sharply demarcated, and has a thicker feel in relation to surrounding skin.

History and physical examination

Ask the patient when he first noticed the butterfly rash and if he has recently been exposed to the sun. Has he noticed a rash elsewhere on his body? Also ask about recent weight or hair loss. Does he have a family history of lupus? Is he taking hydralazine or procainamide (common causes of drug-induced lupus erythematosus)?

Inspect the rash, noting macules, papules, pustules, and scaling. Is the rash edematous? Are areas of hypopigmentation or hyperpigmentation present? Look for blisters or ulcers in the mouth, and note inflamed lesions. Check for rashes elsewhere on the body.

Rare in pediatric patients, a butterfly rash may occur as part of an infectious disease such as erythema infectiosum, or "slapped cheek syndrome."

Recognizing butterfly rash

In classic butterfly rash, lesions appear on the cheeks and the bridge of the nose, creating a characteristic butterfly pattern. The rash may vary in severity from malar erythema to discoid lesions (plaques).

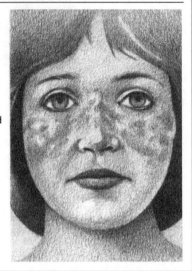

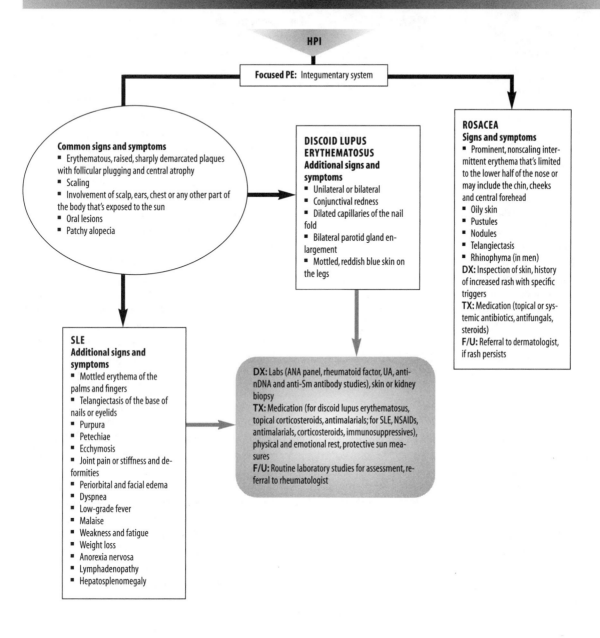

HPI

Focused PE: Integumentary system

Common signs and symptoms
- Erythematous, raised, sharply demarcated plaques with follicular plugging and central atrophy
- Scaling
- Involvement of scalp, ears, chest or any other part of the body that's exposed to the sun
- Oral lesions
- Patchy alopecia

DISCOID LUPUS ERYTHEMATOSUS
Additional signs and symptoms
- Unilateral or bilateral
- Conjunctival redness
- Dilated capillaries of the nail fold
- Bilateral parotid gland enlargement
- Mottled, reddish blue skin on the legs

ROSACEA
Signs and symptoms
- Prominent, nonscaling intermittent erythema that's limited to the lower half of the nose or may include the chin, cheeks and central forehead
- Oily skin
- Pustules
- Nodules
- Telangiectasis
- Rhinophyma (in men)

DX: Inspection of skin, history of increased rash with specific triggers
TX: Medication (topical or systemic antibiotics, antifungals, steroids)
F/U: Referral to dermatologist, if rash persists

SLE
Additional signs and symptoms
- Mottled erythema of the palms and fingers
- Telangiectasis of the base of nails or eyelids
- Purpura
- Petechiae
- Ecchymosis
- Joint pain or stiffness and deformities
- Periorbital and facial edema
- Dyspnea
- Low-grade fever
- Malaise
- Weakness and fatigue
- Weight loss
- Anorexia nervosa
- Lymphadenopathy
- Hepatosplenomegaly

DX: Labs (ANA panel, rheumatoid factor, UA, anti-nDNA and anti-Sm antibody studies), skin or kidney biopsy
TX: Medication (for discoid lupus erythematosus, topical corticosteroids, antimalarials; for SLE, NSAIDs, antimalarials, corticosteroids, immunosuppressives), physical and emotional rest, protective sun measures
F/U: Routine laboratory studies for assessment, referral to rheumatologist

Additional differential diagnoses: polymorphous light eruption ■ seborrheic dermatitis

Other causes: hydralazine ■ procainamide

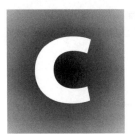

Chest expansion, asymmetrical

Asymmetrical chest expansion is the uneven extension of portions of the chest wall during inspiration. During normal respiration, the thorax uniformly expands upward and outward and then contracts downward and inward. When this process is disrupted, breathing becomes uncoordinated, resulting in asymmetrical chest expansion.

Asymmetrical chest expansion may develop suddenly or gradually and may affect one or both sides of the chest wall. It may occur as delayed expiration (chest lag); as abnormal movement during inspiration (for example, intercostal retractions, paradoxical movement, or chest-abdomen asynchrony); or as unilateral absence of movement. This sign usually results from pleural disorders, such as life-threatening hemothorax or tension pneumothorax. However, it can also result from musculoskeletal or urologic disorders, airway obstruction, or trauma. Regardless of its underlying cause, asymmetrical chest expansion produces rapid and shallow or deep respirations that increase the work of breathing.

History and physical examination

If you don't suspect flail chest, and if the patient isn't experiencing acute respiratory distress, obtain a brief history. Asymmetrical chest expansion commonly results from mechanical airflow obstruction, so find out if the patient is experiencing dyspnea or pain during breathing. If so, does he feel short of breath constantly or intermittently? Does the pain worsen his feeling of breathlessness? Does repositioning, coughing, or any other activity relieve or worsen the patient's dyspnea or pain? Is the pain more noticeable during inspiration or expiration? Can he inhale deeply?

Ask if the patient has a history of pulmonary or systemic illness, such as frequent upper respiratory infections, asthma, tuberculosis, pneumonia, or cancer. Has he had thoracic surgery? (This typically produces asymmetrical chest expansion on the affected side.) Also ask about blunt or penetrating chest trauma, which may have caused pulmonary injury. Obtain an occupational history to find out if the patient may have inhaled toxic fumes or aspirated a toxic substance.

Next, perform a physical examination. Inspect the neck for ecchymosis, swelling, or hematomas. Look for facial swelling. Listen for noisy air movement. These signs may indicate a mediastinal, esophageal, or tracheobronchial injury. Inspect the jugular veins for distention, which may indicate increased intrathoracic pressure as a result of tension pneumothorax. Then gently palpate the trachea for midline positioning. (Deviation of the trachea usually indicates an acute problem requiring immediate intervention.) Examine the posterior chest wall for areas of tenderness or deformity. Palpating the chest wall may indicate fractured ribs or sternum.

To evaluate the extent of asymmetrical chest expansion, place your hands — with fingers together and thumbs abducted toward the spine — flat on both sections of the lower posterior chest wall. Position your thumbs at the 10th rib, and grasp the lateral rib cage with your hands. As the patient inhales, note the uneven separation of your thumbs and gauge the distance between them. Then repeat this technique on the upper posterior chest wall. Next, use the ulnar surface of your hand to palpate for vocal or tactile fremitus on both sides of the chest.

To check for vocal fremitus, ask the patient to repeat "99" as you proceed. Note any asymmetrical vibrations and areas of enhanced, diminished, or absent fremitus. Then percuss and auscultate to detect air and fluid in the lungs and pleural spaces. Finally, auscultate all lung fields for normal and adventitious breath sounds. Examine the patient's anterior chest wall, using the same assessment techniques.

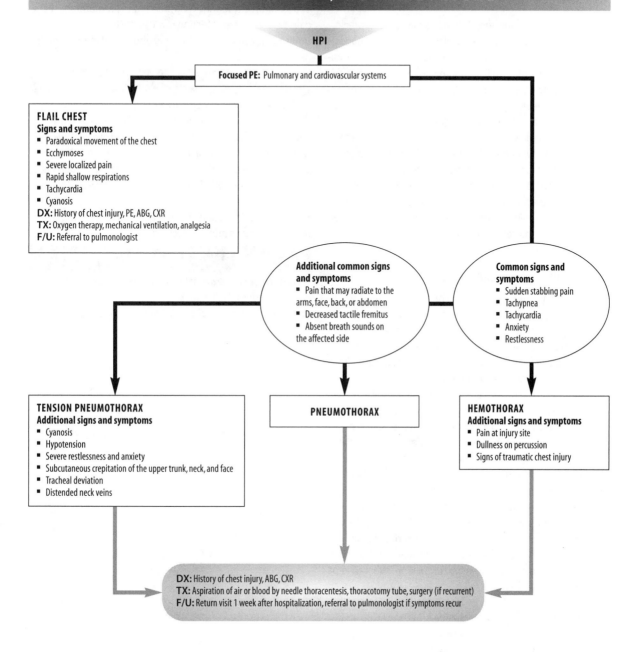

HPI

Focused PE: Pulmonary and cardiovascular systems

FLAIL CHEST
Signs and symptoms
- Paradoxical movement of the chest
- Ecchymoses
- Severe localized pain
- Rapid shallow respirations
- Tachycardia
- Cyanosis

DX: History of chest injury, PE, ABG, CXR
TX: Oxygen therapy, mechanical ventilation, analgesia
F/U: Referral to pulmonologist

Additional common signs and symptoms
- Pain that may radiate to the arms, face, back, or abdomen
- Decreased tactile fremitus
- Absent breath sounds on the affected side

Common signs and symptoms
- Sudden stabbing pain
- Tachypnea
- Tachycardia
- Anxiety
- Restlessness

TENSION PNEUMOTHORAX
Additional signs and symptoms
- Cyanosis
- Hypotension
- Severe restlessness and anxiety
- Subcutaneous crepitation of the upper trunk, neck, and face
- Tracheal deviation
- Distended neck veins

PNEUMOTHORAX

HEMOTHORAX
Additional signs and symptoms
- Pain at injury site
- Dullness on percussion
- Signs of traumatic chest injury

DX: History of chest injury, ABG, CXR
TX: Aspiration of air or blood by needle thoracentesis, thoracotomy tube, surgery (if recurrent)
F/U: Return visit 1 week after hospitalization, referral to pulmonologist if symptoms recur

Additional differential diagnoses: bronchial obstruction ▪ kyphoscoliosis ▪ myasthenia gravis ▪ phrenic nerve dysfunction ▪ pleural effusion ▪ pneumonia ▪ poliomyelitis ▪ pulmonary embolism

Other causes: pneumonectomy ▪ surgery ▪ intubation of a mainstem bronchus

Chest pain

Chest pain usually results from disorders that affect thoracic or abdominal organs — the heart, pleurae, lungs, esophagus, rib cage, gallbladder, pancreas, or stomach. An important indicator of several acute and life-threatening cardiopulmonary and GI disorders, chest pain can also result from musculoskeletal and hematologic disorders, anxiety, and drug therapy.

Chest pain can arise suddenly or gradually, and its cause may be difficult to ascertain initially. The pain can radiate to the arms, neck, jaw, or back. It can be steady or intermittent, mild or acute. It can range in character from a sharp shooting sensation to a dull, achy pain, a feeling of heaviness, a feeling of fullness, or even indigestion. It can occur at rest or be provoked or aggravated by stress, anxiety, physical exertion, deep breathing, or eating certain foods.

History and physical examination

Ask the patient when his chest pain began. Did it develop suddenly or gradually? Is it more severe or frequent now than when it first started? Does anything relieve the pain? Ask the patient about associated symptoms. Sudden, severe chest pain requires prompt evaluation and treatment because it may herald a life-threatening disorder.

If the chest pain isn't severe, proceed with the history. Ask if the patient feels diffuse pain or can point to the painful area. Sometimes a patient won't perceive the sensation he's feeling as pain, so ask whether he has any discomfort radiating to his neck, jaw, arms, or back. If he does, ask him to describe it. Is it a dull, aching, pressurelike sensation? A sharp, stabbing, knifelike pain? Does he feel it on the surface or deep inside? Find out whether it's constant or intermittent. If it's intermittent, how long does it last? Ask if movement, exertion, breathing, position changes, or eating certain foods worsens or helps relieve the pain. Does he have any belching? Does anything in particular seem to bring it on? What time of day does the pain occur?

Review the patient's history for cardiac or pulmonary disease, chest trauma, psychiatric disorders, GI disease, or sickle cell anemia. Find out what medications he's taking, if any, and ask about recent dosage or schedule changes. Ask about a history of smoking and about cholesterol levels. Assess family history for hypertension, coronary artery disease, myocardial infarction, or diabetes mellitus.

Take the patient's vital signs, noting tachypnea, fever, tachycardia, pulsus paradoxus, and hypertension or hypotension. Also look for jugular vein distention and peripheral edema. Observe the patient's breathing pattern, and inspect his chest for asymmetrical expansion. Auscultate his lungs for pleural friction rub, crackles, rhonchi, wheezing, or diminished or absent breath sounds. Next, auscultate for murmurs, clicks, gallops, or pericardial friction rub. Palpate for lifts, heaves, thrills, gallops, tactile fremitus, and abdominal mass or tenderness.

PEDIATRIC POINTERS

- *Even children old enough to talk may have difficulty describing chest pain, so be alert for nonverbal clues, such as restlessness, facial grimaces, or holding of the painful area. Ask the child to first point to the painful area and then to point to where the pain goes. Determine the pain's severity by asking the parents if the pain interferes with the child's normal activities and behavior.*
- *A child may complain of chest pain in an attempt to get attention or to avoid attending school.*

ELDER CARE CUE

Because older people are at higher risk for developing life-threatening conditions, such as MI, angina, and aortic dissection, you must carefully evaluate chest pain in an elderly patient.

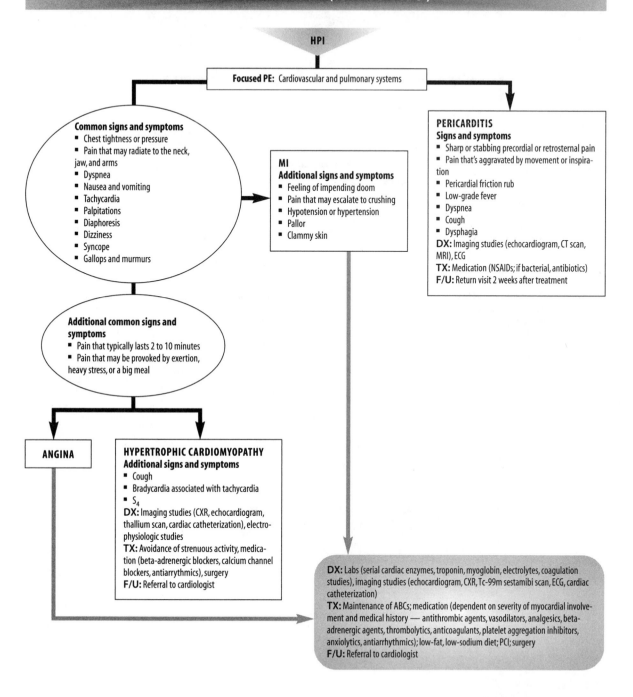

HPI

Focused PE: Cardiovascular and pulmonary systems

Common signs and symptoms
- Chest tightness or pressure
- Pain that may radiate to the neck, jaw, and arms
- Dyspnea
- Nausea and vomiting
- Tachycardia
- Palpitations
- Diaphoresis
- Dizziness
- Syncope
- Gallops and murmurs

MI
Additional signs and symptoms
- Feeling of impending doom
- Pain that may escalate to crushing
- Hypotension or hypertension
- Pallor
- Clammy skin

PERICARDITIS
Signs and symptoms
- Sharp or stabbing precordial or retrosternal pain
- Pain that's aggravated by movement or inspiration
- Pericardial friction rub
- Low-grade fever
- Dyspnea
- Cough
- Dysphagia
DX: Imaging studies (echocardiogram, CT scan, MRI), ECG
TX: Medication (NSAIDs; if bacterial, antibiotics)
F/U: Return visit 2 weeks after treatment

Additional common signs and symptoms
- Pain that typically lasts 2 to 10 minutes
- Pain that may be provoked by exertion, heavy stress, or a big meal

ANGINA

HYPERTROPHIC CARDIOMYOPATHY
Additional signs and symptoms
- Cough
- Bradycardia associated with tachycardia
- S_4
DX: Imaging studies (CXR, echocardiogram, thallium scan, cardiac catheterization), electro-physiologic studies
TX: Avoidance of strenuous activity, medication (beta-adrenergic blockers, calcium channel blockers, antiarrythmics), surgery
F/U: Referral to cardiologist

DX: Labs (serial cardiac enzymes, troponin, myoglobin, electrolytes, coagulation studies), imaging studies (echocardiogram, CXR, Tc-99m sestamibi scan, ECG, cardiac catheterization)
TX: Maintenance of ABCs; medication (dependent on severity of myocardial involvement and medical history — antithrombic agents, vasodilators, analgesics, beta-adrenergic agents, thrombolytics, anticoagulants, platelet aggregation inhibitors, anxiolytics, antiarrhythmics); low-fat, low-sodium diet; PCI; surgery
F/U: Referral to cardiologist

Additional differential diagnoses: aortic aneurysm (dissecting) ▪ costochondritis ▪ mediastinitis

Other causes: beta-adrenergic blockers (abrupt withdrawal can cause rebound angina in patients with coronary heart disease) ▪ Chinese restaurant syndrome

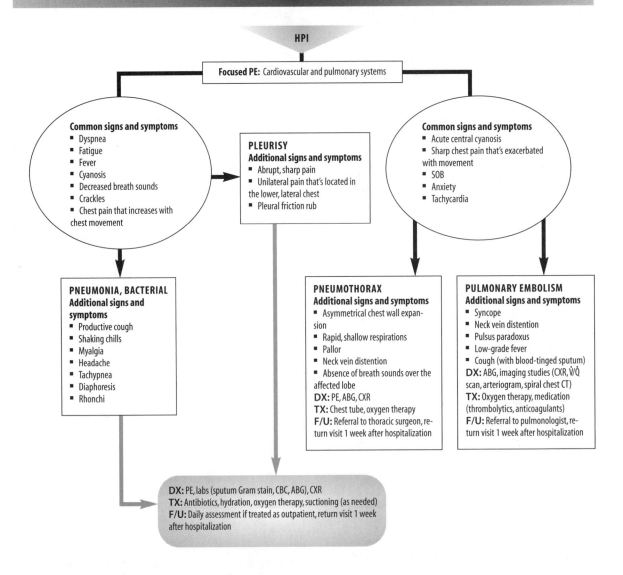

HPI

Focused PE: Cardiovascular and pulmonary systems

Common signs and symptoms
- Dyspnea
- Fatigue
- Fever
- Cyanosis
- Decreased breath sounds
- Crackles
- Chest pain that increases with chest movement

PLEURISY
Additional signs and symptoms
- Abrupt, sharp pain
- Unilateral pain that's located in the lower, lateral chest
- Pleural friction rub

Common signs and symptoms
- Acute central cyanosis
- Sharp chest pain that's exacerbated with movement
- SOB
- Anxiety
- Tachycardia

PNEUMONIA, BACTERIAL
Additional signs and symptoms
- Productive cough
- Shaking chills
- Myalgia
- Headache
- Tachypnea
- Diaphoresis
- Rhonchi

PNEUMOTHORAX
Additional signs and symptoms
- Asymmetrical chest wall expansion
- Rapid, shallow respirations
- Pallor
- Neck vein distention
- Absence of breath sounds over the affected lobe
DX: PE, ABG, CXR
TX: Chest tube, oxygen therapy
F/U: Referral to thoracic surgeon, return visit 1 week after hospitalization

PULMONARY EMBOLISM
Additional signs and symptoms
- Syncope
- Neck vein distention
- Pulsus paradoxus
- Low-grade fever
- Cough (with blood-tinged sputum)
DX: ABG, imaging studies (CXR, V̇/Q̇ scan, arteriogram, spiral chest CT)
TX: Oxygen therapy, medication (thrombolytics, anticoagulants)
F/U: Referral to pulmonologist, return visit 1 week after hospitalization

DX: PE, labs (sputum Gram stain, CBC, ABG), CXR
TX: Antibiotics, hydration, oxygen therapy, suctioning (as needed)
F/U: Daily assessment if treated as outpatient, return visit 1 week after hospitalization

Additional differential diagnoses: blastomycosis ▪ bronchitis ▪ coccidioidomycosis ▪ interstitial lung disease ▪ lung abscess ▪ lung cancer ▪ pulmonary actinomycosis ▪ pulmonary hypertension ▪ tuberculosis

HPI

Focused PE: Mental health, musculoskeletal and GI systems

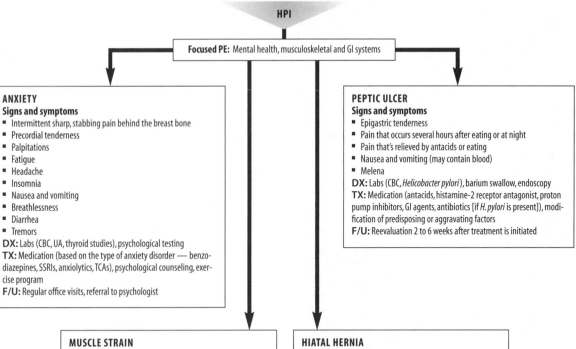

ANXIETY
Signs and symptoms
- Intermittent sharp, stabbing pain behind the breast bone
- Precordial tenderness
- Palpitations
- Fatigue
- Headache
- Insomnia
- Nausea and vomiting
- Breathlessness
- Diarrhea
- Tremors

DX: Labs (CBC, UA, thyroid studies), psychological testing
TX: Medication (based on the type of anxiety disorder — benzo-diazepines, SSRIs, anxiolytics, TCAs), psychological counseling, exercise program
F/U: Regular office visits, referral to psychologist

PEPTIC ULCER
Signs and symptoms
- Epigastric tenderness
- Pain that occurs several hours after eating or at night
- Pain that's relieved by antacids or eating
- Nausea and vomiting (may contain blood)
- Melena

DX: Labs (CBC, *Helicobacter pylori*), barium swallow, endoscopy
TX: Medication (antacids, histamine-2 receptor antagonist, proton pump inhibitors, GI agents, antibiotics [if *H. pylori* is present]), modification of predisposing or aggravating factors
F/U: Reevaluation 2 to 6 weeks after treatment is initiated

MUSCLE STRAIN
Signs and symptoms
- Superficial or continuous ache or "pulling" sensation that's located in the chest
- Pain that's aggravated by lifting, pulling, or pushing heavy objects
- Pain that increases with palpation
ACUTE
- Fatigue
- Swelling of the affected area
- Weakness

DX: History of excessive muscle use, PE, ECG
TX: NSAIDs, rest or avoidance of increased muscle use
F/U: Reevaluation in 2 weeks (if pain persists or increases)

HIATAL HERNIA
Signs and symptoms
- Chest pain or pressure after meals
- Dysphagia
- Belching
- Hiccups

DX: Labs (CBC, cardiac enzymes, LFT, amylase, lipase), imaging studies (CXR, barium swallow), ECG, endoscopy
TX: Antacids, diet and activity modification, surgery (rare)
F/U: Reevaluation as needed (based on symptoms and lifestyle modifications)

Additional differential diagnoses: esophageal spasm ▪ GERD ▪ herpes zoster ▪ norcardiosis ▪ pancreatitis ▪ rib fracture ▪ sickle cell crisis ▪ thoracic outlet syndrome

Cheyne-Stokes respirations

The most common pattern of periodic breathing, Cheyne-Stokes respirations are characterized by a waxing and waning period of hyperpnea that alternates with a shorter period of apnea. This pattern can occur normally in patients with heart or lung disease. It usually indicates increased intracranial pressure (ICP) from a deep cerebral or brain stem lesion or a metabolic disturbance in the brain.

Cheyne-Stokes respirations may indicate a major change in the patient's condition — usually for the worse. For example, in a patient who has had head trauma or brain surgery, Cheyne-Stokes respirations may signal increasing ICP.

History and physical examination

If you detect Cheyne-Stokes respirations in a patient with a history of head trauma, recent brain surgery, or another brain insult, quickly take his vital signs. Keep his head elevated 30 degrees, and perform a rapid neurologic examination to obtain baseline data. Reevaluate the patient's neurologic status frequently. If ICP continues to rise, you'll detect changes in the patient's level of consciousness, pupillary reactions, and ability to move his extremities.

Time the periods of hyperpnea and apnea for 3 or 4 minutes to evaluate respirations and to obtain baseline data. Be alert for prolonged periods of apnea. Frequently check blood pressure; also check skin color to detect signs of hypoxemia. Maintain airway patency and institute emergency measures, if necessary.

If the patient's condition permits, obtain a brief history. Ask especially about drug use — large doses of narcotics, hypnotics, or barbiturates can precipitate Cheyne-Stokes respirations.

PEDIATRIC POINTER	

Cheyne-Stokes respirations rarely occur in children, except during late-stage heart failure.

ELDER CARE CUE	

Subtle evidence of Cheyne-Stokes respirations can occur normally in elderly patients during sleep.

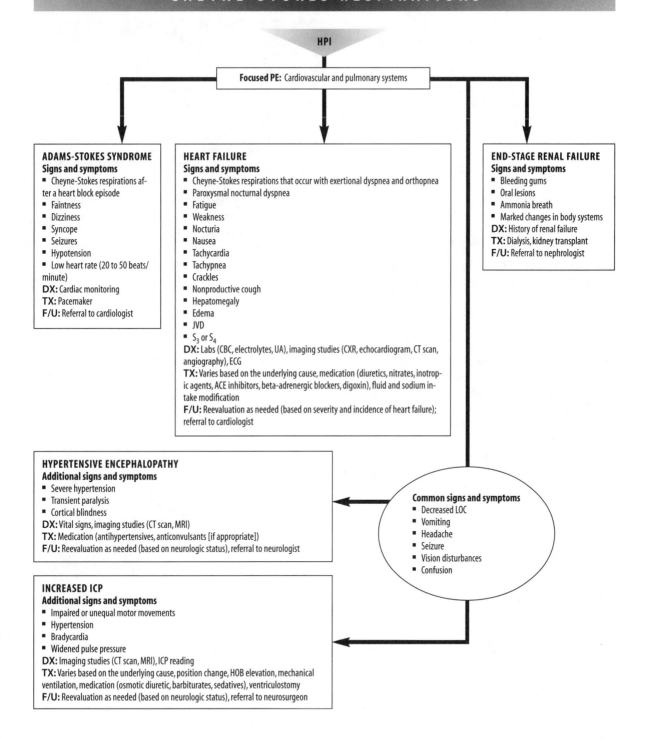

HPI

Focused PE: Cardiovascular and pulmonary systems

ADAMS-STOKES SYNDROME
Signs and symptoms
- Cheyne-Stokes respirations after a heart block episode
- Faintness
- Dizziness
- Syncope
- Seizures
- Hypotension
- Low heart rate (20 to 50 beats/minute)

DX: Cardiac monitoring
TX: Pacemaker
F/U: Referral to cardiologist

HEART FAILURE
Signs and symptoms
- Cheyne-Stokes respirations that occur with exertional dyspnea and orthopnea
- Paroxysmal nocturnal dyspnea
- Fatigue
- Weakness
- Nocturia
- Nausea
- Tachycardia
- Tachypnea
- Crackles
- Nonproductive cough
- Hepatomegaly
- Edema
- JVD
- S_3 or S_4

DX: Labs (CBC, electrolytes, UA), imaging studies (CXR, echocardiogram, CT scan, angiography), ECG
TX: Varies based on the underlying cause, medication (diuretics, nitrates, inotropic agents, ACE inhibitors, beta-adrenergic blockers, digoxin), fluid and sodium intake modification
F/U: Reevaluation as needed (based on severity and incidence of heart failure); referral to cardiologist

END-STAGE RENAL FAILURE
Signs and symptoms
- Bleeding gums
- Oral lesions
- Ammonia breath
- Marked changes in body systems

DX: History of renal failure
TX: Dialysis, kidney transplant
F/U: Referral to nephrologist

HYPERTENSIVE ENCEPHALOPATHY
Additional signs and symptoms
- Severe hypertension
- Transient paralysis
- Cortical blindness

DX: Vital signs, imaging studies (CT scan, MRI)
TX: Medication (antihypertensives, anticonvulsants [if appropriate])
F/U: Reevaluation as needed (based on neurologic status), referral to neurologist

Common signs and symptoms
- Decreased LOC
- Vomiting
- Headache
- Seizure
- Vision disturbances
- Confusion

INCREASED ICP
Additional signs and symptoms
- Impaired or unequal motor movements
- Hypertension
- Bradycardia
- Widened pulse pressure

DX: Imaging studies (CT scan, MRI), ICP reading
TX: Varies based on the underlying cause, position change, HOB elevation, mechanical ventilation, medication (osmotic diuretic, barbiturates, sedatives), ventriculostomy
F/U: Reevaluation as needed (based on neurologic status), referral to neurosurgeon

Other causes: large doses of hypnotics, narcotics, or barbiturates

Chills

Chills (rigors) are extreme, involuntary muscle contractions with characteristic paroxysms of violent shivering and teeth chattering. Commonly accompanied by fever, chills tend to arise suddenly, usually heralding the onset of infection. Certain diseases, such as pneumococcal pneumonia, produce only a single, shaking chill. Other diseases, such as malaria, produce intermittent chills with recurring high fever. Still others produce continuous chills for up to 1 hour, precipitating a high fever.

Chills can also result from lymphomas, transfusion reactions, and certain drugs. Chills without fever occur as a normal response to exposure to cold. (See *Rare causes of chills*.)

History and physical examination

Ask the patient when the chills began and if they're continuous or intermittent. Because fever commonly accompanies or follows chills, take his temperature to obtain a baseline reading. Then check his temperature often to monitor fluctuations and to determine his temperature curve. Typically, a localized infection produces sudden onset of shaking chills, sweats, and high fever. A systemic infection produces intermittent chills with recurring episodes of high fever or continuous chills that may last up to 1 hour and precipitate a high fever.

Ask about related signs and symptoms, such as headache, dysuria, diarrhea, confusion, chest pain, abdominal pain, cough, sore throat, or nausea. Does the patient have any known allergies, an infection, or a recent history of an infectious disorder? Find out what medications he's taking and if any drug has improved or worsened his symptoms. Has he received any treatment that may predispose him to an infection (such as chemotherapy)? Ask about recent exposure to farm animals, guinea pigs, hamsters, dogs, and such birds as pigeons, parrots, and parakeets. Also ask about recent insect or animal bites, travel to foreign countries, and contact with a person who has an active infection.

Rare causes of chills

Chills can result from disorders that rarely occur in the United States but may be fairly common worldwide. So, remember to ask about recent foreign travel when you obtain a patient's history. Keep in mind this partial list of rare disorders that produce chills:

- brucellosis (undulant fever)
- dengue (breakbone fever)
- epidemic typhus (louse-borne typhus)
- leptospirosis
- lymphocytic choriomeningitis
- plague
- pulmonary tularemia
- rat bite fever
- relapsing fever.

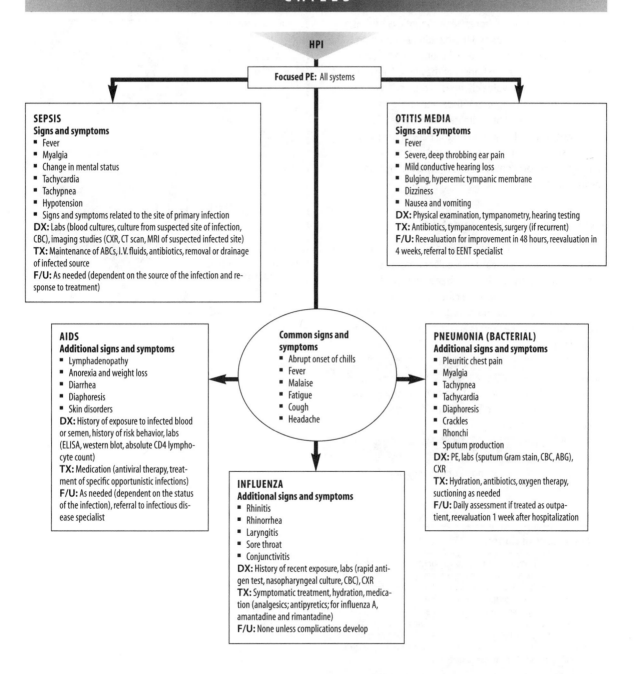

HPI

Focused PE: All systems

SEPSIS
Signs and symptoms
- Fever
- Myalgia
- Change in mental status
- Tachycardia
- Tachypnea
- Hypotension
- Signs and symptoms related to the site of primary infection

DX: Labs (blood cultures, culture from suspected site of infection, CBC), imaging studies (CXR, CT scan, MRI of suspected infected site)
TX: Maintenance of ABCs, I.V. fluids, antibiotics, removal or drainage of infected source
F/U: As needed (dependent on the source of the infection and response to treatment)

OTITIS MEDIA
Signs and symptoms
- Fever
- Severe, deep throbbing ear pain
- Mild conductive hearing loss
- Bulging, hyperemic tympanic membrane
- Dizziness
- Nausea and vomiting

DX: Physical examination, tympanometry, hearing testing
TX: Antibiotics, tympanocentesis, surgery (if recurrent)
F/U: Reevaluation for improvement in 48 hours, reevaluation in 4 weeks, referral to EENT specialist

AIDS
Additional signs and symptoms
- Lymphadenopathy
- Anorexia and weight loss
- Diarrhea
- Diaphoresis
- Skin disorders

DX: History of exposure to infected blood or semen, history of risk behavior, labs (ELISA, western blot, absolute CD4 lymphocyte count)
TX: Medication (antiviral therapy, treatment of specific opportunistic infections)
F/U: As needed (dependent on the status of the infection), referral to infectious disease specialist

Common signs and symptoms
- Abrupt onset of chills
- Fever
- Malaise
- Fatigue
- Cough
- Headache

PNEUMONIA (BACTERIAL)
Additional signs and symptoms
- Pleuritic chest pain
- Myalgia
- Tachypnea
- Tachycardia
- Diaphoresis
- Crackles
- Rhonchi
- Sputum production

DX: PE, labs (sputum Gram stain, CBC, ABG), CXR
TX: Hydration, antibiotics, oxygen therapy, suctioning as needed
F/U: Daily assessment if treated as outpatient, reevaluation 1 week after hospitalization

INFLUENZA
Additional signs and symptoms
- Rhinitis
- Rhinorrhea
- Laryngitis
- Sore throat
- Conjunctivitis

DX: History of recent exposure, labs (rapid antigen test, nasopharyngeal culture, CBC), CXR
TX: Symptomatic treatment, hydration, medication (analgesics; antipyretics; for influenza A, amantadine and rimantadine)
F/U: None unless complications develop

Additional differential diagnoses: bacteremia ▪ cholangitis (gram-negative) ▪ hemolytic anemia ▪ hepatic abscess ▪ Hodgkin's disease ▪ infective endocarditis ▪ lung abscess ▪ Lyme disease ▪ lymphangitis ▪ lymphogranuloma venereum ▪ malaria ▪ miliary tuberculosis ▪ PID ▪ peritonitis ▪ puerperal or postabortal sepsis ▪ pyelonephritis ▪ renal abscess ▪ Rocky Mountain spotted fever ▪ septic arthritis ▪ sinusitis ▪ snake bite

---

Other causes: amphotericin B ▪ hemolytic reaction ▪ infection at I.V. insertion site ▪ I.V. bleomycin ▪ I.V. therapy ▪ nonhemolytic febrile reaction ▪ oral antipyretics ▪ phenytoin ▪ transfusion reaction

Clubbing

A nonspecific sign of pulmonary and cyanotic cardiovascular disorders, cirrhosis, colitis and thyroid disease, clubbing is the painless, usually bilateral increase in soft tissue around the terminal phalanges of the fingers or toes. (See *Rare causes of clubbing*.) It doesn't involve changes in the underlying bone. In early clubbing, the normal 160-degree angle between the nail and the nail base approximates 180 degrees. As clubbing progresses, this angle widens and the base of the nail becomes visibly swollen. In late clubbing, the angle where the nail meets the now-convex nail base extends more than halfway up the nail.

History and physical examination

You'll probably detect clubbing while evaluating other signs of known pulmonary or cardiovascular disease. Ask about a history of alcohol use or thyroid disease. Review the patient's current treatment plan because clubbing may resolve with correction of the underlying disorder. Also, evaluate the extent of clubbing in the fingers and toes. (See *Evaluating clubbed fingers*.)

> **PEDIATRIC POINTER**
>
> *In children, clubbing occurs most commonly in cyanotic congenital heart disease and cystic fibrosis. Surgical correction of heart defects may reverse clubbing.*

> **ELDER CARE CUE**
>
> *Arthritic deformities of the fingers or toes may disguise the presence of clubbing.*

Rare causes of clubbing

Clubbing is typically a sign of pulmonary or cardiovascular disease, but it can also result from certain hepatic and GI disorders, such as cirrhosis, Crohn's disease, and ulcerative colitis. Clubbing occurs only rarely in these disorders, however, so first check for more common signs and symptoms. For example, a patient with cirrhosis usually experiences right-upper-quadrant pain and hepatomegaly. A patient with Crohn's disease typically has abdominal cramping and tenderness. A patient with ulcerative colitis may develop diffuse abdominal pain and blood-streaked diarrhea.

Evaluating clubbed fingers

To quickly examine a patient's fingers for early clubbing, gently palpate the bases of his nails. Normally, they feel firm; however, in early clubbing, nail bases feel springy when palpated. To evaluate late clubbing, have the patient place the first phalanges of the forefingers together, as shown. Normal nail bases are concave and create a small space when the first phalanges are opposed (as shown above right).

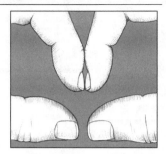

In late clubbing, however, the now-convex nail bases can touch without leaving a space (as shown below right).

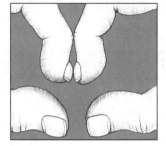

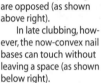

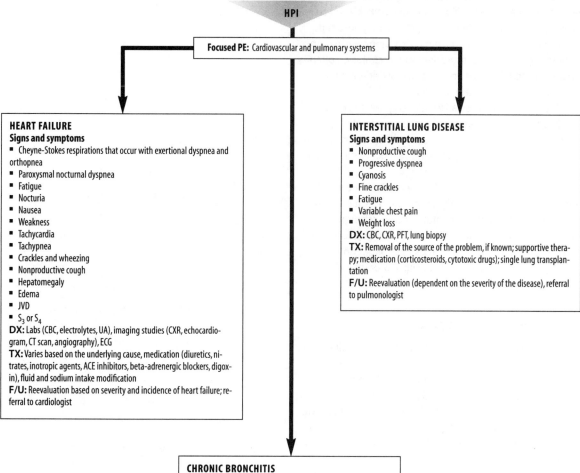

HPI

Focused PE: Cardiovascular and pulmonary systems

HEART FAILURE
Signs and symptoms
- Cheyne-Stokes respirations that occur with exertional dyspnea and orthopnea
- Paroxysmal nocturnal dyspnea
- Fatigue
- Nocturia
- Nausea
- Weakness
- Tachycardia
- Tachypnea
- Crackles and wheezing
- Nonproductive cough
- Hepatomegaly
- Edema
- JVD
- S_3 or S_4

DX: Labs (CBC, electrolytes, UA), imaging studies (CXR, echocardiogram, CT scan, angiography), ECG
TX: Varies based on the underlying cause, medication (diuretics, nitrates, inotropic agents, ACE inhibitors, beta-adrenergic blockers, digoxin), fluid and sodium intake modification
F/U: Reevaluation based on severity and incidence of heart failure; referral to cardiologist

INTERSTITIAL LUNG DISEASE
Signs and symptoms
- Nonproductive cough
- Progressive dyspnea
- Cyanosis
- Fine crackles
- Fatigue
- Variable chest pain
- Weight loss

DX: CBC, CXR, PFT, lung biopsy
TX: Removal of the source of the problem, if known; supportive therapy; medication (corticosteroids, cytotoxic drugs); single lung transplantation
F/U: Reevaluation (dependent on the severity of the disease), referral to pulmonologist

CHRONIC BRONCHITIS
Signs and symptoms
- Barrel chest
- Cough
- Dyspnea
- Tachypnea
- Cyanosis
- Pursed-lip breathing
- Anorexia
- Malaise
- Diminished breath sounds
- Use of accessory muscles of respiration

DX: Labs (CBC, ABG), CXR, PFT
TX: Smoking cessation program, medication (bronchodilators, sympathomimetics, anticholinergics, corticosteroids), surgery (in selected cases)
F/U: Reevaluation once per month if severe, biannually if stable

---

Additional differential diagnoses: bronchiectasis ▪ emphysema ▪ endocarditis ▪ lung abscess ▪ lung and pleural cancer

Confusion

An umbrella term for puzzling or inappropriate behavior or responses, *confusion* is the inability to think quickly and coherently. Depending on its cause, confusion may arise suddenly or gradually and may be temporary or irreversible. Aggravated by stress and sensory deprivation, confusion often occurs in hospitalized patients — especially elderly patients, in whom it may be mistaken for senility.

When severe confusion arises suddenly and the patient also has hallucinations and psychomotor hyperactivity, his condition is classified as *delirium*. Long-term, progressive confusion with deterioration of all cognitive functions is classified as *dementia*.

Confusion can result from a fluid and electrolyte imbalance or hypoxemia due to pulmonary disorders. It can also have a metabolic, neurologic, cardiovascular, cerebrovascular, or nutritional origin or can result from a severe systemic infection or the effects of toxins, drugs, or alcohol. Confusion may signal worsening of an underlying and, perhaps, irreversible disease.

History and physical examination

When you take the patient's history, ask him to describe what's bothering him. He may not report confusion as his chief complaint but instead may complain of memory loss, persistent apprehension, or inability to concentrate. He may be unable to respond logically to direct questions. Check with a family member or friend about onset and frequency. Find out if the patient has a history of head trauma or a cardiopulmonary, metabolic, cerebrovascular, or neurologic disorder. What medication is he taking, if any? Ask about changes in eating or sleeping habits and in drug or alcohol use.

Perform an assessment to determine the presence of systemic disorders. Check vital signs and assess for changes in blood pressure, temperature, and pulse.

Next, perform a neurologic assessment to establish the patient's level of consciousness. Also perform a Mini–Mental Status Examination.

PEDIATRIC POINTERS

- *Confusion can't be determined in infants and young children.*
- *Older children with acute febrile illnesses commonly experience transient delirium or acute confusion.*

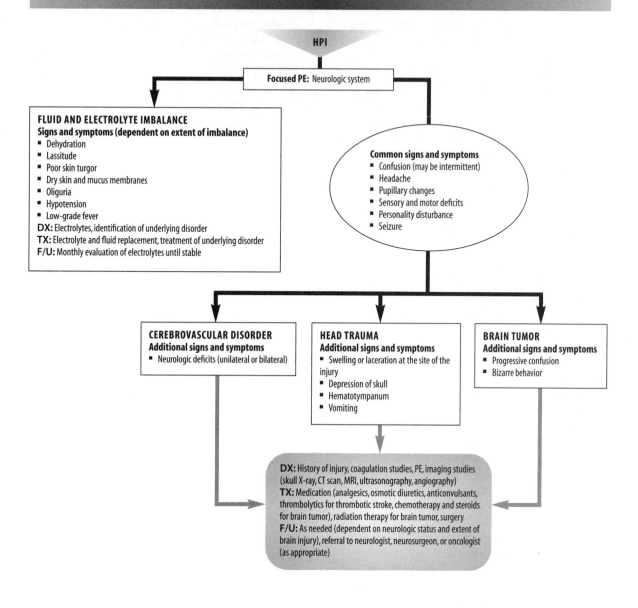

HPI

Focused PE: Neurologic system

FLUID AND ELECTROLYTE IMBALANCE
Signs and symptoms (dependent on extent of imbalance)
- Dehydration
- Lassitude
- Poor skin turgor
- Dry skin and mucus membranes
- Oliguria
- Hypotension
- Low-grade fever

DX: Electrolytes, identification of underlying disorder
TX: Electrolyte and fluid replacement, treatment of underlying disorder
F/U: Monthly evaluation of electrolytes until stable

Common signs and symptoms
- Confusion (may be intermittent)
- Headache
- Pupillary changes
- Sensory and motor deficits
- Personality disturbance
- Seizure

CEREBROVASCULAR DISORDER
Additional signs and symptoms
- Neurologic deficits (unilateral or bilateral)

HEAD TRAUMA
Additional signs and symptoms
- Swelling or laceration at the site of the injury
- Depression of skull
- Hematotympanum
- Vomiting

BRAIN TUMOR
Additional signs and symptoms
- Progressive confusion
- Bizarre behavior

DX: History of injury, coagulation studies, PE, imaging studies (skull X-ray, CT scan, MRI, ultrasonography, angiography)
TX: Medication (analgesics, osmotic diuretics, anticonvulsants, thrombolytics for thrombotic stroke, chemotherapy and steroids for brain tumor), radiation therapy for brain tumor, surgery
F/U: As needed (dependent on neurologic status and extent of brain injury), referral to neurologist, neurosurgeon, or oncologist (as appropriate)

Additional differential diagnoses: decreased cerebral perfusion ▪ heatstroke ▪ heavy metal poisoning ▪ hypothermia ▪ hypoxemia ▪ metabolic encephalapathy ▪ nutritional deficiencies ▪ seizure disorders ▪ thyroid hormone disorders

Other causes: alcohol intoxication ▪ alcohol withdrawal ▪ drugs ▪ herbal medicines

Conjunctival injection

A common ocular sign associated with inflammation, conjunctival injection is nonuniform redness of the conjunctiva from hyperemia. This redness can be diffuse, localized, or peripheral, or it may encircle a clear cornea.

Conjunctival injection usually results from bacterial or viral conjunctivitis, but it can also signal a severe ocular disorder that, if untreated, may lead to permanent blindness. In particular, conjunctival injection is an early sign of trachoma, a leading cause of blindness in Third World countries and among Native Americans living in the southwestern United States.

Conjunctival injection can also result from minor eye irritation due to inadequate sleep, overuse of contact lenses, environmental irritants, and excessive eye rubbing.

History and physical examination

If the patient with conjunctival injection reports a chemical splash to the eye, quickly irrigate the eye with copious amounts of normal saline solution. (Remember to remove contact lenses first.) Evert the lids and wipe the fornices with a cotton-tipped applicator to remove any foreign body particles and as much of the chemical as possible.

When you take the patient's history, always ask if he has any associated pain. If so, when did the pain begin and where is it located? Is it constant or intermittent? Also ask about itching, burning, photophobia, blurred vision, halo vision, excessive tearing, or a foreign body sensation in the eye. Does the patient have a history of eye disease, allergies, or trauma? If he has suffered ocular trauma, avoid touching the affected eye. Test his visual acuity and intraocular pressure (IOP) only if his eyelids can be opened without applying pressure. Place a metal shield over the affected eye to protect it, if necessary.

If the patient's condition permits, examine the affected eye. First, determine the location and severity of conjunctival injection. Is it circumoral or localized? Peripheral or diffuse? Note any conjunctival or lid edema, ocular deviation, conjunctival follicles, ptosis, or exophthalmos. Also note the type and amount of any discharge.

Test the patient's visual acuity to establish a baseline. Note if the patient has had vision changes. Is his vision blurred or his visual acuity markedly decreased? Next, test pupillary reaction to light.

Perform IOP measurements. To gauge increased IOP without a tonometer, gently place your index finger over the closed eyelid; if the globe feels rock-hard, IOP is elevated.

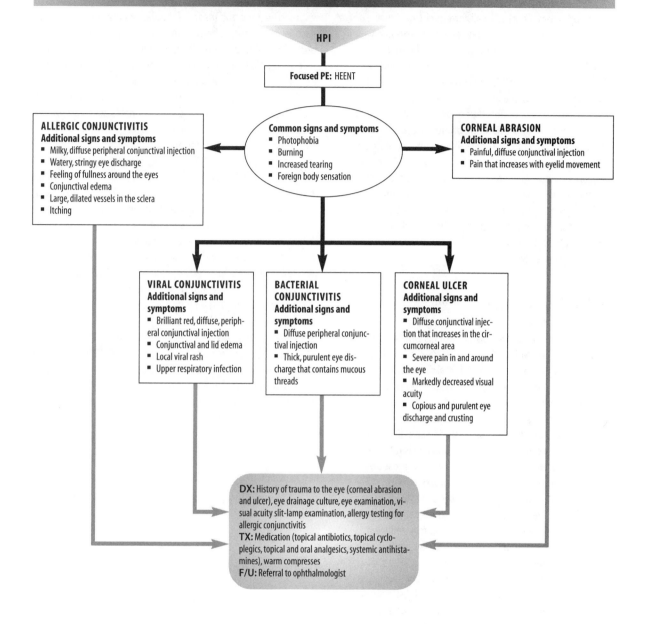

HPI

Focused PE: HEENT

Common signs and symptoms
- Photophobia
- Burning
- Increased tearing
- Foreign body sensation

ALLERGIC CONJUNCTIVITIS
Additional signs and symptoms
- Milky, diffuse peripheral conjunctival injection
- Watery, stringy eye discharge
- Feeling of fullness around the eyes
- Conjunctival edema
- Large, dilated vessels in the sclera
- Itching

CORNEAL ABRASION
Additional signs and symptoms
- Painful, diffuse conjunctival injection
- Pain that increases with eyelid movement

VIRAL CONJUNCTIVITIS
Additional signs and symptoms
- Brilliant red, diffuse, peripheral conjunctival injection
- Conjunctival and lid edema
- Local viral rash
- Upper respiratory infection

BACTERIAL CONJUNCTIVITIS
Additional signs and symptoms
- Diffuse peripheral conjunctival injection
- Thick, purulent eye discharge that contains mucous threads

CORNEAL ULCER
Additional signs and symptoms
- Diffuse conjunctival injection that increases in the circumcorneal area
- Severe pain in and around the eye
- Markedly decreased visual acuity
- Copious and purulent eye discharge and crusting

DX: History of trauma to the eye (corneal abrasion and ulcer), eye drainage culture, eye examination, visual acuity slit-lamp examination, allergy testing for allergic conjunctivitis
TX: Medication (topical antibiotics, topical cycloplegics, topical and oral analgesics, systemic antihistamines), warm compresses
F/U: Referral to ophthalmologist

Additional differential diagnoses: blepharitis ▪ chemical burn ▪ corneal erosion ▪ dacryoadenitis ▪ episcleritis ▪ foreign body ▪ glaucoma ▪ hyphema ▪ iritis ▪ keratoconjunctivitis sicca ▪ ocular laceration ▪ ocular tumor ▪ Stevens-Johnson syndrome ▪ uveitis

Constipation

Constipation is defined as small, infrequent, or difficult bowel movements. Because normal bowel movements can vary in frequency and from individual to individual, constipation must be determined in relation to the patient's normal elimination pattern. Constipation may be a minor annoyance or, uncommonly, a sign of a life-threatening disorder such as acute intestinal obstruction. If untreated, constipation can lead to headache, anorexia, and abdominal discomfort and can adversely affect the patient's lifestyle and well-being.

Constipation most commonly occurs when the urge to defecate is suppressed and the muscles associated with bowel movements remain contracted. Because the autonomic nervous system controls bowel movements — by sensing rectal distention from fecal contents and by stimulating the external sphincter — any factor that influences this system may cause bowel dysfunction.

History and physical examination

Ask the patient to describe the frequency of his bowel movements and the size and consistency of his stools. How long has he had constipation? Acute constipation usually has an organic cause, such as an anal or rectal disorder. In a patient over age 45, recent onset of constipation may be an early sign of colorectal cancer. Conversely, chronic constipation typically has a functional cause and may be related to stress.

Does the patient have pain related to constipation? If so, when did he first notice the pain and where is it located? Cramping abdominal pain and distention suggest obstipation — extreme, persistent constipation due to intestinal tract obstruction. Ask the patient if defecation worsens or helps relieve the pain. Defecation usually worsens pain but, in disorders such as irritable bowel syndrome, it may relieve it.

Ask the patient to describe a typical day's menu; estimate his daily fiber and fluid intake. Ask him about any changes in eating habits, in medication or alcohol use, or in physical activity. Has he experienced recent emotional distress? Has constipation affected his family life or social contacts? Also, ask about his job. A sedentary or stressful job can contribute to constipation.

Find out whether the patient has a history of GI, rectoanal, neurologic, or metabolic disorders; abdominal surgery; or radiation therapy. Then ask about the medications he's taking, including over-the-counter preparations, such as laxatives, mineral oil, stool softeners, and enemas.

Inspect the abdomen for distention or scars from previous surgery. Then auscultate for bowel sounds, and characterize their motility. Percuss all four quadrants, and gently palpate for abdominal tenderness, a palpable mass, and hepatomegaly. Next, examine the patient's rectum. Spread his buttocks to expose the anus, and inspect for inflammation, lesions, scars, fissures, and external hemorrhoids. Use a disposable glove and lubricant to palpate the anal sphincter for laxity or stricture. Also palpate for rectal masses and fecal impaction. Finally, obtain a stool sample and test it for occult blood.

As you assess the patient, remember that constipation can result from several life-threatening disorders, such as acute intestinal obstruction and mesenteric artery ischemia, but it doesn't herald these conditions.

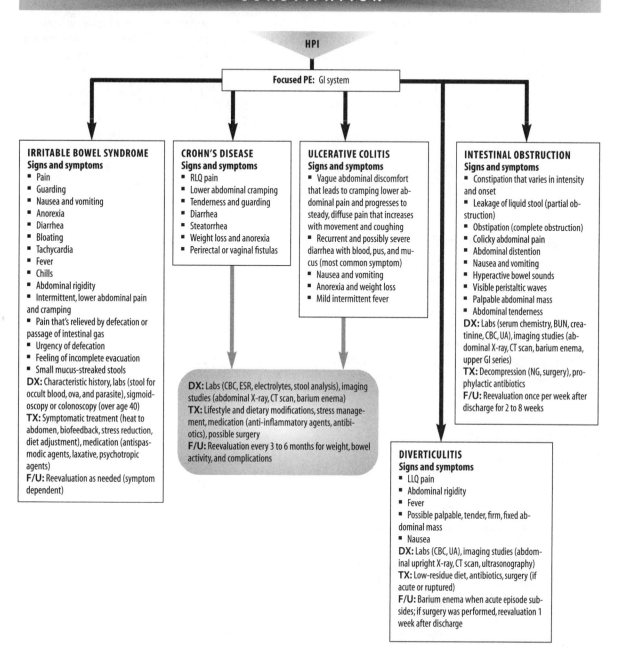

HPI

Focused PE: GI system

IRRITABLE BOWEL SYNDROME
Signs and symptoms
- Pain
- Guarding
- Nausea and vomiting
- Anorexia
- Diarrhea
- Bloating
- Tachycardia
- Fever
- Chills
- Abdominal rigidity
- Intermittent, lower abdominal pain and cramping
- Pain that's relieved by defecation or passage of intestinal gas
- Urgency of defecation
- Feeling of incomplete evacuation
- Small mucus-streaked stools

DX: Characteristic history, labs (stool for occult blood, ova, and parasite), sigmoidoscopy or colonoscopy (over age 40)
TX: Symptomatic treatment (heat to abdomen, biofeedback, stress reduction, diet adjustment), medication (antispasmodic agents, laxative, psychotropic agents)
F/U: Reevaluation as needed (symptom dependent)

CROHN'S DISEASE
Signs and symptoms
- RLQ pain
- Lower abdominal cramping
- Tenderness and guarding
- Diarrhea
- Steatorrhea
- Weight loss and anorexia
- Perirectal or vaginal fistulas

ULCERATIVE COLITIS
Signs and symptoms
- Vague abdominal discomfort that leads to cramping lower abdominal pain and progresses to steady, diffuse pain that increases with movement and coughing
- Recurrent and possibly severe diarrhea with blood, pus, and mucus (most common symptom)
- Nausea and vomiting
- Anorexia and weight loss
- Mild intermittent fever

DX: Labs (CBC, ESR, electrolytes, stool analysis), imaging studies (abdominal X-ray, CT scan, barium enema)
TX: Lifestyle and dietary modifications, stress management, medication (anti-inflammatory agents, antibiotics), possible surgery
F/U: Reevaluation every 3 to 6 months for weight, bowel activity, and complications

INTESTINAL OBSTRUCTION
Signs and symptoms
- Constipation that varies in intensity and onset
- Leakage of liquid stool (partial obstruction)
- Obstipation (complete obstruction)
- Colicky abdominal pain
- Abdominal distention
- Nausea and vomiting
- Hyperactive bowel sounds
- Visible peristaltic waves
- Palpable abdominal mass
- Abdominal tenderness

DX: Labs (serum chemistry, BUN, creatinine, CBC, UA), imaging studies (abdominal X-ray, CT scan, barium enema, upper GI series)
TX: Decompression (NG, surgery), prophylactic antibiotics
F/U: Reevaluation once per week after discharge for 2 to 8 weeks

DIVERTICULITIS
Signs and symptoms
- LLQ pain
- Abdominal rigidity
- Fever
- Possible palpable, tender, firm, fixed abdominal mass
- Nausea

DX: Labs (CBC, UA), imaging studies (abdominal upright X-ray, CT scan, ultrasonography)
TX: Low-residue diet, antibiotics, surgery (if acute or ruptured)
F/U: Barium enema when acute episode subsides; if surgery was performed, reevaluation 1 week after discharge

---

Additional differential diagnoses: anal fissure ▪ anorectal abscess ▪ cirrhosis ▪ diabetic neuropathy ▪ diverticulosis ▪ hemorrhoids ▪ hepatic porphyria ▪ hypercalcemia ▪ hypothyroidism ▪ ischemia ▪ mesenteric artery ▪ multiple sclerosis ▪ paraplegia ▪ Parkinson's disease ▪ spinal cord lesion ▪ tabes dorsalis ▪ ulcerative proctitis

Other causes: barium retention (from GI study) ▪ drugs (narcotic analgesics, excessive use of laxatives or enemas) ▪ surgery ▪ radiation therapy

Corneal reflex, absent

The corneal reflex is tested bilaterally by drawing a fine-pointed wisp of sterile cotton from a corner of each eye to the cornea. Normally, even though only one eye is tested at a time, the patient blinks bilaterally each time either cornea is touched — this is the corneal reflex. When this reflex is absent, neither eyelid closes when the cornea of one is touched. (See *Eliciting the corneal reflex.*)

The site of the afferent fibers for this reflex is in the ophthalmic branch of the trigeminal nerve (cranial nerve V); the efferent fibers are located in the facial nerve (cranial nerve VII). Unilateral or bilateral absence of the corneal reflex may result from damage to these nerves.

History and physical examination

If you're unable to elicit the corneal reflex, look for other signs of trigeminal nerve dysfunction. To test the three sensory portions of the nerve, touch each side of the patient's face on the brow, cheek, and jaw with a cotton wisp and ask him to compare the sensations.

If you suspect facial nerve involvement, note if the upper face (brow and eyes) and lower face (cheek, mouth, and chin) are weak bilaterally. Lower-motor-neuron facial weakness affects the face on the same side as the lesion, whereas upper-motor-neuron weakness affects the side opposite the lesion — predominantly the lower facial muscles.

Because an absent corneal reflex may signify such progressive neurologic disorders as Guillain-Barré syndrome, ask the patient about associated symptoms (facial pain, dysphagia, limb weakness).

PEDIATRIC POINTERS

- *Brain stem lesions and injuries are the most common causes of absent corneal reflexes in children; Guillain-Barré syndrome and trigeminal neuralgia are less common.*
- *Infants, especially those born prematurely, may have an absent corneal reflex due to anoxic damage to the brain stem.*

Eliciting the corneal reflex

To elicit the corneal reflex, have the patient turn her eyes away from you to avoid involuntary blinking during the procedure. Then approach the patient from the opposite side, out of her line of vision, and brush the cornea lightly with a fine wisp of sterile cotton. Repeat the procedure on the other eye.

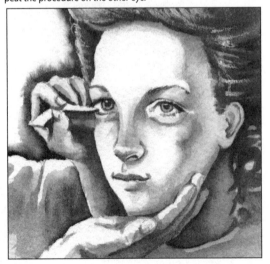

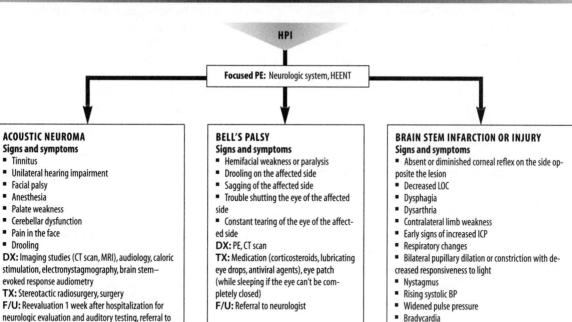

HPI

Focused PE: Neurologic system, HEENT

ACOUSTIC NEUROMA
Signs and symptoms
- Tinnitus
- Unilateral hearing impairment
- Facial palsy
- Anesthesia
- Palate weakness
- Cerebellar dysfunction
- Pain in the face
- Drooling

DX: Imaging studies (CT scan, MRI), audiology, caloric stimulation, electronystagmography, brain stem—evoked response audiometry
TX: Stereotactic radiosurgery, surgery
F/U: Reevaluation 1 week after hospitalization for neurologic evaluation and auditory testing, referral to otolaryngologist

---

BELL'S PALSY
Signs and symptoms
- Hemifacial weakness or paralysis
- Drooling on the affected side
- Sagging of the affected side
- Trouble shutting the eye of the affected side
- Constant tearing of the eye of the affected side

DX: PE, CT scan
TX: Medication (corticosteroids, lubricating eye drops, antiviral agents), eye patch (while sleeping if the eye can't be completely closed)
F/U: Referral to neurologist

BRAIN STEM INFARCTION OR INJURY
Signs and symptoms
- Absent or diminished corneal reflex on the side opposite the lesion
- Decreased LOC
- Dysphagia
- Dysarthria
- Contralateral limb weakness
- Early signs of increased ICP
- Respiratory changes
- Bilateral pupillary dilation or constriction with decreased responsiveness to light
- Nystagmus
- Rising systolic BP
- Widened pulse pressure
- Bradycardia
- Coma

DX: Imaging studies (skull X-ray, CT scan, MRI, angiography), EEG, ICP monitoring
TX: Medication (if embolic event, anticoagulants; antihypertensives; corticosteroids; if increased ICP, osmotic diuretics)
F/U: Referral to neurologist

Additional differential diagnoses: Guillain-Barré syndrome ▪ herpetic keratoconjunctivitis ▪ trigeminal neuralgia (tic douloureux)

Cough

Resonant, brassy, and harsh, a *barking cough* indicates edema of the larynx and surrounding tissue. Because children's airways are smaller in diameter than those of adults, edema can rapidly lead to airway occlusion — a life-threatening emergency.

A *nonproductive cough* is a noisy, forceful expulsion of air from the lungs that doesn't yield sputum or blood. A nonproductive cough isn't only ineffective but can also cause damage, such as airway collapse or rupture of alveoli or blebs. A nonproductive cough that later becomes productive is a classic sign of progressive respiratory disease.

A nonproductive cough may occur in paroxysms and can worsen by becoming more frequent. An acute cough has a sudden onset and may be self-limiting; a cough that persists beyond 3 months is considered chronic and, in many cases, results from cigarette smoking.

Productive coughing is a sudden, forceful, noisy expulsion of air that contains sputum, blood, or both. (The sputum's color, consistency, and odor provide important clues about the patient's condition.) Productive coughing can occur as a single cough or as paroxysmal coughing and can be voluntarily induced, although it's usually a reflexive response to stimulation of the airway mucosa.

Productive coughing commonly results from an acute or a chronic cardiovascular or respiratory infection that causes inflammation, edema, and increased mucus production in the airways. The most common cause of chronic productive coughing is cigarette smoking, which produces mucoid sputum ranging in color from clear to yellow to brown.

History and physical examination

Ask the patient when the cough began and whether body position, time of day, or specific activity affects it. How does the cough sound — harsh, brassy, dry, hacking? Try to determine if the cough is related to smoking or an environmental irritant. Next, ask about the frequency and intensity of coughing. If he has pain associated with coughing, breathing, or activity, when did it begin? Where is it located? If the patient is a child, ask the parents when the barking cough began and what signs and symptoms accompanied it. Has he had previous episodes of coughing? Did his condition improve with exposure to cold air?

Ask the patient about recent or chronic illness (especially cardiovascular, pulmonary, or GI disorders), allergies, cancer, surgery, or trauma. Also ask about hypersensitivity to drugs, foods, pets, dust, or pollen. Find out what medications the patient takes, and ask about recent changes in schedule or dosages. Also ask about recent changes in appetite, weight, exercise tolerance, or energy level and recent exposure to irritating fumes, chemicals, smoke, or infectious persons.

As you're taking his history, you can begin the physical examination. Observe the patient's general appearance and manner: Is he agitated, restless, or lethargic; pale, diaphoretic, or flushed; anxious, confused, or nervous? Also note whether he's cyanotic or has clubbed fingers or peripheral edema.

Take the patient's vital signs. Check the depth and rhythm of his respirations, and note if wheezing or "crowing" noises occur with breathing. Feel the patient's skin: Is it cold or warm, clammy or dry? Check his nose and mouth for congestion, inflammation, drainage, or signs of infection or allergies. Inspect his neck for distended veins and tracheal deviation, and palpate for masses or enlarged lymph nodes.

Examine his chest, observing its configuration and looking for abnormal chest wall motion. Do you note retractions or accessory muscle use? Percuss for dullness, tympany, or flatness. Auscultate for wheezing, crackles, rhonchi, pleural friction rubs, and decreased or absent breath sounds. Finally, examine his abdomen for distention, tenderness, masses, or abnormal bowel sounds.

If the patient has a productive cough, find out how much sputum he's coughing up each day. At what time of day does he cough up the most sputum? Does his sputum production have any relationship to what or when he eats or to his activities or environment? Ask him if he has noticed an increase in sputum production since his coughing began. Also ask about the color, odor, and consistency of the sputum.

PEDIATRIC POINTERS

- *Sudden onset of paroxysmal nonproductive coughing may indicate aspiration of a foreign body — a common danger in children, especially those between ages 6 months and 4 years.*
- *Causes of nonproductive coughing in infants and children include asthma, bacterial pneumonia, acute bronchiolitis, acute otitis media, measles, cystic fibrosis, life-threatening pertussis, and airway hyperactivity, stress, emotional stimulation, or attention-seeking behavior.*
- *Because a child's airway is narrow, a productive cough can quickly cause airway occlusion and respiratory distress from thick or excessive secretions.*
- *Causes of productive cough in children include asthma, bronchiectasis, bronchitis, acute bronchiolitis, cystic fibrosis, and pertussis.*

ELDER CARE CUE

Always ask an elderly patient about a cough because it may be an indication of serious acute or chronic illness.

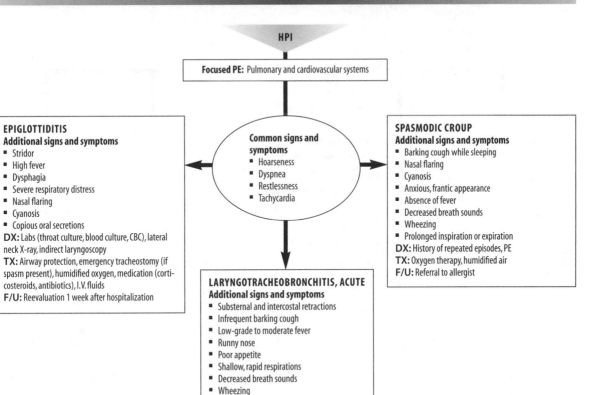

HPI

Focused PE: Pulmonary and cardiovascular systems

Common signs and symptoms
- Hoarseness
- Dyspnea
- Restlessness
- Tachycardia

EPIGLOTTIDITIS
Additional signs and symptoms
- Stridor
- High fever
- Dysphagia
- Severe respiratory distress
- Nasal flaring
- Cyanosis
- Copious oral secretions

DX: Labs (throat culture, blood culture, CBC), lateral neck X-ray, indirect laryngoscopy
TX: Airway protection, emergency tracheostomy (if spasm present), humidified oxygen, medication (corticosteroids, antibiotics), I.V. fluids
F/U: Reevaluation 1 week after hospitalization

SPASMODIC CROUP
Additional signs and symptoms
- Barking cough while sleeping
- Nasal flaring
- Cyanosis
- Anxious, frantic appearance
- Absence of fever
- Decreased breath sounds
- Wheezing
- Prolonged inspiration or expiration

DX: History of repeated episodes, PE
TX: Oxygen therapy, humidified air
F/U: Referral to allergist

LARYNGOTRACHEOBRONCHITIS, ACUTE
Additional signs and symptoms
- Substernal and intercostal retractions
- Infrequent barking cough
- Low-grade to moderate fever
- Runny nose
- Poor appetite
- Shallow, rapid respirations
- Decreased breath sounds
- Wheezing
- Prolonged inspiration or expiration
- Red epiglottis

DX: PE, neck X-ray
TX: Warm or cool humidified air, oxygen therapy, antibiotics
F/U: Reevaluation 1 week after the beginning of treatment (unless condition worsens) or 1 week after hospitalization

Additional differential diagnosis: aspiration of foreign body

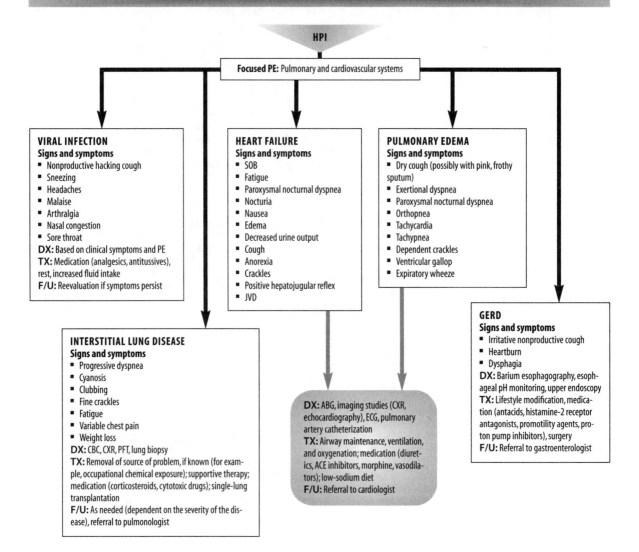

HPI

Focused PE: Pulmonary and cardiovascular systems

VIRAL INFECTION
Signs and symptoms
- Nonproductive hacking cough
- Sneezing
- Headaches
- Malaise
- Arthralgia
- Nasal congestion
- Sore throat

DX: Based on clinical symptoms and PE
TX: Medication (analgesics, antitussives), rest, increased fluid intake
F/U: Reevaluation if symptoms persist

HEART FAILURE
Signs and symptoms
- SOB
- Fatigue
- Paroxysmal nocturnal dyspnea
- Nocturia
- Nausea
- Edema
- Decreased urine output
- Cough
- Anorexia
- Crackles
- Positive hepatojugular reflex
- JVD

PULMONARY EDEMA
Signs and symptoms
- Dry cough (possibly with pink, frothy sputum)
- Exertional dyspnea
- Paroxysmal nocturnal dyspnea
- Orthopnea
- Tachycardia
- Tachypnea
- Dependent crackles
- Ventricular gallop
- Expiratory wheeze

GERD
Signs and symptoms
- Irritative nonproductive cough
- Heartburn
- Dysphagia

DX: Barium esophagography, esophageal pH monitoring, upper endoscopy
TX: Lifestyle modification, medication (antacids, histamine-2 receptor antagonists, promotility agents, proton pump inhibitors), surgery
F/U: Referral to gastroenterologist

INTERSTITIAL LUNG DISEASE
Signs and symptoms
- Progressive dyspnea
- Cyanosis
- Clubbing
- Fine crackles
- Fatigue
- Variable chest pain
- Weight loss

DX: CBC, CXR, PFT, lung biopsy
TX: Removal of source of problem, if known (for example, occupational chemical exposure); supportive therapy; medication (corticosteroids, cytotoxic drugs); single-lung transplantation
F/U: As needed (dependent on the severity of the disease), referral to pulmonologist

DX: ABG, imaging studies (CXR, echocardiography), ECG, pulmonary artery catheterization
TX: Airway maintenance, ventilation, and oxygenation; medication (diuretics, ACE inhibitors, morphine, vasodilators); low-sodium diet
F/U: Referral to cardiologist

Additional differential diagnoses: airway occlusion (partial) ▪ aortic aneurysm (thoracic) ▪ asthma ▪ atelectasis ▪ bronchogenic carcinoma ▪ Hantavirus pulmonary syndrome ▪ laryngeal tumor ▪ laryngitis ▪ Legionnaire's disease ▪ pleural effusion ▪ sarcoidosis ▪ sinusitis (chronic)

Other causes: bronchoscopy ▪ PFTs ▪ tracheal suctioning ▪ inhalants ▪ intermittent positive-pressure breathing

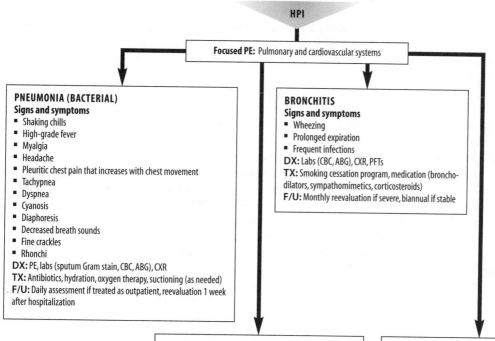

HPI

Focused PE: Pulmonary and cardiovascular systems

PNEUMONIA (BACTERIAL)
Signs and symptoms
- Shaking chills
- High-grade fever
- Myalgia
- Headache
- Pleuritic chest pain that increases with chest movement
- Tachypnea
- Dyspnea
- Cyanosis
- Diaphoresis
- Decreased breath sounds
- Fine crackles
- Rhonchi

DX: PE, labs (sputum Gram stain, CBC, ABG), CXR
TX: Antibiotics, hydration, oxygen therapy, suctioning (as needed)
F/U: Daily assessment if treated as outpatient, reevaluation 1 week after hospitalization

BRONCHITIS
Signs and symptoms
- Wheezing
- Prolonged expiration
- Frequent infections

DX: Labs (CBC, ABG), CXR, PFTs
TX: Smoking cessation program, medication (bronchodilators, sympathomimetics, corticosteroids)
F/U: Monthly reevaluation if severe, biannual if stable

PULMONARY TUBERCULOSIS
Signs and symptoms
- Mild to severe productive cough
- Hemoptysis
- Malaise
- Dyspnea
- Pleuritic chest pain
- Night sweats
- Tendency to become fatigued
- Weight loss
- Amphoric breath sounds
- Chest dullness on percussion
- Increased fremitus with crackles after coughing

DX: Tuberculin skin test, sputum for AFB, CXR, bronchoscopy, open lung biopsy
TX: Medication (antitubercular drugs, specific drugs for resistant strains)
F/U: Referral to pulmonologist

LUNG CANCER
Signs and symptoms
- Chronic cough that produces small amounts of purulent, blood-streaked sputum (bronchogenic carcinoma)
- Cough that produces large amounts of frothy sputum (bronchoalveolar carcinoma)
- Dyspnea
- Anorexia
- Fatigue
- Weight loss
- Chest pain
- Fever
- Diaphoresis
- Wheezing
- Clubbing

DX: Imaging studies (CXR, CT scan, MRI), bronchoscopy, needle biopsy, open lung biopsy
TX: Varies (dependent on the type and stage of the cancer), medication (chemotherapy, analgesia), radiation therapy, surgery
F/U: Referral to oncologist and surgeon

Additional differential diagnoses: actinomycosis ▪ aspiration pneumonitis ▪ asthma (acute) ▪ bronchiectasis ▪ chemical pneumonitis ▪ nocardiosis ▪ psittacosis ▪ pulmonary edema ▪ silicosis

Other causes: bronchoscopy ▪ PFTs ▪ drugs (expectorants) ▪ respiratory treatments

Crackles

A common finding in certain cardiovascular and pulmonary disorders, crackles are nonmusical clicking or rattling noises heard during auscultation of breath sounds. Also known as rales or crepitations, crackles usually occur during inspiration and recur constantly from one respiratory cycle to the next. They can be unilateral or bilateral, moist or dry. They're characterized by their pitch, loudness, location, persistence, and occurrence during the respiratory cycle.

Crackles indicate abnormal movement of air through fluid-filled airways. They can be irregularly dispersed, as in pneumonia, or localized, as in bronchiectasis. (A few basilar crackles can be heard in normal lungs after prolonged shallow breathing. These normal crackles clear with a few deep breaths.) Usually, though, crackles indicate the degree of an underlying illness. When crackles result from a generalized disorder, they usually occur in the less distended and more dependent areas of the lungs, such as the lung bases when the patient is standing. Crackles due to air passing through inflammatory exudate may not be audible if the involved portion of the lung isn't being ventilated because of shallow respirations.

History and physical examination

Quickly take the patient's vital signs and examine him for signs of respiratory distress or airway obstruction. Check the depth and rhythm of respirations. Is he struggling to breathe? Check for increased accessory muscle use and chest wall motion, retractions, stridor, or nasal flaring. Institute emergency measures if necessary.

If the patient also has a cough, ask when it began and if it's constant or intermittent. Find out what the cough sounds like and whether he's coughing up sputum or blood. If the cough is productive, determine the sputum's consistency, amount, odor, and color.

Ask the patient if he has any pain. If so, where is it located? When did he first notice it? Does it radiate to other areas? Also ask the patient if movement, coughing, or breathing worsens or helps relieve his pain. Note the patient's position: Is he lying still or moving about restlessly?

Obtain a brief medical history. Does the patient have cancer or any known respiratory or cardiovascular problems? Ask if he has had any recent surgery, trauma, or illness and whether he smokes or drinks alcohol. Is he experiencing hoarseness or difficulty swallowing? Find out which medications he's taking. Also ask about recent weight loss, anorexia, nausea, vomiting, fatigue, weakness, vertigo, and syncope. Has the patient been exposed to irritants, such as vapors, fumes, or smoke?

Next, perform a physical examination. Examine the patient's nose and mouth for signs of infection, such as inflammation or increased secretions. Note his breath odor: Halitosis could indicate pulmonary infection. Check his neck for masses, tenderness, swelling, lymphadenopathy, or venous distention.

Inspect the patient's chest for abnormal configuration or uneven expansion. Percuss for dullness, tympany, or flatness. Auscultate his lungs for other abnormal, diminished, or absent breath sounds. Listen to his heart for abnormal sounds, and check his hands and feet for edema or clubbing.

PEDIATRIC POINTERS

- *Crackles in an infant or child may indicate a serious cardiovascular or respiratory disorder.*
- *Pneumonias produce diffuse, sudden crackles in children.*
- *Esophageal atresia and tracheoesophageal fistula can cause bubbling, moist crackles due to aspiration of food or secretions into the lungs — especially in newborn infants.*
- *Pulmonary edema causes fine crackles at the bases of the lungs, and bronchiectasis produces moist crackles.*
- *Cystic fibrosis produces widespread, fine to coarse inspiratory crackles and wheezing in infants.*
- *Sickle cell anemia may produce crackles when it causes pulmonary infarction or infection.*

ELDER CARE CUES

- *Crackles that clear after deep breathing may indicate mild basilar atelectasis.*
- *In older patients, auscultate lung bases before and after auscultating apices.*

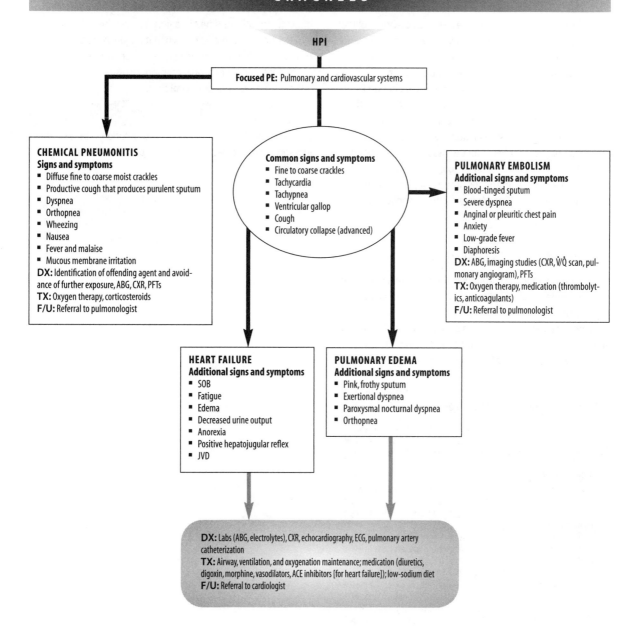

HPI

Focused PE: Pulmonary and cardiovascular systems

CHEMICAL PNEUMONITIS
Signs and symptoms
- Diffuse fine to coarse moist crackles
- Productive cough that produces purulent sputum
- Dyspnea
- Orthopnea
- Wheezing
- Nausea
- Fever and malaise
- Mucous membrane irritation

DX: Identification of offending agent and avoidance of further exposure, ABG, CXR, PFTs
TX: Oxygen therapy, corticosteroids
F/U: Referral to pulmonologist

Common signs and symptoms
- Fine to coarse crackles
- Tachycardia
- Tachypnea
- Ventricular gallop
- Cough
- Circulatory collapse (advanced)

PULMONARY EMBOLISM
Additional signs and symptoms
- Blood-tinged sputum
- Severe dyspnea
- Anginal or pleuritic chest pain
- Anxiety
- Low-grade fever
- Diaphoresis

DX: ABG, imaging studies (CXR, V̇/Q̇ scan, pulmonary angiogram), PFTs
TX: Oxygen therapy, medication (thrombolytics, anticoagulants)
F/U: Referral to pulmonologist

HEART FAILURE
Additional signs and symptoms
- SOB
- Fatigue
- Edema
- Decreased urine output
- Anorexia
- Positive hepatojugular reflex
- JVD

PULMONARY EDEMA
Additional signs and symptoms
- Pink, frothy sputum
- Exertional dyspnea
- Paroxysmal nocturnal dyspnea
- Orthopnea

DX: Labs (ABG, electrolytes), CXR, echocardiography, ECG, pulmonary artery catheterization
TX: Airway, ventilation, and oxygenation maintenance; medication (diuretics, digoxin, morphine, vasodilators, ACE inhibitors [for heart failure]); low-sodium diet
F/U: Referral to cardiologist

Additional differential diagnoses: ARDS ▪ asthma (acute) ▪ bronchiectasis ▪ bronchitis (chronic) ▪ interstitial fibrosis of the lungs ▪ Legionnaire's disease ▪ lung abscess ▪ pneumonia ▪ psittacosis ▪ pulmonary tuberculosis ▪ sarcoidosis ▪ silicosis ▪ tracheobronchitis

Crepitation, subcutaneous

When bubbles of air or other gases (such as carbon dioxide) are trapped in subcutaneous tissue, palpation or stroking of the skin produces a crackling sound called *subcutaneous crepitation*. The bubbles feel like small, unstable nodules and aren't painful, even though subcutaneous crepitation is often associated with painful disorders. Usually, the affected tissue is visibly edematous; this can lead to life-threatening airway occlusion if the edema affects the neck or upper chest.

The air or gas bubbles enter the tissues through open wounds, from the action of anaerobic microorganisms, or from traumatic or spontaneous rupture or perforation of pulmonary or GI organs. (See *Managing subcutaneous crepitation*.)

History and physical examination

Because subcutaneous crepitation can indicate a life-threatening disorder, you'll need to perform a rapid initial evaluation and intervene if necessary.

When the patient's condition permits, palpate the affected skin to evaluate the location and extent of subcutaneous crepitation and to obtain baseline information. Repalpate frequently to determine if the subcutaneous crepitation is increasing. Ask the patient if he's experiencing pain or having difficulty breathing. If he's in pain, find out where the pain is located, how severe it is, and when it began. Ask about recent thoracic surgery, diagnostic tests, and respiratory therapy or a history of trauma or chronic pulmonary disease. Check the patient's temperature and vital signs.

Children may develop subcutaneous crepitation in the neck from ingestion of corrosive substances that perforate the esophagus.

Managing subcutaneous crepitation

Subcutaneous crepitation occurs when air or gas bubbles escape into tissues. It may signal life-threatening rupture of an air-filled or gas-producing organ or a fulminating anaerobic infection.

ORGAN RUPTURE
If the patient shows signs of respiratory distress — such as severe dyspnea, tachypnea, accessory muscle use, nasal flaring, air hunger, or tachycardia — quickly test for Hamman's sign to detect trapped air bubbles in the mediastinum.

To test for Hamman's sign, help the patient assume a left-lateral recumbent position. Then place your stethoscope over the precordium. If you hear a loud crunching sound that synchronizes with his heartbeat, the patient has a positive Hamman's sign.

Depending on which organ is ruptured, be prepared for endotracheal intubation, an emergency tracheotomy, or chest tube insertion. Start administering supplemental oxygen immediately. Start an I.V. to administer fluids and medication, and connect the patient to a cardiac monitor.

ANAEROBIC INFECTION
If the patient has an open wound with a foul odor and local swelling and discoloration, you must act quickly. Take the patient's vital signs, checking especially for fever, tachycardia, hypotension, and tachypnea. Next, start an I.V. line to administer fluids and medication, and provide supplemental oxygen.

In addition, be prepared for emergency surgery to drain and debride the wound. If the patient's condition is life-threatening, you may need to prepare him for transfer to a facility with a hyperbaric chamber.

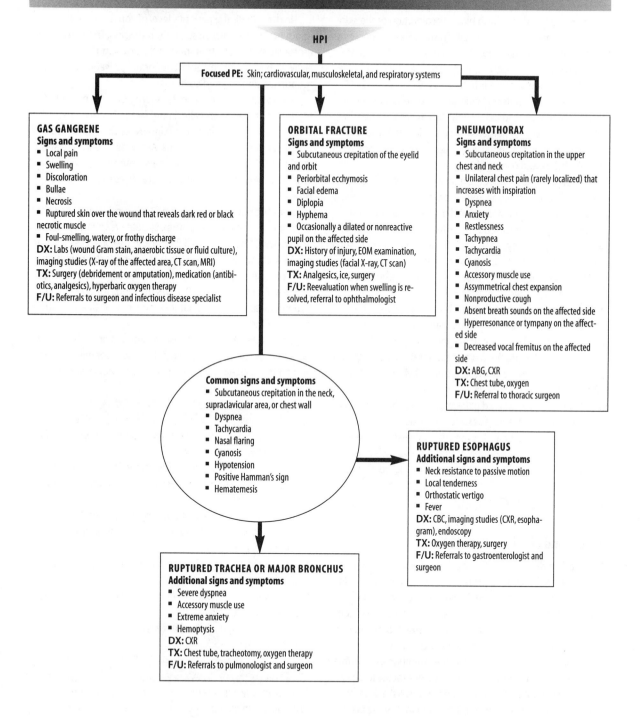

HPI

Focused PE: Skin; cardiovascular, musculoskeletal, and respiratory systems

GAS GANGRENE
Signs and symptoms
- Local pain
- Swelling
- Discoloration
- Bullae
- Necrosis
- Ruptured skin over the wound that reveals dark red or black necrotic muscle
- Foul-smelling, watery, or frothy discharge

DX: Labs (wound Gram stain, anaerobic tissue or fluid culture), imaging studies (X-ray of the affected area, CT scan, MRI)
TX: Surgery (debridement or amputation), medication (antibiotics, analgesics), hyperbaric oxygen therapy
F/U: Referrals to surgeon and infectious disease specialist

ORBITAL FRACTURE
Signs and symptoms
- Subcutaneous crepitation of the eyelid and orbit
- Periorbital ecchymosis
- Facial edema
- Diplopia
- Hyphema
- Occasionally a dilated or nonreactive pupil on the affected side

DX: History of injury, EOM examination, imaging studies (facial X-ray, CT scan)
TX: Analgesics, ice, surgery
F/U: Reevaluation when swelling is resolved, referral to ophthalmologist

PNEUMOTHORAX
Signs and symptoms
- Subcutaneous crepitation in the upper chest and neck
- Unilateral chest pain (rarely localized) that increases with inspiration
- Dyspnea
- Anxiety
- Restlessness
- Tachypnea
- Tachycardia
- Cyanosis
- Accessory muscle use
- Assymmetrical chest expansion
- Nonproductive cough
- Absent breath sounds on the affected side
- Hyperresonance or tympany on the affected side
- Decreased vocal fremitus on the affected side

DX: ABG, CXR
TX: Chest tube, oxygen
F/U: Referral to thoracic surgeon

Common signs and symptoms
- Subcutaneous crepitation in the neck, supraclavicular area, or chest wall
- Dyspnea
- Tachycardia
- Nasal flaring
- Cyanosis
- Hypotension
- Positive Hamman's sign
- Hematemesis

RUPTURED ESOPHAGUS
Additional signs and symptoms
- Neck resistance to passive motion
- Local tenderness
- Orthostatic vertigo
- Fever

DX: CBC, imaging studies (CXR, esophagram), endoscopy
TX: Oxygen therapy, surgery
F/U: Referrals to gastroenterologist and surgeon

RUPTURED TRACHEA OR MAJOR BRONCHUS
Additional signs and symptoms
- Severe dyspnea
- Accessory muscle use
- Extreme anxiety
- Hemoptysis

DX: CXR
TX: Chest tube, tracheotomy, oxygen therapy
F/U: Referrals to pulmonologist and surgeon

Other causes: bronchoscopy ▪ intermittent positive-pressure breathing ▪ mechanical ventilation ▪ respiratory treatments ▪ thoracic surgery ▪ upper GI tract endoscopy

Cyanosis

Cyanosis — a bluish or bluish black discoloration of the skin and mucous membranes — results from excessive concentration of unoxygenated hemoglobin in the blood. This common sign may develop abruptly or gradually. It can be classified as central or peripheral, although the two types may coexist.

Central cyanosis reflects inadequate oxygenation of systemic arterial blood caused by right-to-left cardiac shunting, pulmonary disease, or hematologic disorders. It may occur anywhere on the skin and also on the mucous membranes of the mouth, lips, and conjunctiva.

Peripheral cyanosis reflects sluggish peripheral circulation caused by vasoconstriction, reduced cardiac output, or vascular occlusion. It may be widespread or may occur locally in one extremity; however, it doesn't affect mucous membranes. Typically, peripheral cyanosis appears on exposed areas, such as the fingers, nail beds, feet, nose, and ears.

Although cyanosis is an important sign of cardiovascular and pulmonary disorders, it isn't always an accurate gauge of oxygenation. Several factors contribute to its development: hemoglobin concentration and oxygen saturation, cardiac output, and partial pressure of oxygen (PO_2). Cyanosis is usually undetectable until the oxygen saturation of hemoglobin falls below 80%. Severe cyanosis is quite obvious, whereas mild cyanosis is more difficult to detect, even in natural, bright light. In dark-skinned patients, cyanosis is most apparent in the mucous membranes and nail beds.

Transient, nonpathologic cyanosis may result from environmental factors. For example, peripheral cyanosis may result from cutaneous vasoconstriction following brief exposure to cold air or water. Central cyanosis may result from reduced PO_2 at high altitudes.

History and physical examination

If the patient displays sudden, localized cyanosis and other signs of arterial occlusion, protect the affected limb from injury; however, don't massage the limb. If you see central cyanosis stemming from a pulmonary disorder or shock, perform a rapid evaluation. Take immediate steps to maintain an airway, assist breathing, and monitor circulation.

If cyanosis accompanies less-acute conditions, perform a thorough examination. Begin with a history, focusing on cardiac, pulmonary, and hematologic disorders. Ask about previous surgery. Then begin the physical examination by taking vital signs. Inspect the skin and mucous membranes to determine the extent of cyanosis. Ask the patient when he first noticed the cyanosis. Does it subside and recur? Is it aggravated by cold, smoking, or stress? Alleviated by massage or rewarm-

ing? Check the skin for coolness, pallor, redness, pain, and ulceration. Also note clubbing.

Next, evaluate the patient's level of consciousness. Ask about headaches, dizziness, or blurred vision. Then test his motor strength. Ask about pain in the arms and legs (especially with walking) and about abnormal sensations, such as numbness, tingling, and coldness.

Ask about chest pain and its severity. Can the patient identify any aggravating and alleviating factors? Palpate peripheral pulses and test capillary refill time. Note the temperature of the extremities. Also note edema. Auscultate heart rate and rhythm, noting especially gallops and murmurs. Also auscultate the abdominal aorta and femoral arteries to detect any bruits.

Does the patient have a cough? Is it productive? If so, have the patient describe the sputum. Evaluate respiratory rate and rhythm. Check for nasal flaring and use of accessory muscles. Ask about sleep apnea. Does the patient sleep with his head propped up on pillows? Inspect for asymmetrical chest expansion or barrel chest. Percuss the lungs for dullness or hyperresonance, and auscultate for decreased or adventitious breath sounds.

Inspect the abdomen for ascites, and test for shifting dullness or fluid wave. Percuss and palpate for liver enlargement and tenderness. Also, ask about nausea, anorexia, and weight loss.

PEDIATRIC POINTERS

- *Many pulmonary disorders responsible for cyanosis in adults also cause cyanosis in children.*
- *Central cyanosis may result from cystic fibrosis, asthma, airway obstruction by a foreign body, acute laryngotracheobronchitis, and epiglottiditis.*
- *Cyanosis may also result from congenital heart defects, such as transposition of the great vessels, that cause right-to-left intracardiac shunting.*
- *In children, circumoral cyanosis may precede generalized cyanosis.*
- *Acrocyanosis may occur in infants because of excessive crying or exposure to cold.*
- *Exercise and agitation enhance cyanosis, so provide comfort and regular rest periods.*

ELDER CARE CUE

Because elderly patients have reduced tissue perfusion, peripheral cyanosis can present even with a slight decrease in cardiac output or systemic blood pressure.

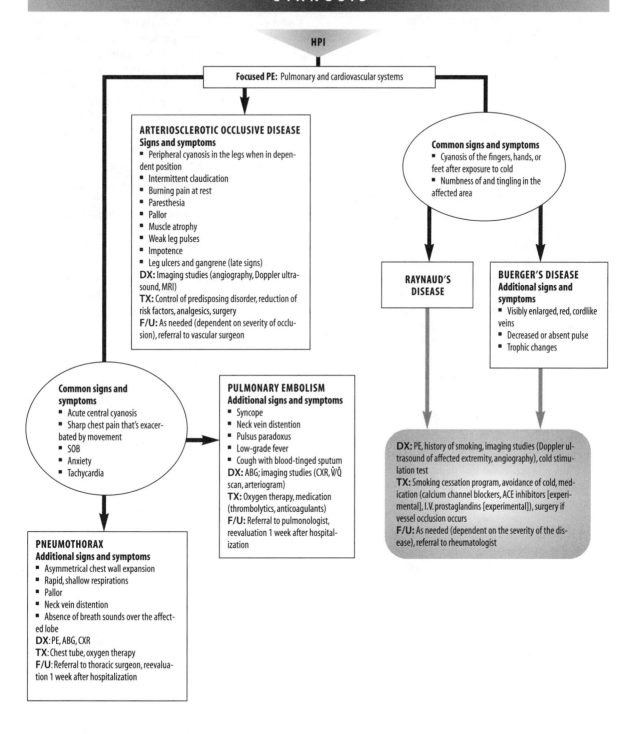

HPI

Focused PE: Pulmonary and cardiovascular systems

ARTERIOSCLEROTIC OCCLUSIVE DISEASE
Signs and symptoms
- Peripheral cyanosis in the legs when in dependent position
- Intermittent claudication
- Burning pain at rest
- Paresthesia
- Pallor
- Muscle atrophy
- Weak leg pulses
- Impotence
- Leg ulcers and gangrene (late signs)
DX: Imaging studies (angiography, Doppler ultrasound, MRI)
TX: Control of predisposing disorder, reduction of risk factors, analgesics, surgery
F/U: As needed (dependent on severity of occlusion), referral to vascular surgeon

Common signs and symptoms
- Cyanosis of the fingers, hands, or feet after exposure to cold
- Numbness of and tingling in the affected area

RAYNAUD'S DISEASE

BUERGER'S DISEASE
Additional signs and symptoms
- Visibly enlarged, red, cordlike veins
- Decreased or absent pulse
- Trophic changes

Common signs and symptoms
- Acute central cyanosis
- Sharp chest pain that's exacerbated by movement
- SOB
- Anxiety
- Tachycardia

PULMONARY EMBOLISM
Additional signs and symptoms
- Syncope
- Neck vein distention
- Pulsus paradoxus
- Low-grade fever
- Cough with blood-tinged sputum
DX: ABG; imaging studies (CXR, V̇/Q̇ scan, arteriogram)
TX: Oxygen therapy, medication (thrombolytics, anticoagulants)
F/U: Referral to pulmonologist, reevaluation 1 week after hospitalization

DX: PE, history of smoking, imaging studies (Doppler ultrasound of affected extremity, angiography), cold stimulation test
TX: Smoking cessation program, avoidance of cold, medication (calcium channel blockers, ACE inhibitors [experimental], I.V. prostaglandins [experimental]), surgery if vessel occlusion occurs
F/U: As needed (dependent on the severity of the disease), referral to rheumatologist

PNEUMOTHORAX
Additional signs and symptoms
- Asymmetrical chest wall expansion
- Rapid, shallow respirations
- Pallor
- Neck vein distention
- Absence of breath sounds over the affected lobe
DX: PE, ABG, CXR
TX: Chest tube, oxygen therapy
F/U: Referral to thoracic surgeon, reevaluation 1 week after hospitalization

Additional differential diagnoses: bronchiectasis ▪ COPD ▪ DVT ▪ heart failure ▪ lung cancer ▪ lupus erythematosus ▪ peripheral arterial occlusion (acute) ▪ pneumonia ▪ polycythemia vera ▪ pulmonary edema ▪ pulmonary embolism ▪ shock ▪ sleep apnea

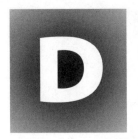

Decerebrate posture

Decerebrate posture (decerebrate rigidity, abnormal extensor reflex) is characterized by adduction and extension of the arms, with the wrists pronated and the fingers flexed. The legs are stiffly extended, with plantar flexion of the feet. In severe cases, the back is acutely arched (opisthotonos). (See *Recognizing decerebrate posture.*) This sign indicates upper brain stem damage, which may result from primary lesions, such as infarction, hemorrhage, or tumor; metabolic encephalopathy; head injury; or brain stem compression associated with increased intracranial pressure (ICP).

Decerebrate posture may be elicited by noxious stimuli or may occur spontaneously. It may be unilateral or bilateral. In concurrent brain stem and cerebral damage, decerebrate posture may affect only the arms, while the legs may remain flaccid. Alternatively, decerebrate posture may affect one side of the body and decorticate posture the other. The two postures may also alternate as the patient's neurologic status fluctuates. Generally, the duration of each posturing episode correlates with the severity of brain stem damage.

History and physical examination

Your first priority is to ensure a patent airway. Insert an artificial airway, elevate the head of the bed, and turn the patient's head to the side to prevent aspiration. (Don't disrupt spinal alignment if you suspect spinal cord injury.)

Next, examine spontaneous respirations. Institute emergency measures if necessary.

After taking vital signs, determine the patient's level of consciousness (LOC); use the Glasgow Coma Scale as a reference. Then evaluate the pupils for size, equality, and response to light. Assess deep tendon and cranial nerve reflexes, and test for doll's eye sign.

Next, explore the history of the patient's coma. If you can't obtain this information, look for clues to the causative disorder, such as hepatomegaly, cyanosis, diabetic skin changes, needle tracks, or obvious trauma. If a family member is available, find out when the patient's LOC began deteriorating. Did it occur abruptly? What did the patient complain of before he lost consciousness? Does he have a history of diabetes, liver disease, cancer, blood clots, or aneurysm? Ask about any accident or trauma responsible for the coma.

PEDIATRIC POINTERS

- *Children under age 2 may not display decerebrate posture because of nervous system immaturity. However, if the posture does occur, it's usually the more severe opisthotonos. In fact, opisthotonos is more common in infants and young children than in adults and is usually a terminal sign.*
- *In children, the most common cause of decerebrate posture is head injury. It also occurs in Reye's syndrome — the result of increased ICP causing brain stem compression.*

Recognizing decerebrate posture

Decerebrate posture results from damage to the upper brain stem. In this posture the arms are adducted and extended, with the wrists pronated and the fingers flexed. The legs are stiffly extended, with plantar flexion of the feet.

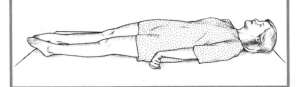

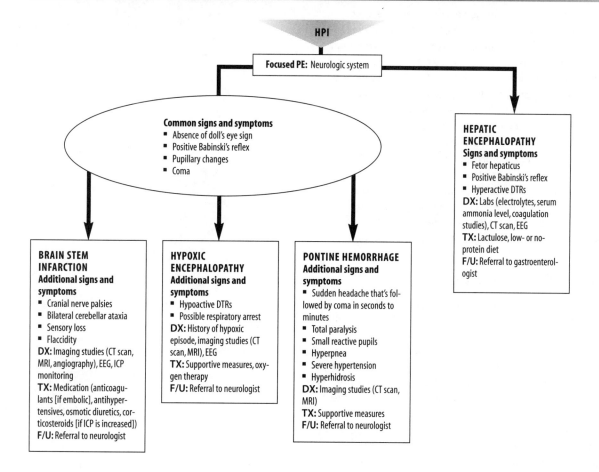

HPI

Focused PE: Neurologic system

Common signs and symptoms
- Absence of doll's eye sign
- Positive Babinski's reflex
- Pupillary changes
- Coma

HEPATIC ENCEPHALOPATHY
Signs and symptoms
- Fetor hepaticus
- Positive Babinski's reflex
- Hyperactive DTRs

DX: Labs (electrolytes, serum ammonia level, coagulation studies), CT scan, EEG
TX: Lactulose, low- or no-protein diet
F/U: Referral to gastroenterologist

BRAIN STEM INFARCTION
Additional signs and symptoms
- Cranial nerve palsies
- Bilateral cerebellar ataxia
- Sensory loss
- Flaccidity

DX: Imaging studies (CT scan, MRI, angiography), EEG, ICP monitoring
TX: Medication (anticoagulants [if embolic], antihypertensives, osmotic diuretics, corticosteroids [if ICP is increased])
F/U: Referral to neurologist

HYPOXIC ENCEPHALOPATHY
Additional signs and symptoms
- Hypoactive DTRs
- Possible respiratory arrest

DX: History of hypoxic episode, imaging studies (CT scan, MRI), EEG
TX: Supportive measures, oxygen therapy
F/U: Referral to neurologist

PONTINE HEMORRHAGE
Additional signs and symptoms
- Sudden headache that's followed by coma in seconds to minutes
- Total paralysis
- Small reactive pupils
- Hyperpnea
- Severe hypertension
- Hyperhidrosis

DX: Imaging studies (CT scan, MRI)
TX: Supportive measures
F/U: Referral to neurologist

Additional differential diagnoses: brain stem tumor ▪ cerebral lesion ▪ hypoglycemic encephalopathy ▪ posterior fossa hemorrhage

---

Other cause: lumbar puncture

Decorticate posture

A sign of corticospinal damage, decorticate posture (decorticate rigidity, abnormal flexor response) is characterized by adduction of the arms and flexion of the elbows, with wrists and fingers flexed on the chest. The legs are extended and internally rotated, with plantar flexion of the feet. This posture may occur unilaterally or bilaterally. (See *Recognizing decorticate posture.*) It usually results from stroke or head injury. It may be elicited by noxious stimuli or may occur spontaneously. The intensity of the required stimulus, the duration of the posture, and the frequency of spontaneous episodes vary with the severity and location of cerebral injury.

Although a serious sign, decorticate posture carries a more favorable prognosis than decerebrate posture. However, if the causative disorder extends lower in the brain stem, decorticate posture may progress to decerebrate posture.

History and physical examination

Obtain vital signs and evaluate the patient's level of consciousness. If his consciousness is impaired, insert an oropharyngeal airway, elevate the patient's head 30 degrees, and turn the patient's head to the side to prevent aspiration (unless spinal cord injury is suspected). Evaluate the patient's respiratory rate, rhythm, and depth. Prepare to institute emergency measures if necessary. In addition, institute seizure precautions.

Test the patient's motor and sensory functions. Evaluate pupil size, equality, and response to light. Then test cranial nerve and deep tendon reflexes. Ask about headache, dizziness, nausea, abnormal vision, and numbness or tingling. When did the patient first notice these symptoms? Is his family aware of any behavior changes? Also ask about a history of cerebrovascular disease, cancer, meningitis, encephalitis, upper respiratory infection, or recent trauma.

Recognizing decorticate posture

Decorticate posture results from damage to one or both corticospinal tracts. In this posture, the arms are adducted and flexed, with the wrists and fingers flexed on the chest. The legs are usually extended and internally rotated, with plantar flexion of the feet.

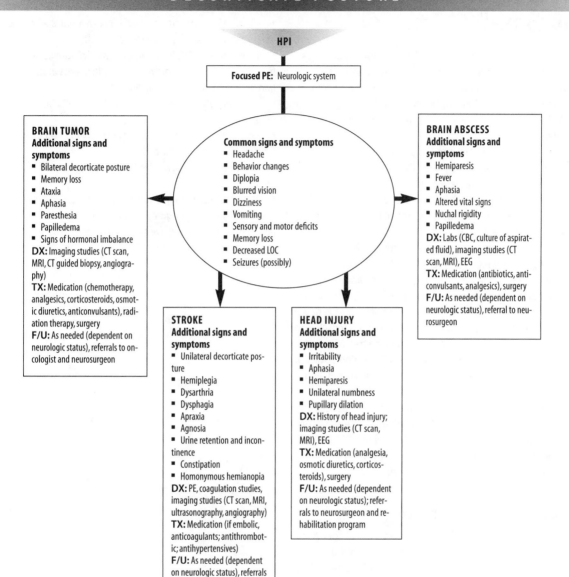

HPI

Focused PE: Neurologic system

BRAIN TUMOR
Additional signs and symptoms
- Bilateral decorticate posture
- Memory loss
- Ataxia
- Aphasia
- Paresthesia
- Papilledema
- Signs of hormonal imbalance

DX: Imaging studies (CT scan, MRI, CT guided biopsy, angiography)
TX: Medication (chemotherapy, analgesics, corticosteroids, osmotic diuretics, anticonvulsants), radiation therapy, surgery
F/U: As needed (dependent on neurologic status), referrals to oncologist and neurosurgeon

Common signs and symptoms
- Headache
- Behavior changes
- Diplopia
- Blurred vision
- Dizziness
- Vomiting
- Sensory and motor deficits
- Memory loss
- Decreased LOC
- Seizures (possibly)

BRAIN ABSCESS
Additional signs and symptoms
- Hemiparesis
- Fever
- Aphasia
- Altered vital signs
- Nuchal rigidity
- Papilledema

DX: Labs (CBC, culture of aspirated fluid), imaging studies (CT scan, MRI), EEG
TX: Medication (antibiotics, anticonvulsants, analgesics), surgery
F/U: As needed (dependent on neurologic status), referral to neurosurgeon

STROKE
Additional signs and symptoms
- Unilateral decorticate posture
- Hemiplegia
- Dysarthria
- Dysphagia
- Apraxia
- Agnosia
- Urine retention and incontinence
- Constipation
- Homonymous hemianopia

DX: PE, coagulation studies, imaging studies (CT scan, MRI, ultrasonography, angiography)
TX: Medication (if embolic, anticoagulants; antithrombotic; antihypertensives)
F/U: As needed (dependent on neurologic status), referrals to neurologist and rehabilitation program

HEAD INJURY
Additional signs and symptoms
- Irritability
- Aphasia
- Hemiparesis
- Unilateral numbness
- Pupillary dilation

DX: History of head injury; imaging studies (CT scan, MRI), EEG
TX: Medication (analgesia, osmotic diuretics, corticosteroids), surgery
F/U: As needed (dependent on neurologic status); referrals to neurosurgeon and rehabilitation program

Deep tendon reflexes, abnormal

A *hyperactive deep tendon reflex* (DTR) is an abnormally brisk muscle contraction that occurs in response to a sudden stretch induced by sharply tapping the muscle's tendon of insertion. This elicited sign may be graded as brisk or pathologically hyperactive. Hyperactive DTRs are commonly accompanied by clonus.

The corticospinal tract and other descending tracts govern the reflex arc — the relay cycle that produces any reflex response. A corticospinal lesion above the level of the reflex arc being tested may result in hyperactive DTRs. Abnormal neuromuscular transmission at the end of the reflex arc may also cause hyperactive DTRs. For example, a deficiency of calcium or magnesium may cause hyperactive DTRs because these electrolytes regulate neuromuscular excitability.

Although hyperactive DTRs frequently accompany other neurologic findings, they may be of specific diagnostic value. For example, they're an early, cardinal sign of hypocalcemia.

A *hypoactive DTR* is an abnormally diminished muscle contraction that occurs in response to a sudden stretch induced by sharply tapping the muscle's tendon of insertion. It may be graded as minimal (+) or absent (0). Symmetrically reduced (+) reflexes may be normal.

Hypoactive DTRs may result from damage to the reflex arc involving the specific muscle, the peripheral nerve, the nerve roots, or the spinal cord at that level. Hypoactive DTRs are an important sign of many disorders, especially when they appear with other neurologic signs and symptoms.

History and physical examination

After eliciting abnormal DTRs, take the patient's history. Ask about spinal cord injury or other trauma and about prolonged exposure to cold, wind, or water. Could the patient be pregnant? A positive response to any of these questions requires prompt evaluation to rule out life-threatening autonomic hyperreflexia, tetanus, preeclampsia, or hypothermia. Ask about the onset and progression of associated signs and symptoms.

Next, perform a neurologic examination. Evaluate level of consciousness, and test motor and sensory function in the limbs. Ask about paresthesia. Check for ataxia or tremors and for speech and vision deficits. Test for Chvostek's and Trousseau's signs and for carpopedal spasm. Ask about vomiting or altered bladder habits. Be sure to take the patient's vital signs.

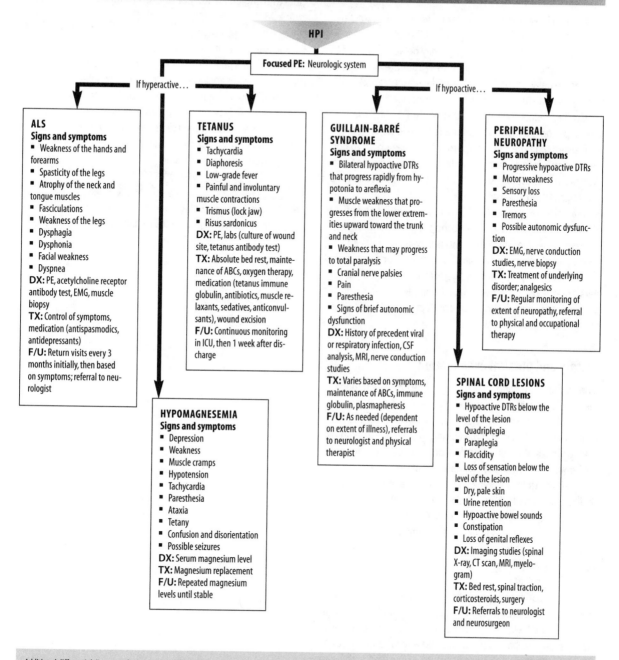

HPI

Focused PE: Neurologic system

If hyperactive...

If hypoactive...

ALS
Signs and symptoms
- Weakness of the hands and forearms
- Spasticity of the legs
- Atrophy of the neck and tongue muscles
- Fasciculations
- Weakness of the legs
- Dysphagia
- Dysphonia
- Facial weakness
- Dyspnea

DX: PE, acetylcholine receptor antibody test, EMG, muscle biopsy
TX: Control of symptoms, medication (antispasmodics, antidepressants)
F/U: Return visits every 3 months initially, then based on symptoms; referral to neurologist

TETANUS
Signs and symptoms
- Tachycardia
- Diaphoresis
- Low-grade fever
- Painful and involuntary muscle contractions
- Trismus (lock jaw)
- Risus sardonicus

DX: PE, labs (culture of wound site, tetanus antibody test)
TX: Absolute bed rest, maintenance of ABCs, oxygen therapy, medication (tetanus immune globulin, antibiotics, muscle relaxants, sedatives, anticonvulsants), wound excision
F/U: Continuous monitoring in ICU, then 1 week after discharge

HYPOMAGNESEMIA
Signs and symptoms
- Depression
- Weakness
- Muscle cramps
- Hypotension
- Tachycardia
- Paresthesia
- Ataxia
- Tetany
- Confusion and disorientation
- Possible seizures

DX: Serum magnesium level
TX: Magnesium replacement
F/U: Repeated magnesium levels until stable

GUILLAIN-BARRÉ SYNDROME
Signs and symptoms
- Bilateral hypoactive DTRs that progress rapidly from hypotonia to areflexia
- Muscle weakness that progresses from the lower extremities upward toward the trunk and neck
- Weakness that may progress to total paralysis
- Cranial nerve palsies
- Pain
- Paresthesia
- Signs of brief autonomic dysfunction

DX: History of precedent viral or respiratory infection, CSF analysis, MRI, nerve conduction studies
TX: Varies based on symptoms, maintenance of ABCs, immune globulin, plasmapheresis
F/U: As needed (dependent on extent of illness), referrals to neurologist and physical therapist

PERIPHERAL NEUROPATHY
Signs and symptoms
- Progressive hypoactive DTRs
- Motor weakness
- Sensory loss
- Paresthesia
- Tremors
- Possible autonomic dysfunction

DX: EMG, nerve conduction studies, nerve biopsy
TX: Treatment of underlying disorder; analgesics
F/U: Regular monitoring of extent of neuropathy, referral to physical and occupational therapy

SPINAL CORD LESIONS
Signs and symptoms
- Hypoactive DTRs below the level of the lesion
- Quadriplegia
- Paraplegia
- Flaccidity
- Loss of sensation below the level of the lesion
- Dry, pale skin
- Urine retention
- Hypoactive bowel sounds
- Constipation
- Loss of genital reflexes

DX: Imaging studies (spinal X-ray, CT scan, MRI, myelogram)
TX: Bed rest, spinal traction, corticosteroids, surgery
F/U: Referrals to neurologist and neurosurgeon

Additional differential diagnoses for hyperactive reflexes: brain tumor ▪ hepatic encephalopathy ▪ hypocalcemia ▪ hypothermia ▪ multiple sclerosis ▪ preeclampsia ▪ spinal cord lesion ▪ stroke

---

Additional differential diagnoses for hypoactive reflexes: botulism ▪ cerebellar dysfunction ▪ Eaton-Lambert syndrome ▪ polymyositis ▪ syringomyelia ▪ tabes dorsalis

---

Other causes for hypoactive reflexes: barbiturates and paralyzants (such as pancuronium and curare)

Depression

Depression is a mental state of depressed mood characterized by feelings of sadness, despair, and loss of interest or pleasure in activities. These feelings may be accompanied by somatic complaints, such as changes in appetite, sleep disturbances, restlessness or lethargy, and decreased concentration. Thoughts of death or suicide may also occur.

Clinical depression must be distinguished from "the blues," periodic bouts of dysphoria that are less persistent and severe than the clinical disorder. The criterion for major depression is one or more episodes of depressed mood, or decreased interest or the ability to take pleasure in all or most activities, lasting at least 2 weeks.

Major depression strikes 10% to 15% of adults and affects all racial, ethnic, age, and socioeconomic groups. It's twice as common in women as in men and is especially prevalent among adolescents. Depression has numerous causes, including genetic and family history, medical and psychiatric disorders, and the use of certain drugs. A complete psychiatric and physical examination should be conducted to exclude possible medical causes.

History and physical examination

During the examination, try to determine how the patient feels about herself, her family, and her environment. Your goal is to explore the nature of her depression, the extent to which other factors affect it, and her coping mechanisms. Begin by asking what's bothering her. How does her current mood differ from her usual mood? Then ask her to describe the way she feels about herself. What are her plans and dreams? How realistic are they? Is she generally satisfied with what she has accomplished in her work, relationships, and other interests? Ask about any changes in her social interactions, sleep patterns, normal activities, or ability to make decisions and concentrate. Explore drug and alcohol use. Listen for clues that she may be suicidal.

Ask the patient about her family — its patterns of interaction and characteristic responses to success and failure. What part does she feel she plays in her family life? Find out if other family members have been depressed, and whether anyone important to the patient has been sick or has died in the past year. Finally, ask the patient about her environment. Has her lifestyle changed in the past month? Six months? Year? When she's feeling blue, where does she go and what does she do to feel better? Find out how she feels about her role in the community and the resources that are available to her. Try to determine if she has an adequate support network to help her cope with her depression.

Always ask patients with depressive symptoms about suicidal thinking and history of suicide attempts.

WOMEN'S HEALTH TIPS

- *Because emotional lability is normal in adolescence, depression can be difficult to assess and diagnose in teenagers. Clues to underlying depression may include somatic complaints, sexual promiscuity, poor grades, and abuse of alcohol or drugs.*
- *Use of a family systems model often helps determine the cause of depression in adolescents. Once family roles are determined, family therapy or group therapy with peers may help the patient overcome her depression.*

ELDER CARE CUE

Depressed older adults at highest risk for suicide are those who are age 85 or older, have high self-esteem, and need to be in control.

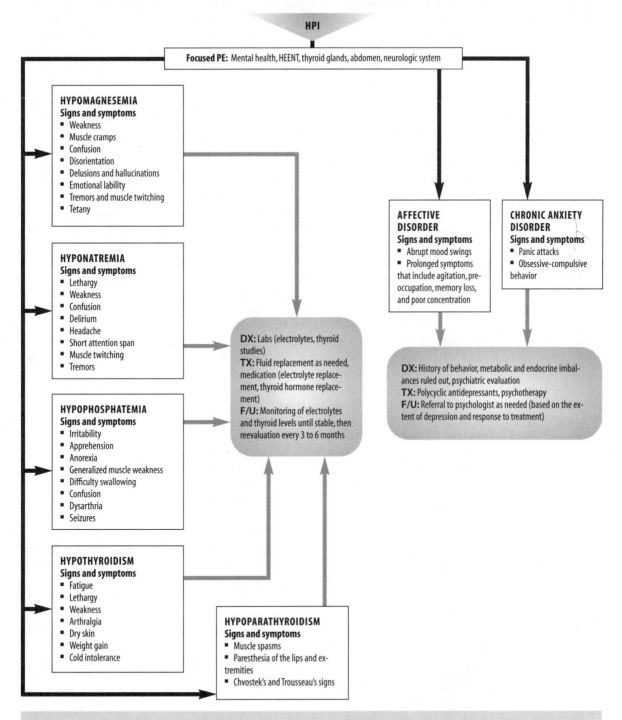

HPI

Focused PE: Mental health, HEENT, thyroid glands, abdomen, neurologic system

HYPOMAGNESEMIA
Signs and symptoms
- Weakness
- Muscle cramps
- Confusion
- Disorientation
- Delusions and hallucinations
- Emotional lability
- Tremors and muscle twitching
- Tetany

HYPONATREMIA
Signs and symptoms
- Lethargy
- Weakness
- Confusion
- Delirium
- Headache
- Short attention span
- Muscle twitching
- Tremors

HYPOPHOSPHATEMIA
Signs and symptoms
- Irritability
- Apprehension
- Anorexia
- Generalized muscle weakness
- Difficulty swallowing
- Confusion
- Dysarthria
- Seizures

HYPOTHYROIDISM
Signs and symptoms
- Fatigue
- Lethargy
- Weakness
- Arthralgia
- Dry skin
- Weight gain
- Cold intolerance

HYPOPARATHYROIDISM
Signs and symptoms
- Muscle spasms
- Paresthesia of the lips and extremities
- Chvostek's and Trousseau's signs

DX: Labs (electrolytes, thyroid studies)
TX: Fluid replacement as needed, medication (electrolyte replacement, thyroid hormone replacement)
F/U: Monitoring of electrolytes and thyroid levels until stable, then reevaluation every 3 to 6 months

AFFECTIVE DISORDER
Signs and symptoms
- Abrupt mood swings
- Prolonged symptoms that include agitation, preoccupation, memory loss, and poor concentration

CHRONIC ANXIETY DISORDER
Signs and symptoms
- Panic attacks
- Obsessive-compulsive behavior

DX: History of behavior, metabolic and endocrine imbalances ruled out, psychiatric evaluation
TX: Polycyclic antidepressants, psychotherapy
F/U: Referral to psychologist as needed (based on the extent of depression and response to treatment)

Other causes: alcohol abuse ▪ antiarrhythmics (such as disopyramide) ▪ anticonvulsants (such as diazepam) ▪ antiparkinsonian drugs ▪ barbiturates ▪ beta-adrenergic blockers (such as propranolol) ▪ levodopa ▪ indomethacin ▪ cycloserine ▪ corticosteroids ▪ centrally-acting antihypertensives (such as reserpine [common in high dosages], methyldopa, and clonidine) ▪ chemotherapeutics (such as asparaginase) ▪ digoxin ▪ NSAIDs ▪ oral contraceptives

Diaphoresis

Diaphoresis is profuse sweating — at times, amounting to more than 1 L (1.1 qt) of sweat per hour. This sign represents an autonomic nervous system response to physical or psychogenic stress or to fever or high environmental temperature. When caused by stress, diaphoresis may be generalized or limited to the palms of the hands, soles of the feet, and forehead. When caused by fever or high environmental temperature, it's usually generalized.

Diaphoresis usually begins abruptly and may be accompanied by other autonomic system signs, such as tachycardia and increased blood pressure. However, this sign also varies with age because sweat glands function immaturely in infants and are less active in elderly patients. As a result, these age-groups may fail to display diaphoresis associated with its common causes. Intermittent diaphoresis may accompany chronic disorders characterized by recurrent fever; isolated diaphoresis may mark an episode of acute pain or fever. Night sweats may characterize intermittent fever because body temperature tends to return to normal between 2 a.m. and 4 a.m. before rising again. (Temperature is usually lowest around 6 a.m.)

When caused by high external temperature, diaphoresis is a normal response. Acclimatization usually requires several days of exposure to high temperatures; during this process, diaphoresis helps maintain normal body temperature. Diaphoresis also commonly occurs during menopause, preceded by a sensation of intense heat (a hot flash). Other causes include exercise or exertion that accelerates metabolism, creating internal heat, and mild to moderate anxiety that helps initiate the fight-or-flight response.

History and physical examination

If the patient is diaphoretic, quickly rule out the possibility of a life-threatening cause, such as hypoglycemia or myocardial infarction. Begin the history by having the patient describe his chief complaint. Then explore associated signs and symptoms. Note general fatigue and weakness. Does the patient have insomnia, headache, and changes in vision or hearing? Is he often dizzy? Does he have palpitations? Ask about pleuritic pain, cough, sputum, difficulty breathing, nausea, vomiting, abdominal pain, and altered bowel or bladder habits. Ask the female patient about amenorrhea and changes in her menstrual cycle. Is she menopausal? Ask about paresthesia, muscle cramps or stiffness, and joint pain. Has she noticed any changes in elimination habits? Note any weight loss or gain. Has the patient had to change her glove or shoe size lately?

Complete the history by asking about travel to tropical countries. Note recent exposure to high environmental temperatures or to pesticides. Did the patient recently experience an insect bite? Check for a history of partial gastrectomy or of drug or alcohol abuse. Finally, obtain a thorough drug history.

Next, perform a physical examination. First, determine the extent of diaphoresis by inspecting the trunk and extremities as well as the palms, soles, and forehead. Also, check the patient's clothing for dampness. Ask whether diaphoresis occurs during the day or at night. Observe for flushing, abnormal skin texture or lesions, and an increased amount of coarse body hair. Note poor skin turgor and dry mucous membranes. Check for splinter hemorrhages and Plummer's nails (separation of the fingernail ends from the nail beds).

Then evaluate the patient's mental status and take his vital signs. Observe for fasciculations and flaccid paralysis. Be alert for seizures. Note the patient's facial expression and examine the eyes for pupillary dilation or constriction, exophthalmos, and excessive tearing. Test visual fields. Also check for hearing loss and for tooth or gum disease. Percuss the lungs for dullness and auscultate for crackles, diminished or bronchial breath sounds, and increased vocal fremitus. Look for decreased respiratory excursion. Palpate for lymphadenopathy and hepatosplenomegaly.

HPI

Focused PE: All systems

MI
Signs and symptoms
- Chest tightness or pressure
- Pain that may radiate to the neck, jaw, and arms
- Dyspnea
- Nausea and vomiting
- Tachycardia
- Palpitations
- Dizziness
- Syncope
- Gallops and murmurs
- Feeling of impending doom
- Pain that may escalate to crushing
- Hypotension or hypertension
- Pallor
- Clammy skin

DX: Labs (serial cardiac enzymes, troponin, myoglobin, electrolytes), imaging studies (echocardiogram, CXR, Tc-99m sestamibi scan), ECG, cardiac catheterization
TX: Maintenance of ABCs; oxygen therapy; medication (based on severity of myocardial involvement and medical history — antithrombic agents, vasodilators, analgesics, beta-adrenergic agents, thrombolytics, anticoagulants, platelet aggregation inhibitors, anxiolytics, antiarrhythmics); low-fat, low-sodium diet; PCI; surgery
F/U: Referral to cardiologist

Common signs and symptoms
- Profuse diaphoresis that leads to dry skin
- Ashen appearance
- Poor skin turgor
- Dry mucus membranes
- Severe thirst
- Headache
- Nausea and vomiting

HEATSTROKE
Additional signs and symptoms
- Exhaustion
- Confusion and disorientation
- Extremely hot, flushed skin
- Coma
- Circulatory collapse
- Core temperature > 105° F (40.6° C)
- Irrational and agitated behavior
- Aggressive behavior
- Seizure

HEAT EXHAUSTION
Additional signs and symptoms
- Core temperature that's elevated but < 103° F (39.4° C)

DX: PE, temperature, labs (electrolytes, BUN, creatinine)
TX: I.V. hydration, careful electrolyte monitoring, maintenance of ABCs, hemodynamic monitoring, rapid cooling with ice packs, cooling blanket
F/U: Reevaluation 1 week after hospitalization; investigation of underlying cause

PNEUMONIA
Signs and symptoms
- Intermittent diaphoresis
- Fever
- Productive cough
- Pleuritic pain
- Headache
- Fatigue
- Myalgia
- Bronchial breath sounds

DX: Labs (sputum culture, CBC), CXR
TX: Increased fluid intake, medication (antibiotics, antipyretics, analgesics)
F/U: Reevaluation 48 to 72 hours, then on completion of treatment

HYPOGLYCEMIA
Signs and symptoms
- Slow mentation
- Irritability
- Tremors
- Hypotension
- Dizziness
- Blurred vision
- Complaint of hunger
- Decreased LOC

DX: PE, history of insulin use, serum glucose
TX: Orange juice, I.V. 50% dextrose
F/U: Referral to endocrinologist

AUTONOMIC HYPERREFLEXIA
Signs and symptoms
- Loss of motor tone
- Blurred vision
- Pounding headache
- Dramatically elevated BP
- Goose pimples
- Bradycardia

DX: PE, identification of stimulus
TX: Management of cause, maintenance of ABCs
F/U: Reevaluation as needed (based on cause), monitoring of patient with spinal cord injury and teaching of methods to treat stimulus

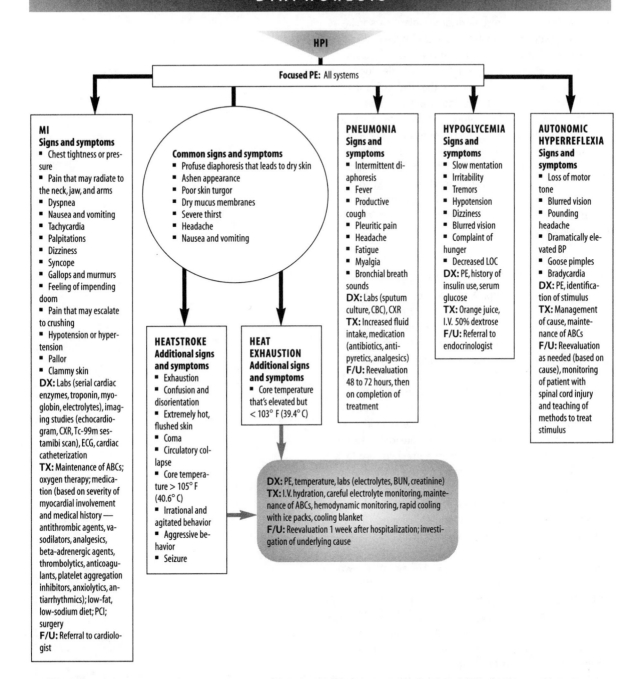

Additional differential diagnoses: acromegaly ▪ AIDS ▪ anxiety disorders ▪ drug and alcohol withdrawal syndromes ▪ empyema ▪ envenomation ▪ heart failure ▪ Hodgkin's disease ▪ immunoblastic lymphadenopathy ▪ infective endocarditis ▪ liver or lung abscess ▪ malaria ▪ Ménière's disease ▪ pheochromocytoma ▪ relapsing fever ▪ tetanus ▪ thyrotoxicosis ▪ tuberculosis

Other causes: acetaminophen and aspirin poisoning ▪ antipsychotics ▪ antipyretics ▪ dumping syndrome ▪ pesticide poisoning ▪ sympathomimetics ▪ thyroid hormone

Diarrhea

Usually a chief sign of intestinal disorders, diarrhea is an increase in the volume of stools compared with the patient's normal bowel habits. It varies in severity and may be acute or chronic. Acute diarrhea may result from acute infection, food sensitivities, stress, fecal impaction, or the effects of drugs. Chronic diarrhea may result from food allergies, chronic infection, obstructive and inflammatory bowel disease, malabsorption syndromes, certain endocrine disorders, and the effects of GI surgery. Periodic diarrhea may result from food intolerance or from ingestion of spicy or high-fiber foods or caffeine.

One or more pathophysiologic mechanisms may contribute to diarrhea. The fluid and electrolyte imbalances it produces may precipitate life-threatening arrhythmias or hypovolemic shock.

History and physical examination

If the patient's diarrhea is profuse, check for signs of shock — tachycardia, hypotension, and cool, pale, clammy skin. Check for electrolyte imbalances, and look for an irregular pulse, muscle weakness, anorexia, and nausea and vomiting. Keep emergency resuscitation equipment handy.

If the patient isn't in shock, proceed with a brief physical examination. Check the patient's weight. Evaluate hydration, check skin turgor, and take blood pressure with the patient lying, sitting, and standing. Inspect the abdomen for diffuse distention. Auscultate bowel sounds and palpate for tenderness. Take the patient's temperature and note any chills. Also, look for a rash. Conduct a rectal examination and a pelvic examination if indicated.

Explore signs and symptoms associated with diarrhea. Does the patient have abdominal pain and cramps? Difficulty breathing? Is he weak or fatigued? Find out his drug history. Has he had GI surgery or radiation therapy recently? Ask the patient to briefly describe his diet. Does he have any known food allergies? Lastly, find out if he's under unusual stress.

PEDIATRIC POINTERS

- *Diarrhea in children frequently results from infection, although chronic diarrhea may result from malabsorption syndrome, anatomic defects, or allergies.*
- *Because dehydration and electrolyte imbalance occur rapidly in children, diarrhea can be life-threatening.*

ELDER CARE CUE

In the elderly patient with new-onset segmental colitis, always consider ischemia before diagnosing the patient as having Crohn's disease.

DIARRHEA

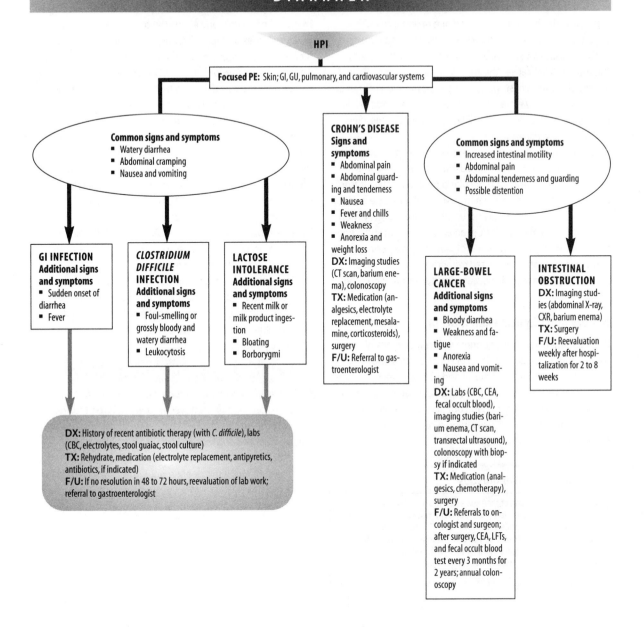

HPI

Focused PE: Skin; GI, GU, pulmonary, and cardiovascular systems

Common signs and symptoms
- Watery diarrhea
- Abdominal cramping
- Nausea and vomiting

CROHN'S DISEASE
Signs and symptoms
- Abdominal pain
- Abdominal guarding and tenderness
- Nausea
- Fever and chills
- Weakness
- Anorexia and weight loss

DX: Imaging studies (CT scan, barium enema), colonoscopy
TX: Medication (analgesics, electrolyte replacement, mesalamine, corticosteroids), surgery
F/U: Referral to gastroenterologist

Common signs and symptoms
- Increased intestinal motility
- Abdominal pain
- Abdominal tenderness and guarding
- Possible distention

GI INFECTION
Additional signs and symptoms
- Sudden onset of diarrhea
- Fever

CLOSTRIDIUM DIFFICILE INFECTION
Additional signs and symptoms
- Foul-smelling or grossly bloody and watery diarrhea
- Leukocytosis

LACTOSE INTOLERANCE
Additional signs and symptoms
- Recent milk or milk product ingestion
- Bloating
- Borborygmi

LARGE-BOWEL CANCER
Additional signs and symptoms
- Bloody diarrhea
- Weakness and fatigue
- Anorexia
- Nausea and vomiting

DX: Labs (CBC, CEA, fecal occult blood), imaging studies (barium enema, CT scan, transrectal ultrasound), colonoscopy with biopsy if indicated
TX: Medication (analgesics, chemotherapy), surgery
F/U: Referrals to oncologist and surgeon; after surgery, CEA, LFTs, and fecal occult blood test every 3 months for 2 years; annual colonoscopy

INTESTINAL OBSTRUCTION
DX: Imaging studies (abdominal X-ray, CXR, barium enema)
TX: Surgery
F/U: Reevaluation weekly after hospitalization for 2 to 8 weeks

DX: History of recent antibiotic therapy (with *C. difficile*), labs (CBC, electrolytes, stool guaiac, stool culture)
TX: Rehydrate, medication (electrolyte replacement, antipyretics, antibiotics, if indicated)
F/U: If no resolution in 48 to 72 hours, reevaluation of lab work; referral to gastroenterologist

---

Additional differential diagnoses: acute appendicitis ▪ carcinoid syndrome ▪ irritable bowel syndrome ▪ ischemic bowel disease ▪ lead poisoning ▪ malabsorption syndrome ▪ pseudomembranous enterocolitis ▪ rotavirus gastroenteritis ▪ thyrotoxicosis

---

Other causes: antibiotics (ampicillin, cephalosporins, tetracyclines, clindamycin) ▪ colchicine ▪ dantrolene ▪ dehydration ▪ digoxin and quinidine (in high doses) ▪ ethacrynic acid ▪ gastrectomy ▪ gastroenterostomy ▪ guanethidine ▪ herbal medicines (ginkgo biloba, ginseng, licorice) ▪ high-dose radiation therapy ▪ lactulose ▪ laxative abuse ▪ magnesium-containing antacids ▪ mefenamic acid ▪ methotrexate ▪ metyrosine ▪ pyloroplasty

Diplopia

Diplopia is double vision — seeing one object as two. This symptom results when extraocular muscles fail to work together, causing images to fall on noncorresponding parts of the retinas. What causes this muscle incoordination? Orbital lesions, the effects of surgery, or impaired function of cranial nerves that supply extraocular muscles (oculomotor, CN III; trochlear, CN IV; abducens, CN VI) may be responsible. (See *Testing extraocular muscles*.)

Diplopia usually begins intermittently and affects near or far vision exclusively. It can be classified as monocular or binocular. More common binocular diplopia may result from ocular deviation or displacement, extraocular muscle palsies, or psychoneurosis, or it may occur after retinal surgery. Monocular diplopia may result from an early cataract, retinal edema or scarring, iridodialysis, a subluxated lens, a poorly fitting contact lens, or an uncorrected refractive error such as astigmatism. Diplopia may also occur in hysteria or malingering.

History and physical examination

If the patient complains of double vision, first check his neurologic status. Evaluate his level of consciousness, pupil size and response to light, and motor and sensory function. Then take his vital signs. Briefly ask about associated symptoms, especially a severe headache. Find out about associated neurologic symptoms first because diplopia can accompany serious disorders.

Next, continue with a more detailed examination. Find out when the patient first noticed diplopia. Are the images side-by-side (horizontal), one above the other (vertical), or a combination? Does diplopia affect near or far vision? Does it affect certain directions of gaze? Ask if diplopia has worsened, remained the same, or subsided. Does its severity change throughout the day? Diplopia that worsens or appears in the evening may indicate myasthenia gravis. Find out if the patient can correct diplopia by tilting his head. If so, ask him to show you. (If the patient has a fourth nerve lesion, tilting of the head toward the opposite shoulder causes compensatory tilting of the unaffected eye. If he has incomplete sixth nerve palsy, tilting of the head toward the side of the paralyzed muscle may relax the affected lateral rectus muscle.)

Explore associated symptoms such as eye pain. Ask about hypertension, diabetes mellitus, allergies, and thyroid, neurologic, or muscular disorders. Also, note a history of extraocular muscle disorders, trauma, or eye surgery.

Observe the patient for ocular deviation, ptosis, proptosis, lid edema, and conjunctival injection. Distinguish monocular from binocular diplopia by asking the patient to occlude one eye. If he still sees double, he has monocular diplopia. Test visual acuity and extraocular muscles.

PEDIATRIC POINTERS

- *Strabismus, which can be congenital or acquired at an early age, produces diplopia; however, in young children, the brain rapidly compensates for double vision by suppressing one image, so diplopia is a rare complaint.*
- *School-age children who complain of double vision require a careful examination to rule out serious disorders such as brain tumor.*

Testing extraocular muscles

The coordinated action of six muscles controls eyeball movements. To test the function of each muscle and the cranial nerve (CN) that innervates it, ask the patient to look in the direction controlled by that muscle. The six directions you can test make up the *cardinal fields of gaze*. The patient's inability to turn the eye in the designated direction indicates muscle weakness or paralysis.

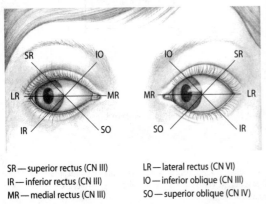

SR — superior rectus (CN III)
IR — inferior rectus (CN III)
MR — medial rectus (CN III)
LR — lateral rectus (CN VI)
IO — inferior oblique (CN III)
SO — superior oblique (CN IV)

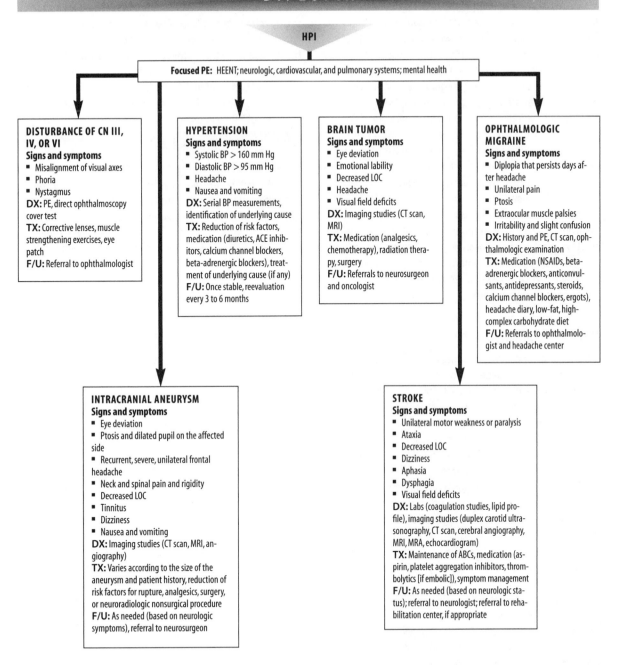

HPI

Focused PE: HEENT; neurologic, cardiovascular, and pulmonary systems; mental health

DISTURBANCE OF CN III, IV, OR VI
Signs and symptoms
- Misalignment of visual axes
- Phoria
- Nystagmus

DX: PE, direct ophthalmoscopy cover test
TX: Corrective lenses, muscle strengthening exercises, eye patch
F/U: Referral to ophthalmologist

HYPERTENSION
Signs and symptoms
- Systolic BP > 160 mm Hg
- Diastolic BP > 95 mm Hg
- Headache
- Nausea and vomiting

DX: Serial BP measurements, identification of underlying cause
TX: Reduction of risk factors, medication (diuretics, ACE inhibitors, calcium channel blockers, beta-adrenergic blockers), treatment of underlying cause (if any)
F/U: Once stable, reevaluation every 3 to 6 months

BRAIN TUMOR
Signs and symptoms
- Eye deviation
- Emotional lability
- Decreased LOC
- Headache
- Visual field deficits

DX: Imaging studies (CT scan, MRI)
TX: Medication (analgesics, chemotherapy), radiation therapy, surgery
F/U: Referrals to neurosurgeon and oncologist

OPHTHALMOLOGIC MIGRAINE
Signs and symptoms
- Diplopia that persists days after headache
- Unilateral pain
- Ptosis
- Extraocular muscle palsies
- Irritability and slight confusion

DX: History and PE, CT scan, ophthalmologic examination
TX: Medication (NSAIDs, beta-adrenergic blockers, anticonvulsants, antidepressants, steroids, calcium channel blockers, ergots), headache diary, low-fat, high-complex carbohydrate diet
F/U: Referrals to ophthalmologist and headache center

INTRACRANIAL ANEURYSM
Signs and symptoms
- Eye deviation
- Ptosis and dilated pupil on the affected side
- Recurrent, severe, unilateral frontal headache
- Neck and spinal pain and rigidity
- Decreased LOC
- Tinnitus
- Dizziness
- Nausea and vomiting

DX: Imaging studies (CT scan, MRI, angiography)
TX: Varies according to the size of the aneurysm and patient history, reduction of risk factors for rupture, analgesics, surgery, or neuroradiologic nonsurgical procedure
F/U: As needed (based on neurologic symptoms), referral to neurosurgeon

STROKE
Signs and symptoms
- Unilateral motor weakness or paralysis
- Ataxia
- Decreased LOC
- Dizziness
- Aphasia
- Dysphagia
- Visual field deficits

DX: Labs (coagulation studies, lipid profile), imaging studies (duplex carotid ultrasonography, CT scan, cerebral angiography, MRI, MRA, echocardiogram)
TX: Maintenance of ABCs, medication (aspirin, platelet aggregation inhibitors, thrombolytics [if embolic]), symptom management
F/U: As needed (based on neurologic status); referral to neurologist; referral to rehabilitation center, if appropriate

Additional differential diagnoses: alcohol intoxication ▪ botulism ▪ cavernous sinus thrombosis ▪ diabetes mellitus ▪ encephalitis ▪ head injury ▪ multiple sclerosis ▪ myasthenia gravis ▪ orbital blowout fracture ▪ orbital cellulitis ▪ orbital tumors ▪ thyrotoxicosis

Other cause: eye surgery

Dizziness

A common symptom, dizziness is a sensation of imbalance or faintness, sometimes associated with giddiness, weakness, confusion, and blurred or double vision. Episodes of dizziness are usually brief; they may be mild or severe with abrupt or gradual onset. Dizziness may be aggravated by standing up quickly and alleviated by lying down and by rest.

Dizziness typically results from inadequate blood flow and oxygen supply to the cerebrum and spinal cord. It may occur in anxiety, in respiratory and cardiovascular disorders, and in postconcussion syndrome. It's a key symptom in certain serious disorders, such as hypertension and vertebrobasilar artery insufficiency.

Dizziness is often confused with vertigo — a sensation of revolving in space or of surroundings revolving about oneself. However, unlike dizziness, vertigo is often accompanied by nausea, vomiting, nystagmus, staggering gait, and tinnitus or hearing loss. Dizziness and vertigo may occur together, as in postconcussion syndrome.

History and physical examination

If the patient complains of dizziness, first determine its severity and onset. Ask the patient to describe it. Is the dizziness associated with headache or blurred vision? Next, take the patient's vital signs and ask about a history of high blood pressure. Tell the patient to lie down, and recheck his vital signs. Ask about a history of diabetes and cardiovascular disease. Is the patient taking drugs prescribed for high blood pressure? If so, when did he take his last dose?

If the patient's blood pressure is normal, obtain a more complete history. Ask about myocardial infarction, heart failure, or atherosclerosis, which may predispose the patient to cardiac arrhythmias, hypertension, and a transient ischemic attack. Does he have a history of anemia, chronic obstructive pulmonary disease, anxiety disorders, or head injury? Obtain a complete drug history.

Next, explore the patient's dizziness fully. How often does it occur? How long does each episode last? Does the dizziness abate spontaneously? Does it lead to loss of consciousness? Find out if dizziness is triggered by sitting or standing up suddenly or stooping over. Does being in a crowd make the patient feel dizzy? Ask about emotional stress. Has the patient been irritable or anxious lately? Does he have insomnia or difficulty concentrating? During the interview, look for fidgeting and eyelid twitching. Does the patient startle easily? Also, ask about palpitations, chest pain, diaphoresis, shortness of breath, and chronic cough.

Next, perform a physical examination. Begin with a quick neurocheck, assessing level of consciousness, motor and sensory functions, and reflexes. Then inspect for poor skin turgor and dry mucous membranes, signs of dehydration. Auscultate heart rate and rhythm. Inspect for barrel chest, clubbing, cyanosis, and use of accessory muscles. Also auscultate breath sounds. Take the patient's blood pressure while he's lying, sitting, and standing to check for orthostatic hypotension. Test capillary refill time in the extremities, and palpate for edema.

PEDIATRIC POINTERS

- *Dizziness is less common in children than in adults.*
- *Children may have difficulty describing this symptom and instead complain of tiredness, stomachache, or feeling sick. If you suspect dizziness, assess for vertigo as well.*
- *A more common symptom in children, vertigo may result from vision disorders, ear infections, and the effects of antibiotics.*

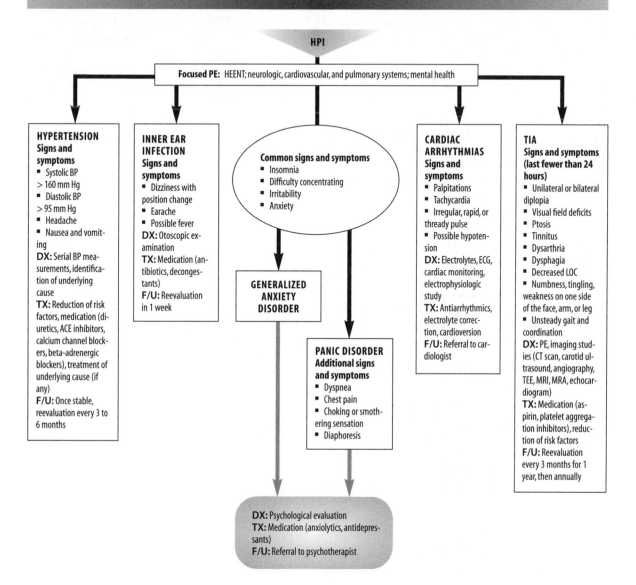

HPI

Focused PE: HEENT; neurologic, cardiovascular, and pulmonary systems; mental health

HYPERTENSION
Signs and symptoms
- Systolic BP > 160 mm Hg
- Diastolic BP > 95 mm Hg
- Headache
- Nausea and vomiting

DX: Serial BP measurements, identification of underlying cause
TX: Reduction of risk factors, medication (diuretics, ACE inhibitors, calcium channel blockers, beta-adrenergic blockers), treatment of underlying cause (if any)
F/U: Once stable, reevaluation every 3 to 6 months

INNER EAR INFECTION
Signs and symptoms
- Dizziness with position change
- Earache
- Possible fever

DX: Otoscopic examination
TX: Medication (antibiotics, decongestants)
F/U: Reevaluation in 1 week

Common signs and symptoms
- Insomnia
- Difficulty concentrating
- Irritability
- Anxiety

GENERALIZED ANXIETY DISORDER

PANIC DISORDER
Additional signs and symptoms
- Dyspnea
- Chest pain
- Choking or smothering sensation
- Diaphoresis

CARDIAC ARRHYTHMIAS
Signs and symptoms
- Palpitations
- Tachycardia
- Irregular, rapid, or thready pulse
- Possible hypotension

DX: Electrolytes, ECG, cardiac monitoring, electrophysiologic study
TX: Antiarrhythmics, electrolyte correction, cardioversion
F/U: Referral to cardiologist

TIA
Signs and symptoms (last fewer than 24 hours)
- Unilateral or bilateral diplopia
- Visual field deficits
- Ptosis
- Tinnitus
- Dysarthria
- Dysphagia
- Decreased LOC
- Numbness, tingling, weakness on one side of the face, arm, or leg
- Unsteady gait and coordination

DX: PE, imaging studies (CT scan, carotid ultrasound, angiography, TEE, MRI, MRA, echocardiogram)
TX: Medication (aspirin, platelet aggregation inhibitors), reduction of risk factors
F/U: Reevaluation every 3 months for 1 year, then annually

DX: Psychological evaluation
TX: Medication (anxiolytics, antidepressants)
F/U: Referral to psychotherapist

Additional differential diagnoses: carotid sinus hypersensitivity ▪ emphysema ▪ hyperventilation syndrome ▪ orthostatic hypotension ▪ postconcussion syndrome

Other causes: antianxiety drugs ▪ antihistamines ▪ antihypertensives ▪ CNS depressants ▪ decongestants ▪ narcotics ▪ St. John's wort ▪ vasodilators

Doll's eye sign, absent

An indicator of brain stem dysfunction, the absence of the doll's eye sign is detected by rapid, gentle turning of the patient's head from side to side. The eyes remain fixed in midposition, instead of moving laterally toward the side opposite the direction the head is turned. (See *Testing for absent doll's eye sign.*)

The absence of doll's eye sign, also known as negative oculocephalic reflex, indicates injury to the midbrain or pons, involving cranial nerves III, VI, and VIII. It typically accompanies coma caused by lesions of the cerebellum and brain stem. This sign usually can't be relied upon in a conscious patient because he can control eye movements voluntarily. Absent doll's eye sign is necessary for a diagnosis of brain death.

A variant of absent doll's eye sign that develops gradually is known as *abnormal doll's eye sign:* Because conjugate eye movement is lost, one eye may move laterally while the other remains fixed or moves in the opposite direction. An abnormal doll's eye sign usually accompanies metabolic coma or increased intracranial pressure (ICP). Associated brain stem dysfunction may be reversible or may progress to deeper coma with absent doll's eye sign.

History and physical examination

After detecting an absent doll's eye sign, perform a neurologic examination. First, evaluate the patient's level of consciousness, using the Glasgow Coma Scale. Note decerebrate or decorticate posture. Examine the pupils for size, equality, and response to light. Check for signs of increased ICP — increased blood pressure, increasing pulse pressure, and bradycardia.

Testing for absent doll's eye sign

To evaluate the patient's oculocephalic reflex, hold her upper eyelids open and quickly (but gently) turn her head from side to side, noting eye movements with each head turn.

In absent doll's eye sign, the eyes remain fixed in midposition.

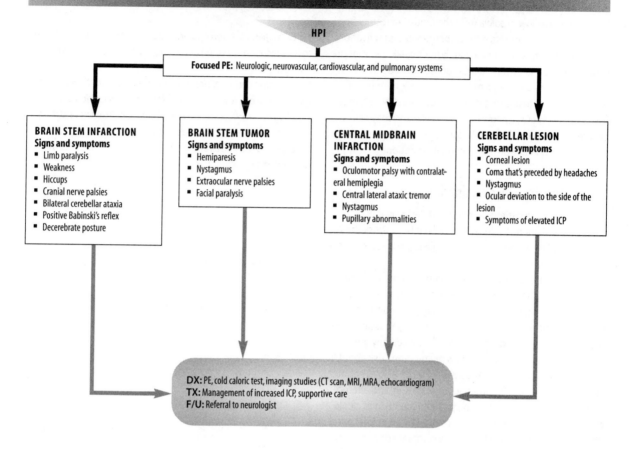

HPI

Focused PE: Neurologic, neurovascular, cardiovascular, and pulmonary systems

BRAIN STEM INFARCTION
Signs and symptoms
- Limb paralysis
- Weakness
- Hiccups
- Cranial nerve palsies
- Bilateral cerebellar ataxia
- Positive Babinski's reflex
- Decerebrate posture

BRAIN STEM TUMOR
Signs and symptoms
- Hemiparesis
- Nystagmus
- Extraocular nerve palsies
- Facial paralysis

CENTRAL MIDBRAIN INFARCTION
Signs and symptoms
- Oculomotor palsy with contralateral hemiplegia
- Central lateral ataxic tremor
- Nystagmus
- Pupillary abnormalities

CEREBELLAR LESION
Signs and symptoms
- Corneal lesion
- Coma that's preceded by headaches
- Nystagmus
- Ocular deviation to the side of the lesion
- Symptoms of elevated ICP

DX: PE, cold caloric test, imaging studies (CT scan, MRI, MRA, echocardiogram)
TX: Management of increased ICP, supportive care
F/U: Referral to neurologist

Other cause: barbiturates

Drooling

Drooling — the flow of saliva from the mouth — results from a failure to swallow or retain saliva, or from excess salivation. It may stem from facial muscle paralysis or weakness that prevents mouth closure, from neuromuscular disorders or local pain that causes dysphagia or, less commonly, from the effects of drugs or toxins that induce salivation. Drooling may be scant or copious (up to 1 L [1.1 qt] daily) and may cause circumoral irritation. Because it signals an inability to handle secretions, drooling warns of potential aspiration.

History and physical examination

If you observe the patient drooling, first determine its amount. Is it scant or copious? When did it begin? Ask the patient if his pillow is wet in the morning. Also, inspect for circumoral irritation.

Then explore associated signs and symptoms. Ask about sore throat and difficulty swallowing, chewing, speaking, or breathing. Have the patient describe any pain, numbness, tingling, or stiffness in the face and neck and any muscle weakness in the face and extremities. Has he noticed any mental status changes, such as drowsiness or agitation? Ask about changes in vision, hearing, and sense of taste. Also ask about anorexia, weight loss, fatigue, nausea, vomiting, and altered bowel or bladder habits. Has the patient recently had a cold or other infection? Was he recently bitten by an animal or exposed to pesticides? Finally, obtain a complete drug history.

Next, perform a physical examination. Take vital signs. Inspect for signs of facial paralysis or abnormal expression. Examine the mouth and neck for swelling, the throat for edema and redness, and the tonsils for exudate. Note foul breath odor. Examine the tongue for bilateral furrowing (trident tongue). Look for pallor and skin lesions and for frontal baldness. Carefully assess any bite or puncture marks.

Assess cranial nerves II through VII, IX, and X. Then check pupillary size and response to light. Assess the patient's speech. Evaluate muscle strength and palpate for tenderness or atrophy. Also palpate for lymphadenopathy, especially in the cervical area. Test for poor balance, hyperreflexia, and positive Babinski's reflex. Also assess sensory function for paresthesia.

PEDIATRIC POINTERS

- *Normally, an infant can't control saliva flow until about age 1, when muscular reflexes that initiate swallowing and lip closure mature.*

- *Salivation and drooling typically increase with teething, which begins at about the fifth month and continues until about age 2.*
- *Excessive salivation and drooling may also occur in response to hunger or anticipation of feeding, and in association with nausea.*
- *Common causes of drooling include epiglottiditis, retropharyngeal abscess, severe tonsillitis, stomatitis, herpetic lesions, esophageal atresia, cerebral palsy, mental deficiency, and drug withdrawal in neonates of addicted mothers.*
- *Drooling may also result from a foreign body in the esophagus, causing dysphagia.*

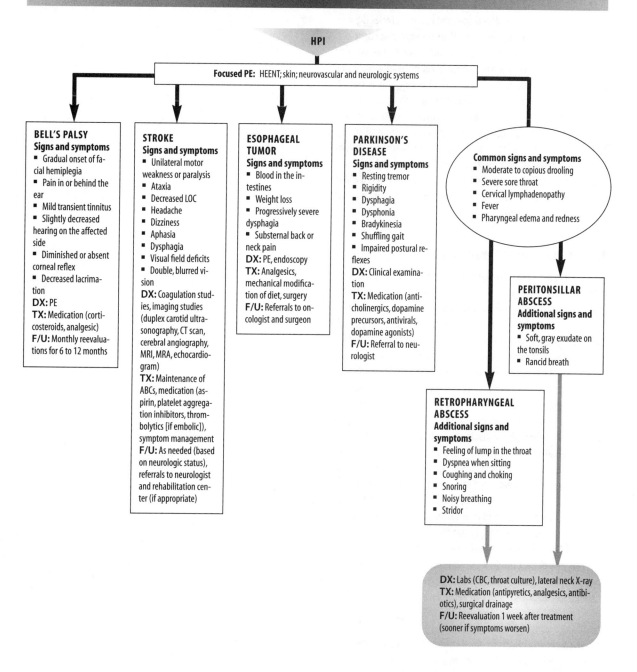

HPI

Focused PE: HEENT; skin; neurovascular and neurologic systems

BELL'S PALSY
Signs and symptoms
- Gradual onset of facial hemiplegia
- Pain in or behind the ear
- Mild transient tinnitus
- Slightly decreased hearing on the affected side
- Diminished or absent corneal reflex
- Decreased lacrimation
DX: PE
TX: Medication (corticosteroids, analgesic)
F/U: Monthly reevaluations for 6 to 12 months

STROKE
Signs and symptoms
- Unilateral motor weakness or paralysis
- Ataxia
- Decreased LOC
- Headache
- Dizziness
- Aphasia
- Dysphagia
- Visual field deficits
- Double, blurred vision
DX: Coagulation studies, imaging studies (duplex carotid ultrasonography, CT scan, cerebral angiography, MRI, MRA, echocardiogram)
TX: Maintenance of ABCs, medication (aspirin, platelet aggregation inhibitors, thrombolytics [if embolic]), symptom management
F/U: As needed (based on neurologic status), referrals to neurologist and rehabilitation center (if appropriate)

ESOPHAGEAL TUMOR
Signs and symptoms
- Blood in the intestines
- Weight loss
- Progressively severe dysphagia
- Substernal back or neck pain
DX: PE, endoscopy
TX: Analgesics, mechanical modification of diet, surgery
F/U: Referrals to oncologist and surgeon

PARKINSON'S DISEASE
Signs and symptoms
- Resting tremor
- Rigidity
- Dysphagia
- Dysphonia
- Bradykinesia
- Shuffling gait
- Impaired postural reflexes
DX: Clinical examination
TX: Medication (anticholinergics, dopamine precursors, antivirals, dopamine agonists)
F/U: Referral to neurologist

Common signs and symptoms
- Moderate to copious drooling
- Severe sore throat
- Cervical lymphadenopathy
- Fever
- Pharyngeal edema and redness

PERITONSILLAR ABSCESS
Additional signs and symptoms
- Soft, gray exudate on the tonsils
- Rancid breath

RETROPHARYNGEAL ABSCESS
Additional signs and symptoms
- Feeling of lump in the throat
- Dyspnea when sitting
- Coughing and choking
- Snoring
- Noisy breathing
- Stridor

DX: Labs (CBC, throat culture), lateral neck X-ray
TX: Medication (antipyretics, analgesics, antibiotics), surgical drainage
F/U: Reevaluation 1 week after treatment (sooner if symptoms worsen)

Additional differential diagnoses: achalasia ▪ acoustic neuroma ▪ ALS ▪ diphtheria ▪ envenomation ▪ glossopharyngeal neuralgia ▪ Guillain-Barré syndrome ▪ hypocalcemia ▪ Ludwig's angina ▪ paralytic poliomyelitis ▪ pesticide poisoning ▪ rabies

Other causes: clonazepam ▪ ethionamide ▪ haloperidol

Dysarthria

Dysarthria (poorly articulated speech) is characterized by slurring and labored, irregular rhythm. It may be accompanied by nasal voice tone caused by palate weakness. Whether it occurs abruptly or gradually, dysarthria is usually evident in ordinary conversation. It's confirmed by asking the patient to produce a few simple sounds and words, such as "ba," "sh," and "cat." However, dysarthria is occasionally confused with aphasia, loss of the ability to produce or comprehend speech.

Dysarthria results from damage to the brain stem that affects cranial nerves IX, X, or XI. Degenerative neurologic disorders commonly cause dysarthria. In fact, dysarthria is a chief sign of olivopontocerebellar degeneration. It may also result from ill-fitting dentures.

History and physical examination

If the patient displays dysarthria, ask him about associated difficulty swallowing. Then determine respiratory rate and depth. Measure vital capacity with a Wright respirometer, if available. Assess blood pressure and heart rate. Usually, tachycardia, slightly increased blood pressure, and shortness of breath are early signs of respiratory muscle weakness.

Ensure a patent airway. Place the patient in Fowler's position. Keep emergency resuscitation equipment nearby.

If dysarthria is not accompanied by respiratory muscle weakness and dysphagia, continue to assess for other neurologic deficits. Compare muscle strength and tone in the limbs. Then evaluate tactile sensation. Ask the patient about numbness or tingling. Test deep tendon reflexes and note gait ataxia. Next, test visual fields and ask about double vision. Check for signs of facial weakness, such as ptosis. Finally, determine level of consciousness and mental status.

Explore dysarthria fully. When did it begin? Has it improved? Speech improves with resolution of a transient ischemic attack, but not in a completed stroke. Ask if dysarthria worsens during the day. Then obtain a drug and alcohol history. Also ask about a history of seizures.

PEDIATRIC POINTERS

- *Dysarthria in children usually results from brain stem glioma, a slow-growing tumor that primarily affects children.*
- *It may also result from cerebral palsy.*
- *Dysarthria may be difficult to detect, especially in an infant or a young child who hasn't perfected speech. Be sure to look for other neurologic deficits, too.*

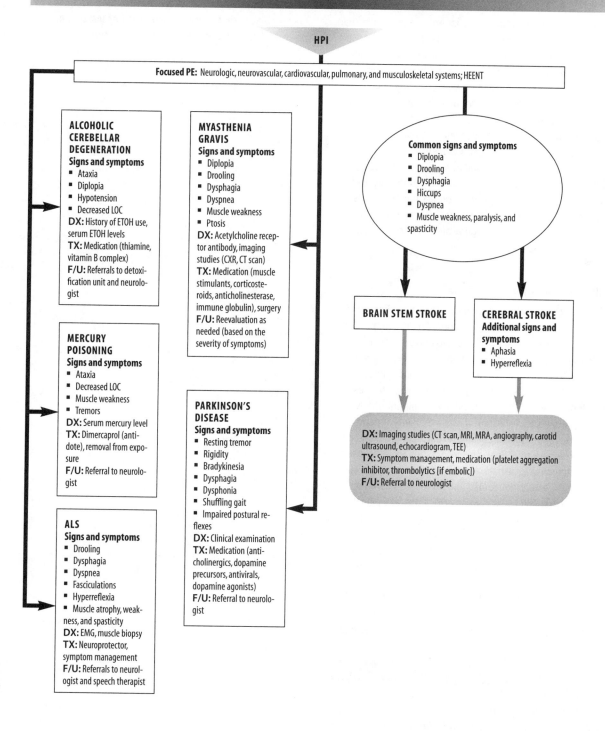

HPI

Focused PE: Neurologic, neurovascular, cardiovascular, pulmonary, and musculoskeletal systems; HEENT

ALCOHOLIC CEREBELLAR DEGENERATION
Signs and symptoms
- Ataxia
- Diplopia
- Hypotension
- Decreased LOC

DX: History of ETOH use, serum ETOH levels
TX: Medication (thiamine, vitamin B complex)
F/U: Referrals to detoxification unit and neurologist

MERCURY POISONING
Signs and symptoms
- Ataxia
- Decreased LOC
- Muscle weakness
- Tremors

DX: Serum mercury level
TX: Dimercaprol (antidote), removal from exposure
F/U: Referral to neurologist

ALS
Signs and symptoms
- Drooling
- Dysphagia
- Dyspnea
- Fasciculations
- Hyperreflexia
- Muscle atrophy, weakness, and spasticity

DX: EMG, muscle biopsy
TX: Neuroprotector, symptom management
F/U: Referrals to neurologist and speech therapist

MYASTHENIA GRAVIS
Signs and symptoms
- Diplopia
- Drooling
- Dysphagia
- Dyspnea
- Muscle weakness
- Ptosis

DX: Acetylcholine receptor antibody, imaging studies (CXR, CT scan)
TX: Medication (muscle stimulants, corticosteroids, anticholinesterase, immune globulin), surgery
F/U: Reevaluation as needed (based on the severity of symptoms)

PARKINSON'S DISEASE
Signs and symptoms
- Resting tremor
- Rigidity
- Bradykinesia
- Dysphagia
- Dysphonia
- Shuffling gait
- Impaired postural reflexes

DX: Clinical examination
TX: Medication (anticholinergics, dopamine precursors, antivirals, dopamine agonists)
F/U: Referral to neurologist

Common signs and symptoms
- Diplopia
- Drooling
- Dysphagia
- Hiccups
- Dyspnea
- Muscle weakness, paralysis, and spasticity

BRAIN STEM STROKE

CEREBRAL STROKE
Additional signs and symptoms
- Aphasia
- Hyperreflexia

DX: Imaging studies (CT scan, MRI, MRA, angiography, carotid ultrasound, echocardiogram, TEE)
TX: Symptom management, medication (platelet aggregation inhibitor, thrombolytics [if embolic])
F/U: Referral to neurologist

Other causes: anticonvulsants ▪ barbiturates

Dysmenorrhea

Dysmenorrhea — painful menstruation — affects more than 50% of menstruating women; in fact, it's the leading cause of lost time from school and work among women of childbearing age. Dysmenorrhea may involve sharp, intermittent pain or dull, aching pain. It's usually characterized by mild to severe cramping or colicky pain in the pelvis or lower abdomen that may radiate to the thighs and lower sacrum. This pain may precede menstruation by several days or may accompany it. The pain gradually subsides as bleeding tapers off.

Dysmenorrhea may be idiopathic, as in premenstrual syndrome and primary dysmenorrhea. It commonly results from endometriosis and other pelvic disorders. It may also result from structural abnormalities such as an imperforate hymen. Stress and poor health may aggravate dysmenorrhea; rest and mild exercise may relieve it.

History and physical examination

If the patient complains of dysmenorrhea, have her describe it fully. Is it intermittent or continuous? Sharp, cramping, or aching? Ask where the pain is located and whether it's bilateral. How long has she been experiencing it? When does the pain begin and end, and when is it severe? Does it radiate to the back? Explore associated symptoms, such as nausea and vomiting, altered bowel or urinary habits, bloating, pelvic or rectal pressure, and unusual fatigue, irritability, or depression.

Then obtain a menstrual and sexual history. Ask the patient if her menstrual flow is heavy or scant. Have her describe any vaginal discharge between menses. Does she experience pain during sexual intercourse, and does it occur with menses? Find out what relieves her cramps. Does she take pain medication? Is it effective? Note her method of contraception, and ask about a history of pelvic infection. Does she have any signs and symptoms of urinary system obstruction, such as pyuria, urine retention, or incontinence? Determine how she copes with stress.

Next, perform a focused physical examination. Take vital signs, noting fever and accompanying chills. Inspect the abdomen for distention, and palpate for tenderness and masses. Note costovertebral angle tenderness.

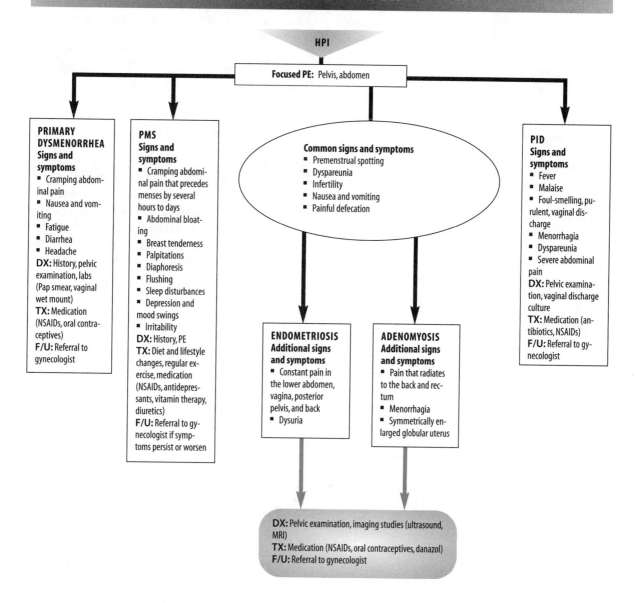

HPI

Focused PE: Pelvis, abdomen

PRIMARY DYSMENORRHEA
Signs and symptoms
- Cramping abdominal pain
- Nausea and vomiting
- Fatigue
- Diarrhea
- Headache

DX: History, pelvic examination, labs (Pap smear, vaginal wet mount)
TX: Medication (NSAIDs, oral contraceptives)
F/U: Referral to gynecologist

PMS
Signs and symptoms
- Cramping abdominal pain that precedes menses by several hours to days
- Abdominal bloating
- Breast tenderness
- Palpitations
- Diaphoresis
- Flushing
- Sleep disturbances
- Depression and mood swings
- Irritability

DX: History, PE
TX: Diet and lifestyle changes, regular exercise, medication (NSAIDs, antidepressants, vitamin therapy, diuretics)
F/U: Referral to gynecologist if symptoms persist or worsen

Common signs and symptoms
- Premenstrual spotting
- Dyspareunia
- Infertility
- Nausea and vomiting
- Painful defecation

PID
Signs and symptoms
- Fever
- Malaise
- Foul-smelling, purulent, vaginal discharge
- Menorrhagia
- Dyspareunia
- Severe abdominal pain

DX: Pelvic examination, vaginal discharge culture
TX: Medication (antibiotics, NSAIDs)
F/U: Referral to gynecologist

ENDOMETRIOSIS
Additional signs and symptoms
- Constant pain in the lower abdomen, vagina, posterior pelvis, and back
- Dysuria

ADENOMYOSIS
Additional signs and symptoms
- Pain that radiates to the back and rectum
- Menorrhagia
- Symmetrically enlarged globular uterus

DX: Pelvic examination, imaging studies (ultrasound, MRI)
TX: Medication (NSAIDs, oral contraceptives, danazol)
F/U: Referral to gynecologist

Other cause: intrauterine devices

Dyspareunia

A major obstacle to sexual enjoyment, dyspareunia is painful or difficult coitus. Although most sexually active women occasionally experience mild dyspareunia, persistent or severe dyspareunia is cause for concern. Dyspareunia may occur with attempted penetration or during or after coitus. It may stem from friction of the penis against perineal tissue or from jarring of deeper adnexal structures. The location of pain helps determine its cause.

Dyspareunia frequently accompanies pelvic disorders. However, it may also result from diminished vaginal lubrication associated with aging, the effects of drugs, and psychological factors — most notably, fear of pain or injury. A cycle of fear, pain, and tension may become established in which repeated episodes of painful coitus condition the patient to anticipate pain, causing fear, which prevents sexual arousal and adequate vaginal lubrication. Contraction of the pubococcygeus muscle also occurs, making penetration still more difficult and traumatic.

Other psychological factors include guilt feelings about sex, fear of pregnancy or of injury to the fetus during pregnancy, and anxiety caused by a disrupted sexual relationship or by a new sexual partner. Inadequate vaginal lubrication associated with insufficient foreplay and mental or physical fatigue may also cause dyspareunia.

History and physical examination

Begin by asking the patient to describe the pain. Does it occur with attempted penetration or deep thrusting? How long does it last? Is the pain intermittent or does it always accompany intercourse? Ask whether changing coital position relieves the pain.

Next, ask about a history of pelvic, vaginal, or urinary infection. Does the patient have signs and symptoms of a current infection? Have her describe any discharge. Also ask about malaise, fever, headache, fatigue, abdominal or back pain, nausea and vomiting, and diarrhea or constipation.

Obtain a sexual and menstrual history. Determine whether dyspareunia is related to the patient's menstrual cycle. Are her cycles regular? Ask about dysmenorrhea and metrorrhagia. Has the patient had a baby? If so, did she have an episiotomy? Note whether she's breast-feeding. Ask about previous pregnancy, sexual abuse, or pelvic surgery. Also find out what contraceptive method the patient uses. Then try to determine her attitude toward sexual intimacy. Does she feel tense during coitus? Is she satisfied with the length of foreplay? Does she usually achieve orgasm? Ask about a history of rape, incest, or sexual abuse as a child.

Next, perform a physical examination. Take vital signs. Palpate the abdomen for tenderness, pain, or masses and for inguinal lymphadenopathy. Finally, inspect the genitalia for lesions and vaginal discharge.

PEDIATRIC POINTER

Dyspareunia can also be an adolescent problem. Although about 40% of adolescents are sexually active by the age of 19, most are reluctant to initiate a frank sexual discussion. Obtain a thorough sexual history by asking the patient direct but nonjudgmental questions.

WOMEN'S HEALTH TIP

In postmenopausal women, the absence of estrogen reduces vaginal diameter and elasticity, which causes tearing of the vaginal mucosa during intercourse. These tears, as well as inflammatory reactions to bacterial invasion, cause fibrous adhesions that occlude the vagina. Dyspareunia can result from any or all of these conditions.

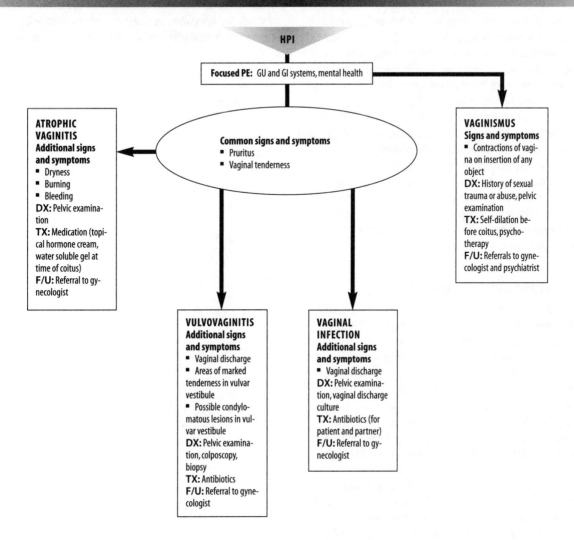

HPI

Focused PE: GU and GI systems, mental health

Common signs and symptoms
- Pruritus
- Vaginal tenderness

ATROPHIC VAGINITIS
Additional signs and symptoms
- Dryness
- Burning
- Bleeding

DX: Pelvic examination
TX: Medication (topical hormone cream, water soluble gel at time of coitus)
F/U: Referral to gynecologist

VAGINISMUS
Signs and symptoms
- Contractions of vagina on insertion of any object

DX: History of sexual trauma or abuse, pelvic examination
TX: Self-dilation before coitus, psychotherapy
F/U: Referrals to gynecologist and psychiatrist

VULVOVAGINITIS
Additional signs and symptoms
- Vaginal discharge
- Areas of marked tenderness in vulvar vestibule
- Possible condylomatous lesions in vulvar vestibule

DX: Pelvic examination, colposcopy, biopsy
TX: Antibiotics
F/U: Referral to gynecologist

VAGINAL INFECTION
Additional signs and symptoms
- Vaginal discharge

DX: Pelvic examination, vaginal discharge culture
TX: Antibiotics (for patient and partner)
F/U: Referral to gynecologist

Other causes: diaphragms ▪ douches ▪ intrauterine devices ▪ spermicidal jellies ▪ vaginal creams and deodorants

Dyspepsia

Dyspepsia refers to an uncomfortable fullness after meals that's associated with epigastric gnawing pain, nausea, belching, heartburn, and abdominal cramping and distention. Typically aggravated by spicy, fatty, or high-fiber foods and by excess caffeine intake, dyspepsia without other pathology indicates impaired digestive function.

Dyspepsia is caused by GI disorders (such as ulcers) and, to a lesser extent, by cardiac, pulmonary, and renal disorders and adverse drug effects. It results when altered gastric secretions lead to excess stomach acidity. This symptom may also result from stress, overly rapid eating, or improper chewing. It usually occurs a few hours after eating and lasts for a variable period of time. Its severity depends on the amount and type of food eaten and on GI motility. Additional food or antacids may relieve the discomfort.

History and physical examination

If the patient complains of dyspepsia, begin by obtaining a complete history of the symptom, asking him to describe it fully. How often and when does it occur, specifically in relation to meals? Do any drugs or activities relieve or aggravate it? Is there associated nausea, vomiting, melena, hematemesis, cough, or chest pain? Inquire what drugs he's currently taking, especially over-the-counter drugs. Ask about recent surgery, medical, social, or work related problems. Does he have a history of renal, cardiovascular, or pulmonary disease? Has he noticed any change in the amount or color of his urine?

Focus the physical examination on the abdomen. Inspect for distention, ascites, scars, jaundice, uremic frost, and bruising. Auscultate for bowel sounds and characterize the motility. Palpate and percuss the abdomen, noting any tenderness, pain, guarding, rebound, organ enlargement, or tympany.

Finally, examine other body systems. Auscultate for gallops and crackles. Percuss the lungs to detect consolidation. Note peripheral edema and any swelling of lymph nodes.

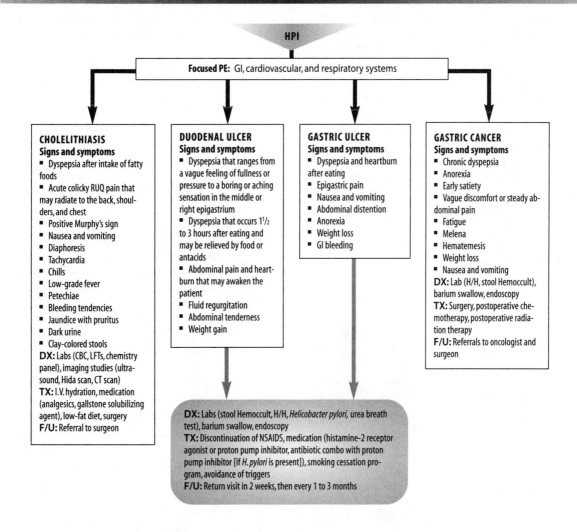

HPI

Focused PE: GI, cardiovascular, and respiratory systems

CHOLELITHIASIS
Signs and symptoms
- Dyspepsia after intake of fatty foods
- Acute colicky RUQ pain that may radiate to the back, shoulders, and chest
- Positive Murphy's sign
- Nausea and vomiting
- Diaphoresis
- Tachycardia
- Chills
- Low-grade fever
- Petechiae
- Bleeding tendencies
- Jaundice with pruritus
- Dark urine
- Clay-colored stools

DX: Labs (CBC, LFTs, chemistry panel), imaging studies (ultrasound, Hida scan, CT scan)
TX: I.V. hydration, medication (analgesics, gallstone solubilizing agent), low-fat diet, surgery
F/U: Referral to surgeon

DUODENAL ULCER
Signs and symptoms
- Dyspepsia that ranges from a vague feeling of fullness or pressure to a boring or aching sensation in the middle or right epigastrium
- Dyspepsia that occurs 1½ to 3 hours after eating and may be relieved by food or antacids
- Abdominal pain and heartburn that may awaken the patient
- Fluid regurgitation
- Abdominal tenderness
- Weight gain

GASTRIC ULCER
Signs and symptoms
- Dyspepsia and heartburn after eating
- Epigastric pain
- Nausea and vomiting
- Abdominal distention
- Anorexia
- Weight loss
- GI bleeding

GASTRIC CANCER
Signs and symptoms
- Chronic dyspepsia
- Anorexia
- Early satiety
- Vague discomfort or steady abdominal pain
- Fatigue
- Melena
- Hematemesis
- Weight loss
- Nausea and vomiting

DX: Lab (H/H, stool Hemoccult), barium swallow, endoscopy
TX: Surgery, postoperative chemotherapy, postoperative radiation therapy
F/U: Referrals to oncologist and surgeon

DX: Labs (stool Hemoccult, H/H, *Helicobacter pylori*, urea breath test), barium swallow, endoscopy
TX: Discontinuation of NSAIDS, medication (histamine-2 receptor agonist or proton pump inhibitor, antibiotic combo with proton pump inhibitor [if *H. pylori* is present]), smoking cessation program, avoidance of triggers
F/U: Return visit in 2 weeks, then every 1 to 3 months

Additional differential diagnoses: gastric dilatation (acute) ▪ gastritis (chronic) ▪ heart failure ▪ hepatitis ▪ pancreatitis (chronic) ▪ pulmonary embolus ▪ pulmonary tuberculosis ▪ uremia

Other causes: anti-inflammatory drugs ▪ aspirin ▪ diuretics ▪ antibiotics ▪ antihypertensives ▪ surgery

Dysphagia

Dysphagia — difficulty swallowing — is a common symptom that's usually easy to localize. It may be constant or intermittent and is classified by the phase of swallowing it affects. (See *Classifying dysphagia*.) Among the factors that interfere with swallowing are severe pain, obstruction, abnormal peristalsis, impaired gag reflex, and excessive, scanty, or thick oral secretions.

Dysphagia is the most common — and sometimes the *only* — symptom of esophageal disorders. However, it may also result from oropharyngeal, respiratory, neurologic, and collagen disorders or from the effects of toxins and treatments. Dysphagia increases the risk of choking and aspiration and may lead to malnutrition and dehydration.

Classifying dysphagia

Because swallowing occurs in three distinct phases, dysphagia can be classified by the phase that it affects. Each phase suggests a specific pathology for dysphagia.

PHASE 1
Swallowing begins in the *transfer phase* with chewing and moistening of food with saliva. The tongue presses against the hard palate to transfer the chewed food to the back of the throat; the fifth cranial nerve then stimulates the swallowing reflex. Phase 1 dysphagia typically results from a neuromuscular disorder.

PHASE 2
In the *transport phase,* the soft palate closes against the pharyngeal wall to prevent nasal regurgitation. At the same time, the larynx rises and the vocal cords close to keep food out of the lungs; breathing stops momentarily as the throat muscles constrict to move food into the esophagus. Phase 2 dysphagia usually indicates spasm or cancer.

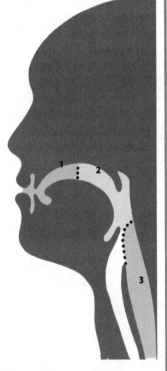

PHASE 3
Peristalsis and gravity work together in the *entrance phase* to move food through the esophageal sphincter and into the stomach. Phase 3 dysphagia results from lower esophageal narrowing by diverticula, esophagitis, and other disorders.

History and physical examination

If the patient suddenly complains of dysphagia and displays signs of respiratory distress, such as dyspnea and stridor, suspect an airway obstruction and quickly perform abdominal thrusts. Initiate emergency measures if necessary.

If the patient's dysphagia doesn't suggest airway obstruction, begin with a health history. Ask the patient if swallowing is painful. If so, is the pain constant or intermittent? Have the patient point to where dysphagia feels most intense. Does eating alleviate or aggravate the symptom? Are solids or liquids more difficult to swallow? If the answer is liquids, ask if hot, cold, and lukewarm fluids affect him differently? Does the symptom disappear after several attempts to swallow a few times? Is swallowing easier in different positions? Ask if he has recently experienced any vomiting, regurgitation, weight loss, anorexia, hoarseness, dyspnea, or a cough.

To evaluate the patient's swallowing reflex, place your finger along the thyroid notch and instruct him to swallow. If you feel the larynx rise, the reflex is intact. Next, have the patient cough to assess cough reflex. Check gag reflex if you're sure the patient has a good swallow and cough reflex. Listen closely to his speech for signs of muscle weakness. Does he have aphasia or dysarthria? Is his voice nasal, hoarse, or breathy? Assess the patient's mouth carefully, check for dry mucous membranes and thick, sticky secretions. Observe for tongue and facial weakness. Assess for disorientation, which may make him neglect to swallow.

PEDIATRIC POINTERS

- *In looking for dysphagia in an infant or a small child, be sure to pay close attention to his sucking and swallowing ability. Coughing, choking, or regurgitation during feeding suggests dysphagia.*
- *Corrosive esophagitis and esophageal obstruction by a foreign body are more common causes of dysphagia in children than in adults.*
- *Dysphagia may result from congenital anomalies, such as annular stenosis, dysphagia lusoria, and esophageal atresia.*

ELDER CARE CUE

In patients older than age 50, dysphagia is often the presenting complaint in cases of head or neck cancer. The incidence of such cancers increases markedly in this age-group.

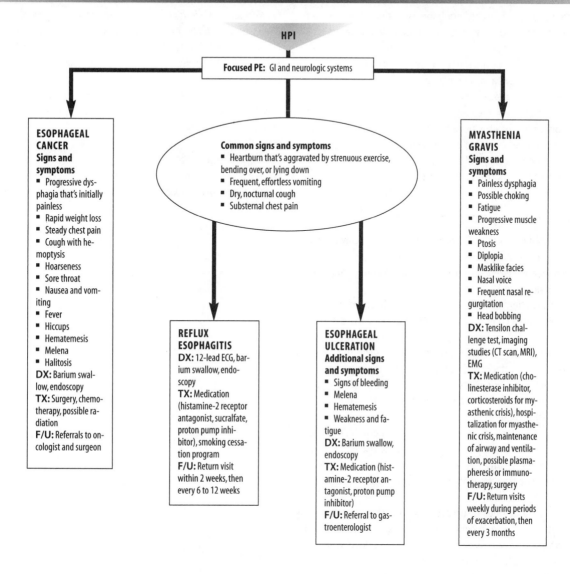

HPI

Focused PE: GI and neurologic systems

ESOPHAGEAL CANCER
Signs and symptoms
- Progressive dysphagia that's initially painless
- Rapid weight loss
- Steady chest pain
- Cough with hemoptysis
- Hoarseness
- Sore throat
- Nausea and vomiting
- Fever
- Hiccups
- Hematemesis
- Melena
- Halitosis
DX: Barium swallow, endoscopy
TX: Surgery, chemotherapy, possible radiation
F/U: Referrals to oncologist and surgeon

Common signs and symptoms
- Heartburn that's aggravated by strenuous exercise, bending over, or lying down
- Frequent, effortless vomiting
- Dry, nocturnal cough
- Substernal chest pain

MYASTHENIA GRAVIS
Signs and symptoms
- Painless dysphagia
- Possible choking
- Fatigue
- Progressive muscle weakness
- Ptosis
- Diplopia
- Masklike facies
- Nasal voice
- Frequent nasal regurgitation
- Head bobbing
DX: Tensilon challenge test, imaging studies (CT scan, MRI), EMG
TX: Medication (cholinesterase inhibitor, corticosteroids for myasthenic crisis), hospitalization for myasthenic crisis, maintenance of airway and ventilation, possible plasmapheresis or immunotherapy, surgery
F/U: Return visits weekly during periods of exacerbation, then every 3 months

REFLUX ESOPHAGITIS
DX: 12-lead ECG, barium swallow, endoscopy
TX: Medication (histamine-2 receptor antagonist, sucralfate, proton pump inhibitor), smoking cessation program
F/U: Return visit within 2 weeks, then every 6 to 12 weeks

ESOPHAGEAL ULCERATION
Additional signs and symptoms
- Signs of bleeding
- Melena
- Hematemesis
- Weakness and fatigue
DX: Barium swallow, endoscopy
TX: Medication (histamine-2 receptor antagonist, proton pump inhibitor)
F/U: Referral to gastroenterologist

Additional differential diagnoses: achalasia ▪ airway obstruction ▪ ALS ▪ bulbar paralysis ▪ dysphagia lusoria ▪ esophageal compression (external) ▪ esophageal diverticulum ▪ esophageal leiomyoma ▪ esophageal obstruction by foreign body ▪ esophageal spasm ▪ esophagitis ▪ gastric carcinoma ▪ hypocalcemia ▪ laryngeal cancer (extrinsic) ▪ laryngeal nerve damage ▪ lead poisoning ▪ mediastinitis ▪ oral cavity tumor ▪ Parkinson's disease ▪ pharyngitis (chronic) ▪ Plummer-Vinson syndrome ▪ progressive systemic sclerosis ▪ SLE

Other causes: radiation therapy ▪ surgery (such as recent tracheostomy)

Dyspnea

Often a symptom of cardiopulmonary dysfunction, dyspnea is the sensation of difficult or uncomfortable breathing. It's usually reported as shortness of breath. The severity varies greatly and may be unrelated to the severity of the underlying cause. Dyspnea may be of sudden or gradual onset.

Most people experience dyspnea when they overexert themselves, but the severity depends on their overall physical condition. In a healthy person dyspnea is quickly relieved by rest. Pathologic causes of dyspnea include pulmonary, cardiac, neuromuscular, and allergic disorders. In addition, anxiety may cause shortness of breath.

History and physical examination

If a patient complains of shortness of breath, quickly look for signs of respiratory distress, such as tachypnea, cyanosis, restlessness, and accessory muscle use. Initiate emergency measures if necessary.

If the patient can answer questions without increasing his distress, take a complete history. Ask if the shortness of breath began suddenly or gradually. Is it constant or intermittent? Does it occur during activity or while at rest? Has the patient had dyspneic attacks before? Have the attacks increased in severity? What aggravates or alleviates these attacks? Does the patient have a productive or nonproductive cough or chest pain? Is there any history of recent trauma, upper respiratory tract infections, deep vein phlebitis, immobility, or other disorders? Ask the patient about tobacco use and exposure to occupational irritants or toxic fumes. Find out if he also has orthopnea, paroxysmal nocturnal dyspnea, or progressive fatigue.

Because dyspnea is subjective and may be exacerbated by anxiety, patients from cultures that are highly emotional may complain of shortness of breath sooner than those who are more stoic about symptoms of illness.

During the physical examination, look for signs of chronic dyspnea, such as accessory muscle hypertrophy (especially in the shoulders and neck). Also look for pursed-lip exhalation, finger clubbing, peripheral edema, barrel chest, diaphoresis, and distended neck veins.

Check blood pressure and auscultate for crackles, abnormal heart sounds or rhythms, egophony, bronchophony, and whispered pectoriloquy. Finally, palpate the abdomen for hepatomegaly.

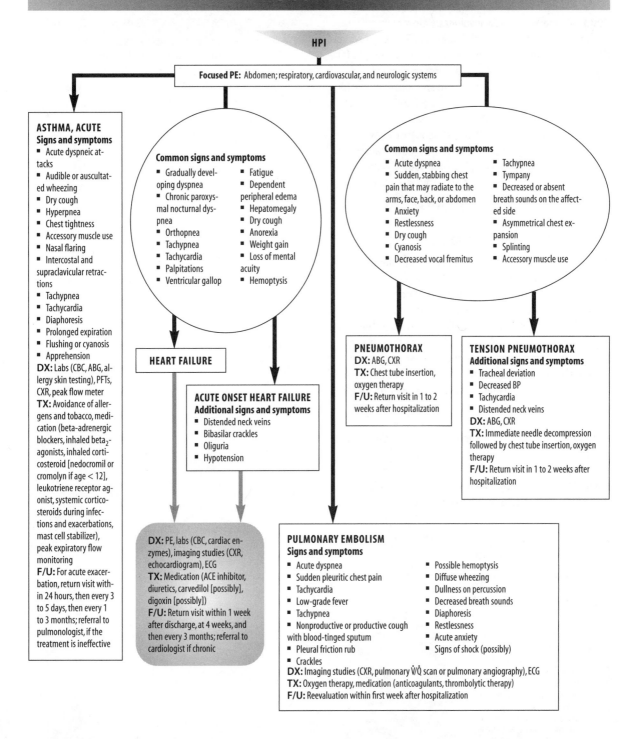

HPI

Focused PE: Abdomen; respiratory, cardiovascular, and neurologic systems

ASTHMA, ACUTE
Signs and symptoms
- Acute dyspneic attacks
- Audible or auscultated wheezing
- Dry cough
- Hyperpnea
- Chest tightness
- Accessory muscle use
- Nasal flaring
- Intercostal and supraclavicular retractions
- Tachypnea
- Tachycardia
- Diaphoresis
- Prolonged expiration
- Flushing or cyanosis
- Apprehension

DX: Labs (CBC, ABG, allergy skin testing), PFTs, CXR, peak flow meter
TX: Avoidance of allergens and tobacco, medication (beta-adrenergic blockers, inhaled beta$_2$-agonists, inhaled corticosteroid [nedocromil or cromolyn if age < 12], leukotriene receptor agonist, systemic corticosteroids during infections and exacerbations, mast cell stabilizer), peak expiratory flow monitoring
F/U: For acute exacerbation, return visit within 24 hours, then every 3 to 5 days, then every 1 to 3 months; referral to pulmonologist, if the treatment is ineffective

Common signs and symptoms
- Gradually developing dyspnea
- Chronic paroxysmal nocturnal dyspnea
- Orthopnea
- Tachypnea
- Tachycardia
- Palpitations
- Ventricular gallop
- Fatigue
- Dependent peripheral edema
- Hepatomegaly
- Dry cough
- Anorexia
- Weight gain
- Loss of mental acuity
- Hemoptysis

HEART FAILURE

ACUTE ONSET HEART FAILURE
Additional signs and symptoms
- Distended neck veins
- Bibasilar crackles
- Oliguria
- Hypotension

DX: PE, labs (CBC, cardiac enzymes), imaging studies (CXR, echocardiogram), ECG
TX: Medication (ACE inhibitor, diuretics, carvedilol [possibly], digoxin [possibly])
F/U: Return visit within 1 week after discharge, at 4 weeks, and then every 3 months; referral to cardiologist if chronic

Common signs and symptoms
- Acute dyspnea
- Sudden, stabbing chest pain that may radiate to the arms, face, back, or abdomen
- Anxiety
- Restlessness
- Dry cough
- Cyanosis
- Decreased vocal fremitus
- Tachypnea
- Tympany
- Decreased or absent breath sounds on the affected side
- Asymmetrical chest expansion
- Splinting
- Accessory muscle use

PNEUMOTHORAX
DX: ABG, CXR
TX: Chest tube insertion, oxygen therapy
F/U: Return visit in 1 to 2 weeks after hospitalization

TENSION PNEUMOTHORAX
Additional signs and symptoms
- Tracheal deviation
- Decreased BP
- Tachycardia
- Distended neck veins

DX: ABG, CXR
TX: Immediate needle decompression followed by chest tube insertion, oxygen therapy
F/U: Return visit in 1 to 2 weeks after hospitalization

PULMONARY EMBOLISM
Signs and symptoms
- Acute dyspnea
- Sudden pleuritic chest pain
- Tachycardia
- Low-grade fever
- Tachypnea
- Nonproductive or productive cough with blood-tinged sputum
- Pleural friction rub
- Crackles
- Possible hemoptysis
- Diffuse wheezing
- Dullness on percussion
- Decreased breath sounds
- Diaphoresis
- Restlessness
- Acute anxiety
- Signs of shock (possibly)

DX: Imaging studies (CXR, pulmonary V̇/Q̇ scan or pulmonary angiography), ECG
TX: Oxygen therapy, medication (anticoagulants, thrombolytic therapy)
F/U: Reevaluation within first week after hospitalization

Additional differential diagnoses: anemia ▪ ARDS ▪ aspiration of a foreign body ▪ cardiac arrhythmias ▪ COPD ▪ cor pulmonale ▪ emphysema ▪ flail chest ▪ inhalation injury ▪ interstitial fibrosis ▪ lung cancer ▪ MI ▪ pleural effusion ▪ pneumonia ▪ pulmonary edema ▪ tuberculosis

Dystonia

Dystonia is marked by slow, involuntary movements of large-muscle groups in the limbs, trunk, and neck. This extrapyramidal sign may involve flexion of the foot, hyperextension of the legs, extension and pronation of the arms, arching of the back, and extension and rotation of the neck (spasmodic torticollis). It's typically aggravated by walking and emotional stress and relieved by sleep.

Dystonia may be intermittent — lasting just a few minutes — or continuous and painful. Occasionally, it causes permanent contractures, resulting in a grotesque posture. Although dystonia may be hereditary or idiopathic, it usually results from extrapyramidal disorders or adverse drug effects.

History and physical examination

If possible, include the patient's family in obtaining the history. The family may be more aware of behavior changes than the patient. Begin by asking when dystonia occurs. Is it aggravated by emotional upset? Does it disappear during sleep? Is there a family history of dystonia? Obtain a drug history, noting especially the use of phenothiazines or antipsychotics. Dystonia is a common adverse effect of these drugs, and dosage adjustments may be needed to minimize this effect.

Next, examine the patient's coordination and voluntary muscle movement. Observe the patients gait as he walks across the room; then have him squeeze your fingers to assess muscle strength. (See *Recognizing dystonia.*) Check coordination by having him touch your fingertip and then his nose repeatedly. Follow this by testing gross motor movement of the leg by placing his heel on one knee, sliding it down his shin, then returning it to his knee. Finally, assess fine-motor movement by asking the patient to touch each finger to his thumb in succession.

- *Children don't exhibit dystonia until after they can walk; it rarely occurs until after age 10.*
- *Common causes include Fahr's syndrome, dystonia musculorum deformans, athetoid cerebral palsy, and the residual effects of anoxia at birth.*

Recognizing dystonia

Dystonia, chorea, and athetosis may occur simultaneously. To differentiate between them, keep the following points in mind:

- *Dystonic movements* are slow and twisting and involve large muscle groups in the head, neck (as shown at right), trunk, and limbs. They may be intermittent or continuous.
- *Choreiform movements* are rapid, highly complex, and jerky.
- *Athetoid movements* are slow, sinuous, and writhing but always continuous; they typically affect the hands and extremities.

DYSTONIA OF THE NECK (SPASMODIC TORTICOLLIS)

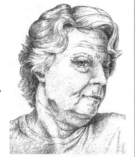

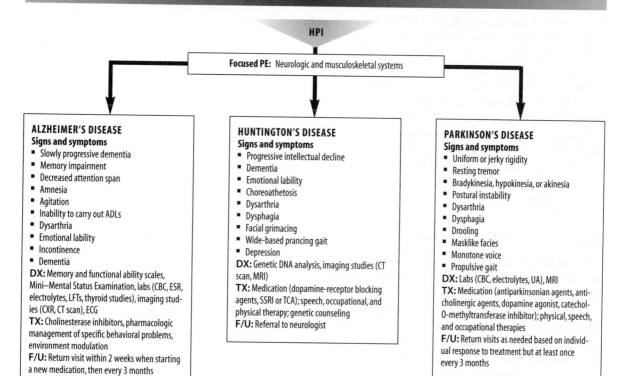

HPI

Focused PE: Neurologic and musculoskeletal systems

ALZHEIMER'S DISEASE
Signs and symptoms
- Slowly progressive dementia
- Memory impairment
- Decreased attention span
- Amnesia
- Agitation
- Inability to carry out ADLs
- Dysarthria
- Emotional lability
- Incontinence
- Dementia

DX: Memory and functional ability scales, Mini–Mental Status Examination, labs (CBC, ESR, electrolytes, LFTs, thyroid studies), imaging studies (CXR, CT scan), ECG

TX: Cholinesterase inhibitors, pharmacologic management of specific behavioral problems, environment modulation

F/U: Return visit within 2 weeks when starting a new medication, then every 3 months

HUNTINGTON'S DISEASE
Signs and symptoms
- Progressive intellectual decline
- Dementia
- Emotional lability
- Choreoathetosis
- Dysarthria
- Dysphagia
- Facial grimacing
- Wide-based prancing gait
- Depression

DX: Genetic DNA analysis, imaging studies (CT scan, MRI)

TX: Medication (dopamine-receptor blocking agents, SSRI or TCA); speech, occupational, and physical therapy; genetic counseling

F/U: Referral to neurologist

PARKINSON'S DISEASE
Signs and symptoms
- Uniform or jerky rigidity
- Resting tremor
- Bradykinesia, hypokinesia, or akinesia
- Postural instability
- Dysarthria
- Dysphagia
- Drooling
- Masklike facies
- Monotone voice
- Propulsive gait

DX: Labs (CBC, electrolytes, UA), MRI

TX: Medication (antiparkinsonian agents, anticholinergic agents, dopamine agonist, catechol-O-methyltransferase inhibitor); physical, speech, and occupational therapies

F/U: Return visits as needed based on individual response to treatment but at least once every 3 months

Additional differential diagnoses: dystonia musculorum deformans ▪ Hallervorden-Spatz disease ▪ olivopontocerebellar atrophy ▪ Pick's disease ▪ supranuclear ophthalmoplegia (Steele-Richardson-Olszewski syndrome) ▪ Wilson's disease

Other causes: phenothiazines ▪ haloperidol, loxapine, and other antipsychotics ▪ antiemetic doses of metoclopramide, risperidone, and metyrosine ▪ excessive doses of levodopa

Dysuria

Dysuria — painful or difficult urination — is often accompanied by urinary frequency, urgency, or hesitancy. This symptom usually reflects lower urinary tract infection — a common disorder, especially in women.

Dysuria results from lower urinary tract irritation or inflammation, which stimulates nerve endings in the bladder and urethra. The pain's onset provides clues to its cause; for example, pain just *before* voiding usually indicates bladder irritation or distention, whereas pain at the *start* of urination typically results from bladder outlet irritation. Pain at the *end* of voiding may signal bladder spasms; in women, it may indicate vaginal candidiasis.

History and physical examination

If the patient complains of dysuria, have him describe its severity and location. When did he first notice it? Did anything precipitate it? Does anything aggravate or alleviate it?

Next, ask about previous urinary or genital tract infections. Has the patient recently undergone invasive procedures, such as cystoscopy or urethral dilatation? Also ask if he has a history of intestinal disease. Ask the female patient about menstrual disorders and use of products that irritate the urinary tract, such as bubble bath salts, feminine deodorants, contraceptive gels, or perineal lotions. Also ask her about vaginal discharge or pruritus.

During the physical examination, inspect the urethral meatus for discharge, irritation, or other abnormalities. A pelvic or rectal examination may be necessary.

WOMEN'S HEALTH TIPS

- *The perineum should be wiped from front to back after urination and defecation to prevent contamination with fecal material.*
- *Feminine deodorants, douches, bubble baths, and similar irritants may cause dysuria.*

ELDER CARE CUE

Be aware that elderly people tend to under-report their symptoms even though older men have an increased incidence of nonsexually-related urinary tract infections and postmenopausal women have an increased incidence of noninfectious dysuria.

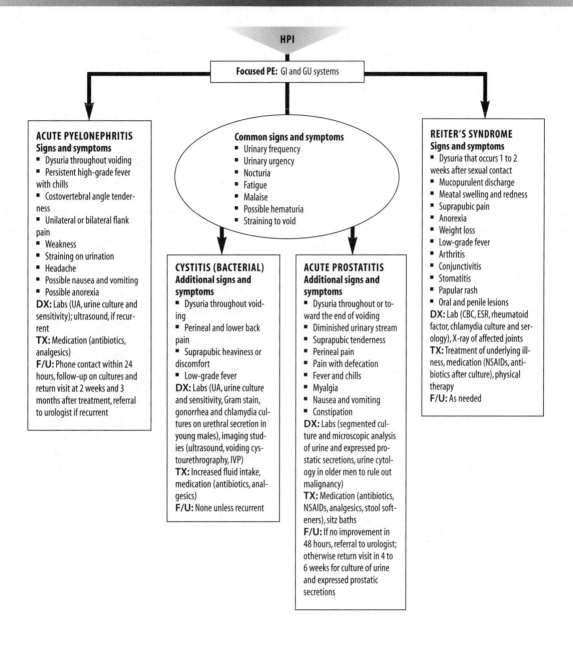

HPI

Focused PE: GI and GU systems

ACUTE PYELONEPHRITIS
Signs and symptoms
- Dysuria throughout voiding
- Persistent high-grade fever with chills
- Costovertebral angle tenderness
- Unilateral or bilateral flank pain
- Weakness
- Straining on urination
- Headache
- Possible nausea and vomiting
- Possible anorexia

DX: Labs (UA, urine culture and sensitivity); ultrasound, if recurrent
TX: Medication (antibiotics, analgesics)
F/U: Phone contact within 24 hours, follow-up on cultures and return visit at 2 weeks and 3 months after treatment, referral to urologist if recurrent

Common signs and symptoms
- Urinary frequency
- Urinary urgency
- Nocturia
- Fatigue
- Malaise
- Possible hematuria
- Straining to void

CYSTITIS (BACTERIAL)
Additional signs and symptoms
- Dysuria throughout voiding
- Perineal and lower back pain
- Suprapubic heaviness or discomfort
- Low-grade fever

DX: Labs (UA, urine culture and sensitivity, Gram stain, gonorrhea and chlamydia cultures on urethral secretion in young males), imaging studies (ultrasound, voiding cystourethrography, IVP)
TX: Increased fluid intake, medication (antibiotics, analgesics)
F/U: None unless recurrent

ACUTE PROSTATITIS
Additional signs and symptoms
- Dysuria throughout or toward the end of voiding
- Diminished urinary stream
- Suprapubic tenderness
- Perineal pain
- Pain with defecation
- Fever and chills
- Myalgia
- Nausea and vomiting
- Constipation

DX: Labs (segmented culture and microscopic analysis of urine and expressed prostatic secretions, urine cytology in older men to rule out malignancy)
TX: Medication (antibiotics, NSAIDs, analgesics, stool softeners), sitz baths
F/U: If no improvement in 48 hours, referral to urologist; otherwise return visit in 4 to 6 weeks for culture of urine and expressed prostatic secretions

REITER'S SYNDROME
Signs and symptoms
- Dysuria that occurs 1 to 2 weeks after sexual contact
- Mucopurulent discharge
- Meatal swelling and redness
- Suprapubic pain
- Anorexia
- Weight loss
- Low-grade fever
- Arthritis
- Conjunctivitis
- Stomatitis
- Papular rash
- Oral and penile lesions

DX: Lab (CBC, ESR, rheumatoid factor, chlamydia culture and serology), X-ray of affected joints
TX: Treatment of underlying illness, medication (NSAIDs, antibiotics after culture), physical therapy
F/U: As needed

Additional differential diagnoses: appendicitis ▪ bladder cancer ▪ chemical irritant ▪ chronic prostatitis ▪ cystitis ▪ diverticulitis ▪ paraurethral gland inflammation ▪ urethral syndrome ▪ urethritis ▪ urinary system obstruction ▪ vaginitis

Other causes: MAO inhibitors ▪ metyrosine

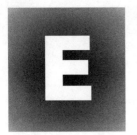

Earache

Earaches (otalgia) usually result from disorders of the external and middle ear associated with infection, obstruction, or trauma. Their severity ranges from a feeling of fullness or blockage to deep, boring pain; at times, they may be difficult to localize precisely. This common symptom may be intermittent or continuous and may develop suddenly or gradually.

History and physical examination

Ask the patient to characterize his earache. How long has he had it? Is it intermittent or continuous? Is it painful or slightly annoying? Can he localize the site of ear pain? Does he have pain in any other areas, such as the jaw?

Ask about recent ear injury or other trauma. Does swimming or showering trigger ear discomfort? Has he been swimming lately in a lake or river? Is discomfort associated with itching? If so, find out where the itching is most intense and when it began. Ask about ear drainage and, if present, have the patient characterize it. Does he hear ringing or noise in his ears? Ask about dizziness or vertigo. Does the earache

worsen when the patient changes position? Does he have difficulty swallowing, hoarseness, neck pain, or pain when he opens his mouth?

Find out if the patient has recently had a head cold or problems with his eyes, mouth, teeth, jaws, sinuses, or throat. Disorders in these areas may refer pain to the ear along the cranial nerves.

Begin your physical examination by inspecting the external ear for redness, drainage, swelling, or deformity. Then apply pressure to the mastoid process and tragus to elicit any tenderness. Using an otoscope, examine the external auditory canal for lesions, bleeding or discharge, impacted cerumen, foreign bodies, tenderness, or swelling. Examine the tympanic membrane. Is it intact? Is it pearly gray (normal)? Look for tympanic membrane landmarks: the cone of light, umbo, pars tensa, and the handle and short process of the malleus. (See *Using an otoscope correctly*.) Perform the watch tick, whispered voice, Rinne, and Weber's tests to assess for hearing loss.

PEDIATRIC POINTERS

- *Common causes of earache in children are acute otitis media and insertion of foreign bodies that become lodged or infected.*
- *Be alert for crying or ear-tugging in a young child — nonverbal clues to earache.*
- *To examine the child's ears, place him supine with his arms extended and held securely by his parent. Then hold the otoscope with the handle pointing toward the top of the child's head and brace it against him using one or two fingers.*
- *Because an ear examination may upset the child with an earache, save it for the end of your physical examination.*

Using an otoscope correctly

When the patient reports an earache, use an otoscope to inspect ear structures closely. Follow these techniques to obtain the best view and ensure patient safety.

CHILD
To inspect an infant's or a young child's ear, grasp the *lower part* of the auricle and pull it *down and back* to straighten the upward S-curve of the external canal. Then gently insert the speculum into the canal no more than 1.2 cm (1/2").

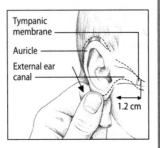

Tympanic membrane
Auricle
External ear canal
1.2 cm

ADULT
To inspect an adult's ear, grasp the *upper part* of the auricle and pull it *up and back* to straighten the external canal. Then insert the speculum about 2.5 cm (1"). Also use this technique for children over age 3.

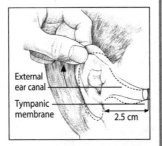

External ear canal
Tympanic membrane
2.5 cm

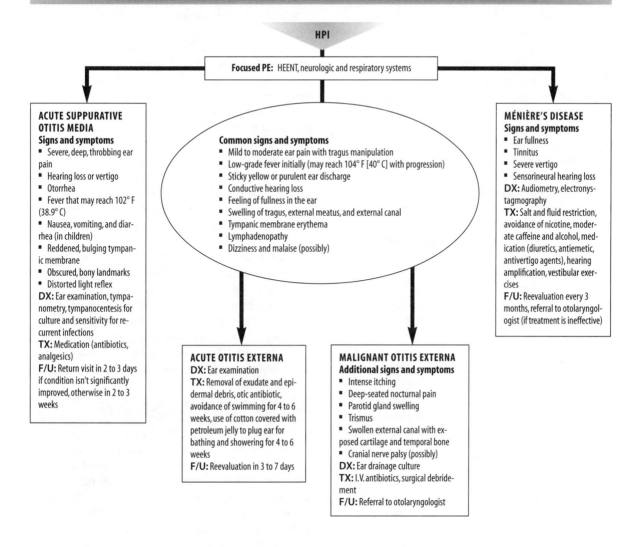

HPI

Focused PE: HEENT, neurologic and respiratory systems

ACUTE SUPPURATIVE OTITIS MEDIA
Signs and symptoms
- Severe, deep, throbbing ear pain
- Hearing loss or vertigo
- Otorrhea
- Fever that may reach 102° F (38.9° C)
- Nausea, vomiting, and diarrhea (in children)
- Reddened, bulging tympanic membrane
- Obscured, bony landmarks
- Distorted light reflex

DX: Ear examination, tympanometry, tympanocentesis for culture and sensitivity for recurrent infections
TX: Medication (antibiotics, analgesics)
F/U: Return visit in 2 to 3 days if condition isn't significantly improved, otherwise in 2 to 3 weeks

Common signs and symptoms
- Mild to moderate ear pain with tragus manipulation
- Low-grade fever initially (may reach 104° F [40° C] with progression)
- Sticky yellow or purulent ear discharge
- Conductive hearing loss
- Feeling of fullness in the ear
- Swelling of tragus, external meatus, and external canal
- Tympanic membrane erythema
- Lymphadenopathy
- Dizziness and malaise (possibly)

MÉNIÈRE'S DISEASE
Signs and symptoms
- Ear fullness
- Tinnitus
- Severe vertigo
- Sensorineural hearing loss

DX: Audiometry, electronystagmography
TX: Salt and fluid restriction, avoidance of nicotine, moderate caffeine and alcohol, medication (diuretics, antiemetic, antivertigo agents), hearing amplification, vestibular exercises
F/U: Reevaluation every 3 months, referral to otolaryngologist (if treatment is ineffective)

ACUTE OTITIS EXTERNA
DX: Ear examination
TX: Removal of exudate and epidermal debris, otic antibiotic, avoidance of swimming for 4 to 6 weeks, use of cotton covered with petroleum jelly to plug ear for bathing and showering for 4 to 6 weeks
F/U: Reevaluation in 3 to 7 days

MALIGNANT OTITIS EXTERNA
Additional signs and symptoms
- Intense itching
- Deep-seated nocturnal pain
- Parotid gland swelling
- Trismus
- Swollen external canal with exposed cartilage and temporal bone
- Cranial nerve palsy (possibly)

DX: Ear drainage culture
TX: I.V. antibiotics, surgical debridement
F/U: Referral to otolaryngologist

Additional differential diagnoses: abscess (extradural) ▪ barotrauma (acute) ▪ cerumen impaction ▪ chondrodermatitis nodularis chronica helicis ▪ ear canal obstruction by insect ▪ frostbite ▪ furunculosis ▪ herpes zoster oticus (Ramsay Hunt syndrome) ▪ keratosis obturans ▪ mastoiditis (acute) ▪ middle ear tumor ▪ myringitis bullosa ▪ otitis media ▪ perichondritis ▪ petrositis ▪ TMJ infection

Edema

A common sign in severely ill patients, *generalized edema* is the excessive accumulation of interstitial fluid throughout the body. Its severity varies widely; slight edema may be difficult to detect, especially if the patient is obese, whereas massive edema is immediately apparent.

Generalized edema is typically chronic and progressive. It may result from cardiac, renal, endocrine, or hepatic disorders as well as from severe burns, malnutrition, or the effects of certain drugs and treatments.

Facial edema refers to either localized swelling — around the eyes, for instance — or more generalized facial swelling that may extend to the neck and upper arms. Occasionally painful, this sign may develop gradually or abruptly. Sometimes it precedes onset of peripheral or generalized edema. Mild edema may be difficult to detect; the patient or someone who is familiar with his appearance may report it before it's noticed during assessment.

Leg edema results when excess interstitial fluid accumulates in one or both legs. It may affect just the foot and ankle or extend to the thigh, and may be slight or dramatic, pitting or nonpitting.

Leg edema may result from venous disorders, trauma, and certain bone and cardiac disorders that disturb normal fluid balance. However, several nonpathologic mechanisms may also cause leg edema. For example, prolonged sitting, standing, or immobility may cause bilateral orthostatic edema.

History and physical examination

Quickly determine the edema's severity, including the degree of pitting. If the patient has severe generalized edema, promptly take his vital signs, and check for distended neck veins and cyanotic lips. Auscultate the lungs and heart. Be alert for signs of cardiac failure or pulmonary congestion, such as crackles or ventricular gallop. Facial edema may affect the upper airway, causing life-threatening obstruction. Initiate emergency measures if necessary.

Obtain a complete medical history. First, note when the edema began. Does it move throughout the course of the day — for example, from the upper extremities to the lower, periorbitally, or within the sacral area? Is the edema worse in the morning or at the end of the day? Is it affected by position changes? Is it accompanied by shortness of breath or pain in the arms or legs? Find out how much weight the patient has gained. Has his urine output changed?

Next, ask about previous cardiac, renal, hepatic, endocrine, or GI disorders. Have the patient describe his diet so you can assess for protein malnutrition. Explore his drug history and note recent I.V. therapy.

Begin the physical examination by comparing the arms and legs for symmetrical edema. Also, note ecchymoses and cyanosis. Assess the back, sacrum, and hips of the bedridden patient for dependent edema. Palpate peripheral pulses, noting whether hands and feet feel cold. Finally, perform a complete cardiac and respiratory assessment.

If facial edema is present, ask if it developed suddenly or gradually. Is it more prominent in the early morning, or does it worsen throughout the day? Has the patient noticed any weight gain? If so, how much and over what length of time? Has he noticed a change in his urine color or output? In his appetite? Take a drug history and ask about recent facial trauma. Examine the oral cavity to evaluate dental hygiene and look for signs of infection. Visualize the oropharynx and look for soft-tissue swelling.

Examine each leg for pitting edema. Because leg edema may compromise arterial blood flow, palpate peripheral pulses to detect any insufficiency. Observe leg color and look for unusual vein patterns. Then palpate for warmth, tenderness, and cords, and gently squeeze the calf muscle against the tibia to check for deep pain. If leg edema is unilateral, dorsiflex the foot to look for Homans' sign, which is indicated by calf pain. Finally, note skin thickening or ulceration in the edematous areas.

PEDIATRIC POINTERS

- *Renal failure in children commonly causes generalized edema.*
- *Kwashiorkor — protein-deficiency malnutrition — is more common in children than adults and causes anasarca.*
- *Children are more likely to develop periorbital edema because periorbital tissue pressure is lower in children than adults.*
- *Periorbital edema is more common than peripheral edema in children with such disorders as heart failure and acute glomerulonephritis. Pertussis may also cause periorbital edema.*
- *Uncommon in children, leg edema may result from osteomyelitis, leg trauma or, rarely, heart failure.*

ELDER CARE CUES

- *Elderly patients are more likely to develop edema for several reasons, including decreased cardiac and renal function and, in some cases, poor nutritional status.*
- *Use caution when giving older patients I.V. fluids or medications that can raise sodium levels and thereby increase fluid retention.*

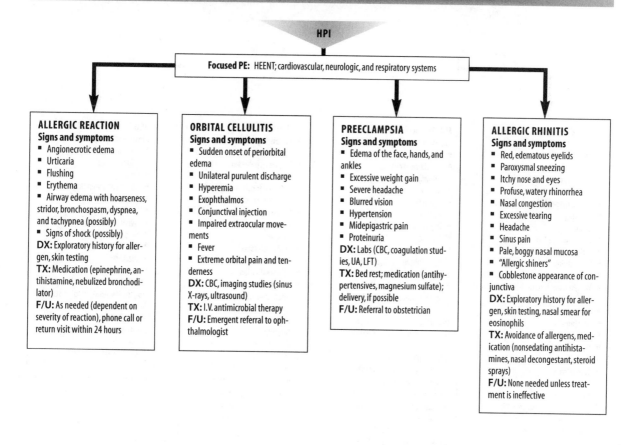

HPI

Focused PE: HEENT; cardiovascular, neurologic, and respiratory systems

ALLERGIC REACTION
Signs and symptoms
- Angionecrotic edema
- Urticaria
- Flushing
- Erythema
- Airway edema with hoarseness, stridor, bronchospasm, dyspnea, and tachypnea (possibly)
- Signs of shock (possibly)

DX: Exploratory history for allergen, skin testing
TX: Medication (epinephrine, antihistamine, nebulized bronchodilator)
F/U: As needed (dependent on severity of reaction), phone call or return visit within 24 hours

ORBITAL CELLULITIS
Signs and symptoms
- Sudden onset of periorbital edema
- Unilateral purulent discharge
- Hyperemia
- Exophthalmos
- Conjunctival injection
- Impaired extraocular movements
- Fever
- Extreme orbital pain and tenderness

DX: CBC, imaging studies (sinus X-rays, ultrasound)
TX: I.V. antimicrobial therapy
F/U: Emergent referral to ophthalmologist

PREECLAMPSIA
Signs and symptoms
- Edema of the face, hands, and ankles
- Excessive weight gain
- Severe headache
- Blurred vision
- Hypertension
- Midepigastric pain
- Proteinuria

DX: Labs (CBC, coagulation studies, UA, LFT)
TX: Bed rest; medication (antihypertensives, magnesium sulfate); delivery, if possible
F/U: Referral to obstetrician

ALLERGIC RHINITIS
Signs and symptoms
- Red, edematous eyelids
- Paroxysmal sneezing
- Itchy nose and eyes
- Profuse, watery rhinorrhea
- Nasal congestion
- Excessive tearing
- Headache
- Sinus pain
- Pale, boggy nasal mucosa
- "Allergic shiners"
- Cobblestone appearance of conjunctiva

DX: Exploratory history for allergen, skin testing, nasal smear for eosinophils
TX: Avoidance of allergens, medication (nonsedating antihistamines, nasal decongestant, steroid sprays)
F/U: None needed unless treatment is ineffective

Additional differential diagnoses: abscess (peritonsillar or periodontal) ▪ cavernous sinus thrombosis ▪ chalazion ▪ conjunctivitis ▪ corneal ulcers (fungal) ▪ dacryoadenitis ▪ dacryocystitis ▪ dermatomyositis ▪ facial burns ▪ facial trauma ▪ frontal sinus cancer ▪ generalized edema ▪ herpes zoster ophthalmicus (shingles) ▪ hordeolum (stye) ▪ malnutrition ▪ Melkersson's syndrome ▪ myxedema ▪ nephrotic syndrome ▪ osteomyelitis ▪ sinusitis ▪ superior vena cava syndrome ▪ trachoma ▪ richinosis

Other causes: drugs ▪ long-term use of glucocorticoids ▪ drugs that cause allergic reactions (aspirin, antipyretics, penicillin, sulfa preparations) ▪ allergic reaction to contrast medium ▪ cranial, nasal, or jaw surgery

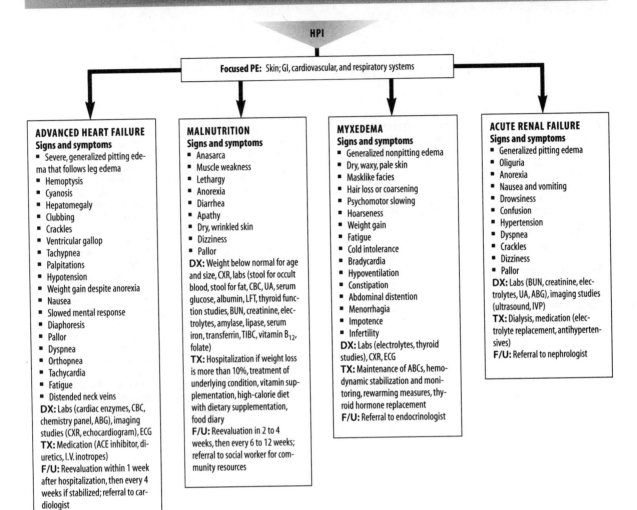

HPI

Focused PE: Skin; GI, cardiovascular, and respiratory systems

ADVANCED HEART FAILURE
Signs and symptoms
- Severe, generalized pitting edema that follows leg edema
- Hemoptysis
- Cyanosis
- Hepatomegaly
- Clubbing
- Crackles
- Ventricular gallop
- Tachypnea
- Palpitations
- Hypotension
- Weight gain despite anorexia
- Nausea
- Slowed mental response
- Diaphoresis
- Pallor
- Dyspnea
- Orthopnea
- Tachycardia
- Fatigue
- Distended neck veins

DX: Labs (cardiac enzymes, CBC, chemistry panel, ABG), imaging studies (CXR, echocardiogram), ECG
TX: Medication (ACE inhibitor, diuretics, I.V. inotropes)
F/U: Reevaluation within 1 week after hospitalization, then every 4 weeks if stabilized; referral to cardiologist

MALNUTRITION
Signs and symptoms
- Anasarca
- Muscle weakness
- Lethargy
- Anorexia
- Diarrhea
- Apathy
- Dry, wrinkled skin
- Dizziness
- Pallor

DX: Weight below normal for age and size, CXR, labs (stool for occult blood, stool for fat, CBC, UA, serum glucose, albumin, BUN, creatinine, electrolytes, amylase, lipase, serum iron, transferrin, TIBC, vitamin B_{12}, folate)
TX: Hospitalization if weight loss is more than 10%, treatment of underlying condition, vitamin supplementation, high-calorie diet with dietary supplementation, food diary
F/U: Reevaluation in 2 to 4 weeks, then every 6 to 12 weeks; referral to social worker for community resources

MYXEDEMA
Signs and symptoms
- Generalized nonpitting edema
- Dry, waxy, pale skin
- Masklike facies
- Hair loss or coarsening
- Psychomotor slowing
- Hoarseness
- Weight gain
- Fatigue
- Cold intolerance
- Bradycardia
- Hypoventilation
- Constipation
- Abdominal distention
- Menorrhagia
- Impotence
- Infertility

DX: Labs (electrolytes, thyroid studies), CXR, ECG
TX: Maintenance of ABCs, hemodynamic stabilization and monitoring, rewarming measures, thyroid hormone replacement
F/U: Referral to endocrinologist

ACUTE RENAL FAILURE
Signs and symptoms
- Generalized pitting edema
- Oliguria
- Anorexia
- Nausea and vomiting
- Drowsiness
- Confusion
- Hypertension
- Dyspnea
- Crackles
- Dizziness
- Pallor

DX: Labs (BUN, creatinine, electrolytes, UA, ABG), imaging studies (ultrasound, IVP)
TX: Dialysis, medication (electrolyte replacement, antihypertensives)
F/U: Referral to nephrologist

Additional differential diagnoses: angioneurotic edema ▪ burns ▪ cirrhosis ▪ nephrotic syndrome ▪ pericardial effusion ▪ pericarditis (chronic constrictive) ▪ protein-losing enteropathy ▪ renal failure (chronic) ▪ septic shock

---

Other causes: drugs that cause sodium retention (antihypertensives, corticosteroids, androgenic and anabolic steroids, estrogens, NSAIDs) ▪ I.V. saline solution infusions ▪ enteral feedings

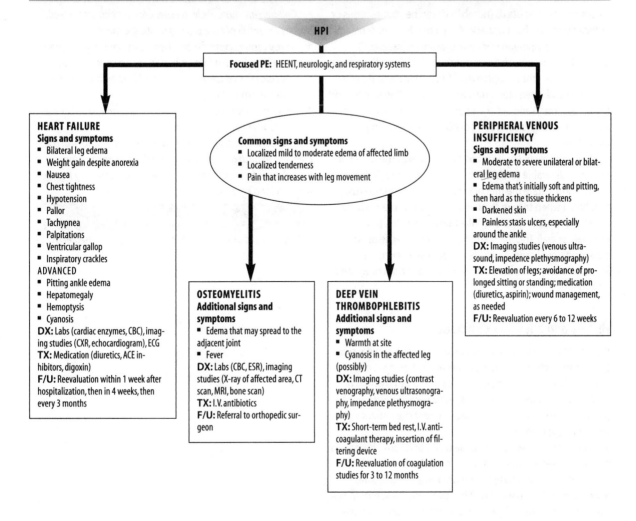

HPI

Focused PE: HEENT, neurologic, and respiratory systems

HEART FAILURE
Signs and symptoms
- Bilateral leg edema
- Weight gain despite anorexia
- Nausea
- Chest tightness
- Hypotension
- Pallor
- Tachypnea
- Palpitations
- Ventricular gallop
- Inspiratory crackles
ADVANCED
- Pitting ankle edema
- Hepatomegaly
- Hemoptysis
- Cyanosis

DX: Labs (cardiac enzymes, CBC), imaging studies (CXR, echocardiogram), ECG
TX: Medication (diuretics, ACE inhibitors, digoxin)
F/U: Reevaluation within 1 week after hospitalization, then in 4 weeks, then every 3 months

Common signs and symptoms
- Localized mild to moderate edema of affected limb
- Localized tenderness
- Pain that increases with leg movement

OSTEOMYELITIS
Additional signs and symptoms
- Edema that may spread to the adjacent joint
- Fever

DX: Labs (CBC, ESR), imaging studies (X-ray of affected area, CT scan, MRI, bone scan)
TX: I.V. antibiotics
F/U: Referral to orthopedic surgeon

DEEP VEIN THROMBOPHLEBITIS
Additional signs and symptoms
- Warmth at site
- Cyanosis in the affected leg (possibly)

DX: Imaging studies (contrast venography, venous ultrasonography, impedance plethysmography)
TX: Short-term bed rest, I.V. anticoagulant therapy, insertion of filtering device
F/U: Reevaluation of coagulation studies for 3 to 12 months

PERIPHERAL VENOUS INSUFFICIENCY
Signs and symptoms
- Moderate to severe unilateral or bilateral leg edema
- Edema that's initially soft and pitting, then hard as the tissue thickens
- Darkened skin
- Painless stasis ulcers, especially around the ankle

DX: Imaging studies (venous ultrasound, impedence plethysmography)
TX: Elevation of legs; avoidance of prolonged sitting or standing; medication (diuretics, aspirin); wound management, as needed
F/U: Reevaluation every 6 to 12 weeks

Additional differential diagnoses: burns ▪ envenomation ▪ leg trauma ▪ peripheral vascular disease ▪ phlegmasia cerulea dolens ▪ superficial vein thrombophlebitis

Epistaxis

A common sign, epistaxis (nosebleed) can be spontaneous or induced from the front or back of the nose. Most nosebleeds occur in the anterior-inferior nasal septum (Kiesselbach's plexus), but they may also occur at the point where the inferior turbinates meet the nasopharynx. Usually unilateral, they seem bilateral when blood runs from the bleeding side behind the nasal septum and out the opposite side. Epistaxis ranges from mild oozing to severe — possibly life-threatening — blood loss.

A rich supply of fragile blood vessels makes the nose particularly vulnerable to bleeding. Air moving through the nose can dry and irritate the mucous membranes, forming crusts that bleed when they're removed; dry mucous membranes are also more susceptible to infections, which can produce epistaxis as well. Trauma is another common cause of epistaxis. Additional causes include septal deviations; hematologic, coagulation, renal, and GI disorders; and certain drugs and treatments.

History and physical examination

If your patient has severe epistaxis, quickly take his vital signs. Be alert for tachypnea, hypotension, and other signs of hypovolemic shock. Attempt to control bleeding by pinching the nares closed. (However, if you suspect a nasal fracture, *don't* pinch the nares. Instead, place gauze under the patient's nose to absorb the blood.)

Have a hypovolemic patient lie down and turn his head to the side to prevent blood from draining down the back of his throat, which could cause aspiration or vomiting of swallowed blood. If the patient isn't hypovolemic, have him sit upright and tilt his head forward. Constantly check airway patency. Initiate emergency measures if necessary.

If your patient isn't in distress, take a history. Does he have a history of recent trauma? How often has he had nosebleeds in the past? Have the nosebleeds been long or unusually severe? Has the patient recently had surgery in the sinus area? Ask about a history of hypertension, bleeding or liver disorders, and other recent illnesses. Ask if the patient bruises easily. Find out what drugs he uses, especially anti-inflammatories, such as aspirin, and anticoagulants, such as warfarin sodium. Question if there's use of cocaine or other illicit drug use nasally.

Begin the physical examination by inspecting the patient's skin for other signs of bleeding, such as ecchymoses and petechiae, and noting any jaundice, pallor, or other abnormalities. When examining a trauma patient, look for associated injuries, such as eye trauma or facial fractures.

PEDIATRIC POINTERS

- *Children are more likely to experience anterior nosebleeds, usually the result of nose picking or allergic rhinitis.*
- *Biliary atresia, cystic fibrosis, hereditary afibrinogenemia, and nasal trauma due to a foreign body can also cause epistaxis.*
- *Rubeola may cause an oozing nosebleed along with the characteristic maculopapular rash.*
- *Two rare childhood diseases — pertussis and diphtheria — can also cause oozing epistaxis.*
- *Suspect a bleeding disorder if you see excess umbilical cord bleeding at birth or profuse bleeding during circumcision.*
- *Epistaxis frequently begins at puberty in hereditary hemorrhagic telangiectasia.*

ELDER CARE CUE

Elderly patients are more likely to have posterior nosebleeds.

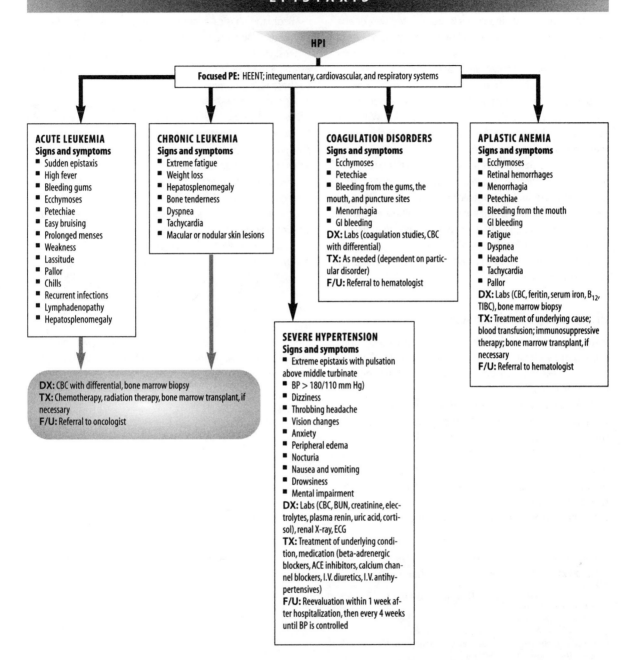

HPI

Focused PE: HEENT; integumentary, cardiovascular, and respiratory systems

ACUTE LEUKEMIA
Signs and symptoms
- Sudden epistaxis
- High fever
- Bleeding gums
- Ecchymoses
- Petechiae
- Easy bruising
- Prolonged menses
- Weakness
- Lassitude
- Pallor
- Chills
- Recurrent infections
- Lymphadenopathy
- Hepatosplenomegaly

CHRONIC LEUKEMIA
Signs and symptoms
- Extreme fatigue
- Weight loss
- Hepatosplenomegaly
- Bone tenderness
- Dyspnea
- Tachycardia
- Macular or nodular skin lesions

COAGULATION DISORDERS
Signs and symptoms
- Ecchymoses
- Petechiae
- Bleeding from the gums, the mouth, and puncture sites
- Menorrhagia
- GI bleeding
DX: Labs (coagulation studies, CBC with differential)
TX: As needed (dependent on particular disorder)
F/U: Referral to hematologist

APLASTIC ANEMIA
Signs and symptoms
- Ecchymoses
- Retinal hemorrhages
- Menorrhagia
- Petechiae
- Bleeding from the mouth
- GI bleeding
- Fatigue
- Dyspnea
- Headache
- Tachycardia
- Pallor
DX: Labs (CBC, feritin, serum iron, B$_{12}$, TIBC), bone marrow biopsy
TX: Treatment of underlying cause; blood transfusion; immunosuppressive therapy; bone marrow transplant, if necessary
F/U: Referral to hematologist

DX: CBC with differential, bone marrow biopsy
TX: Chemotherapy, radiation therapy, bone marrow transplant, if necessary
F/U: Referral to oncologist

SEVERE HYPERTENSION
Signs and symptoms
- Extreme epistaxis with pulsation above middle turbinate
- BP > 180/110 mm Hg)
- Dizziness
- Throbbing headache
- Vision changes
- Anxiety
- Peripheral edema
- Nocturia
- Nausea and vomiting
- Drowsiness
- Mental impairment
DX: Labs (CBC, BUN, creatinine, electrolytes, plasma renin, uric acid, cortisol), renal X-ray, ECG
TX: Treatment of underlying condition, medication (beta-adrenergic blockers, ACE inhibitors, calcium channel blockers, I.V. diuretics, I.V. antihypertensives)
F/U: Reevaluation within 1 week after hospitalization, then every 4 weeks until BP is controlled

Additional differential diagnoses: angiofibroma (juvenile) ▪ barotrauma ▪ biliary obstruction ▪ cirrhosis ▪ glomerulonephritis (chronic) ▪ hepatitis ▪ hereditary hemorrhagic telangiectasia (Rendu-Osler-Weber syndrome) ▪ infectious mononucleosis ▪ influenza ▪ maxillofacial injury ▪ nasal fracture ▪ nasal tumor ▪ orbital floor fracture ▪ polycythemia vera ▪ renal failure ▪ sarcoidosis ▪ scleroma ▪ sinusitis (acute) ▪ skull fracture ▪ SLE ▪ syphilis ▪ typhoid fever

Other causes: anticoagulants (such as coumadin) ▪ anti-inflammatories (such as aspirin) ▪ chemical irritants ▪ facial and nasal surgery (rare), including septoplasty, rhinoplasty, antrostomy, endoscopic sinus procedures, orbital decompression, and dental extraction ▪ habitual illicit drug use, especially cocaine

Erythema

Dilated or congested blood vessels produce red skin, or erythema, the most common sign of skin inflammation or irritation. Erythema may be localized or generalized and may occur suddenly or gradually. Skin color can range from bright red in acute conditions to pale violet or brown in chronic problems. Erythema must be differentiated from purpura, which causes redness from bleeding into the skin. When pressure is applied directly to the skin, erythema blanches momentarily, but purpura doesn't.

Erythema usually results from changes in the arteries, veins, and small vessels that lead to increased small-vessel perfusion. Drugs and neurogenic mechanisms can also allow extra blood to enter the small vessels. In addition, erythema can result from trauma and tissue damage as well as from changes in supporting tissues, which increase vessel visibility. A number of rare disorders can also cause this sign. (See *Rare causes of erythema*.)

History and physical examination

If your patient has sudden progressive erythema with rapid pulse, dyspnea, hoarseness, and agitation, quickly take his vital signs. These may be signs of anaphylactic shock. Initiate emergency measures if necessary.

If erythema isn't associated with anaphylaxis, obtain a detailed health history. Find out how long the patient has had the erythema and where it first began. Has he had associated pain or itching? Has he recently had a fever, upper respiratory infection, or joint pain? Does he have a history of skin disease or other illness? Does he or anyone in his family have allergies, asthma, or eczema? Find out if he has been exposed to someone who has had a similar rash or who is now ill.

Obtain a complete drug history, including recent immunizations. Ask about food intake and exposure to chemicals.

Begin the physical examination by assessing the extent, distribution, and intensity of erythema. Look for edema and other skin lesions, such as hives, scales, papules, and purpura. Examine the affected area for warmth, and gently palpate it to check for tenderness or crepitus.

PEDIATRIC POINTERS

- *Normally, newborn rash (erythema toxicum neonatorum), a pink papular rash, develops during the first 4 days after birth and spontaneously disappears by the 10th day.*
- *Newborns and infants can also develop erythema from infections and other disorders. For instance, candidiasis can produce thick, white lesions over an erythematous base on the oral mucosa, as well as diaper rash with beefy red erythema.*
- *Roseola, rubeola, scarlet fever, granuloma annulare, and cutis marmorata also cause erythema in children.*

ELDER CARE CUE

Elderly patients commonly have well-demarcated purple macules or patches, usually on the back of the hands and on the forearms. Known as actinic purpura, this condition results from blood leaking through fragile capillaries. The lesions disappear spontaneously.

Rare causes of erythema

In exceptional cases, your patient's erythema may be caused by one of these rare disorders:
- *acute febrile neutrophilic dermatosis,* which produces erythematous lesions on the face, neck, and extremities after a high fever
- *erythema ab igne,* which produces lacy erythema and telangiectases after exposure to radiant heat
- *erythema chronicum migrans,* which produces erythematous macules and papules on the trunk, upper arms, or thighs after a tick bite
- *erythema gyratum repens,* which produces wavy bands of erythema and is often associated with internal malignancy
- *toxic epidermal necrolysis,* which causes severe, widespread erythema, tenderness, and skin loss related to staphylococci or, possibly, to the use of certain drugs.

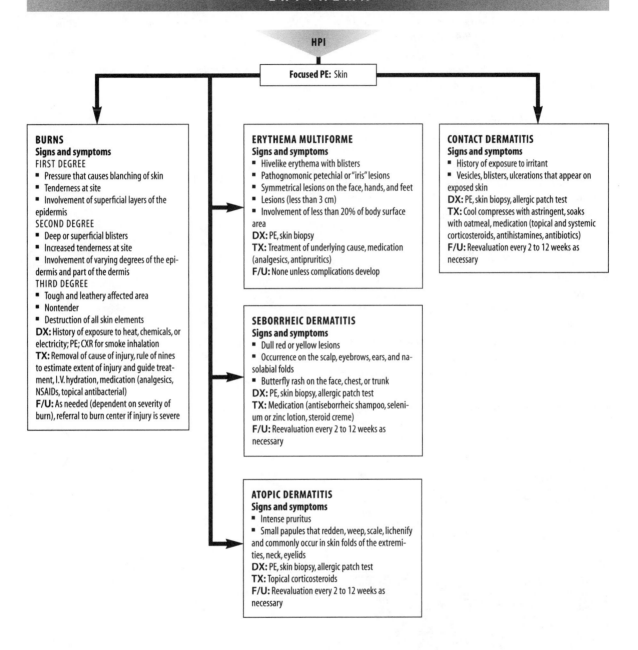

HPI

Focused PE: Skin

BURNS
Signs and symptoms
FIRST DEGREE
- Pressure that causes blanching of skin
- Tenderness at site
- Involvement of superficial layers of the epidermis
SECOND DEGREE
- Deep or superficial blisters
- Increased tenderness at site
- Involvement of varying degrees of the epidermis and part of the dermis
THIRD DEGREE
- Tough and leathery affected area
- Nontender
- Destruction of all skin elements
DX: History of exposure to heat, chemicals, or electricity; PE; CXR for smoke inhalation
TX: Removal of cause of injury, rule of nines to estimate extent of injury and guide treatment, I.V. hydration, medication (analgesics, NSAIDs, topical antibacterial)
F/U: As needed (dependent on severity of burn), referral to burn center if injury is severe

ERYTHEMA MULTIFORME
Signs and symptoms
- Hivelike erythema with blisters
- Pathognomonic petechial or "iris" lesions
- Symmetrical lesions on the face, hands, and feet
- Lesions (less than 3 cm)
- Involvement of less than 20% of body surface area
DX: PE, skin biopsy
TX: Treatment of underlying cause, medication (analgesics, antipruritics)
F/U: None unless complications develop

SEBORRHEIC DERMATITIS
Signs and symptoms
- Dull red or yellow lesions
- Occurrence on the scalp, eyebrows, ears, and nasolabial folds
- Butterfly rash on the face, chest, or trunk
DX: PE, skin biopsy, allergic patch test
TX: Medication (antiseborrheic shampoo, selenium or zinc lotion, steroid creme)
F/U: Reevaluation every 2 to 12 weeks as necessary

ATOPIC DERMATITIS
Signs and symptoms
- Intense pruritus
- Small papules that redden, weep, scale, lichenify and commonly occur in skin folds of the extremities, neck, eyelids
DX: PE, skin biopsy, allergic patch test
TX: Topical corticosteroids
F/U: Reevaluation every 2 to 12 weeks as necessary

CONTACT DERMATITIS
Signs and symptoms
- History of exposure to irritant
- Vesicles, blisters, ulcerations that appear on exposed skin
DX: PE, skin biopsy, allergic patch test
TX: Cool compresses with astringent, soaks with oatmeal, medication (topical and systemic corticosteroids, antihistamines, antibiotics)
F/U: Reevaluation every 2 to 12 weeks as necessary

Additional differential diagnoses: allergic reaction ▪ candidiasis ▪ chronic liver disease ▪ dermatomyositis ▪ erysipelas ▪ erythema annulare centrifugum ▪ erythema marginatum rheumaticum ▪ erythema nodosum ▪ frostbite ▪ intertrigo ▪ necrotizing fasciitis ▪ polymorphous light eruption ▪ psoriasis ▪ Raynaud's disease ▪ rheumatoid arthritis ▪ rosacea ▪ rubella ▪ SLE ▪ thrombophlebitis ▪ toxic shock syndrome

Other causes: drugs ▪ ingestion of ginkgo biloba fruit pulp ▪ St. John's wort ▪ radiation therapy

Exophthalmos

Exophthalmos (proptosis) — the abnormal protrusion of one or both eyeballs — may result from hemorrhage, edema, or inflammation behind the eye; extraocular muscle relaxation; or space-occupying intraorbital lesions and metastatic tumors. This sign may occur suddenly or gradually, causing mild to dramatic protrusion. Occasionally, the affected eye also pulsates. The most common cause of exophthalmos in adults is dysthyroid eye disease.

Exophthalmos is usually easily observed. However, lid retraction may mimic exophthalmos even when protrusion is absent. Similarly, ptosis in one eye may make the other eye appear exophthalmic by comparison. An exophthalmometer can differentiate these signs by measuring ocular protrusion.

History and physical examination

Begin by asking when the patient first noticed exophthalmos. Is it associated with pain in or around the eye? If so, ask him how severe it is and how long he has had it. Then ask about recent sinus infection or vision problems. Take the patient's vital signs, noting fever, which may accompany eye infection. Next, evaluate the severity of exophthalmos with an exophthalmometer. (See *Detecting unilateral exophthalmos.*) If the eyes bulge severely, look for cloudiness on the cornea, which may indicate ulcer formation. Describe any eye discharge and observe for ptosis. Then check visual acuity, with and without correction, and evaluate extraocular movements.

- *In children around age 5, a rare tumor — optic nerve glioma — may cause exophthalmos.*
- *Rhabdomyosarcoma, a more common tumor, usually affects children between ages 4 and 12 and produces rapid onset of exophthalmos.*

Detecting unilateral exophthalmos

If one of the patient's eyes seems more prominent than the other, examine both eyes from above the patient's head. Look down across his face, gently draw his lids up, and compare the relationship of the corneas to the lower lids. Abnormal protrusion of one eye suggests unilateral exophthalmos. *Remember:* Don't perform this test if you suspect eye trauma.

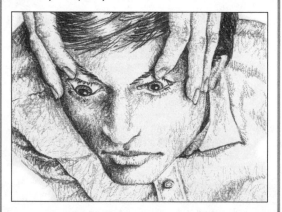

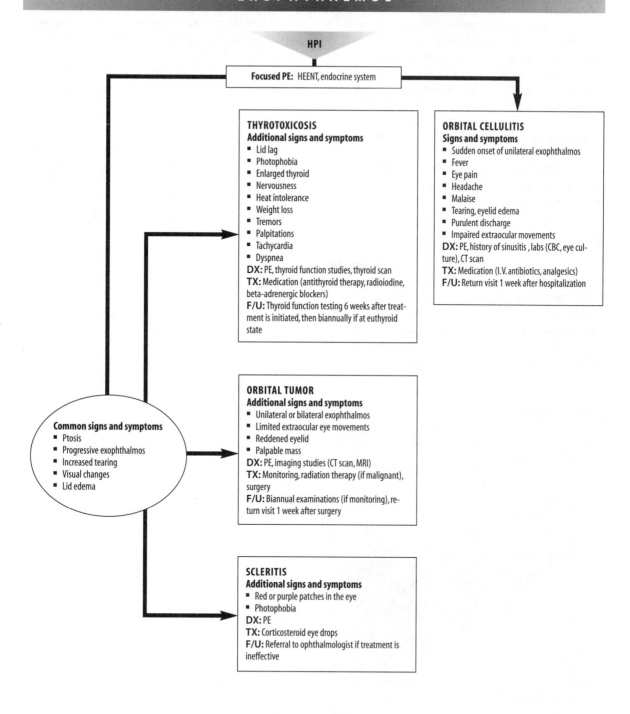

HPI

Focused PE: HEENT, endocrine system

THYROTOXICOSIS
Additional signs and symptoms
- Lid lag
- Photophobia
- Enlarged thyroid
- Nervousness
- Heat intolerance
- Weight loss
- Tremors
- Palpitations
- Tachycardia
- Dyspnea

DX: PE, thyroid function studies, thyroid scan
TX: Medication (antithyroid therapy, radioiodine, beta-adrenergic blockers)
F/U: Thyroid function testing 6 weeks after treatment is initiated, then biannually if at euthyroid state

ORBITAL CELLULITIS
Signs and symptoms
- Sudden onset of unilateral exophthalmos
- Fever
- Eye pain
- Headache
- Malaise
- Tearing, eyelid edema
- Purulent discharge
- Impaired extraocular movements

DX: PE, history of sinusitis , labs (CBC, eye culture), CT scan
TX: Medication (I.V. antibiotics, analgesics)
F/U: Return visit 1 week after hospitalization

ORBITAL TUMOR
Additional signs and symptoms
- Unilateral or bilateral exophthalmos
- Limited extraocular eye movements
- Reddened eyelid
- Palpable mass

DX: PE, imaging studies (CT scan, MRI)
TX: Monitoring, radiation therapy (if malignant), surgery
F/U: Biannual examinations (if monitoring), return visit 1 week after surgery

Common signs and symptoms
- Ptosis
- Progressive exophthalmos
- Increased tearing
- Visual changes
- Lid edema

SCLERITIS
Additional signs and symptoms
- Red or purple patches in the eye
- Photophobia

DX: PE
TX: Corticosteroid eye drops
F/U: Referral to ophthalmologist if treatment is ineffective

Additional differential diagnoses: cavernous sinus thrombosis ▪ dacryoadenitis ▪ foreign body ▪ Hodgkin's disease ▪ lacrimal gland tumor ▪ leiomyosarcoma ▪ leukemia ▪ lymphangioma ▪ ocular tuberculosis ▪ optic nerve meningioma ▪ orbital choristoma ▪ orbital emphysema ▪ orbital pseudotumor ▪ parasite infestation

Eye discharge

Usually associated with conjunctivitis, an eye discharge is the excretion of any substance other than tears. This common sign may occur in one or both eyes, producing scant to copious discharge. The discharge may be purulent, frothy, mucoid, cheesy, serous, clear, or stringy and white Sometimes, the discharge can be expressed by applying pressure to the tear sac, punctum, meibomian glands, or canaliculus.

An eye discharge commonly results from inflammatory and infectious eye disorders but may also occur in certain systemic disorders. (See *Sources of eye discharge*.) Because this sign may accompany a disorder that threatens vision, it must be assessed and treated immediately.

History and physical examination

Begin your evaluation by finding out when the discharge began. Does it occur at certain times of day or in connection with certain activities? If the patient complains of pain, ask him to show you its exact location and to describe its character. Is the pain dull, continuous, sharp, or stabbing? Do his eyes itch or burn? Do they tear excessively? Are they sensitive to light? Does he feel like something is in them?

After taking vital signs, carefully inspect the eye discharge. Note its amount and consistency. Then test visual acuity, with and without correction. Examine external eye structures, beginning with the unaffected eye to prevent cross-contamination. Observe for eyelid edema, entropion, crusts, lesions, and trichiasis. Next, ask the patient to blink as you watch for impaired lid movement. If the eyes seem to bulge, measure them with an exophthalmometer. Test the six cardinal fields of gaze. Examine for conjunctival injection and follicles and for corneal cloudiness or white lesions.

PEDIATRIC POINTERS

- *In infants, prophylactic eye medication (silver nitrate) may cause eye irritation and discharge.*
- *In children, discharges usually result from eye trauma, eye infection, or upper respiratory infection.*

Sources of eye discharge

An eye discharge can come from the tear sac, punctum, meibomian glands, or canaliculi. If the patient reports a discharge that's not immediately apparent, you can express a sample by pressing your fingertip lightly over these structures. Then characterize the discharge and note its source.

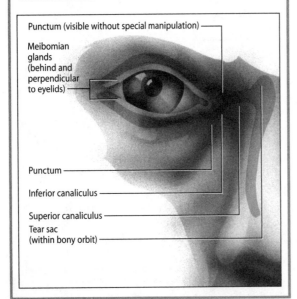

Punctum (visible without special manipulation)

Meibomian glands (behind and perpendicular to eyelids)

Punctum

Inferior canaliculus

Superior canaliculus

Tear sac (within bony orbit)

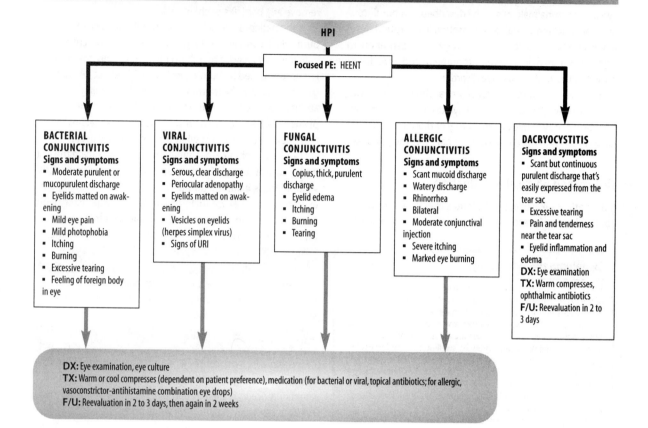

HPI

Focused PE: HEENT

BACTERIAL CONJUNCTIVITIS
Signs and symptoms
- Moderate purulent or mucopurulent discharge
- Eyelids matted on awakening
- Mild eye pain
- Mild photophobia
- Itching
- Burning
- Excessive tearing
- Feeling of foreign body in eye

VIRAL CONJUNCTIVITIS
Signs and symptoms
- Serous, clear discharge
- Periocular adenopathy
- Eyelids matted on awakening
- Vesicles on eyelids (herpes simplex virus)
- Signs of URI

FUNGAL CONJUNCTIVITIS
Signs and symptoms
- Copius, thick, purulent discharge
- Eyelid edema
- Itching
- Burning
- Tearing

ALLERGIC CONJUNCTIVITIS
Signs and symptoms
- Scant mucoid discharge
- Watery discharge
- Rhinorrhea
- Bilateral
- Moderate conjunctival injection
- Severe itching
- Marked eye burning

DACRYOCYSTITIS
Signs and symptoms
- Scant but continuous purulent discharge that's easily expressed from the tear sac
- Excessive tearing
- Pain and tenderness near the tear sac
- Eyelid inflammation and edema
DX: Eye examination
TX: Warm compresses, ophthalmic antibiotics
F/U: Reevaluation in 2 to 3 days

DX: Eye examination, eye culture
TX: Warm or cool compresses (dependent on patient preference), medication (for bacterial or viral, topical antibiotics; for allergic, vasoconstrictor-antihistamine combination eye drops)
F/U: Reevaluation in 2 to 3 days, then again in 2 weeks

Additional differential diagnoses: canaliculitis ▪ corneal ulcer ▪ dacryoadenitis ▪ erythema multiforme major ▪ herpes zoster ophthalmicus ▪ meibomianitis ▪ orbital cellulitis ▪ pemphigus ▪ psoriasis vulgaris ▪ trachoma

Eye pain

Eye pain (ophthalmalgia) may be described as a burning, throbbing, aching, or stabbing sensation in or around the eye. It may also be characterized as a foreign-body sensation. This sign varies from mild to severe; its duration and exact location provide clues to the causative disorder.

Eye pain usually results from corneal abrasion, but it may also be due to glaucoma or other eye disorders, trauma, and neurologic or systemic disorders. Any of these may stimulate nerve endings in the cornea or external eye, producing pain.

History and physical examination

If the patient's eye pain results from a chemical burn, remove contact lenses, if present, and irrigate the eye with at least 1 L (1.1 qt) of normal saline solution over 10 minutes. Evert the lids and wipe the fornices with a cotton-tipped applicator to remove any particles or chemicals.

If the patient's eye pain doesn't result from a chemical burn, take a complete history. Have the patient describe the pain fully. Is it an ache or a sharp pain? How long does it last? Is it accompanied by burning or itching? Find out when it began. Is it worse in the morning or late in the evening? Ask about recent trauma or surgery, especially if the patient complains of sudden, severe pain. Does he have headaches? If so, find out how often and at what time of day they occur.

During the physical examination, *don't* manipulate the eye if you suspect trauma. Carefully assess the lids and conjunctiva for redness, inflammation, and swelling. Then examine the eyes for ptosis or exophthalmos. Finally, test visual acuity with and without correction, and assess extraocular movements. Characterize any discharge. (See *Examining the external eye*.)

PEDIATRIC POINTER

Trauma and infection are the most common causes of eye pain in children. Be alert for nonverbal clues to pain, such as tightly shutting or frequently rubbing the eyes.

ELDER CARE CUE

Glaucoma, which can cause eye pain, is usually a disease of older patients, becoming clinically significant after age 40. It most commonly occurs bilaterally and leads to slowly progressive visual loss, especially in peripheral visual fields.

Examining the external eye

For patients with eye pain or other ocular symptoms, examination of the external eye forms an important part of the ocular assessment. Here's how to examine the external eye.

First, inspect the eyelids for ptosis and incomplete closure. Also, observe the lids for edema, erythema, cyanosis, hematoma, and masses. Evaluate skin lesions, growths, swelling, and tenderness by gross palpation. Are the lids everted or inverted? Do the eyelashes turn inward? Have some of them been lost? Do the lashes adhere to one another or contain a discharge? Next, examine the lid margins, noting especially any debris, scaling, lesions, or unusual secretions. Also, watch for eyelid spasms.

Now gently retract the eyelid with your thumb and forefinger, and assess the conjunctiva for redness, cloudiness, follicles, and blisters or other lesions. Check for chemosis by pressing the lower lid against the eyeball and noting any bulging above this compression point. Observe the sclera, noting any change from its normal white color.

Next, shine a light across the cornea to detect scars, abrasions, or ulcers. Note any color changes, dots, or opaque or cloudy areas. Also, assess the anterior eye chamber, which should be clean, deep, shadow-free, and filled with clear aqueous humor.

Inspect the color, shape, texture, and pattern of the iris. Then assess the pupils' size, shape, and equality. Finally, evaluate their response to light. Are they sluggish, fixed, or unresponsive? Does pupil dilation or constriction occur only on one side?

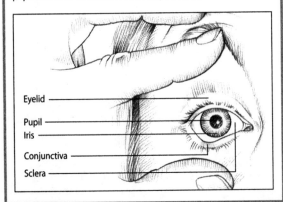

Eyelid

Pupil

Iris

Conjunctiva

Sclera

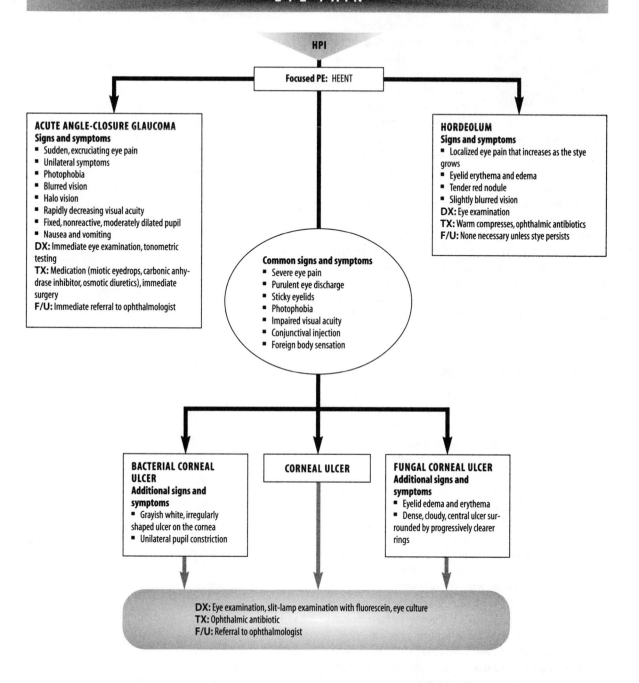

HPI

Focused PE: HEENT

ACUTE ANGLE-CLOSURE GLAUCOMA
Signs and symptoms
- Sudden, excruciating eye pain
- Unilateral symptoms
- Photophobia
- Blurred vision
- Halo vision
- Rapidly decreasing visual acuity
- Fixed, nonreactive, moderately dilated pupil
- Nausea and vomiting

DX: Immediate eye examination, tonometric testing
TX: Medication (miotic eyedrops, carbonic anhydrase inhibitor, osmotic diuretics), immediate surgery
F/U: Immediate referral to ophthalmologist

HORDEOLUM
Signs and symptoms
- Localized eye pain that increases as the stye grows
- Eyelid erythema and edema
- Tender red nodule
- Slightly blurred vision

DX: Eye examination
TX: Warm compresses, ophthalmic antibiotics
F/U: None necessary unless stye persists

Common signs and symptoms
- Severe eye pain
- Purulent eye discharge
- Sticky eyelids
- Photophobia
- Impaired visual acuity
- Conjunctival injection
- Foreign body sensation

BACTERIAL CORNEAL ULCER
Additional signs and symptoms
- Grayish white, irregularly shaped ulcer on the cornea
- Unilateral pupil constriction

CORNEAL ULCER

FUNGAL CORNEAL ULCER
Additional signs and symptoms
- Eyelid edema and erythema
- Dense, cloudy, central ulcer surrounded by progressively clearer rings

DX: Eye examination, slit-lamp examination with fluorescein, eye culture
TX: Ophthalmic antibiotic
F/U: Referral to ophthalmologist

Additional differential diagnoses: astigmatism ▪ blepharitis ▪ burns ▪ chalazion ▪ conjunctivitis ▪ corneal abrasion ▪ corneal erosion ▪ dacryoadenitis ▪ dacryocystitis ▪ episcleritis ▪ foreign body ▪ glaucoma ▪ herpes zoster ophthalmicus ▪ hyphema ▪ interstitial keratitis ▪ iritis (acute) ▪ keratoconjunctivitis sicca ▪ lacrimal gland tumor ▪ migraine headache ▪ optic neuritis ▪ orbital cellulitis ▪ pemphigus ▪ scleritis ▪ sclerokeratitis ▪ trachoma ▪ uveitis

Other causes: contact lenses ▪ ocular surgery

Fasciculations

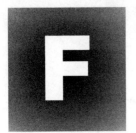

Fasciculations are local muscle contractions representing the spontaneous discharge of a muscle fiber bundle innervated by a single motor nerve filament. These contractions cause visible dimpling or wavelike twitching of the skin, but they aren't strong enough to produce joint movement. They occur irregularly at frequencies ranging from once every several seconds to two or three times per second; infrequently, myokymia — continuous, rapid fasciculations that cause a rippling effect — may occur. Because fasciculations are brief and painless, they may go undetected or are ignored.

Benign, nonpathologic fasciculations are common and normal. They may occur in tense, anxious, or overtired people and commonly affect the eyelid, thumb, or calf. However, fasciculations may also indicate a severe neurologic disorder, most notably a diffuse motor neuron disorder that causes loss of control over muscle fiber discharge. They're also early signs of pesticide poisoning.

History and physical examination

Begin by asking the patient about the nature, onset, and duration of the fasciculations. If the onset was sudden, ask about precipitating events such as exposure to pesticides. *Note:* Pesticide poisoning, although uncommon, is a medical emergency requiring prompt and vigorous intervention. Institute emergency measures, if necessary.

If the patient isn't in severe distress, find out if he has experienced sensory changes, such as paresthesia, or difficulty speaking, swallowing, breathing, or controlling bowel or bladder function. Ask him if he's in pain.

Explore the patient's medical history for neurologic disorders, cancer, and recent infections. Also ask about his lifestyle, especially stress at home, on the job, or at school.

Perform a physical examination, looking for fasciculations while the affected muscle is at rest. Observe and test for motor and sensory abnormalities, particularly muscle atrophy and weakness, and decreased deep tendon reflexes. If you note these signs, suspect motor neuron disease, and perform a comprehensive neurologic examination.

PEDIATRIC POINTER

Fasciculations, particularly of the tongue, are an important early sign of Werdnig-Hoffmann disease.

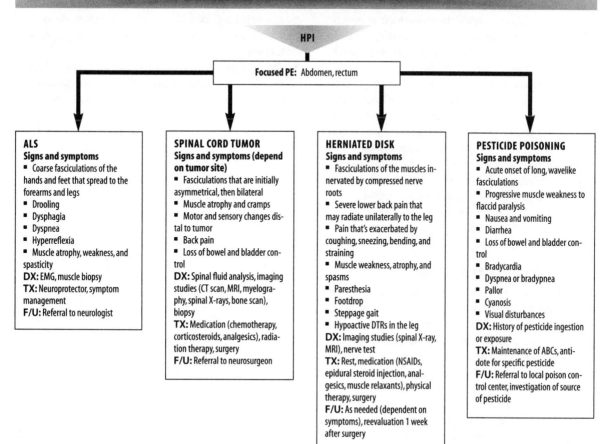

HPI

Focused PE: Abdomen, rectum

ALS
Signs and symptoms
- Coarse fasciculations of the hands and feet that spread to the forearms and legs
- Drooling
- Dysphagia
- Dyspnea
- Hyperreflexia
- Muscle atrophy, weakness, and spasticity
DX: EMG, muscle biopsy
TX: Neuroprotector, symptom management
F/U: Referral to neurologist

SPINAL CORD TUMOR
Signs and symptoms (depend on tumor site)
- Fasciculations that are initially asymmetrical, then bilateral
- Muscle atrophy and cramps
- Motor and sensory changes distal to tumor
- Back pain
- Loss of bowel and bladder control
DX: Spinal fluid analysis, imaging studies (CT scan, MRI, myelography, spinal X-rays, bone scan), biopsy
TX: Medication (chemotherapy, corticosteroids, analgesics), radiation therapy, surgery
F/U: Referral to neurosurgeon

HERNIATED DISK
Signs and symptoms
- Fasciculations of the muscles innervated by compressed nerve roots
- Severe lower back pain that may radiate unilaterally to the leg
- Pain that's exacerbated by coughing, sneezing, bending, and straining
- Muscle weakness, atrophy, and spasms
- Paresthesia
- Footdrop
- Steppage gait
- Hypoactive DTRs in the leg
DX: Imaging studies (spinal X-ray, MRI), nerve test
TX: Rest, medication (NSAIDs, epidural steroid injection, analgesics, muscle relaxants), physical therapy, surgery
F/U: As needed (dependent on symptoms), reevaluation 1 week after surgery

PESTICIDE POISONING
Signs and symptoms
- Acute onset of long, wavelike fasciculations
- Progressive muscle weakness to flaccid paralysis
- Nausea and vomiting
- Diarrhea
- Loss of bowel and bladder control
- Bradycardia
- Dyspnea or bradypnea
- Pallor
- Cyanosis
- Visual disturbances
DX: History of pesticide ingestion or exposure
TX: Maintenance of ABCs, antidote for specific pesticide
F/U: Referral to local poison control center, investigation of source of pesticide

---

Additional differential diagnoses: Guillain-Barré syndrome ▪ poliomyelitis ▪ syringomyelia

Fatigue

Fatigue is a feeling of excessive tiredness, lack of energy, or exhaustion accompanied by a strong desire to rest or sleep. This common symptom is distinct from weakness, which involves the muscles, but may occur with it.

Fatigue is a normal and important response to physical overexertion, prolonged emotional stress, and sleep deprivation. However, it can also be a nonspecific symptom of a psychological or physiologic disorder — especially viral infection and endocrine, cardiovascular, or neurologic disease.

Fatigue reflects hypermetabolic and hypometabolic states in which nutrients needed for cellular energy and growth are lacking because of overly rapid depletion, impaired replacement mechanisms, insufficient hormone production, or inadequate nutrient intake or metabolism.

History and physical examination

Obtain a careful history to identify the patient's fatigue pattern. Fatigue that worsens with activity and improves with rest generally indicates a physical disorder; the opposite pattern, a psychological disorder. Fatigue that lasts longer than 4 months, constant fatigue that's unrelieved by rest, and transient exhaustion that quickly gives way to bursts of energy are other findings associated with psychological disorders.

Ask about related symptoms and any recent viral illness or stressful changes in lifestyle. Explore nutritional habits and appetite or weight changes. Carefully review the patient's medical and psychiatric history for chronic disorders that commonly produce fatigue. Ask about a family history of such disorders.

Observe the patient's general appearance for overt signs of depression or organic illness. Is he unkempt or expressionless? Does he appear tired or sickly, or have a slumped posture? If warranted, evaluate his mental status, noting especially mental clouding, attention deficits, agitation, psychomotor retardation, or depression.

FATIGUE

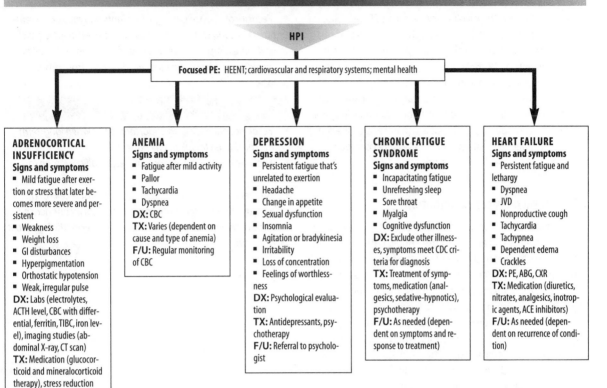

HPI

Focused PE: HEENT; cardiovascular and respiratory systems; mental health

ADRENOCORTICAL INSUFFICIENCY
Signs and symptoms
- Mild fatigue after exertion or stress that later becomes more severe and persistent
- Weakness
- Weight loss
- GI disturbances
- Hyperpigmentation
- Orthostatic hypotension
- Weak, irregular pulse

DX: Labs (electrolytes, ACTH level, CBC with differential, ferritin, TIBC, iron level), imaging studies (abdominal X-ray, CT scan)

TX: Medication (glucocorticoid and mineralocorticoid therapy), stress reduction

F/U: Regular monitoring of therapy

ANEMIA
Signs and symptoms
- Fatigue after mild activity
- Pallor
- Tachycardia
- Dyspnea

DX: CBC

TX: Varies (dependent on cause and type of anemia)

F/U: Regular monitoring of CBC

DEPRESSION
Signs and symptoms
- Persistent fatigue that's unrelated to exertion
- Headache
- Change in appetite
- Sexual dysfunction
- Insomnia
- Agitation or bradykinesia
- Irritability
- Loss of concentration
- Feelings of worthlessness

DX: Psychological evaluation

TX: Antidepressants, psychotherapy

F/U: Referral to psychologist

CHRONIC FATIGUE SYNDROME
Signs and symptoms
- Incapacitating fatigue
- Unrefreshing sleep
- Sore throat
- Myalgia
- Cognitive dysfunction

DX: Exclude other illnesses, symptoms meet CDC criteria for diagnosis

TX: Treatment of symptoms, medication (analgesics, sedative-hypnotics), psychotherapy

F/U: As needed (dependent on symptoms and response to treatment)

HEART FAILURE
Signs and symptoms
- Persistent fatigue and lethargy
- Dyspnea
- JVD
- Nonproductive cough
- Tachycardia
- Tachypnea
- Dependent edema
- Crackles

DX: PE, ABG, CXR

TX: Medication (diuretics, nitrates, analgesics, inotropic agents, ACE inhibitors)

F/U: As needed (dependent on recurrence of condition)

Additional differential diagnoses: AIDS ▪ anxiety ▪ cancer ▪ cirrhosis ▪ hypercortisolism ▪ hypopituitarism ▪ hypothyroidism ▪ infection ▪ Lyme disease ▪ malnutrition ▪ myasthenia gravis ▪ MI ▪ renal failure ▪ restrictive lung disease ▪ rheumatoid arthritis ▪ SLE ▪ sleep apnea ▪ thyrotoxicosis ▪ valvular heart disease

---

Other causes: antihypertensives ▪ sedatives ▪ cardiac glycosides ▪ surgery

Fecal incontinence

Fecal incontinence, the involuntary passage of feces, follows loss or impairment of external anal sphincter control. It can result from various GI, neurologic, and psychological disorders; the effects of drugs; and surgery. In some patients, it may even be a purposeful manipulative behavior.

Fecal incontinence may be temporary or permanent; its onset may be gradual, as in dementia, or sudden, as in spinal cord trauma. Although usually not a sign of severe illness, it can greatly affect the patient's physical and psychological well-being. (See *Bowel retraining tips*.)

History and physical examination

Ask the patient with fecal incontinence about its onset, duration, and severity and about any discernible pattern — for instance, at night or with diarrhea. Note the frequency, consistency, and volume of stools passed within the last 24 hours and obtain a stool sample. Focus your history taking on GI, neurologic, and psychological disorders.

Let the history guide your physical examination. If you suspect a brain or spinal cord lesion, perform a complete neurologic examination. If a GI disturbance seems likely, inspect the abdomen for distention, auscultate for bowel sounds, and percuss and palpate for a mass. Inspect the anal area for signs of excoriation or infection. If not contraindicated, check for fecal impaction, which may be associated with incontinence.

Bowel retraining tips

You can help your patient control fecal incontinence by instituting a bowel retraining program. Here's how:
- Begin by establishing a specific time for defecation. A typical schedule is once a day or once every other day after a meal, usually breakfast. However, be flexible when establishing a schedule, and consider the patient's normal habits and preferences.
- If necessary, help ensure regularity by administering a suppository, either glycerin or bisacodyl, about 30 minutes before the scheduled defecation time. Avoid the routine use of enemas or laxatives because they can cause dependence.
- Provide privacy and a relaxed environment to encourage regularity. If "accidents" occur, assure the patient that they're normal and don't mean that he has failed in the program.
- Adjust the patient's diet to provide adequate bulk and fiber; encourage him to eat more raw fruits and vegetables and whole grains. Ensure a fluid intake of at least 1,000 ml/day.
- If appropriate, encourage the patient to exercise regularly to help stimulate peristalsis.
- Be sure to keep accurate intake and elimination records.

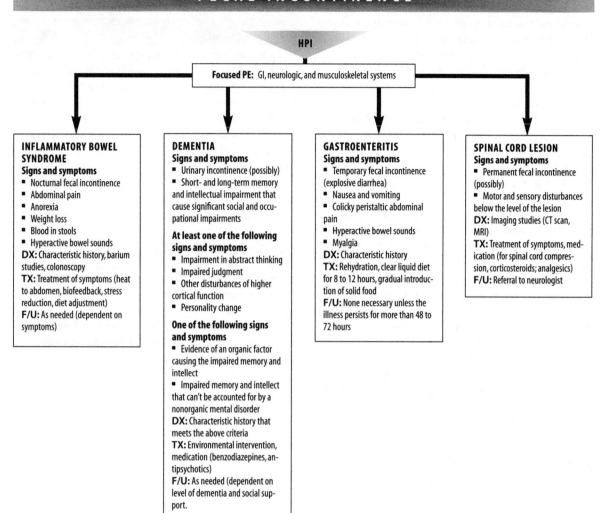

HPI

Focused PE: GI, neurologic, and musculoskeletal systems

INFLAMMATORY BOWEL SYNDROME
Signs and symptoms
- Nocturnal fecal incontinence
- Abdominal pain
- Anorexia
- Weight loss
- Blood in stools
- Hyperactive bowel sounds

DX: Characteristic history, barium studies, colonoscopy

TX: Treatment of symptoms (heat to abdomen, biofeedback, stress reduction, diet adjustment)

F/U: As needed (dependent on symptoms)

DEMENTIA
Signs and symptoms
- Urinary incontinence (possibly)
- Short- and long-term memory and intellectual impairment that cause significant social and occupational impairments

At least one of the following signs and symptoms
- Impairment in abstract thinking
- Impaired judgment
- Other disturbances of higher cortical function
- Personality change

One of the following signs and symptoms
- Evidence of an organic factor causing the impaired memory and intellect
- Impaired memory and intellect that can't be accounted for by a nonorganic mental disorder

DX: Characteristic history that meets the above criteria

TX: Environmental intervention, medication (benzodiazepines, antipsychotics)

F/U: As needed (dependent on level of dementia and social support.

GASTROENTERITIS
Signs and symptoms
- Temporary fecal incontinence (explosive diarrhea)
- Nausea and vomiting
- Colicky peristaltic abdominal pain
- Hyperactive bowel sounds
- Myalgia

DX: Characteristic history

TX: Rehydration, clear liquid diet for 8 to 12 hours, gradual introduction of solid food

F/U: None necessary unless the illness persists for more than 48 to 72 hours

SPINAL CORD LESION
Signs and symptoms
- Permanent fecal incontinence (possibly)
- Motor and sensory disturbances below the level of the lesion

DX: Imaging studies (CT scan, MRI)

TX: Treatment of symptoms, medication (for spinal cord compression, corticosteroids; analgesics)

F/U: Referral to neurologist

Additional differential diagnoses: head trauma ▪ multiple sclerosis ▪ rectovaginal fistula ▪ stroke ▪ tabes dorsalis

Other causes: chronic laxative abuse ▪ pelvic, prostate, or rectal surgery ▪ colostomy ▪ ileostomy

Fever

Fever (pyrexia), a common sign, can arise from disorders affecting virtually every body system. As a result, fever in the absence of other signs usually has little diagnostic significance. A persistent high-grade fever, though, represents an emergency.

Fever can be classified as low-grade (oral reading of 99° to 100.4° F [37.2° to 38° C]), moderate (100.5° to 104° F [38° to 40° C]), or high-grade (above 104° F). Fever over 108° F (42.2° C) causes unconsciousness and, if sustained, leads to permanent brain damage and death.

Fever may also be classified as remittent, intermittent, sustained, relapsing, or undulant. *Remittent fever,* the most common type, is characterized by daily temperature fluctuations above the normal range. *Intermittent fever* is marked by a daily temperature drop into the normal range, then a rise back to above normal. An intermittent fever that fluctuates widely, typically producing chills and sweating, is called *hectic* or *septic fever. Sustained fever* involves persistent temperature elevation with little fluctuation. *Relapsing fever* consists of alternating feverish and afebrile periods. *Undulant fever* refers to a gradual increase in temperature that stays high for a few days and then decreases gradually.

Further classification involves duration — either brief (less than 3 weeks) or prolonged. Prolonged fevers include fever of unknown origin, a classification used when careful examination fails to detect an underlying cause.

History and physical examination

If you detect a fever higher than 106° F (41.1° C), take the patient's other vital signs and determine his level of consciousness. Begin rapid cooling measures: Apply ice packs to the axillae and groin, give tepid sponge baths, or apply a hypothermia blanket. These methods may evoke a *hypothermic* response; to prevent this, constantly monitor the patient's rectal temperature.

If the patient's fever is only mild to moderate, ask him when it began and how high his temperature reached. Did the fever disappear, only to reappear later? Did he experience any other symptoms, such as chills, fatigue, or pain?

Obtain a complete medical history, noting especially immunosuppressive treatments or disorders, infection, trauma, surgery, diagnostic testing, and use of anesthesia or other medications. Ask about recent travel because certain diseases are endemic.

Let the history findings direct your physical examination. Because fever can accompany diverse disorders, the examina-tion may range from a brief evaluation of one body system to a comprehensive review of all systems.

PEDIATRIC POINTERS

- *Infants and young children experience higher and more prolonged fevers, more rapid temperature increases, and greater temperature fluctuations than older children and adults.*
- *Keep in mind that seizures commonly accompany extremely high fever, so take appropriate precautions.*
- *Common pediatric causes of fever include varicella, croup syndrome, dehydration, meningitis, mumps, otitis media, pertussis, roseola infantum, rubella, rubeola, and tonsillitis. Instruct parents not to give aspirin to a child with varicella or flulike symptoms because of the risk of precipitating Reye's syndrome.*
- *Fever can occur as a reaction to immunizations and antibiotics.*

ELDER CARE CUES

- *An elderly person may have an altered sweating mechanism that predisposes them to heatstroke when they're exposed to high temperatures.*
- *An elderly person may also have an impaired thermoregulatory mechanism, making temperature change a less reliable measure of disease severity.*

FEVER

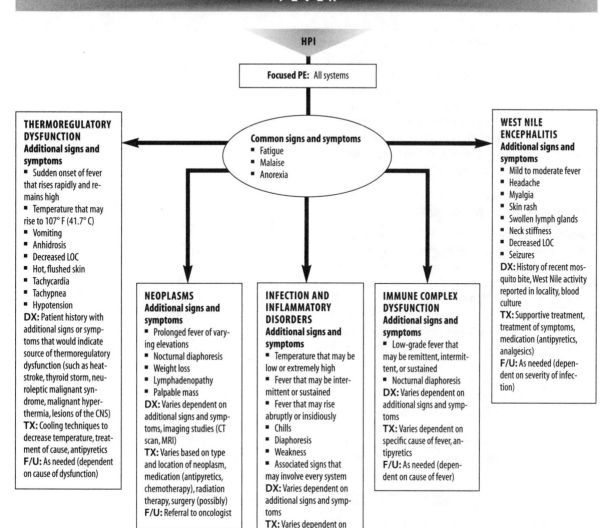

HPI

Focused PE: All systems

Common signs and symptoms
- Fatigue
- Malaise
- Anorexia

THERMOREGULATORY DYSFUNCTION
Additional signs and symptoms
- Sudden onset of fever that rises rapidly and remains high
- Temperature that may rise to 107° F (41.7° C)
- Vomiting
- Anhidrosis
- Decreased LOC
- Hot, flushed skin
- Tachycardia
- Tachypnea
- Hypotension

DX: Patient history with additional signs or symptoms that would indicate source of thermoregulatory dysfunction (such as heatstroke, thyroid storm, neuroleptic malignant syndrome, malignant hyperthermia, lesions of the CNS)
TX: Cooling techniques to decrease temperature, treatment of cause, antipyretics
F/U: As needed (dependent on cause of dysfunction)

NEOPLASMS
Additional signs and symptoms
- Prolonged fever of varying elevations
- Nocturnal diaphoresis
- Weight loss
- Lymphadenopathy
- Palpable mass

DX: Varies dependent on additional signs and symptoms, imaging studies (CT scan, MRI)
TX: Varies based on type and location of neoplasm, medication (antipyretics, chemotherapy), radiation therapy, surgery (possibly)
F/U: Referral to oncologist

INFECTION AND INFLAMMATORY DISORDERS
Additional signs and symptoms
- Temperature that may be low or extremely high
- Fever that may be intermittent or sustained
- Fever that may rise abruptly or insidiously
- Chills
- Diaphoresis
- Weakness
- Associated signs that may involve every system

DX: Varies dependent on additional signs and symptoms
TX: Varies dependent on source of fever, antipyretics
F/U: As needed (dependent on source of infection)

IMMUNE COMPLEX DYSFUNCTION
Additional signs and symptoms
- Low-grade fever that may be remittent, intermittent, or sustained
- Nocturnal diaphoresis

DX: Varies dependent on additional signs and symptoms
TX: Varies dependent on specific cause of fever, antipyretics
F/U: As needed (dependent on cause of fever)

WEST NILE ENCEPHALITIS
Additional signs and symptoms
- Mild to moderate fever
- Headache
- Myalgia
- Skin rash
- Swollen lymph glands
- Neck stiffness
- Decreased LOC
- Seizures

DX: History of recent mosquito bite, West Nile activity reported in locality, blood culture
TX: Supportive treatment, treatment of symptoms, medication (antipyretics, analgesics)
F/U: As needed (dependent on severity of infection)

Other causes: radiographic tests that use contrast medium ▪ hypersensitivity to antifungals, sulfonamides, penicillins, cephalosporins, tetracyclines, barbiturates, phenytoin, quinidine, iodides, phenolphthalein, methyldopa, procainamide, and some antitoxins ▪ chemotherapy (especially with bleomycin, vincristine, and asparaginase) ▪ anticholinergics ▪ phenothiazines ▪ MAO inhibitors ▪ toxic doses of salicylates, amphetamines, and TCAs ▪ inhalant anesthetics ▪ muscle relaxants ▪ surgery ▪ transfusion reactions

Flank pain

Pain in the flank, the area extending from the ribs to the ilium, is a leading indicator of renal and upper urinary tract disease or trauma. Depending on the cause, this symptom may vary from a dull ache to severe stabbing or throbbing pain and may be unilateral or bilateral and constant or intermittent. It's aggravated by costovertebral angle percussion and, in patients with renal or urinary tract obstruction, by increased fluid intake and ingestion of alcohol, caffeine, or diuretic drugs. Unaffected by position changes, flank pain typically responds only to analgesics or to treatment of the underlying disorder.

History and physical examination

If the patient has suffered trauma, quickly look for a visible or palpable flank mass, associated injuries, costovertebral angle pain, hematuria, Turner's sign, and signs of shock (such as tachycardia and cool, clammy skin).

If the patient's condition isn't critical, take a thorough history. Ask about the pain's onset and apparent precipitating events. Have him describe the pain's location, intensity, pattern, and duration. Find out if anything aggravates or alleviates it.

Ask the patient about any changes in his normal pattern of fluid intake and urine output. Explore his history for urinary tract infection or obstruction, renal disease, or recent streptococcal infection.

During the physical examination, palpate the patient's flank area and percuss the costovertebral angle to determine the extent of pain.

PEDIATRIC POINTERS

- *Assessment of flank pain can be difficult if a child can't describe the pain. In such cases, transillumination of the abdomen and flanks may help in assessment of bladder distention and identification of masses.*
- *Common causes of flank pain in children include obstructive uropathy, acute poststreptococcal glomerulonephritis, infantile polycystic kidney disease, and nephroblastoma.*

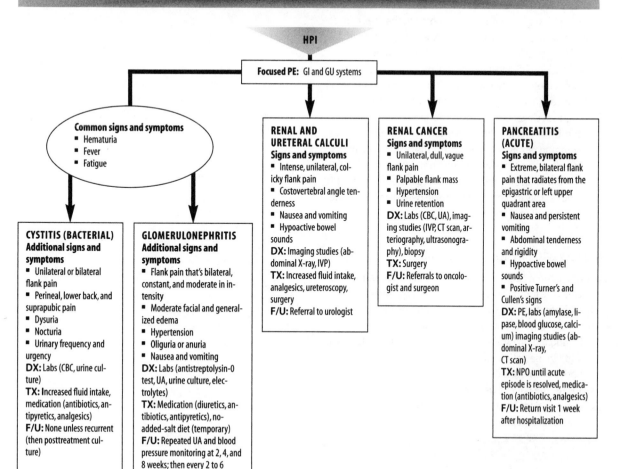

HPI

Focused PE: GI and GU systems

Common signs and symptoms
- Hematuria
- Fever
- Fatigue

CYSTITIS (BACTERIAL)
Additional signs and symptoms
- Unilateral or bilateral flank pain
- Perineal, lower back, and suprapubic pain
- Dysuria
- Nocturia
- Urinary frequency and urgency

DX: Labs (CBC, urine culture)

TX: Increased fluid intake, medication (antibiotics, antipyretics, analgesics)

F/U: None unless recurrent (then posttreatment culture)

GLOMERULONEPHRITIS
Additional signs and symptoms
- Flank pain that's bilateral, constant, and moderate in intensity
- Moderate facial and generalized edema
- Hypertension
- Oliguria or anuria
- Nausea and vomiting

DX: Labs (antistreptolysin-0 test, UA, urine culture, electrolytes)

TX: Medication (diuretics, antibiotics, antipyretics), no-added-salt diet (temporary)

F/U: Repeated UA and blood pressure monitoring at 2, 4, and 8 weeks; then every 2 to 6 months as indicated

RENAL AND URETERAL CALCULI
Signs and symptoms
- Intense, unilateral, colicky flank pain
- Costovertebral angle tenderness
- Nausea and vomiting
- Hypoactive bowel sounds

DX: Imaging studies (abdominal X-ray, IVP)

TX: Increased fluid intake, analgesics, ureteroscopy, surgery

F/U: Referral to urologist

RENAL CANCER
Signs and symptoms
- Unilateral, dull, vague flank pain
- Palpable flank mass
- Hypertension
- Urine retention

DX: Labs (CBC, UA), imaging studies (IVP, CT scan, arteriography, ultrasonography), biopsy

TX: Surgery

F/U: Referrals to oncologist and surgeon

PANCREATITIS (ACUTE)
Signs and symptoms
- Extreme, bilateral flank pain that radiates from the epigastric or left upper quadrant area
- Nausea and persistent vomiting
- Abdominal tenderness and rigidity
- Hypoactive bowel sounds
- Positive Turner's and Cullen's signs

DX: PE, labs (amylase, lipase, blood glucose, calcium) imaging studies (abdominal X-ray, CT scan)

TX: NPO until acute episode is resolved, medication (antibiotics, analgesics)

F/U: Return visit 1 week after hospitalization

Additional differential diagnoses: bladder cancer ▪ cortical necrosis ▪ obstructive neuropathy ▪ papillary necrosis (acute) ▪ perirenal abscess ▪ polycystic kidney disease ▪ pyelonephritis (acute) ▪ renal infarction ▪ renal trauma ▪ renal vein thrombosis

Footdrop

Footdrop — plantar flexion of the foot with the toes bent toward the instep — results from weakness or paralysis of the dorsiflexor muscles of the foot and ankle. A characteristic and important sign of certain peripheral nerve or motor neuron disorders, footdrop may also stem from prolonged immobility when inadequate support, improper positioning, or infrequent passive exercise produces shortening of the Achilles tendon. Unilateral footdrop can result from compression of the common peroneal nerve against the head of the fibula.

Footdrop can range in severity from slight to complete, depending on the extent of muscle weakness or paralysis. It develops slowly in progressive muscle degeneration or suddenly in spinal cord injury.

History and physical examination

Ask the patient about the sign's onset, duration, and character. Does the footdrop fluctuate in severity or remain constant? Does it worsen with fatigue or improve with rest? Ask the patient if he feels weak or tires easily.

During the physical examination, assess muscle tone and strength in the patient's feet and legs, and compare findings on both sides. Assess deep tendon reflexes in both legs as well. Have the patient walk; inspect his shoes for wear and observe the patient for steppage gait — a compensatory response to footdrop.

PEDIATRIC POINTER

Common causes of footdrop in children include spinal birth defects (such as spina bifida) and degenerative disorders (such as muscular dystrophy).

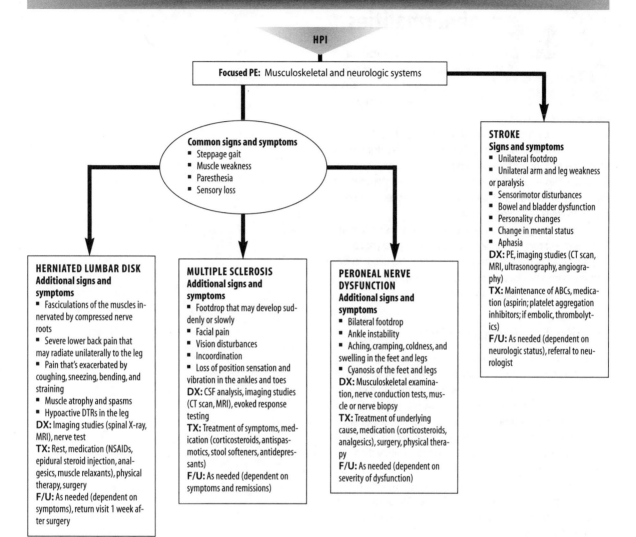

HPI

Focused PE: Musculoskeletal and neurologic systems

Common signs and symptoms
- Steppage gait
- Muscle weakness
- Paresthesia
- Sensory loss

STROKE
Signs and symptoms
- Unilateral footdrop
- Unilateral arm and leg weakness or paralysis
- Sensorimotor disturbances
- Bowel and bladder dysfunction
- Personality changes
- Change in mental status
- Aphasia

DX: PE, imaging studies (CT scan, MRI, ultrasonography, angiography)
TX: Maintenance of ABCs, medication (aspirin; platelet aggregation inhibitors; if embolic, thrombolytics)
F/U: As needed (dependent on neurologic status), referral to neurologist

HERNIATED LUMBAR DISK
Additional signs and symptoms
- Fasciculations of the muscles innervated by compressed nerve roots
- Severe lower back pain that may radiate unilaterally to the leg
- Pain that's exacerbated by coughing, sneezing, bending, and straining
- Muscle atrophy and spasms
- Hypoactive DTRs in the leg

DX: Imaging studies (spinal X-ray, MRI), nerve test
TX: Rest, medication (NSAIDs, epidural steroid injection, analgesics, muscle relaxants), physical therapy, surgery
F/U: As needed (dependent on symptoms), return visit 1 week after surgery

MULTIPLE SCLEROSIS
Additional signs and symptoms
- Footdrop that may develop suddenly or slowly
- Facial pain
- Vision disturbances
- Incoordination
- Loss of position sensation and vibration in the ankles and toes

DX: CSF analysis, imaging studies (CT scan, MRI), evoked response testing
TX: Treatment of symptoms, medication (corticosteroids, antispasmotics, stool softeners, antidepressants)
F/U: As needed (dependent on symptoms and remissions)

PERONEAL NERVE DYSFUNCTION
Additional signs and symptoms
- Bilateral footdrop
- Ankle instability
- Aching, cramping, coldness, and swelling in the feet and legs
- Cyanosis of the feet and legs

DX: Musculoskeletal examination, nerve conduction tests, muscle or nerve biopsy
TX: Treatment of underlying cause, medication (corticosteroids, analgesics), surgery, physical therapy
F/U: As needed (dependent on severity of dysfunction)

Additional differential diagnoses: Guillain-Barré syndrome ▪ myasthenia gravis ▪ poliomyelitis ▪ spinal cord trauma

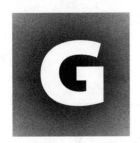

Gag reflex abnormalities

The gag reflex — a protective mechanism that prevents aspiration of food, fluid, and vomitus — normally can be elicited by touching the posterior wall of the oropharynx with a tongue depressor or by suctioning the throat. Prompt elevation of the palate, constriction of the pharyngeal musculature, and a sensation of gagging indicate a normal gag reflex. An abnormal gag reflex — either decreased or absent — interferes with the ability to swallow and, more important, increases susceptibility to life-threatening aspiration.

An impaired gag reflex can result from any lesion that affects its mediators — cranial nerves IX (glossopharyngeal) and X (vagus) or the pons or medulla. It can also occur during a coma, in muscle diseases such as severe myasthenia gravis, or as a temporary result of anesthesia.

History and physical examination

If you detect an abnormal gag reflex, take steps to prevent aspiration by not allowing oral intake. Quickly evaluate level of consciousness. If it's decreased, place the patient in a side-lying position to prevent aspiration; if not, place him in Fowler's position. Ask the patient (or a family member if the patient can't communicate) about the onset and duration of swallowing difficulties. Are liquids more difficult to swallow than solids? Is swallowing more difficult at certain times of the day (as occurs in the bulbar palsy associated with myasthenia gravis)? If the patient also has trouble chewing, suspect more widespread neurologic involvement because chewing involves different cranial nerves.

Explore the patient's medical history for vascular and degenerative disorders. Then assess his respiratory status for evidence of aspiration, and perform a neurologic examination.

PEDIATRIC POINTER

Brain stem glioma is an important cause of abnormal gag reflex in children.

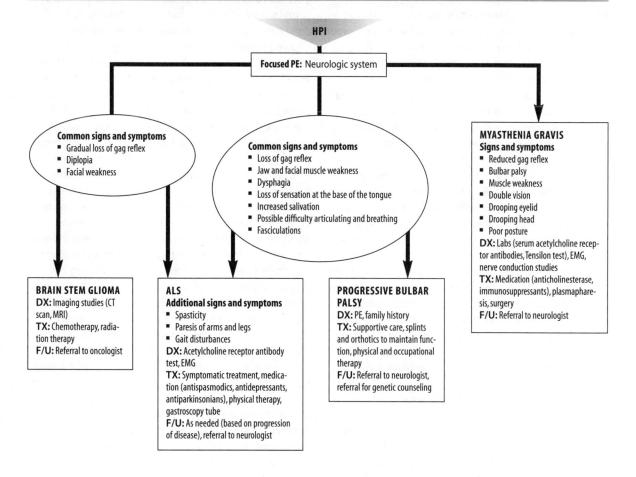

HPI

Focused PE: Neurologic system

Common signs and symptoms
- Gradual loss of gag reflex
- Diplopia
- Facial weakness

Common signs and symptoms
- Loss of gag reflex
- Jaw and facial muscle weakness
- Dysphagia
- Loss of sensation at the base of the tongue
- Increased salivation
- Possible difficulty articulating and breathing
- Fasciculations

MYASTHENIA GRAVIS
Signs and symptoms
- Reduced gag reflex
- Bulbar palsy
- Muscle weakness
- Double vision
- Drooping eyelid
- Drooping head
- Poor posture
DX: Labs (serum acetylcholine receptor antibodies, Tensilon test), EMG, nerve conduction studies
TX: Medication (anticholinesterase, immunosuppressants), plasmapharesis, surgery
F/U: Referral to neurologist

BRAIN STEM GLIOMA
DX: Imaging studies (CT scan, MRI)
TX: Chemotherapy, radiation therapy
F/U: Referral to oncologist

ALS
Additional signs and symptoms
- Spasticity
- Paresis of arms and legs
- Gait disturbances
DX: Acetylcholine receptor antibody test, EMG
TX: Symptomatic treatment, medication (antispasmodics, antidepressants, antiparkinsonians), physical therapy, gastroscopy tube
F/U: As needed (based on progression of disease), referral to neurologist

PROGRESSIVE BULBAR PALSY
DX: PE, family history
TX: Supportive care, splints and orthotics to maintain function, physical and occupational therapy
F/U: Referral to neurologist, referral for genetic counseling

---

Additional differential diagnoses: basilar artery occlusion ▪ cerebrovascular event ▪ compression tumor ▪ multiple sclerosis ▪ Parkinson's disease ▪ radiation injury ▪ Wallenberg's syndrome

---

Other causes: anesthesia (general and local [throat])

Gait, abnormal

A *bizarre gait* has no obvious organic basis; rather, it's produced unconsciously by a person with a somatoform disorder (hysterical neurosis) or consciously by a malingerer. The gait has no consistent pattern. It may mimic an organic impairment but characteristically has a more theatrical or bizarre quality with key elements missing, such as a spastic gait without hip circumduction, or leg "paralysis" with normal reflexes and motor strength. Its manifestations may include wild gyrations, exaggerated stepping, leg dragging, or mimicking unusual walks, such as that of a tightrope walker.

Propulsive gait is characterized by a stooped, rigid posture — the patient's head and neck are bent forward; his flexed, stiffened arms are held away from the body; his fingers are extended; and his knees and hips are stiffly bent. During ambulation, this posture results in a forward shifting of the body's center of gravity and consequent impairment of balance, causing increasingly rapid, short, shuffling steps with involuntary acceleration (festination) and lack of control over forward motion (propulsion) or backward motion (retropulsion).

Propulsive gait is a cardinal sign of advanced Parkinson's disease; it results from progressive degeneration of the ganglia, which are primarily responsible for smooth muscle movement. Because this sign develops gradually and its accompanying effects are often wrongly attributed to aging, propulsive gait often goes unnoticed or unreported until severe disability results.

Spastic gait — sometimes referred to as paretic or weak gait — is a stiff, foot-dragging walk caused by unilateral leg muscle hypertonicity. This gait indicates focal damage to the corticospinal tract. The affected leg becomes rigid, with a marked decrease in flexion at the hip and knee and, possibly, plantar flexion and equinovarus deformity of the foot. Because the patient's leg doesn't swing normally at the hip or knee, his foot tends to drag or shuffle, scraping his toes on the ground. To compensate, the pelvis of the affected side tilts upward in an attempt to lift the toes, causing the patient's leg to abduct and circumduct. Also, arm swing is hindered on the same side as the affected leg.

Spastic gait usually develops after a period of flaccidity (hypotonicity) in the affected leg. Whatever the cause, the gait is usually permanent once it develops.

History and physical examination

Find out when the patient first noticed the gait impairment and whether it developed suddenly or gradually. Ask him if it waxes and wanes or if it has worsened progressively. Does fatigue, hot weather, or warm baths or showers worsen the gait? Such exacerbation typically occurs in multiple sclerosis. Focus your medical history questions on neurologic disorders, recent head trauma, and degenerative diseases.

If you suspect that the patient's gait impairment has no organic cause, begin to investigate other possibilities. Determine if the change in gait coincides with any stressful period or event, such as the death of a loved one or loss of a job. Ask about associated symptoms, and explore any reports of frequent unexplained illnesses and multiple doctor's visits. Subtly try to determine if he'll gain anything from malingering, for instance, added attention or an insurance settlement.

Begin the physical examination by testing the patient's reflexes and sensorimotor function, noting any abnormal response patterns. To quickly check his reports of leg weakness or paralysis, place the patient in the supine position and stand at his feet. Cradle a heel in each of your palms, and rest your hands on the table. Ask the patient to raise the affected leg. In true motor weakness, the heel of the other leg will press downward; in hysteria, this movement will be absent. As a further check, observe the patient for normal movements when he's unaware of being watched. Test and compare strength, range of motion, and sensory function in all limbs. Also, observe and palpate for muscle flaccidity or atrophy.

Also, obtain a thorough drug history, including both medication type and dosage. Ask the patient if he has been taking any tranquilizers, especially phenothiazines. If he knows he has Parkinson's disease and has been taking levodopa, pay particular attention to the dosage because an overdose can cause acute exacerbation of signs and symptoms. If Parkinson's disease isn't a known or suspected diagnosis, ask the patient if he has been acutely or routinely exposed to carbon monoxide or manganese.

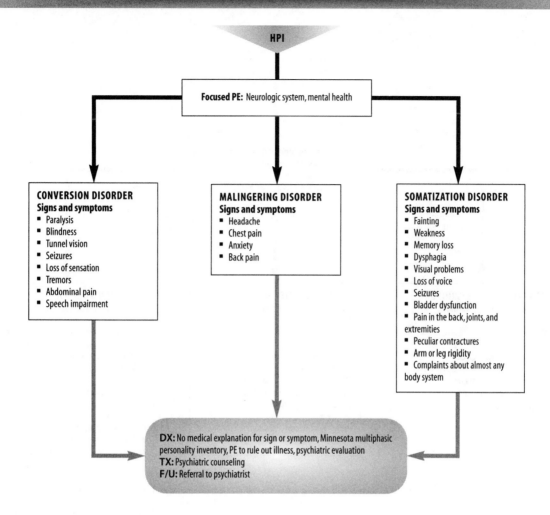

HPI

Focused PE: Neurologic system, mental health

CONVERSION DISORDER
Signs and symptoms
- Paralysis
- Blindness
- Tunnel vision
- Seizures
- Loss of sensation
- Tremors
- Abdominal pain
- Speech impairment

MALINGERING DISORDER
Signs and symptoms
- Headache
- Chest pain
- Anxiety
- Back pain

SOMATIZATION DISORDER
Signs and symptoms
- Fainting
- Weakness
- Memory loss
- Dysphagia
- Visual problems
- Loss of voice
- Seizures
- Bladder dysfunction
- Pain in the back, joints, and extremities
- Peculiar contractures
- Arm or leg rigidity
- Complaints about almost any body system

DX: No medical explanation for sign or symptom, Minnesota multiphasic personality inventory, PE to rule out illness, psychiatric evaluation
TX: Psychiatric counseling
F/U: Referral to psychiatrist

Additional differential diagnoses: orthopedic injury ▪ vestibular defects ▪ visual defects

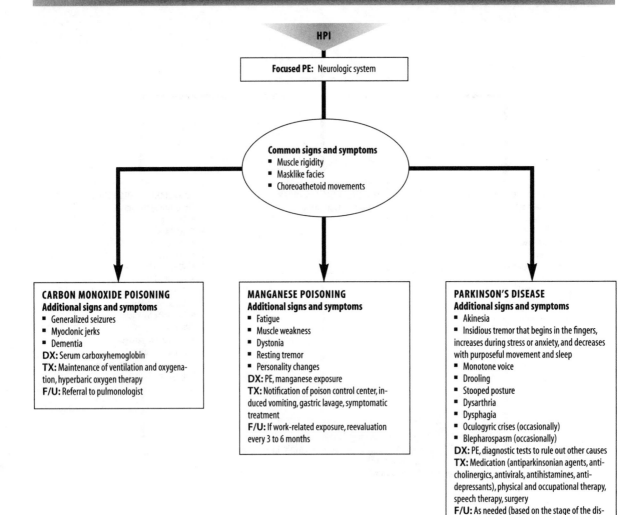

HPI

Focused PE: Neurologic system

Common signs and symptoms
- Muscle rigidity
- Masklike facies
- Choreoathetoid movements

CARBON MONOXIDE POISONING
Additional signs and symptoms
- Generalized seizures
- Myoclonic jerks
- Dementia

DX: Serum carboxyhemoglobin
TX: Maintenance of ventilation and oxygenation, hyperbaric oxygen therapy
F/U: Referral to pulmonologist

MANGANESE POISONING
Additional signs and symptoms
- Fatigue
- Muscle weakness
- Dystonia
- Resting tremor
- Personality changes

DX: PE, manganese exposure
TX: Notification of poison control center, induced vomiting, gastric lavage, symptomatic treatment
F/U: If work-related exposure, reevaluation every 3 to 6 months

PARKINSON'S DISEASE
Additional signs and symptoms
- Akinesia
- Insidious tremor that begins in the fingers, increases during stress or anxiety, and decreases with purposeful movement and sleep
- Monotone voice
- Drooling
- Stooped posture
- Dysarthria
- Dysphagia
- Oculogyric crises (occasionally)
- Blepharospasm (occasionally)

DX: PE, diagnostic tests to rule out other causes
TX: Medication (antiparkinsonian agents, anticholinergics, antivirals, antihistamines, antidepressants), physical and occupational therapy, speech therapy, surgery
F/U: As needed (based on the stage of the disease), referral to neurologist

---

Other causes: antipsychotics (haloperidol, thiothixene, loxapine) ▪ metoclopramide ▪ metyrosine ▪ phenothiazines

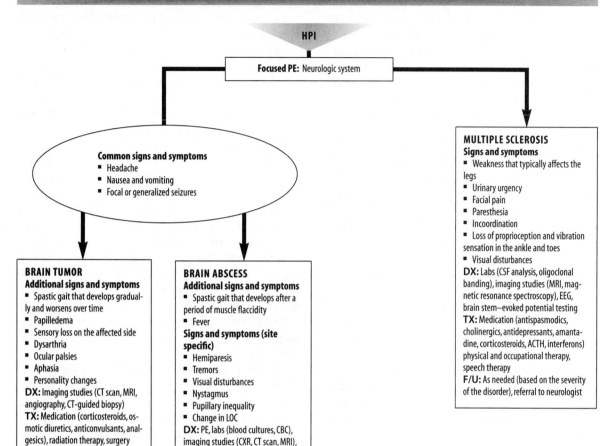

HPI

Focused PE: Neurologic system

Common signs and symptoms
- Headache
- Nausea and vomiting
- Focal or generalized seizures

BRAIN TUMOR
Additional signs and symptoms
- Spastic gait that develops gradually and worsens over time
- Papilledema
- Sensory loss on the affected side
- Dysarthria
- Ocular palsies
- Aphasia
- Personality changes

DX: Imaging studies (CT scan, MRI, angiography, CT-guided biopsy)
TX: Medication (corticosteroids, osmotic diuretics, anticonvulsants, analgesics), radiation therapy, surgery
F/U: As needed (based on neurologic status), referrals to oncologist, neurosurgeon, and rehabilitation program

BRAIN ABSCESS
Additional signs and symptoms
- Spastic gait that develops after a period of muscle flaccidity
- Fever

Signs and symptoms (site specific)
- Hemiparesis
- Tremors
- Visual disturbances
- Nystagmus
- Pupillary inequality
- Change in LOC

DX: PE, labs (blood cultures, CBC), imaging studies (CXR, CT scan, MRI), EEG
TX: Medication (antibiotics, antifungals, antivirals, osmotic diuretics), surgery
F/U: Referrals to neurologist or neurosurgeon and infectious disease specialist

MULTIPLE SCLEROSIS
Signs and symptoms
- Weakness that typically affects the legs
- Urinary urgency
- Facial pain
- Paresthesia
- Incoordination
- Loss of proprioception and vibration sensation in the ankle and toes
- Visual disturbances

DX: Labs (CSF analysis, oligoclonal banding), imaging studies (MRI, magnetic resonance spectroscopy), EEG, brain stem–evoked potential testing
TX: Medication (antispasmodics, cholinergics, antidepressants, amantadine, corticosteroids, ACTH, interferons) physical and occupational therapy, speech therapy
F/U: As needed (based on the severity of the disorder), referral to neurologist

Additional differential diagnoses: arthritis ▪ head trauma ▪ stroke

Other causes: antipsychotics (haloperidol, thiothixene, loxapine) ▪ metoclopramide ▪ metyrosine ▪ phenothiazines

Gallop, atrial or ventricular

An *atrial* or presystolic gallop is an extra heart sound (known as S_4) that's heard or often palpated immediately before the first heart sound (S_1). This low-pitched sound is heard best with the bell of the stethoscope pressed lightly against the cardiac apex. Some clinicians say that an S_4 has the cadence of the "Ten" in Tennessee (Ten = S_4; nes = S_1; see = S_2).

This gallop typically results from hypertension, conduction defects, valvular disorders, or other problems such as ischemia. It results from abnormal forceful atrial contraction caused by augmented ventricular filling or by decreased left ventricular compliance. An atrial gallop usually originates from left atrial contraction, is heard at the apex, and doesn't vary with inspiration. It may also originate from right atrial contraction. If so, it's heard best at the lower left sternal border and intensifies with inspiration.

An atrial gallop seldom occurs in normal hearts; however, it may occur in elderly people, in athletes with physiologic hypertrophy of the left ventricle, and in pregnant women because of augmented ventricular filling.

A *ventricular* gallop is a heart sound (known as S_3) associated with rapid ventricular filling in early diastole. Usually palpable, this low-frequency sound occurs about 0.15 second after the second heart sound (S_2). It may originate in either the left or right ventricle. A right-sided gallop usually sounds louder on inspiration and is heard best along the lower left sternal border or over the xiphoid region. A left-sided gallop usually sounds louder on expiration and is heard best at the apex.

Ventricular gallops are easily overlooked because they're usually faint. For better detection, auscultate in a quiet environment; examine the patient in the supine, left lateral, and semi-Fowler's positions; and have the patient cough or raise his legs to augment the sound.

A physiologic ventricular gallop normally occurs in children and young adults; however, most people lose this S_3 by age 40. This gallop may also occur during the third trimester of pregnancy. Although the physiologic S_3 has the same timing as the pathologic S_3, its intensity waxes and wanes with respiration. It's also heard more faintly if the patient is sitting or standing.

A pathologic ventricular gallop may be one of the earliest signs of ventricular failure. It may result from one of two mechanisms: rapid deceleration of blood entering a stiff, non-compliant ventricle, or rapid acceleration of blood associated with increased flow into the ventricle. A gallop that persists despite therapy indicates a poor prognosis.

Patients with cardiomyopathy or heart failure may develop both a ventricular gallop and an atrial gallop — a condition known as a summation gallop.

History and physical examination

Suspect myocardial ischemia if you auscultate an atrial gallop in a patient with chest pain. Take the patient's vital signs and quickly look for signs of heart failure, such as dyspnea, crackles, and distended neck veins. If you detect these signs, connect the patient to a cardiac monitor and obtain an electrocardiogram. If the patient has dyspnea, elevate the head of the bed. Then auscultate for abnormal breath sounds. Be prepared to administer emergency measures.

When the patient's condition permits, ask about a history of hypertension, angina, valvular stenosis, or cardiomyopathy. If appropriate, have him describe the frequency and severity of anginal attacks.

After auscultating a ventricular gallop, focus your history and examination on the cardiovascular system. Begin the history by asking the patient if he has had any chest pain. If so, have him describe its character, location, frequency, duration, and any alleviating or aggravating factors. Also, ask about palpitations, dizziness, or syncope. Does the patient have difficulty breathing after exertion? While lying down? At rest? Does he have a cough? Ask about a history of cardiac disorders. Is the patient currently receiving any treatment for heart failure? If so, which medications is he taking?

During the physical examination, carefully auscultate for murmurs or abnormalities in the S_1 and S_2. Then listen for pulmonary crackles. Next, assess peripheral pulses, noting pulsus alternans, an alternating strong and weak pulse. Finally, palpate the liver to detect enlargement or tenderness and assess for neck vein distention and peripheral edema.

PEDIATRIC POINTERS

- *Atrial gallop may occur normally in children, especially after exercise. Ventricular gallop is also normally heard in children.*
- *Atrial gallop may also result from congenital heart diseases, such as atrial septal defect, ventricular septal defect, patent ductus arteriosus, and severe pulmonary valvular stenosis.*
- *Ventricular gallop may accompany congenital abnormalities associated with heart failure, such as large ventricular septal defect and patent ductus arteriosus.*
- *A ventricular gallop may also result from sickle cell anemia.*

ELDER CARE CUE

Because the absolute intensity of an atrial gallop doesn't decrease with age, as it does with an S_1, the relative intensity of an S_4 increases compared with an S_1. This explains the increased frequency of an audible S_4 in elderly patients and why this sound may be considered a normal finding in older patients.

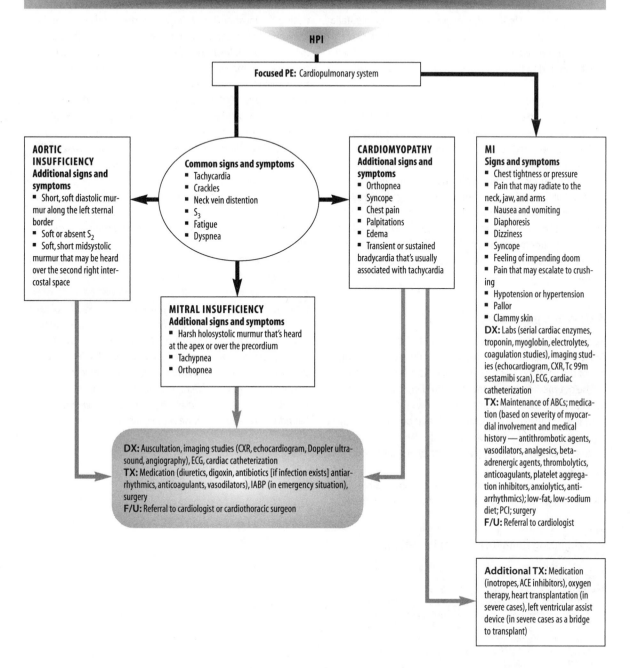

HPI

Focused PE: Cardiopulmonary system

Common signs and symptoms
- Tachycardia
- Crackles
- Neck vein distention
- S_3
- Fatigue
- Dyspnea

AORTIC INSUFFICIENCY
Additional signs and symptoms
- Short, soft diastolic murmur along the left sternal border
- Soft or absent S_2
- Soft, short midsystolic murmur that may be heard over the second right intercostal space

MITRAL INSUFFICIENCY
Additional signs and symptoms
- Harsh holosystolic murmur that's heard at the apex or over the precordium
- Tachypnea
- Orthopnea

CARDIOMYOPATHY
Additional signs and symptoms
- Orthopnea
- Syncope
- Chest pain
- Palpitations
- Edema
- Transient or sustained bradycardia that's usually associated with tachycardia

MI
Signs and symptoms
- Chest tightness or pressure
- Pain that may radiate to the neck, jaw, and arms
- Nausea and vomiting
- Diaphoresis
- Dizziness
- Syncope
- Feeling of impending doom
- Pain that may escalate to crushing
- Hypotension or hypertension
- Pallor
- Clammy skin

DX: Labs (serial cardiac enzymes, troponin, myoglobin, electrolytes, coagulation studies), imaging studies (echocardiogram, CXR, Tc 99m sestamibi scan), ECG, cardiac catheterization
TX: Maintenance of ABCs; medication (based on severity of myocardial involvement and medical history — antithrombotic agents, vasodilators, analgesics, beta-adrenergic agents, thrombolytics, anticoagulants, platelet aggregation inhibitors, anxiolytics, antiarrhythmics); low-fat, low-sodium diet; PCI; surgery
F/U: Referral to cardiologist

DX: Auscultation, imaging studies (CXR, echocardiogram, Doppler ultrasound, angiography), ECG, cardiac catheterization
TX: Medication (diuretics, digoxin, antibiotics [if infection exists] antiarrhythmics, anticoagulants, vasodilators), IABP (in emergency situation), surgery
F/U: Referral to cardiologist or cardiothoracic surgeon

Additional TX: Medication (inotropes, ACE inhibitors), oxygen therapy, heart transplantation (in severe cases), left ventricular assist device (in severe cases as a bridge to transplant)

Additional differential diagnoses for atrial gallop: anemia ▪ angina ▪ aortic stenosis ▪ AV block ▪ hypertension ▪ pulmonary embolism

Additional differential diagnoses for ventricular gallop: heart failure ▪ thyrotoxicosis

Genital lesions (male)

Among the diverse lesions that may affect the male genitalia are warts, papules, ulcers, scales, and pustules. These common lesions may be painful or painless, singular or multiple. They may be limited to the genitalia or may also occur elsewhere on the body.

Genital lesions may result from infection, neoplasms, parasites, allergy, or the effects of drugs. These lesions can profoundly affect the patient's self-image. In fact, the patient may hesitate to seek medical attention because he fears cancer or sexually transmitted disease (STD).

Genital lesions that arise from an STD could mean that the patient is at risk for human immunodeficiency virus (HIV). Genital ulcers make HIV transmission between sexual partners more likely. Unfortunately, if the patient is treating himself, he may alter the lesions, making differential diagnosis especially difficult. (See *Recognizing common male genital lesions*.)

History and physical examination

Begin by asking the patient when he noticed the first lesion. Did it erupt after he began taking a new drug or after a trip out of the country? Has he had similar lesions before? If so, did he get medical treatment for them? Find out if he has been treating the lesion himself. If so, how? Does the lesion itch? If so, is the itching constant or does it bother him only at night? Note whether the lesion is painful. Next, take a complete sexual history, noting the frequency of relations and the number of sexual partners.

Before you examine the patient, observe his clothing. Do his pants fit properly? Tight pants or underwear, especially those made of nonabsorbent fabrics, can promote the growth of bacteria and fungi. Examine the entire skin surface, noting the location, size, color, and pattern of the lesions. Do genital lesions resemble lesions on other parts of the body? Palpate for nodules, masses, and tenderness. Also, look for bleeding, edema, or signs of infection, such as erythema. Finally, take the patient's vital signs.

- *In infants, contact dermatitis (diaper rash) may produce minor irritation or bright red, weepy, excoriated lesions. Use of disposable diapers and careful cleaning of the penis and scrotum can help reduce diaper rash.*
- *In children, impetigo may cause pustules with thick, yellow, weepy crusts.*
- *Children with STDs must be evaluated for signs of sexual abuse.*
- *Adolescents ages 15 to 19 have a high incidence of STDs and related genital lesions. Syphilis, however, may also be congenital.*

- *Elderly adults who are sexually active with multiple partners have as high a risk of developing STDs as do younger adults. However, because of decreased immunity, poor hygiene, poor symptom reporting, and possibly several concurrent conditions, they may present with different symptoms.*
- *Seborrheic dermatitis lasts longer and is more extensive in bedridden patients and those with Parkinson's disease.*

Recognizing common male genital lesions

A wide variety of lesions may affect the male genitalia. Some of the more common ones and their causes are discussed here:
- Penile cancer causes a painless ulcerative lesion on the glans penis or foreskin, possibly accompanied by a foul-smelling discharge.
- Genital warts are marked by clusters of flesh-colored papillary growths that may be barely visible or several inches in diameter.
- Tinea cruris (commonly known as jock itch) produces itchy patches of well-defined, slightly raised, scaly lesions that usually affect the inner thighs and groin.
- A fixed drug eruption causes a bright-red to purplish lesion on the glans penis.
- Genital herpes begins as a swollen, slightly pruritic wheal and later becomes a group of small vesicles or blisters on the foreskin, glans penis, or penile shaft.
- Chancroid causes a painful ulcer that's usually less than 2 cm in diameter and bleeds easily. The lesion may be deep and covered by a gray or yellow exudate at its base.

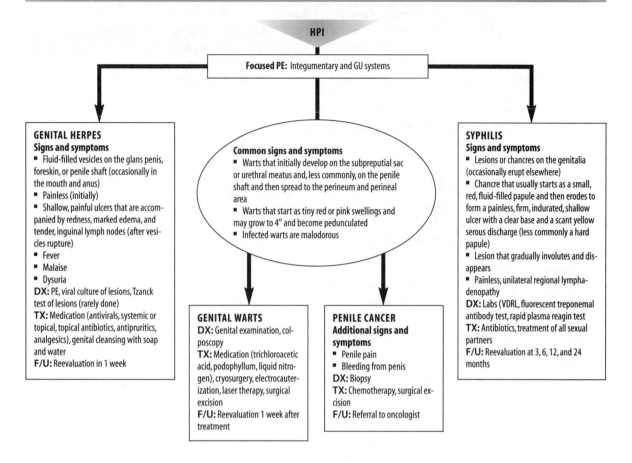

HPI

Focused PE: Integumentary and GU systems

GENITAL HERPES
Signs and symptoms
- Fluid-filled vesicles on the glans penis, foreskin, or penile shaft (occasionally in the mouth and anus)
- Painless (initially)
- Shallow, painful ulcers that are accompanied by redness, marked edema, and tender, inguinal lymph nodes (after vesicles rupture)
- Fever
- Malaise
- Dysuria

DX: PE, viral culture of lesions, Tzanck test of lesions (rarely done)

TX: Medication (antivirals, systemic or topical, topical antibiotics, antipruritics, analgesics), genital cleansing with soap and water

F/U: Reevaluation in 1 week

Common signs and symptoms
- Warts that initially develop on the subpreputial sac or urethral meatus and, less commonly, on the penile shaft and then spread to the perineum and perineal area
- Warts that start as tiny red or pink swellings and may grow to 4" and become pedunculated
- Infected warts are malodorous

GENITAL WARTS
DX: Genital examination, colposcopy
TX: Medication (trichloroacetic acid, podophyllum, liquid nitrogen), cryosurgery, electrocauterization, laser therapy, surgical excision
F/U: Reevaluation 1 week after treatment

PENILE CANCER
Additional signs and symptoms
- Penile pain
- Bleeding from penis

DX: Biopsy
TX: Chemotherapy, surgical excision
F/U: Referral to oncologist

SYPHILIS
Signs and symptoms
- Lesions or chancres on the genitalia (occasionally erupt elsewhere)
- Chancre that usually starts as a small, red, fluid-filled papule and then erodes to form a painless, firm, indurated, shallow ulcer with a clear base and a scant yellow serous discharge (less commonly a hard papule)
- Lesion that gradually involutes and disappears
- Painless, unilateral regional lymphadenopathy

DX: Labs (VDRL, fluorescent treponemal antibody test, rapid plasma reagin test
TX: Antibiotics, treatment of all sexual partners
F/U: Reevaluation at 3, 6, 12, and 24 months

Additional differential diagnoses: balanitis ▪ balanoposthitis ▪ Bowen's disease ▪ candidiasis ▪ chancroid ▪ erythroplasia of Queyrat ▪ folliculitis ▪ Fournier's gangrene ▪ furunculosis ▪ granuloma inguinale ▪ leukoplakia ▪ lichen planus ▪ lymphogranuloma venereum ▪ pediculosis pubis ▪ psoriasis ▪ scabies ▪ seborrheic dermititis ▪ tinea cruris ▪ urticaria

Other causes: phenolphthalein ▪ barbiturates ▪ broad-spectrum antibiotics (tetracycline, sulfonamides)

Gum bleeding

Gum bleeding (gingival bleeding) usually results from dental disorders; less commonly, it may stem from blood dyscrasias or the effects of certain drugs. Physiologic causes of this common sign include pregnancy, which can produce gum swelling in the first or second trimester (pregnancy epulis); atmospheric pressure changes, which usually affect divers and aviators; and oral trauma. Bleeding ranges from slight oozing to life-threatening hemorrhage. It may be spontaneous or may follow trauma. Occasionally, direct pressure can control it.

History and physical examination

If you detect profuse, spontaneous bleeding in the oral cavity, quickly check the patient's airway and look for signs of cardiovascular collapse, such as tachycardia and hypotension. Apply direct pressure to the bleeding site, if able. Be prepared to administer emergency measures.

If gum bleeding isn't an emergency, obtain a history. Find out when the bleeding began. Has it been continuous or intermittent? Does it occur spontaneously or when the patient brushes his teeth? Have the patient show you the site of the bleeding, if possible.

Find out if the patient or any family members have bleeding tendencies; for example, ask about easy bruising and frequent nosebleeds. How much does the patient bleed after a tooth extraction? Does he have a history of liver or spleen disease? Next, check the patient's dental history. Find out how often he brushes his teeth and goes to the dentist. Has he seen a dentist recently? To evaluate nutritional status, have the patient describe his normal diet and intake of alcohol. Finally, note any prescription and over-the-counter drugs he takes.

Next, perform a complete oral examination. If the patient wears dentures, have him remove them. Examine the gums to determine the site and amount of bleeding. Gums normally appear pink and rippled with their margins snugly against the teeth. Check for inflammation, pockets around the teeth, swelling, retraction, hypertrophy, discoloration, and gum hyperplasia. Note obvious decay, discoloration, foreign material such as food, and absence of any teeth.

- *In newborns, bleeding gums may result from vitamin K deficiency associated with a lack of normal intestinal flora or poor maternal nutrition.*

- *In infants who primarily drink cow's milk and don't receive vitamin supplements, bleeding gums can result from vitamin C deficiency.*

In patients who have no teeth, constant gum trauma and bleeding may result from using a dental prosthesis.

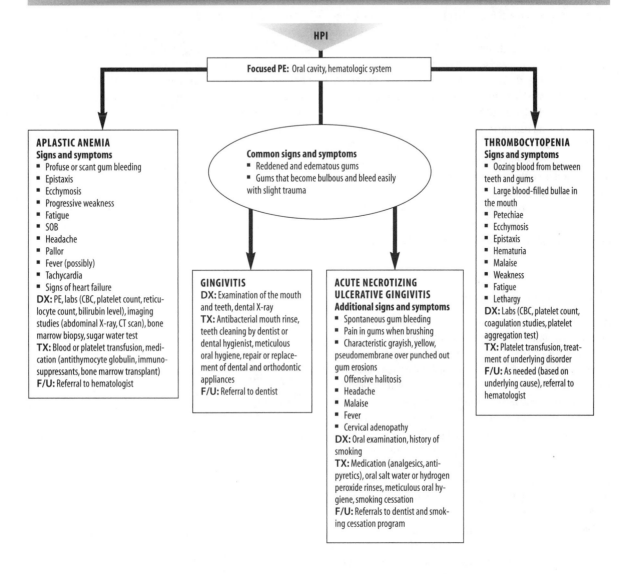

HPI

Focused PE: Oral cavity, hematologic system

APLASTIC ANEMIA
Signs and symptoms
- Profuse or scant gum bleeding
- Epistaxis
- Ecchymosis
- Progressive weakness
- Fatigue
- SOB
- Headache
- Pallor
- Fever (possibly)
- Tachycardia
- Signs of heart failure

DX: PE, labs (CBC, platelet count, reticulocyte count, bilirubin level), imaging studies (abdominal X-ray, CT scan), bone marrow biopsy, sugar water test
TX: Blood or platelet transfusion, medication (antithymocyte globulin, immunosuppressants, bone marrow transplant)
F/U: Referral to hematologist

Common signs and symptoms
- Reddened and edematous gums
- Gums that become bulbous and bleed easily with slight trauma

GINGIVITIS
DX: Examination of the mouth and teeth, dental X-ray
TX: Antibacterial mouth rinse, teeth cleaning by dentist or dental hygienist, meticulous oral hygiene, repair or replacement of dental and orthodontic appliances
F/U: Referral to dentist

ACUTE NECROTIZING ULCERATIVE GINGIVITIS
Additional signs and symptoms
- Spontaneous gum bleeding
- Pain in gums when brushing
- Characteristic grayish, yellow, pseudomembrane over punched out gum erosions
- Offensive halitosis
- Headache
- Malaise
- Fever
- Cervical adenopathy

DX: Oral examination, history of smoking
TX: Medication (analgesics, antipyretics), oral salt water or hydrogen peroxide rinses, meticulous oral hygiene, smoking cessation
F/U: Referrals to dentist and smoking cessation program

THROMBOCYTOPENIA
Signs and symptoms
- Oozing blood from between teeth and gums
- Large blood-filled bullae in the mouth
- Petechiae
- Ecchymosis
- Epistaxis
- Hematuria
- Malaise
- Weakness
- Fatigue
- Lethargy

DX: Labs (CBC, platelet count, coagulation studies, platelet aggregation test)
TX: Platelet transfusion, treatment of underlying disorder
F/U: As needed (based on underlying cause), referral to hematologist

Additional differential diagnoses: agranulocytosis ▪ chemical irritants ▪ cirrhosis ▪ Ehlers-Danlos syndrome ▪ giant cell epulis ▪ hemophilia ▪ hereditary hemorrhagic telangeictasia hypofibrinogenemia ▪ leukemia ▪ malnutrition ▪ pemphigoid (benign mucosal) ▪ periodontal disease ▪ pernicious anemia ▪ polycythemia vera ▪ pyogenic granuloma ▪ thrombasthenia (familial) ▪ thrombocytopenic purpura (idiopathic) ▪ vitamin C deficiency

Other causes: abuse of aspirin and NSAIDs ▪ coumadin ▪ heparin ▪ mucosal "aspirin burn"

Gum swelling

Gum swelling may result from one of two mechanisms: an increase in the size of existing gum cells (hypertrophy) or an increase in their number (hyperplasia). This common sign may involve one or many papillae — the triangular bits of gum between adjacent teeth. Occasionally, the gums swell markedly, obscuring the teeth altogether. Usually, the swelling is most prominent on the labia and bucca.

Gum swelling usually results from the effects of phenytoin; less commonly, from nutritional deficiency and certain systemic disorders. Physiologic gum swelling and bleeding may occur during the first and second trimesters of pregnancy when hormonal changes make the gums highly vascular; even slight irritation causes swelling and gives the papillae a characteristic raspberry hue (pregnancy epulis). Irritating dentures may also cause swelling associated with red, soft, movable masses on the gums.

History and physical examination

After ruling out pregnancy (in a female patient) or the use of phenytoin or similar prescription drugs as the cause of gum swelling, take a history. Have the patient fully describe the swelling. Has he had it before? Is it localized or generalized? Find out when the swelling began, and ask about any aggravating or alleviating factors. Is the swelling painful? Then explore the patient's medical history, focusing on major illnesses, bleeding disorders, and pregnancies (if the patient is female). Also check his dental history. Does he wear dentures? If so, are they new? Ask about use of alcohol and tobacco, which are gum irritants. Then have the patient describe his diet to evaluate nutritional status. Ask about his intake of citrus fruits and vegetables.

Next, inspect the patient's mouth in a good light. If he wears dentures, ask him to remove them before you begin. As you examine the gums, characterize their color and texture, and note any ulcers, lesions, masses, lumps, or debris-filled pockets around the teeth. Then inspect the teeth for discoloration, obvious decay, and looseness.

▪ *Gum swelling may also result from idiopathic fibrous hyperplasia and from inflammatory gum hyperplasia, which is especially common in pubertal girls.*

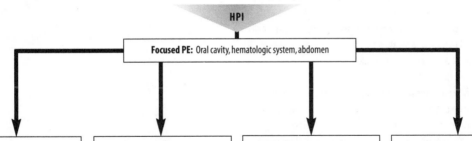

Focused PE: Oral cavity, hematologic system, abdomen

CROHN'S DISEASE
Signs and symptoms
- Granular or cobblestone gum swelling
- Cramping abdominal pain and diarrhea
- Nausea
- Fever
- Tachycardia
- Abdominal distention and pain
- Diarrhea
- Foul-smelling stools
- Weight loss

DX: Fecal occult blood, imaging studies (barium enema, upper GI series, enteroclysis), endoscopy, colonoscopy, sigmoidoscopy with small bowel biopsy
TX: Antibiotics, dietary changes, surgery (if obstruction occurs)
F/U: Referral to gastroenterologist

FIBROUS HYPERPLASIA (IDIOPATHIC)
Signs and symptoms
- Gums that are diffusely enlarged (may cover the teeth)
- Large, firm, painless masses of fibrous tissue that form on the gums
- Lip protrusion
- Difficulty chewing
- Bone pain
- Fractures

DX: PE, X-ray of involved bones
TX: No specific treatment, treatment of bone fractures, monitoring for development of endocrine disorders
F/U: Lab testing every 6 to 12 months, referral to endocrinologist if appropriate

VITAMIN C DEFICIENCY (SCURVY)
Signs and symptoms
- Spongy, tender, edematous gums
- Papillae that appear red or purple
- Gums that bleed easily
- Pockets filled with clotted blood around loose teeth
- Pallor
- Anorexia
- Weakness and lethargy
- Muscle and joint pain
- Insomnia
- Scaly dermatitis
- Skin hemorrhages

DX: Dietary history, labs (serum ascorbic acid levels, WBC ascorbic acid concentration)
TX: Vitamin C (P.O. or I.V.), diet modification
F/U: Monitoring as needed until the condition is improved, referral to dietitian

LEUKEMIA
Signs and symptoms
- Localized, necrotic gum swelling (early sign)
- Tender gums that appear blue and glossy and bleed easily
- High fever
- Sever prostration
- Signs of abnormal bleeding
- Dyspnea
- Tachycardia
- Palpitations
- Abdominal or bone pain

DX: PE, CBC, bone marrow aspiration
TX: Blood or platelet transfusion, chemotherapy, bone marrow transplant
F/U: Referrals to oncologist and hematologist

Additional differential diagnoses: infection ▪ malnutrition ▪ vitamin K deficiency

Other causes: cyclosporine ▪ dentures ▪ phenytoin

Gynecomastia

Occurring only in males, gynecomastia refers to increased breast size due to excessive mammary gland development. This change in breast size may be barely palpable or immediately obvious. Usually bilateral, gynecomastia may be associated with breast tenderness and milk secretion.

Normally, several hormones regulate breast development. Estrogens, growth hormone, and corticosteroids stimulate ductal growth, while progesterone and prolactin stimulate growth of the alveolar lobules. Although the pathophysiology of gynecomastia isn't fully understood, a hormonal imbalance — particularly a change in the estrogen-androgen ratio and an increase in prolactin — is a likely contributing factor. This explains why gynecomastia commonly results from the effects of estrogens and other drugs. It may also result from hormone-secreting tumors and from endocrine, genetic, hepatic, or adrenal disorders. Physiologic gynecomastia may occur in neonatal, pubertal, and geriatric males because of normal fluctuations in hormone levels.

History and physical examination

Begin the history by asking the patient when he first noticed his breast enlargement. How old was he at the time? Since then, have his breasts gotten progressively larger, smaller, or stayed the same? Does he also have breast tenderness or discharge? Next, take a thorough drug history, including prescription, over-the-counter, herbal, and street drugs. Then explore associated signs and symptoms, such as testicular mass or pain, loss of libido, decreased potency, and loss of chest, axillary, or facial hair.

Focus the physical examination on the breasts, testicles, and penis. As you examine the breasts, note any asymmetry, dimpling, abnormal pigmentation, or ulceration. Observe the testicles for size and symmetry. Then palpate them to detect nodules, tenderness, or unusual consistency. Look for normal penile development after puberty, and note hypospadias.

PEDIATRIC POINTERS

- *In newborns, gynecomastia may be associated with galactorrhea. This sign usually disappears within a few weeks but may persist until age 2.*
- *Most males have physiologic gynecomastia at some time during adolescence, usually around age 14. This gynecomastia is usually asymmetrical and tender; it commonly resolves within 2 years and rarely persists beyond age 20.*

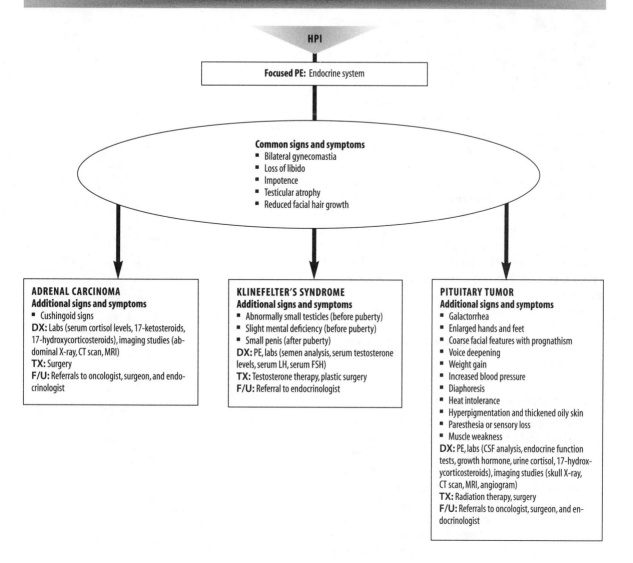

HPI

Focused PE: Endocrine system

Common signs and symptoms
- Bilateral gynecomastia
- Loss of libido
- Impotence
- Testicular atrophy
- Reduced facial hair growth

ADRENAL CARCINOMA
Additional signs and symptoms
- Cushingoid signs

DX: Labs (serum cortisol levels, 17-ketosteroids, 17-hydroxycorticosteroids), imaging studies (abdominal X-ray, CT scan, MRI)
TX: Surgery
F/U: Referrals to oncologist, surgeon, and endocrinologist

KLINEFELTER'S SYNDROME
Additional signs and symptoms
- Abnormally small testicles (before puberty)
- Slight mental deficiency (before puberty)
- Small penis (after puberty)

DX: PE, labs (semen analysis, serum testosterone levels, serum LH, serum FSH)
TX: Testosterone therapy, plastic surgery
F/U: Referral to endocrinologist

PITUITARY TUMOR
Additional signs and symptoms
- Galactorrhea
- Enlarged hands and feet
- Coarse facial features with prognathism
- Voice deepening
- Weight gain
- Increased blood pressure
- Diaphoresis
- Heat intolerance
- Hyperpigmentation and thickened oily skin
- Paresthesia or sensory loss
- Muscle weakness

DX: PE, labs (CSF analysis, endocrine function tests, growth hormone, urine cortisol, 17-hydroxycorticosteroids), imaging studies (skull X-ray, CT scan, MRI, angiogram)
TX: Radiation therapy, surgery
F/U: Referrals to oncologist, surgeon, and endocrinologist

Additional differential diagnoses: breast cancer ▪ cirrhosis ▪ hermaphroditism ▪ hypogonadism ▪ hypothyroidism ▪ liver cancer ▪ lung cancer ▪ malnutrition ▪ obesity ▪ puberty ▪ Reifenstein's syndrome ▪ renal failure (chronic) ▪ testicular failure (secondary) ▪ testicular tumor ▪ thyrotoxicosis

---

Other causes: alcohol ▪ antihypertensives ▪ chlorotrianisene ▪ cardiac glycosides ▪ cimetidine ▪ cyproterone ▪ diethylstilbestrol ▪ estramustine ▪ flutamide ▪ hemodialysis ▪ heroin ▪ human chorionic gonadotropin ▪ ketoconazole ▪ major surgery ▪ marijuana ▪ phenothiazines ▪ spironolactone ▪ testicular irradiation ▪ tricyclic antidepressants

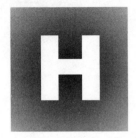

Halo vision

Halo vision refers to seeing rainbowlike, colored rings around lights or bright objects. The rainbowlike effect can be explained by this physical principle: As light passes through water (in the eye, through tears or the cells of various anteretinal media), it breaks up into spectral colors.

Halo vision usually develops suddenly; its duration depends on the causative disorder. This symptom may occur in disorders associated with excessive tearing and corneal epithelial edema. Among these causes, the most common and significant is acute angle-closure glaucoma, which can lead to blindness. In this disorder, increased intraocular pressure (IOP) forces fluid into corneal tissues anterior to Bowman's membrane, causing edema. Halo vision is also an early symptom of cataracts, resulting from dispersion of light by abnormal opacities on the lens.

Nonpathologic causes of excessive tearing associated with halo vision include poorly fitted or overworn contact lenses, emotional extremes, and exposure to intense light, as in snow blindness.

History and physical examination

First, ask the patient how long he has been seeing halos around lights and when he usually sees them. Patients with glaucoma typically see halos in the morning, when IOP is most elevated. Ask the patient if light bothers his eyes. Does he have any eye pain? If so, have him describe it. Remember that halos associated with excruciating eye pain or a severe headache may point to acute angle-closure glaucoma, an ocular emergency. Note a history of glaucoma or cataracts.

Next, examine the patient's eyes, noting conjunctival injection, excessive tearing, and lens changes. Examine pupil size, shape, and response to light. Then test visual acuity by performing an ophthalmoscopic examination.

PEDIATRIC POINTER

Halo vision in a child usually results from congenital cataracts or glaucoma. In a young child, limited verbal ability may make halo vision difficult to assess.

ELDER CARE CUE

Primary glaucoma, the most common cause of halo vision, occurs more frequently in older patients.

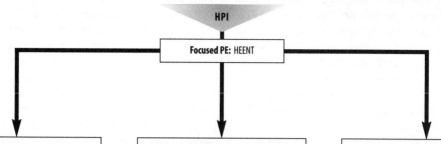

HPI

Focused PE: HEENT

CATARACT
Signs and symptoms
- Blurred vision
- Double vision
- Impaired visual acuity
- Changes in color vision
- Lens opacity

DX: Ophthalmic examination, slit-lamp examination, ultrasonography of the eye
TX: Glasses, magnifying glass, surgery
F/U: Referral to ophthalmologist

CORNEAL ENDOTHELIAL DYSTROPHY
Signs and symptoms
- Impaired visual acuity
- Foreign body sensation
- Eye pain upon wakening

DX: Slit-lamp examination, keratometry, CT scan
TX: Medication (hypertonic drops or ointments, nonhypertonic lubricating drops or ointments), patching (acute episodes of associated corneal erosion), hard or gas permeable contact lenses, surgery
F/U: Referral to ophthalmologist

GLAUCOMA
Signs and symptoms
ACUTE ANGLE CLOSURE
- Blurred vision
- Severe headache
- Excruciating pain in and around the affected eye
- Mild dilated fixed pupil
- Conjunctival injection
- Cloudy cornea
- Impaired visual acuity
- Nausea and vomiting
CHRONIC ANGLE CLOSURE
- Pain and blindness in advanced disease
CHRONIC OPEN-ANGLE
- Mild eye ache
- Peripheral vision loss
- Impaired visual acuity

DX: Ophthalmic examination, slit-lamp examination, tonometry examination, visual field measurement refraction, pupillary reflex response
TX: Medication (beta-adrenergic blocker, ophthalmic drops, epinephrine ophthalmic drops, pilocarpine), surgery for acute angle-closure
F/U: Referral to ophthalmologist

Headache

The most common neurologic symptom, headaches may be localized or generalized, producing mild to severe pain. About 90% of all headaches are benign and can be described as vascular, muscle-contraction, or a combination of both. Occasionally, however, headaches indicate a severe neurologic disorder associated with intracranial inflammation, increased intracranial pressure (ICP), or meningeal irritation. They may also result from ocular or sinus disorders or the effects of drugs, tests, and treatments.

Other causes of headache include fever, eyestrain, dehydration, and systemic febrile illnesses. Headaches may occur in certain metabolic disturbances — such as hypoxemia, hypercapnia, hyperglycemia, and hypoglycemia — but they're not a diagnostic or prominent symptom. Some individuals get headaches after seizures or from coughing, sneezing, heavy lifting, or stooping. (See *Comparing benign headaches*.)

History and physical examination

If the patient reports a headache, ask him to describe its characteristics and location. Is it associated with neck pain? How often does he get a headache? Clarify onset of headaches. Does it awaken him from sleep or recur at certain times of the day? Are there any precipitating symptoms of hunger, elation, or yawning? How long does a typical headache last? Try to identify precipitating factors, such as certain foods and exposure to bright lights. Is the patient under stress? Has he had trouble sleeping?

Take a drug history and ask about head trauma within the last 4 weeks. Has the patient recently experienced nausea, vomiting, photophobia, or visual changes? Does he feel drowsy, confused, or dizzy? Has he recently developed seizures, or does he have a history of seizures?

Begin the physical examination by evaluating the patient's level of consciousness. Then check his vital signs. Be alert for signs of increased ICP — widened pulse pressure, bradycardia, altered respiratory pattern, and increased blood pressure. Check pupil size and response to light, and note any neck stiffness.

PEDIATRIC POINTERS

- *If a child is too young to describe his symptom, suspect a headache if you see him banging or holding his head.*
- *In an infant, a shrill cry or bulging fontanels may indicate increased ICP and headache.*
- *In children over age 3, headache is the most common symptom of a brain tumor.*

Comparing benign headaches

90% of headaches are benign, which may be classified as muscle-contraction (tension), vascular (migraine and cluster), or a combination of both.
As you review the chart below, you'll see that the two major types — muscle-contraction and vascular headaches — are quite different. In a combined headache, features of both appear; this type of headache may affect the patient with a severe muscle-contraction headache or a late-stage migraine. Treatment of a combined headache includes analgesics and sedatives.

CHARACTERISTICS	MUSCLE-CONTRACTION HEADACHES	VASCULAR HEADACHES
Incidence	• Most common type, accounting for 80% of all headaches	• More common in women and those with a family history of migraines • Onset after puberty
Precipitating factors	• Stress, anxiety, tension, improper posture and body alignment • Prolonged muscle contraction without structural damage • Eye, ear, and paranasal sinus disorders that produce reflex muscle contractions	• Hormone fluctuations • Alcohol • Emotional upset • Too little or too much sleep • Foods, such as chocolate, cheese, monosodium glutamate, and cured meats; caffeine withdrawal • Weather changes, such as shifts in barometric pressure
Intensity and duration	• Produce an aching tightness or a band of pain around the head, especially in the neck and in occipital and temporal areas • Occur frequently and usually last for several hours	• May begin with an awareness of an impending migraine or a 5- to 15-minute prodrome of neurologic deficits, such as visual disturbances, dizziness, unsteady gait, or tingling of the face, lips, or hands • Produce severe, constant, throbbing pain that is typically unilateral and may be incapacitating • Last for 4 to 6 hours
Associated signs and symptoms	• Tense neck and facial muscles	• Anorexia, nausea, and vomiting • Occasionally, photophobia, sensitivity to loud noises, weakness, and fatigue • Depending on the type (cluster headache or classic, common, or hemiplegic migraine), possibly chills, depression, eye pain, ptosis, tearing, rhinorrhea, diaphoresis, and facial flushing

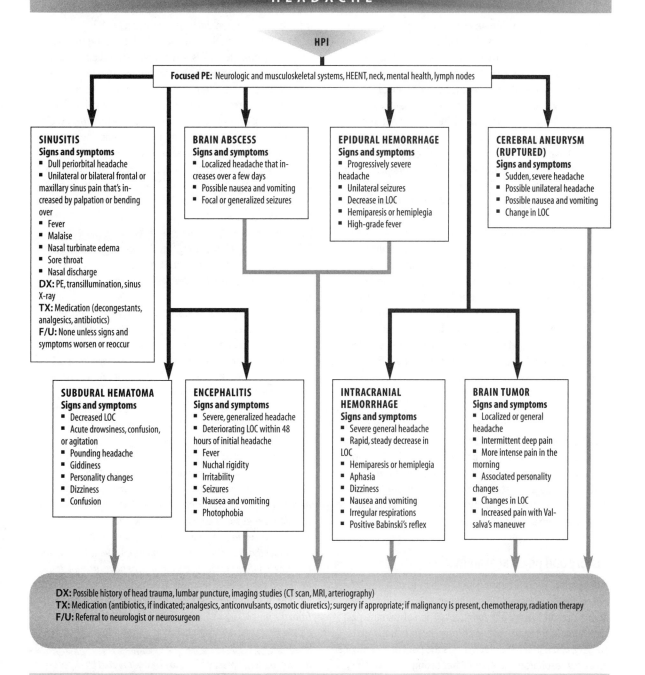

HPI

Focused PE: Neurologic and musculoskeletal systems, HEENT, neck, mental health, lymph nodes

SINUSITIS
Signs and symptoms
- Dull periorbital headache
- Unilateral or bilateral frontal or maxillary sinus pain that's increased by palpation or bending over
- Fever
- Malaise
- Nasal turbinate edema
- Sore throat
- Nasal discharge

DX: PE, transillumination, sinus X-ray
TX: Medication (decongestants, analgesics, antibiotics)
F/U: None unless signs and symptoms worsen or reoccur

BRAIN ABSCESS
Signs and symptoms
- Localized headache that increases over a few days
- Possible nausea and vomiting
- Focal or generalized seizures

EPIDURAL HEMORRHAGE
Signs and symptoms
- Progressively severe headache
- Unilateral seizures
- Decrease in LOC
- Hemiparesis or hemiplegia
- High-grade fever

CEREBRAL ANEURYSM (RUPTURED)
Signs and symptoms
- Sudden, severe headache
- Possible unilateral headache
- Possible nausea and vomiting
- Change in LOC

SUBDURAL HEMATOMA
Signs and symptoms
- Decreased LOC
- Acute drowsiness, confusion, or agitation
- Pounding headache
- Giddiness
- Personality changes
- Dizziness
- Confusion

ENCEPHALITIS
Signs and symptoms
- Severe, generalized headache
- Deteriorating LOC within 48 hours of initial headache
- Fever
- Nuchal rigidity
- Irritability
- Seizures
- Nausea and vomiting
- Photophobia

INTRACRANIAL HEMORRHAGE
Signs and symptoms
- Severe general headache
- Rapid, steady decrease in LOC
- Hemiparesis or hemiplegia
- Aphasia
- Dizziness
- Nausea and vomiting
- Irregular respirations
- Positive Babinski's reflex

BRAIN TUMOR
Signs and symptoms
- Localized or general headache
- Intermittent deep pain
- More intense pain in the morning
- Associated personality changes
- Changes in LOC
- Increased pain with Valsalva's maneuver

DX: Possible history of head trauma, lumbar puncture, imaging studies (CT scan, MRI, arteriography)
TX: Medication (antibiotics, if indicated; analgesics, anticonvulsants, osmotic diuretics); surgery if appropriate; if malignancy is present, chemotherapy, radiation therapy
F/U: Referral to neurologist or neurosurgeon

Additional differential diagnoses: acute angle glaucoma ▪ cervical spine disorder ▪ dental cause ▪ Ebola virus ▪ hantavirus pulmonary syndrome ▪ hypertension ▪ influenza ▪ meningitis ▪ migraine headache ▪ postconcussional syndrome ▪ subarachnoid hemorrhage ▪ temporal arteritis ▪ tension headache ▪ trigeminal neuralgia ▪ West Nile encephalitis

Other causes: cervical traction ▪ herbal medicines, such as St. John's wort, ginseng, and Ephedra ▪ indomethacin ▪ lumbar puncture ▪ myelogram ▪ nitrates ▪ vasodilators ▪ withdrawal from vasopressors, such as caffeine, ergotamine, and sympathomimetic drugs

Hearing loss

Affecting nearly 16 million Americans, hearing loss may be temporary or permanent and partial or complete. This common symptom may involve reception of low-, middle-, or high-frequency tones. If the hearing loss doesn't affect speech frequencies, the patient may be unaware of it.

Normally, sound waves enter the external auditory canal, travel to the middle ear's tympanic membrane and ossicles (incus, malleus, and stapes), and then travel into the inner ear's cochlea. The cochlear division of the eighth cranial (auditory) nerve carries the sound impulse to the brain. This type of sound transmission, called *air conduction,* is normally better than *bone conduction* — sound transmission through bone to the inner ear.

Hearing loss can be classified as conductive, sensorineural, mixed, and functional. *Conductive hearing loss* results from external or middle ear disorders that block sound transmission. This type of hearing loss usually responds to medical or surgical intervention (or in some cases, both). *Sensorineural hearing loss* results from disorders of the inner ear or of the eighth cranial nerve. *Mixed hearing loss* combines aspects of conductive and sensorineural hearing loss. *Functional hearing loss* results from psychological factors rather than identifiable organic damage.

Hearing loss may also result from trauma, infection, allergy, tumors, certain systemic and hereditary disorders, and the effects of ototoxic drugs and treatments. In most cases, however, it results from presbycusis, a type of sensorineural hearing loss that typically affects people over age 50. Other physiologic causes of hearing loss include cerumen impaction; barotitis media associated with descent in an airplane or elevator, diving, or close proximity to an explosion; and chronic exposure to noise over 90 dB.

History and physical examination

If the patient reports hearing loss, ask him to describe it fully. Is it unilateral or bilateral? Continuous or intermittent? Ask about a family history of hearing loss. Then obtain the patient's medical history, noting chronic ear infections, ear surgery, and ear or head trauma. Has the patient recently had an upper respiratory infection? After taking a drug history, have the patient describe his occupation and work environment.

Next, explore associated signs and symptoms. Does the patient have ear pain? If so, is it unilateral or bilateral? Continuous or intermittent? Ask the patient if he has noticed discharge from one or both ears. If so, have him describe its color and consistency and note when it began. Does he hear ringing, buzzing, hissing, or other noises in one or both ears? If so, are the noises constant or intermittent? Does he experience dizziness? If so, when did he first notice it?

Begin the physical examination by inspecting the external ear for inflammation, boils, foreign bodies, and discharge. Then apply pressure to the tragus and mastoid to elicit tenderness. If you detect tenderness or external ear abnormalities, be extra careful with the otoscopic examination. During the examination, note any color change, perforation, bulging, or retraction of the tympanic membrane, which normally looks like a shiny, pearl gray cone.

Next, evaluate the patient's hearing acuity, using the ticking watch and whispered voice tests. Then perform the Weber's and Rinne tests to obtain a preliminary evaluation of the type and degree of hearing loss.

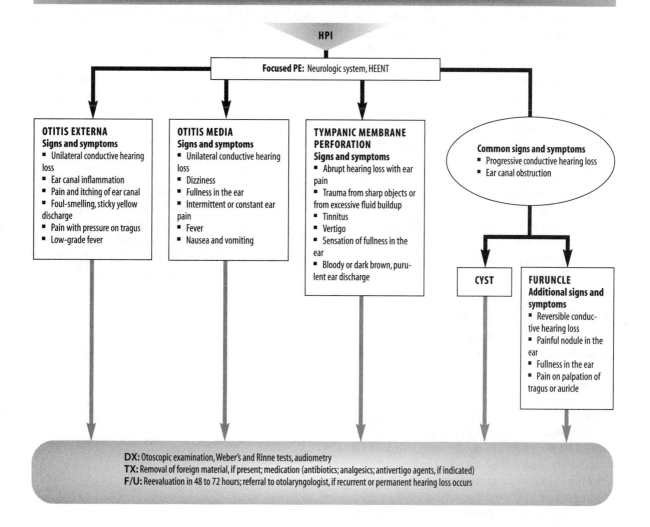

HPI

Focused PE: Neurologic system, HEENT

OTITIS EXTERNA
Signs and symptoms
- Unilateral conductive hearing loss
- Ear canal inflammation
- Pain and itching of ear canal
- Foul-smelling, sticky yellow discharge
- Pain with pressure on tragus
- Low-grade fever

OTITIS MEDIA
Signs and symptoms
- Unilateral conductive hearing loss
- Dizziness
- Fullness in the ear
- Intermittent or constant ear pain
- Fever
- Nausea and vomiting

TYMPANIC MEMBRANE PERFORATION
Signs and symptoms
- Abrupt hearing loss with ear pain
- Trauma from sharp objects or from excessive fluid buildup
- Tinnitus
- Vertigo
- Sensation of fullness in the ear
- Bloody or dark brown, purulent ear discharge

Common signs and symptoms
- Progressive conductive hearing loss
- Ear canal obstruction

CYST

FURUNCLE
Additional signs and symptoms
- Reversible conductive hearing loss
- Painful nodule in the ear
- Fullness in the ear
- Pain on palpation of tragus or auricle

DX: Otoscopic examination, Weber's and Rinne tests, audiometry
TX: Removal of foreign material, if present; medication (antibiotics; analgesics; antivertigo agents, if indicated)
F/U: Reevaluation in 48 to 72 hours; referral to otolaryngologist, if recurrent or permanent hearing loss occurs

Additional differential diagnoses: acoustic neuroma ▪ adenoid hypertrophy ▪ allergies ▪ aural polyps ▪ cerebellopontine tumor ▪ cholesteatoma ▪ external ear canal tumor ▪ glomus jugulare tumor or glomus tympanicum tumor ▪ granuloma ▪ hypothyroidism ▪ Ménière's disease ▪ multiple sclerosis ▪ myringitis nasopharyngeal cancer ▪ osteoma ▪ otosclerosis ▪ Ramsay Hunt syndrome ▪ skull fracture ▪ temporal arteritis ▪ temporal bone fracture ▪ Wegener's granulomatosis

Other causes: head trauma ▪ ototoxic drugs ▪ chloroquine ▪ cisplatin ▪ vancomycin ▪ aminoglycosides (especially neomycin, kanamycin, and amikacin) ▪ loop diuretics, such as furosemide, ethacrynic acid, and bumetanide ▪ quinine ▪ quinidine ▪ high doses of erythromycin or salicylates (such as aspirin) ▪ radiation therapy ▪ myringotomy ▪ myringoplasty ▪ simple or radical mastoidectomy ▪ fenestrations

Hematemesis

Hematemesis, the vomiting of blood, usually indicates GI bleeding above the ligament of Treitz, which suspends the duodenum at its junction with the jejunum. Bright red or blood-streaked vomitus indicates fresh or recent bleeding. Dark red, brown, or black vomitus (the color and consistency of coffee grounds) indicates that blood has been retained in the stomach and partially digested.

Although hematemesis usually results from GI disorders, it may stem from coagulation disorders and from treatments that irritate the GI tract. Swallowed blood from epistaxis or oropharyngeal erosion may also cause bloody vomitus.

Hematemesis is always an important sign, but its severity depends on the amount, source, and rapidity of the bleeding. Massive hematemesis (vomiting of 500 to 1,000 ml of blood) may rapidly be life-threatening. Hematemesis may be precipitated by straining, emotional stress, and the use of anti-inflammatory drugs or alcohol.

History and physical examination

If the patient has massive hematemesis, quickly check his vital signs. If you detect signs of shock, such as tachypnea, hypotension, and tachycardia, place the patient in a supine position and elevate his feet 20 to 30 degrees. Emergency endoscopy may be necessary to locate the source of bleeding. Take measures for the patient to receive emergency care.

If the patient's hematemesis isn't immediately life-threatening, begin with a thorough history. First, have the patient describe the amount, color, and consistency of the vomitus. When did he first notice this sign? Has he ever had hematemesis before? Find out if he also has bloody or black tarry stools. Note whether hematemesis is usually preceded by nausea, flatulence, diarrhea, or weakness. Has he recently had bouts of retching with or without vomiting?

Next, ask about a history of ulcers or of liver or coagulation disorders. Find out how much alcohol the patient drinks, if any. Does he regularly take aspirin or another nonsteroidal anti-inflammatory drug (NSAID), such as phenylbutazone or indomethacin? These drugs may cause erosive gastritis or ulcers.

Begin the physical examination by checking for orthostatic hypotension, an early warning sign of hypovolemia. Take blood pressure and pulse with the patient supine, sitting, then standing. A decrease of 10 mm Hg or more in systolic pressure or an increase of 10 beats/minute or more in pulse rate indicates volume depletion. After obtaining other vital signs, inspect the mucous membranes, nasopharynx, and skin for any signs of bleeding or other abnormalities. Finally, palpate the abdomen for tenderness, pain, or masses. Note lymphadenopathy.

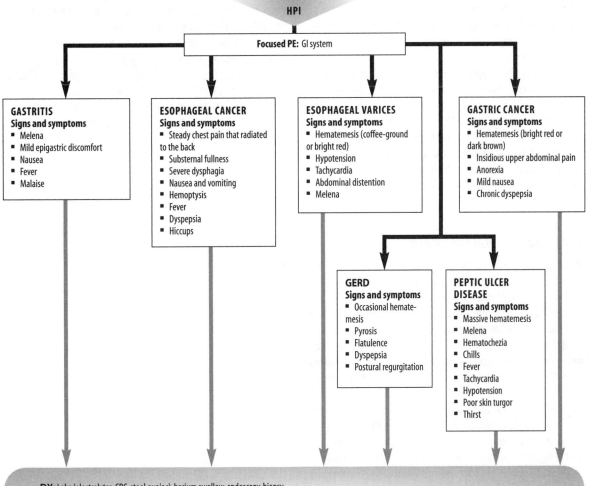

HPI

Focused PE: GI system

GASTRITIS
Signs and symptoms
- Melena
- Mild epigastric discomfort
- Nausea
- Fever
- Malaise

ESOPHAGEAL CANCER
Signs and symptoms
- Steady chest pain that radiated to the back
- Substernal fullness
- Severe dysphagia
- Nausea and vomiting
- Hemoptysis
- Fever
- Dyspepsia
- Hiccups

ESOPHAGEAL VARICES
Signs and symptoms
- Hematemesis (coffee-ground or bright red)
- Hypotension
- Tachycardia
- Abdominal distention
- Melena

GASTRIC CANCER
Signs and symptoms
- Hematemesis (bright red or dark brown)
- Insidious upper abdominal pain
- Anorexia
- Mild nausea
- Chronic dyspepsia

GERD
Signs and symptoms
- Occasional hematemesis
- Pyrosis
- Flatulence
- Dyspepsia
- Postural regurgitation

PEPTIC ULCER DISEASE
Signs and symptoms
- Massive hematemesis
- Melena
- Hematochezia
- Chills
- Fever
- Tachycardia
- Hypotension
- Poor skin turgor
- Thirst

DX: Labs (electrolytes, CBC, stool guaiac), barium swallow, endoscopy, biopsy
TX: Fluid replacement, medication (histamine-2 blockers, antacids, proton pump inhibitors, antibiotics [if indicated]), chemotherapy if appropriate, NG irrigation, blood transfusion, surgery if indicated
F/U: As needed (dependent on diagnosis), referral to gastroenterologist or oncologist if appropriate

Additional differential diagnoses: achalasia ▪ arteriovenous malformation ▪ coagulation disorders ▪ duodenal ulcer ▪ esophageal fistula ▪ esophageal injury ▪ esophageal rupture ▪ GI leiomyoma ▪ Mallory-Weiss syndrome

Other causes: traumatic NG or endotracheal intubation ▪ nose or throat surgery

Hematochezia

The passage of bloody stools, hematochezia usually indicates — and may be the first sign of — GI bleeding below the ligament of Treitz. However, this sign — usually preceded by hematemesis — may also accompany rapid hemorrhage of 1 L or more from the upper GI tract.

Hematochezia ranges from formed, blood-streaked stools to liquid, bloody stools that may be bright red, dark mahogany, or maroon in color (melena). This sign usually develops abruptly and is heralded by abdominal pain.

Although hematochezia commonly is associated with GI disorders, it may also result from coagulation disorders, the effects of toxins, and certain diagnostic tests. Always a significant sign, hematochezia may precipitate life-threatening hypovolemia.

History and physical examination

If the patient has severe hematochezia, quickly check his vital signs. If you detect signs of shock, such as hypotension and tachycardia, place the patient in a supine position and elevate his feet 20 to 30 degrees. Endoscopy may be necessary to detect the source of the bleeding.

If the hematochezia isn't immediately life-threatening, ask the patient to fully describe the amount, color, and consistency of his bloody stools. (If possible, also inspect and characterize the stools yourself.) How long have the stools been bloody? Do they always look the same or does the amount of blood seem to vary? Ask about associated signs and symptoms.

Next, explore the patient's medical history, focusing on GI and coagulation disorders. Ask about use of GI irritants, such as alcohol, aspirin, and other nonsteroidal anti-inflammatory drugs.

Begin the physical examination by checking for orthostatic hypotension, an early sign of shock. Take the patient's blood pressure and pulse while he's lying down, sitting, and standing. If systolic pressure decreases by 10 mm Hg or more, or pulse rate increases by 10 beats/minute or more when he changes position, suspect volume depletion and impending shock.

Examine the skin for petechiae or spider angiomas. Palpate the abdomen for tenderness, pain, or masses. Also, note lymphadenopathy. Finally, a digital rectal examination must be done to rule out any rectal masses.

- *Hematochezia is less common in children than in adults. It may result from structural disorders, such as intussusception and* Meckel's diverticulum, and from inflammatory disorders, such as peptic ulcer disease and ulcerative colitis.
- *In children, ulcerative colitis typically produces chronic, rather than acute, signs and symptoms and may also cause slow growth and maturation related to malnutrition.*
- *Suspect sexual abuse in all cases of rectal bleeding in children.*

Because older people have an increased risk of colon cancer, hematochezia should be evaluated with colonoscopy after perirectal lesions have been ruled out as the cause of bleeding.

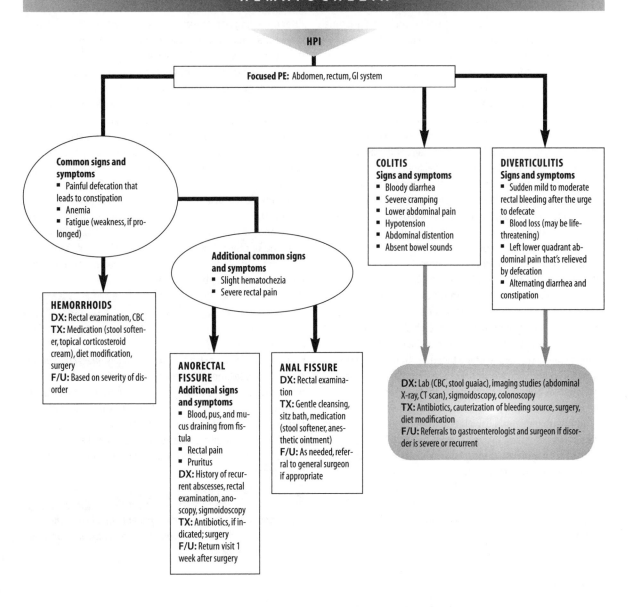

HPI

Focused PE: Abdomen, rectum, GI system

Common signs and symptoms
- Painful defecation that leads to constipation
- Anemia
- Fatigue (weakness, if prolonged)

Additional common signs and symptoms
- Slight hematochezia
- Severe rectal pain

COLITIS
Signs and symptoms
- Bloody diarrhea
- Severe cramping
- Lower abdominal pain
- Hypotension
- Abdominal distention
- Absent bowel sounds

DIVERTICULITIS
Signs and symptoms
- Sudden mild to moderate rectal bleeding after the urge to defecate
- Blood loss (may be life-threatening)
- Left lower quadrant abdominal pain that's relieved by defecation
- Alternating diarrhea and constipation

HEMORRHOIDS
DX: Rectal examination, CBC
TX: Medication (stool softener, topical corticosteroid cream), diet modification, surgery
F/U: Based on severity of disorder

ANORECTAL FISSURE
Additional signs and symptoms
- Blood, pus, and mucus draining from fistula
- Rectal pain
- Pruritus
DX: History of recurrent abscesses, rectal examination, anoscopy, sigmoidoscopy
TX: Antibiotics, if indicated; surgery
F/U: Return visit 1 week after surgery

ANAL FISSURE
DX: Rectal examination
TX: Gentle cleansing, sitz bath, medication (stool softener, anesthetic ointment)
F/U: As needed, referral to general surgeon if appropriate

DX: Lab (CBC, stool guaiac), imaging studies (abdominal X-ray, CT scan), sigmoidoscopy, colonoscopy
TX: Antibiotics, cauterization of bleeding source, surgery, diet modification
F/U: Referrals to gastroenterologist and surgeon if disorder is severe or recurrent

Additional differential diagnoses: amyloidosis • angiodysplasia lesions • arteriovenous malformation • coagulation disorders • colon cancer • colorectal polyps • Crohn's disease • dysentery • esophageal varices • food poisoning • heavy metal poisoning • rectal melanoma • small intestine cancer • typhoid fever • ulcerative proctitis

Other causes: colonoscopy • polypectomy • proctosigmoidoscopy • bowel perforation (rare)

Hematuria

A cardinal sign of renal and urinary tract disorders, hematuria is the abnormal presence of blood in the urine. Strictly defined, it means three or more red blood cells per high-power microscopic field in the urine. Microscopic hematuria is confirmed by an occult blood test, whereas macroscopic hematuria is immediately visible. However, macroscopic hematuria must be distinguished from pseudohematuria. (See *Confirming hematuria*.) Macroscopic hematuria may be continuous or intermittent, is often accompanied by pain, and may be aggravated by prolonged standing or walking.

Hematuria may be classified by the stage of urination it predominantly affects. Bleeding at the start of urination — *initial hematuria* — usually indicates urethral pathology; bleeding at the end of urination — *terminal hematuria* — usually indicates pathology of the bladder neck, posterior urethra, or prostate; bleeding throughout urination — *total hematuria* — usually indicates pathology above the bladder neck.

Hematuria may result from one of two mechanisms: rupture or perforation of vessels in the renal system or urinary tract or impaired glomerular filtration, which allows red blood cells to seep into the urine. The color of the bloody urine provides a clue to the source of the bleeding. Generally, dark or brownish blood indicates renal or upper urinary tract bleeding, whereas bright red blood indicates lower urinary tract bleeding.

Although hematuria usually results from renal and urinary tract disorders, it may also result from certain GI, prostate, vaginal, or coagulation disorders, or from the effects of certain drugs. Invasive therapy and diagnostic tests that involve manipulative instrumentation of the renal and urologic systems may also cause hematuria. Nonpathologic hematuria may result from fever and hypercatabolic states. Transient hematuria may follow strenuous exercise.

History and physical examination

After detecting hematuria, take a pertinent health history. If hematuria is macroscopic, ask the patient when he first noticed blood in his urine. Does it vary in severity between voidings? Is it worse at the beginning, middle, or end of urination? Has it occurred before? Is the patient passing any clots? To rule out artifactitious hematuria, ask about bleeding hemorrhoids or the onset of menses, if appropriate.

Ask about recent abdominal or flank trauma. Has the patient been exercising strenuously? Note a history of renal, urinary, prostatic, or coagulation disorders. Then obtain a drug history.

Begin the physical examination by palpating and percussing the abdomen and flanks. Next, percuss the costovertebral angle to elicit tenderness. Check the urinary meatus for bleeding or other abnormalities. Using a chemical reagent strip, test a urine specimen for protein. A vaginal or digital rectal examination may be necessary.

PEDIATRIC POINTERS

- *Cyclophosphamide is more likely to cause hematuria in children than in adults.*
- *Common causes of hematuria that chiefly affect children include congenital anomalies, such as obstructive uropathy and renal dysplasia; birth trauma; hematologic disorders, such as vitamin K deficiency, hemophilia, and hemolytic uremic syndrome; certain neoplasms, such as Wilms' tumor, bladder cancer, and rhabdomyosarcoma; allergies; foreign bodies in the urinary tract; and venous thrombosis. Artifactual hematuria may result from recent circumcision.*

ELDER CARE CUE

Evaluation of hematuria in elderly patients should include a urine culture, excretory urography or sonography, and consultation with an urologist.

Confirming hematuria

If the patient's urine appears blood-tinged, be sure to rule out pseudohematuria, red or pink urine caused by urinary pigments. First, carefully observe the urine specimen. If it contains a red sediment, it's probably *true* hematuria.

Then check the patient's history for use of drugs associated with pseudohematuria, including rifampin, chlorzoxazone, phenazopyridine, phenothiazines, doxorubicin, phensuximide, phenytoin, daunomycin, and laxatives with phenolphthalein.

Ask about the patient's intake of beets, berries, or foods with red dyes, which may color the urine red. Be aware that porphyrinuria and excess urate excretion can also cause pseudohematuria

Finally, test the urine using a chemical reagent strip. This test can confirm even microscopic hematuria and can also estimate the amount of blood present.

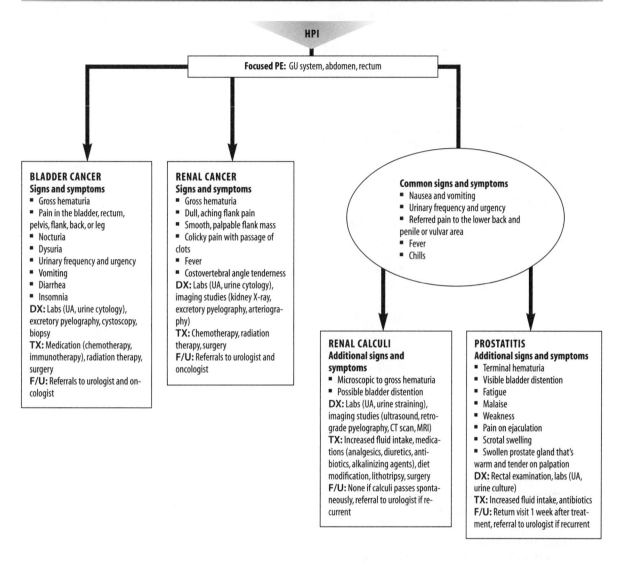

HPI

Focused PE: GU system, abdomen, rectum

BLADDER CANCER
Signs and symptoms
- Gross hematuria
- Pain in the bladder, rectum, pelvis, flank, back, or leg
- Nocturia
- Dysuria
- Urinary frequency and urgency
- Vomiting
- Diarrhea
- Insomnia
DX: Labs (UA, urine cytology), excretory pyelography, cystoscopy, biopsy
TX: Medication (chemotherapy, immunotherapy), radiation therapy, surgery
F/U: Referrals to urologist and oncologist

RENAL CANCER
Signs and symptoms
- Gross hematuria
- Dull, aching flank pain
- Smooth, palpable flank mass
- Colicky pain with passage of clots
- Fever
- Costovertebral angle tenderness
DX: Labs (UA, urine cytology), imaging studies (kidney X-ray, excretory pyelography, arteriography)
TX: Chemotherapy, radiation therapy, surgery
F/U: Referrals to urologist and oncologist

Common signs and symptoms
- Nausea and vomiting
- Urinary frequency and urgency
- Referred pain to the lower back and penile or vulvar area
- Fever
- Chills

RENAL CALCULI
Additional signs and symptoms
- Microscopic to gross hematuria
- Possible bladder distention
DX: Labs (UA, urine straining), imaging studies (ultrasound, retrograde pyelography, CT scan, MRI)
TX: Increased fluid intake, medications (analgesics, diuretics, antibiotics, alkalinizing agents), diet modification, lithotripsy, surgery
F/U: None if calculi passes spontaneously, referral to urologist if recurrent

PROSTATITIS
Additional signs and symptoms
- Terminal hematuria
- Visible bladder distention
- Fatigue
- Malaise
- Weakness
- Pain on ejaculation
- Scrotal swelling
- Swollen prostate gland that's warm and tender on palpation
DX: Rectal examination, labs (UA, urine culture)
TX: Increased fluid intake, antibiotics
F/U: Return visit 1 week after treatment, referral to urologist if recurrent

Additional differential diagnoses: coagulation disorder ▪ cortical necrosis ▪ cystitis ▪ diverticulitis ▪ endocarditis ▪ glomerulonephritis ▪ infection ▪ nephritis ▪ obstructive nephropathy ▪ polycystic kidney disease ▪ prostatic hypertrophy ▪ pyelonephritis ▪ renal infarction ▪ renal papillary necrosis ▪ renal tuberculosis ▪ renal vein thrombosis ▪ schistosomiasis ▪ sickle cell anemia ▪ SLE ▪ vaginitis ▪ vasculitis

Other causes: anticoagulation therapy ▪ bladder, kidney, or urethral trauma ▪ renal biopsy ▪ biopsy or manipulative instrumentation of the urinary tract ▪ analgesics ▪ cyclophosphamide (Cytoxan) ▪ metyrosine ▪ phenylbutazone ▪ penicillin ▪ rifampin ▪ thiabendazole ▪ herbal medicines, such as garlic and ginkgo biloba, when taken with anticoagulants

Hemianopia

Hemianopia is the loss of vision in half the visual field of one or both eyes. However, if the visual field defects are identical in both eyes but affect less than half the field of vision in each eye (incomplete homonymous hemianopia), the lesion may be in the occipital lobe; otherwise, it probably involves the parietal or temporal lobe.

Hemianopia is caused by a lesion affecting the optic chiasm, tract, or radiation. Defects in visual perception due to cerebral lesions are usually associated with impaired color vision.

History and physical examination

Suspect a visual field defect if the patient seems startled when you approach him from one side or if he fails to see objects placed directly in front of him. To help determine the type of defect, compare the patient's visual fields with your own — assuming that yours are normal. First, ask the patient to cover his right eye while you cover your left eye. Then move a pen or similarly shaped object from the periphery of his (and your) uncovered eye into his field of vision. Ask the patient to indicate when he first sees the object. Does he see it at the same time as you? After you? Repeat this test in each quadrant of both eyes. Then, for each eye, plot the defect by shading the area of a circle that corresponds to the area of vision loss.

Next, evaluate the patient's level of consciousness, take his vital signs, and check his pupillary reaction and motor response. Ask if he has recently experienced headache, dysarthria, or seizures. Does he have ptosis or facial or extremity weakness? Hallucinations or loss of color vision? When did neurologic symptoms start? Obtain a medical history, noting especially eye disorders, hypertension, and diabetes mellitus. (See *Recognizing types of hemianopia*.)

PEDIATRIC POINTER

In children, a brain tumor is the most common cause of hemianopia. To help detect this sign, look for nonverbal clues, such as the child reaching for a toy but missing it.

Recognizing types of hemianopia

Lesions of the optic pathways cause visual field defects. The lesion's site determines the type of defect. For example, a lesion of the optic chiasm involving only those fibers that cross over to the opposite side causes bitemporal hemianopia — visual loss in the temporal half of each field. However, a lesion of the optic tract or a complete lesion of the optic radiation produces visual loss in the same half of each field — either left or right homonymous hemianopia.

HEMIANOPIA

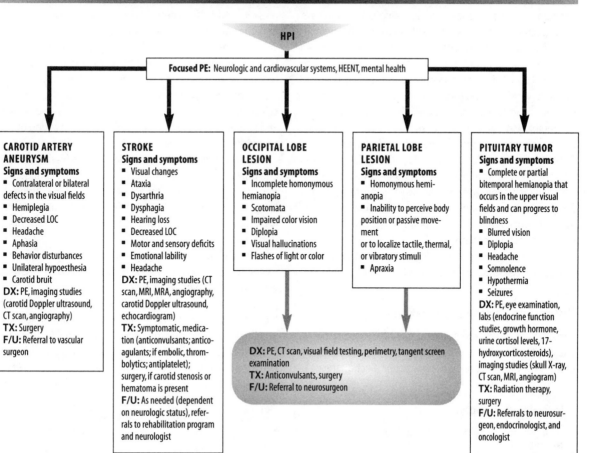

HPI

Focused PE: Neurologic and cardiovascular systems, HEENT, mental health

CAROTID ARTERY ANEURYSM
Signs and symptoms
- Contralateral or bilateral defects in the visual fields
- Hemiplegia
- Decreased LOC
- Headache
- Aphasia
- Behavior disturbances
- Unilateral hypoesthesia
- Carotid bruit

DX: PE, imaging studies (carotid Doppler ultrasound, CT scan, angiography)
TX: Surgery
F/U: Referral to vascular surgeon

STROKE
Signs and symptoms
- Visual changes
- Ataxia
- Dysarthria
- Dysphagia
- Hearing loss
- Decreased LOC
- Motor and sensory deficits
- Emotional lability
- Headache

DX: PE, imaging studies (CT scan, MRI, MRA, angiography, carotid Doppler ultrasound, echocardiogram)
TX: Symptomatic, medication (anticonvulsants; anticoagulants; if embolic, thrombolytics; antiplatelet); surgery, if carotid stenosis or hematoma is present
F/U: As needed (dependent on neurologic status), referrals to rehabilitation program and neurologist

OCCIPITAL LOBE LESION
Signs and symptoms
- Incomplete homonymous hemianopia
- Scotomata
- Impaired color vision
- Diplopia
- Visual hallucinations
- Flashes of light or color

PARIETAL LOBE LESION
Signs and symptoms
- Homonymous hemianopia
- Inability to perceive body position or passive movement or to localize tactile, thermal, or vibratory stimuli
- Apraxia

DX: PE, CT scan, visual field testing, perimetry, tangent screen examination
TX: Anticonvulsants, surgery
F/U: Referral to neurosurgeon

PITUITARY TUMOR
Signs and symptoms
- Complete or partial bitemporal hemianopia that occurs in the upper visual fields and can progress to blindness
- Blurred vision
- Diplopia
- Headache
- Somnolence
- Hypothermia
- Seizures

DX: PE, eye examination, labs (endocrine function studies, growth hormone, urine cortisol levels, 17-hydroxycorticosteroids), imaging studies (skull X-ray, CT scan, MRI, angiogram)
TX: Radiation therapy, surgery
F/U: Referrals to neurosurgeon, endocrinologist, and oncologist

Hemoptysis

Frightening to the patient and often ominous, hemoptysis is the expectoration of blood or bloody sputum from the lungs or tracheobronchial tree. It's sometimes confused with bleeding from the mouth, throat, nasopharynx, or GI tract. Expectoration of 200 ml of blood in a single episode suggests severe bleeding, whereas expectoration of 400 ml in 3 hours or more than 600 ml in 16 hours signals a life-threatening crisis.

Hemoptysis usually results from chronic bronchitis, lung cancer, or bronchiectasis. However, it may also result from inflammatory, infectious, cardiovascular, or coagulation disorders and, rarely, from a ruptured aortic aneurysm. In up to 15% of patients, the cause is unknown. The most common causes of *massive hemoptysis* are lung cancer, bronchiectasis, active tuberculosis, and cavitary pulmonary disease from necrotic infections or tuberculosis.

A number of pathophysiologic processes can cause hemoptysis. (See *Identifying hemoptysis*.)

History and physical examination

If the patient coughs up copious amounts of blood, endotracheal intubation may be required. Massive hemoptysis can cause airway obstruction and asphyxiation. Suction the patient's airway, if possible. An emergency bronchoscopy should be performed to identify the bleeding site. Monitor blood pressure and pulse to detect hypotension and tachycardia until the patient receives emergency care.

If the hemoptysis is mild, ask the patient when it began. Has he ever coughed up blood before? About how much blood is he coughing up now? And how often? Ask about a history of cardiac, pulmonary, or bleeding disorders. If he's receiving anticoagulant therapy, find out the drug, its dosage and schedule, and the duration of therapy. Is he taking other prescription drugs? Does he smoke?

Take the patient's vital signs and examine his nose, mouth, and pharynx for sources of bleeding. Inspect the configuration of his chest and look for abnormal movement during breathing, use of accessory muscles, and retractions. Observe his respiratory rate, depth, and rhythm. Finally, examine his skin for lesions.

Next, palpate the patient's chest for diaphragm level and for tenderness, respiratory excursion, fremitus, and abnormal pulsations; then percuss for flatness, dullness, resonance, hyperresonance, and tympany. Finally, auscultate the lungs, noting especially the quality and intensity of breath sounds. Also auscultate for heart murmurs, bruits, and pleural friction rubs.

Obtain a sputum sample and examine it for overall quantity, for the amount of blood it contains, and for its color, odor, and consistency.

Identifying hemoptysis

These guidelines will help you distinguish hemoptysis from epistaxis, hematemesis, and brown, red, or pink sputum.

HEMOPTYSIS
Often frothy because it's mixed with air, hemoptysis is typically bright-red with an alkaline pH (tested with Nitrazine paper). It's strongly suggested by the presence of respiratory signs and symptoms, including a cough, a tickling sensation in the throat, and blood produced from repeated coughing episodes. (You can rule out epistaxis because the patient's nasal passages and posterior pharynx are usually clear.)

HEMATEMESIS
The usual site of hematemesis is the GI tract; the patient vomits or regurgitates coffee-ground material that contains food particles, tests positive for occult blood, and has an acid pH. But he may vomit bright red blood or may have swallowed blood from the oral cavity and nasopharynx. After an episode of hematemesis, the patient may have stools with traces of blood. Many patients with hematemesis also complain of dyspepsia.

BROWN, RED, OR PINK SPUTUM
Brown, red, or pink sputum can result from oxidation of inhaled bronchodilators. Sputum that looks like old blood may result from the rupture of an amebic abscess into the bronchus. Red or brown sputum may occur in a patient with pneumonia caused by the enterobacterium *Serratia marcescens.* "Currant-jelly" sputum occurs with *Klebsiella* infections.

- *Hemoptysis in children may stem from Goodpasture's syndrome, cystic fibrosis, or (rarely) idiopathic primary pulmonary hemosiderosis.*
- *Sometimes no cause can be found for pulmonary hemorrhage occurring within the first 2 weeks of life; in such cases, the prognosis is poor.*

If the patient is receiving anticoagulants, determine any changes that need to be made in diet or medications (including over-the-counter and natural supplements) because these factors may affect clotting.

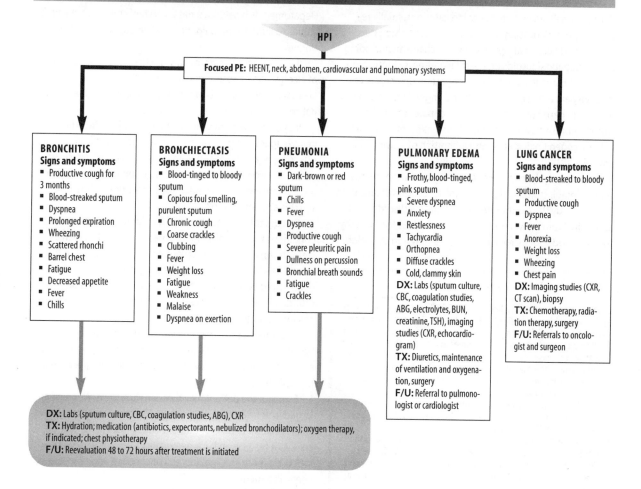

HPI

Focused PE: HEENT, neck, abdomen, cardiovascular and pulmonary systems

BRONCHITIS
Signs and symptoms
- Productive cough for 3 months
- Blood-streaked sputum
- Dyspnea
- Prolonged expiration
- Wheezing
- Scattered rhonchi
- Barrel chest
- Fatigue
- Decreased appetite
- Fever
- Chills

BRONCHIECTASIS
Signs and symptoms
- Blood-tinged to bloody sputum
- Copious foul smelling, purulent sputum
- Chronic cough
- Coarse crackles
- Clubbing
- Fever
- Weight loss
- Fatigue
- Weakness
- Malaise
- Dyspnea on exertion

PNEUMONIA
Signs and symptoms
- Dark-brown or red sputum
- Chills
- Fever
- Dyspnea
- Productive cough
- Severe pleuritic pain
- Dullness on percussion
- Bronchial breath sounds
- Fatigue
- Crackles

PULMONARY EDEMA
Signs and symptoms
- Frothy, blood-tinged, pink sputum
- Severe dyspnea
- Anxiety
- Restlessness
- Tachycardia
- Orthopnea
- Diffuse crackles
- Cold, clammy skin
DX: Labs (sputum culture, CBC, coagulation studies, ABG, electrolytes, BUN, creatinine, TSH), imaging studies (CXR, echocardiogram)
TX: Diuretics, maintenance of ventilation and oxygenation, surgery
F/U: Referral to pulmonologist or cardiologist

LUNG CANCER
Signs and symptoms
- Blood-streaked to bloody sputum
- Productive cough
- Dyspnea
- Fever
- Anorexia
- Weight loss
- Wheezing
- Chest pain
DX: Imaging studies (CXR, CT scan), biopsy
TX: Chemotherapy, radiation therapy, surgery
F/U: Referrals to oncologist and surgeon

DX: Labs (sputum culture, CBC, coagulation studies, ABG), CXR
TX: Hydration; medication (antibiotics, expectorants, nebulized bronchodilators); oxygen therapy, if indicated; chest physiotherapy
F/U: Reevaluation 48 to 72 hours after treatment is initiated

Additional differential diagnoses: aortic aneurysm (ruptured) ▪ bronchial adenoma ▪ coagulation disorder ▪ laryngeal cancer ▪ lung abscess ▪ pulmonary contusion ▪ pulmonary embolism with infarction ▪ pulmonary hypertension ▪ pulmonary tuberculosis ▪ silicosis ▪ SLE ▪ tracheal trauma ▪ Wegener's granulomatosis

Other causes: lung or airway injury from bronchoscopy, laryngoscopy, mediastinoscopy, or lung biopsy

Hepatomegaly

Hepatomegaly, an enlarged liver, indicates potentially reversible primary or secondary liver disease. This sign may stem from diverse pathophysiologic mechanisms, including dilated hepatic sinusoids (in heart failure), persistently high venous pressure leading to liver congestion (in chronic constrictive pericarditis), dysfunction and engorgement of hepatocytes (in hepatitis), fatty infiltration of parenchymal cells causing fibrous tissue (in cirrhosis), distention of liver cells with glycogen (in diabetes), and infiltration of amyloid (in amyloidosis).

Hepatomegaly may be confirmed by palpation, percussion, or imaging studies. It may be mistaken for displacement of the liver by the diaphragm, in a respiratory disorder; by an abdominal tumor; by a spinal deformity such as kyphosis; by the gallbladder; or by fecal material or a tumor in the colon.

Percussing for liver size and position

With your patient supine, begin at the right iliac crest to percuss up the right midclavicular line (MCL), as shown below. The percussion note becomes dull when you reach the liver's inferior border — usually at the costal margin but sometimes at a lower point in a patient with liver disease. Mark this point and then percuss down from the right clavicle, again along the right MCL. The liver's superior border usually lies between the fifth and seventh intercostal spaces. Mark the superior border.

The distance between the two marked points represents the approximate span of the liver's right lobe, which normally ranges from $2\frac{3}{8}''$ to $4\frac{3}{4}''$ (6 to 12 cm).

Next, assess the liver's left lobe similarly, percussing along the sternal midline. Again, mark the points where you hear dull percussion notes. Also, measure the span of the left lobe, which normally ranges from $1\frac{1}{2}''$ to $3\frac{1}{8}''$ (4 to 8 cm). Record your findings for use as a baseline.

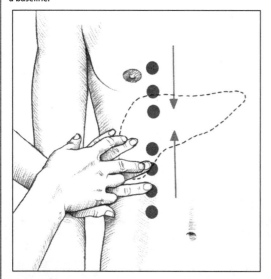

History and physical examination

Hepatomegaly is seldom a patient's chief complaint. It usually comes to light during palpation and percussion of the abdomen.

If you suspect hepatomegaly, ask the patient about his use of alcohol and exposure to hepatitis. Also ask if he's currently ill or taking any prescribed drugs. If he complains of abdominal pain, ask him to locate and describe it.

Inspect the patient's skin and sclera for jaundice, dilated veins (suggesting generalized congestion), scars from previous surgery, and spider angiomas (often occurring in cirrhosis). Next, inspect the contour of his abdomen. Is it protuberant over the liver or distended (possibly from ascites)? Measure his abdominal girth.

Percuss the liver, but be careful to identify structures and conditions that can obscure dull percussion notes, such as the sternum, ribs, breast tissue, pleural effusions, and gas in the colon. (See *Percussing for liver size and position*.) Next, during deep inspiration, palpate the liver's edge; it's tender and rounded in hepatitis and cardiac decompensation, rocklike in carcinoma, and firm in cirrhosis.

Take the patient's baseline vital signs, and assess his nutritional status. An enlarged liver that's functioning poorly causes muscle wasting, exaggerated skeletal prominences, weight loss, thin hair, and edema.

Evaluate the patient's level of consciousness. When an enlarged liver loses its ability to detoxify waste products, the result is accumulation of metabolic substances toxic to brain cells. As a result, watch for personality changes, irritability, agitation, memory loss, inability to concentrate, and — in a severely ill patient — coma.

PEDIATRIC POINTERS

- *Childhood hepatomegaly may stem from Reye's syndrome; biliary atresia; rare disorders such as Wilson's, Gaucher's, and Niemann-Pick diseases; or poorly controlled type I diabetes mellitus.*

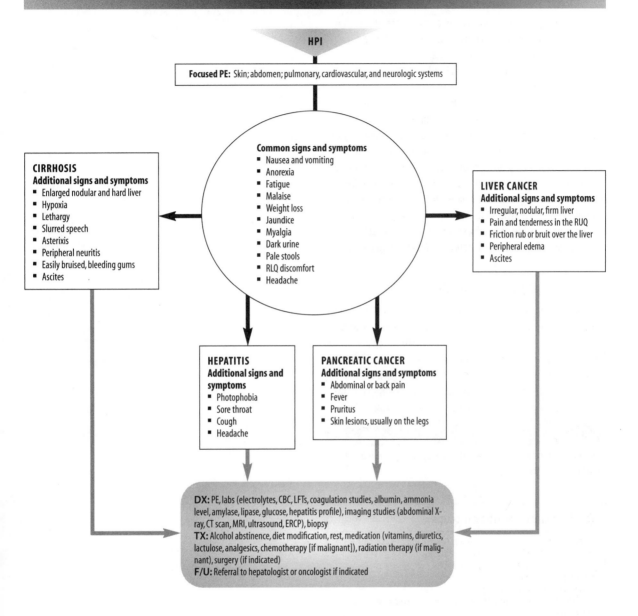

HPI

Focused PE: Skin; abdomen; pulmonary, cardiovascular, and neurologic systems

Common signs and symptoms
- Nausea and vomiting
- Anorexia
- Fatigue
- Malaise
- Weight loss
- Jaundice
- Myalgia
- Dark urine
- Pale stools
- RLQ discomfort
- Headache

CIRRHOSIS
Additional signs and symptoms
- Enlarged nodular and hard liver
- Hypoxia
- Lethargy
- Slurred speech
- Asterixis
- Peripheral neuritis
- Easily bruised, bleeding gums
- Ascites

LIVER CANCER
Additional signs and symptoms
- Irregular, nodular, firm liver
- Pain and tenderness in the RUQ
- Friction rub or bruit over the liver
- Peripheral edema
- Ascites

HEPATITIS
Additional signs and symptoms
- Photophobia
- Sore throat
- Cough
- Headache

PANCREATIC CANCER
Additional signs and symptoms
- Abdominal or back pain
- Fever
- Pruritus
- Skin lesions, usually on the legs

DX: PE, labs (electrolytes, CBC, LFTs, coagulation studies, albumin, ammonia level, amylase, lipase, glucose, hepatitis profile), imaging studies (abdominal X-ray, CT scan, MRI, ultrasound, ERCP), biopsy
TX: Alcohol abstinence, diet modification, rest, medication (vitamins, diuretics, lactulose, analgesics, chemotherapy [if malignant]), radiation therapy (if malignant), surgery (if indicated)
F/U: Referral to hepatologist or oncologist if indicated

Additional differential diagnoses: amyloidosis ▪ diabetes mellitus ▪ granulomatous disorders ▪ hepatic abscess ▪ leukemia ▪ lymphoma ▪ obesity ▪ pericarditis

Hiccups

Hiccups (singultus) occur as a two-stage process: an involuntary, spasmodic contraction of the diaphragm followed by sudden closure of the glottis. Their characteristic sound reflects the vibration of closed vocal cords as air suddenly rushes into the lungs.

Usually benign and transient, hiccups are common and usually subside spontaneously or with simple treatment. However, in a patient with a neurologic disorder, they may indicate increasing intracranial pressure or extension of a brain stem lesion. They may also occur after ingestion of hot or cold liquids or other irritants, after exposure to cold, or with irritation from a drainage tube. Persistent hiccups cause considerable distress and may lead to vomiting. Increased serum levels of carbon dioxide may inhibit hiccups; decreased levels may accentuate them. (See *Treating and preventing hiccups.*)

History and physical examination

Find out when the patient's hiccups began. If he's also vomiting and unconscious, turn him on his side to prevent aspiration.

If the patient is conscious, find out if the hiccups are tiring him. Ask if he has had hiccups before, what caused them, and what made them stop. Also, note whether he has a history of abdominal or thoracic disorders. Base the physical examination on the patient history and associated symptoms.

PEDIATRIC POINTER

In an infant, hiccups usually result from rapid ingestion of liquids without adequate burping.

Treating and preventing hiccups

Hiccups commonly occur without any underlying medical cause. Some home remedies to treat hiccups include:
- holding one's breath as long as possible
- breathing into a paper bag
- ingesting a spoonful of sugar
- drinking cold water from the wrong side of the glass while bending forward.

The following actions may help to prevent hiccups:
- avoiding extremely hot or cold foods
- avoiding spicy foods
- avoiding the use of straws
- burping frequently (for infants).

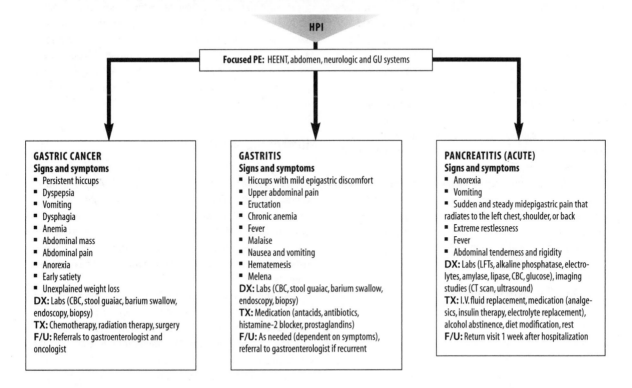

HPI

Focused PE: HEENT, abdomen, neurologic and GU systems

GASTRIC CANCER
Signs and symptoms
- Persistent hiccups
- Dyspepsia
- Vomiting
- Dysphagia
- Anemia
- Abdominal mass
- Abdominal pain
- Anorexia
- Early satiety
- Unexplained weight loss

DX: Labs (CBC, stool guaiac, barium swallow, endoscopy, biopsy)

TX: Chemotherapy, radiation therapy, surgery

F/U: Referrals to gastroenterologist and oncologist

GASTRITIS
Signs and symptoms
- Hiccups with mild epigastric discomfort
- Upper abdominal pain
- Eructation
- Chronic anemia
- Fever
- Malaise
- Nausea and vomiting
- Hematemesis
- Melena

DX: Labs (CBC, stool guaiac, barium swallow, endoscopy, biopsy)

TX: Medication (antacids, antibiotics, histamine-2 blocker, prostaglandins)

F/U: As needed (dependent on symptoms), referral to gastroenterologist if recurrent

PANCREATITIS (ACUTE)
Signs and symptoms
- Anorexia
- Vomiting
- Sudden and steady midepigastric pain that radiates to the left chest, shoulder, or back
- Extreme restlessness
- Fever
- Abdominal tenderness and rigidity

DX: Labs (LFTs, alkaline phosphatase, electrolytes, amylase, lipase, CBC, glucose), imaging studies (CT scan, ultrasound)

TX: I.V. fluid replacement, medication (analgesics, insulin therapy, electrolyte replacement), alcohol abstinence, diet modification, rest

F/U: Return visit 1 week after hospitalization

Additional differential diagnoses: brain stem lesion ▪ increased ICP ▪ pleurisy ▪ pneumonia ▪ renal failure

---

Other causes: abdominal surgery ▪ bloating ▪ hot and spicy foods or liquids ▪ noxious fumes

Hirsutism

Hirsutism is the excessive growth of dark, coarse body hair in females. Excessive androgen production stimulates hair growth on the pubic region, axilla, chin, upper lip, cheeks, anterior neck, sternum, linea alba, forearms, abdomen, back, and upper arms. In *mild hirsutism,* fine and pigmented hair appears on the sides of the face and the chin (but doesn't form a complete beard) and on the extremities, chest, abdomen, and perineum. In *moderate hirsutism,* coarse and pigmented hair appears on the same areas. In *severe hirsutism,* coarse hair also covers the whole beard area, the proximal interphalangeal joints, and the ears and nose.

Depending on the degree of excess androgen production, hirsutism may be associated with acne and increased skin oiliness, increased libido, and menstrual irregularities (including anovulation and amenorrhea). Extremely high androgen levels cause further virilization, including such signs as breast atrophy, loss of female body contour, frontal balding, and deepening of the voice.

Hirsutism may result from endocrine abnormalities and idiopathic causes. It may also occur in pregnancy from transient androgen production by the placenta or corpus luteum, and in menopause from increased androgen and decreased estrogen production. Some patients have a strong familial predisposition to hirsutism, which may be considered normal in the context of their genetic background.

History and physical examination

Begin by asking the patient where on her body she first noticed excessive hair. How old was she then? Where and how quickly did other hirsute areas develop? Does she use any hair removal technique? If so, how often does she use it, and when did she use it last? Next, obtain a menstrual history: the patient's age at menarche, the duration of her menses, the usual amount of blood flow, and the number of days between menses.

Ask about medications. If the patient is taking a drug containing an androgen or progestin compound, or another drug that can cause hirsutism, find out its name, dosage, schedule, and therapeutic aim. Does she sometimes miss doses or take extra ones?

Next, examine the hirsute areas. Does excessive hair appear only on the upper lip or on other body parts as well? Is the hair fine but pigmented or dense and coarse? Is the patient obese? Observe for signs of virilization. (See *Recognizing signs of virilization.*)

PEDIATRIC POINTERS

- *Childhood hirsutism can stem from congenital adrenal hyperplasia. This disorder is almost always detected at birth because affected infants have ambiguous genitalia. Rarely, a mild form becomes apparent after puberty when hirsutism, irregular bleeding or amenorrhea, and signs of virilization appear.*
- *Hirsutism that occurs at or after puberty often results from polycystic ovary disease.*

ELDER CARE CUE

Hirsutism can occur after menopause if peripheral conversion of estrogen is poor.

Recognizing signs of virilization

Excessive androgen levels produce severe hirsutism and other marked signs of virilization, as shown in the figure below.

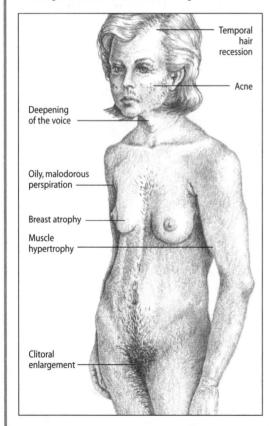

- Temporal hair recession
- Acne
- Deepening of the voice
- Oily, malodorous perspiration
- Breast atrophy
- Muscle hypertrophy
- Clitoral enlargement

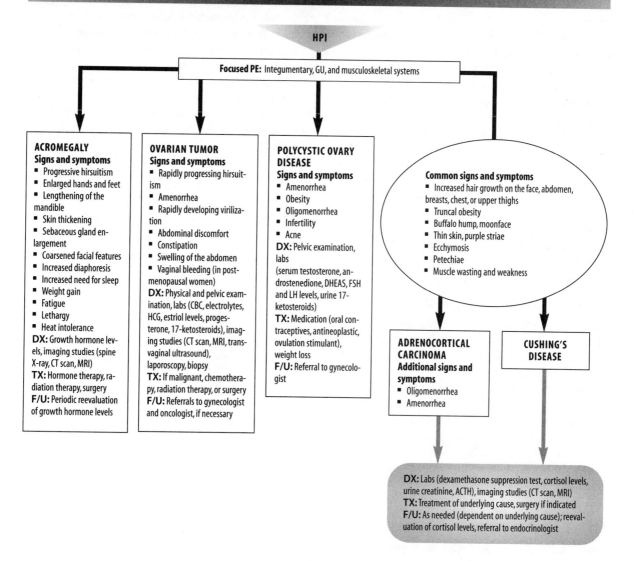

HPI

Focused PE: Integumentary, GU, and musculoskeletal systems

ACROMEGALY
Signs and symptoms
- Progressive hirsutism
- Enlarged hands and feet
- Lengthening of the mandible
- Skin thickening
- Sebaceous gland enlargement
- Coarsened facial features
- Increased diaphoresis
- Increased need for sleep
- Weight gain
- Fatigue
- Lethargy
- Heat intolerance

DX: Growth hormone levels, imaging studies (spine X-ray, CT scan, MRI)
TX: Hormone therapy, radiation therapy, surgery
F/U: Periodic reevaluation of growth hormone levels

OVARIAN TUMOR
Signs and symptoms
- Rapidly progressing hirsutism
- Amenorrhea
- Rapidly developing virilization
- Abdominal discomfort
- Constipation
- Swelling of the abdomen
- Vaginal bleeding (in postmenopausal women)

DX: Physical and pelvic examination, labs (CBC, electrolytes, HCG, estriol levels, progesterone, 17-ketosteroids), imaging studies (CT scan, MRI, transvaginal ultrasound), laporoscopy, biopsy
TX: If malignant, chemotherapy, radiation therapy, or surgery
F/U: Referrals to gynecologist and oncologist, if necessary

POLYCYSTIC OVARY DISEASE
Signs and symptoms
- Amenorrhea
- Obesity
- Oligomenorrhea
- Infertility
- Acne

DX: Pelvic examination, labs (serum testosterone, androstenedione, DHEAS, FSH and LH levels, urine 17-ketosteroids)
TX: Medication (oral contraceptives, antineoplastic, ovulation stimulant), weight loss
F/U: Referral to gynecologist

Common signs and symptoms
- Increased hair growth on the face, abdomen, breasts, chest, or upper thighs
- Truncal obesity
- Buffalo hump, moonface
- Thin skin, purple striae
- Ecchymosis
- Petechiae
- Muscle wasting and weakness

ADRENOCORTICAL CARCINOMA
Additional signs and symptoms
- Oligomenorrhea
- Amenorrhea

CUSHING'S DISEASE

DX: Labs (dexamethasone suppression test, cortisol levels, urine creatinine, ACTH), imaging studies (CT scan, MRI)
TX: Treatment of underlying cause, surgery if indicated
F/U: As needed (dependent on underlying cause); reevaluation of cortisol levels, referral to endocrinologist

Additional differential diagnoses: hyperprolactemia ▪ idiopathic hirsutism

Other causes: drugs containing androgens or progestins ▪ aminoglutethimide ▪ glucocorticoids ▪ metoclopramide ▪ cyclosporine ▪ minoxidil

Hoarseness

Hoarseness — a rough or harsh sound to the voice — can result from infections or inflammatory lesions or exudates of the larynx, from laryngeal edema, and from compression or disruption of the vocal cords or recurrent laryngeal nerve. This common sign can also result from a thoracic aortic aneurysm, vocal cord paralysis, and systemic disorders, such as Sjögren's syndrome and rheumatoid arthritis. It's characteristically worsened by excessive alcohol intake, smoking, inhalation of noxious fumes, excessive talking, and shouting.

Hoarseness can be acute or chronic. For example, chronic hoarseness and laryngitis result when irritating polyps or nodules develop on the vocal cords. Gastroesophageal reflux into the larynx should also be considered as a possible cause of chronic hoarseness. Hoarseness may also result from progressive atrophy of the laryngeal muscles and mucosa due to aging, which leads to diminished control of the vocal cords.

History and physical examination

Obtain a patient history. First, consider his age and sex; laryngeal cancer is most common in men between the ages of 50 and 70. Be sure to ask about the onset of hoarseness. Has the patient been overusing his voice? Has he experienced shortness of breath, a sore throat, dry mouth, a cough, or difficulty swallowing dry food? In addition, ask if he has been in or near a fire within the past 48 hours. Be aware that inhalation injury can cause sudden airway obstruction.

Next, explore associated symptoms. Does the patient have a history of cancer, rheumatoid arthritis, or aortic aneurysm? Does he regularly drink alcohol or smoke?

Inspect the oral cavity and pharynx for redness or exudate, possibly indicating an upper respiratory infection. Palpate the neck for masses and the cervical lymph nodes and the thyroid for enlargement. Palpate the trachea — is it midline? Ask the patient to stick out his tongue; if he can't, he may have paralysis from cranial nerve involvement. Examine the eyes for corneal ulcers and enlarged lacrimal ducts (signs of Sjögren's syndrome). Dilated neck and chest veins may indicate compression by an aortic aneurysm.

Take the patient's vital signs, noting especially fever and bradycardia. Inspect for asymmetrical chest expansion or signs of respiratory distress — nasal flaring, stridor, and intercostal retractions. Then auscultate for crackles, rhonchi, wheezing, and tubular sounds, and percuss for dullness.

HPI

E: HEENT, abdomen, respiratory system

y

tion thera-

gologist

ACUTE LARYNGITIS
Signs and symptoms
- Sudden hoarseness or loss of voice
- Throat pain
- Dysphagia
- Odynophagia
- Cough
- Rhinorrhea
- Diaphoresis
- Fever

DX: Throat culture, laryngoscopy
TX: Rest, increased fluid intake, medication (analgesics; if bacterial, antibiotics)
F/U: Reevaluation 48 to 72 hours after treatment is initiated

THORACIC AORTIC ANEURYSM
Signs and symptoms
- Asymptomatic (possibly)
- Hoarseness
- Severe penetrating pain while supine
- Brassy cough
- Dyspnea
- Wheezing

DX: Radiologic studies (CT scan, MRI, angiography)
TX: Antihypertensives, surgery, aggressive fluid management
F/U: Referral to thoracic surgeon

Additional differential diagnoses: hypothyroidism ▪ laryngeal leukoplakia ▪ rheumatoid arthritis ▪ Sjögren's syndrome ▪ vocal cord polyps or nodules

Other causes: tracheal trauma ▪ vocal cord paralysis ▪ inhalation injury ▪ surgical trauma ▪ prolonged endotracheal intubation

Homans' sign

Homans' sign is positive when deep calf pain results from strong and abrupt dorsiflexion of the ankle. This pain results from venous thrombosis or inflammation of the calf muscles. However, because a positive Homans' sign appears in only 35% of patients with these conditions, it's an unreliable indicator. (See *Eliciting Homans' sign*.) Even when accurate, a positive Homans' sign doesn't indicate the extent of the venous disorder.

This elicited sign may be confused with continuous calf pain, which can result from strains, contusions, cellulitis, or arterial occlusion, or with pain in the posterior ankle or Achilles' tendon (for example, in a woman with Achilles' tendons shortened from wearing high heels).

History and physical examination

When you detect a positive Homans' sign, focus your patient history on signs and symptoms that can accompany deep vein thrombosis (DVT) or thrombophlebitis. These include throbbing, aching, heavy, or tight sensations in the calf and leg pain during or after exercise or routine activity. Also, ask about any shortness of breath or chest pain, which may indicate pulmonary embolism. Be sure to ask about predisposing events, such as leg injury, recent surgery, childbirth, use of contraceptive pills, associated diseases (cancer, nephrosis, hypercoagulable states), and prolonged inactivity.

Next, inspect and palpate the patient's calf for warmth, tenderness, redness, swelling, and the presence of a palpable vein. If you strongly suspect DVT, elicit Homans' sign very carefully to avoid detaching the clot, which could cause pulmonary embolism, a life-threatening condition.

In addition, measure the circumferences of both the patient's calves. The calf with the positive Homans' sign may be larger because of edema and swelling.

PEDIATRIC POINTER

Homans' sign is seldom assessed in children, who rarely have DVT or thrombophlebitis.

Eliciting Homans' sign

To elicit Homans' sign, first support the patient's thigh with one hand and his foot with the other. Bend his leg slightly at the knee; then firmly and abruptly dorsiflex the ankle. Resulting deep calf pain indicates a positive Homans' sign. (The patient may also resist ankle dorsiflexion or flex the knee involuntarily if Homans' sign is positive.)

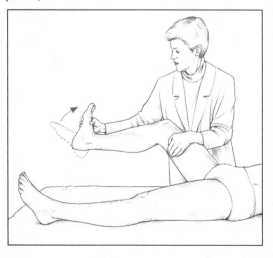

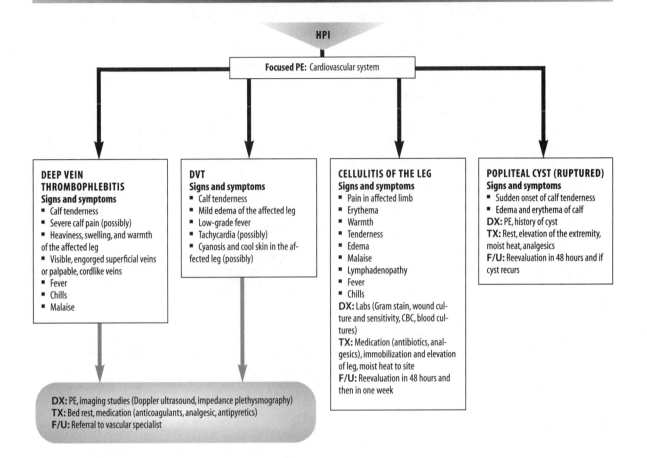

HPI

Focused PE: Cardiovascular system

DEEP VEIN THROMBOPHLEBITIS
Signs and symptoms
- Calf tenderness
- Severe calf pain (possibly)
- Heaviness, swelling, and warmth of the affected leg
- Visible, engorged superficial veins or palpable, cordlike veins
- Fever
- Chills
- Malaise

DVT
Signs and symptoms
- Calf tenderness
- Mild edema of the affected leg
- Low-grade fever
- Tachycardia (possibly)
- Cyanosis and cool skin in the affected leg (possibly)

CELLULITIS OF THE LEG
Signs and symptoms
- Pain in affected limb
- Erythema
- Warmth
- Tenderness
- Edema
- Malaise
- Lymphadenopathy
- Fever
- Chills

DX: Labs (Gram stain, wound culture and sensitivity, CBC, blood cultures)
TX: Medication (antibiotics, analgesics), immobilization and elevation of leg, moist heat to site
F/U: Reevaluation in 48 hours and then in one week

POPLITEAL CYST (RUPTURED)
Signs and symptoms
- Sudden onset of calf tenderness
- Edema and erythema of calf
DX: PE, history of cyst
TX: Rest, elevation of the extremity, moist heat, analgesics
F/U: Reevaluation in 48 hours and if cyst recurs

DX: PE, imaging studies (Doppler ultrasound, impedance plethysmography)
TX: Bed rest, medication (anticoagulants, analgesic, antipyretics)
F/U: Referral to vascular specialist

Hyperpigmentation

Hyperpigmentation, also known as hypermelanosis or excessive skin coloring, usually reflects overproduction, abnormal location, or maldistribution of melanin — the dominant brown or black pigment found in skin, hair, mucous membranes, nails, brain tissue, cardiac muscle, and parts of the eye. This sign can also reflect abnormalities of other skin pigments: carotenoids (yellow), oxyhemoglobin (red), and hemoglobin (blue).

Hyperpigmentation most commonly results from exposure to sunlight. However, it can also result from metabolic, endocrine, neoplastic, and inflammatory disorders; chemical poisoning; drugs; genetic defects; thermal burns; ionizing radiation; and localized activation by sunlight of certain photosensitizing chemicals on the skin.

Many types of benign hyperpigmented lesions occur normally. Some, such as acanthosis nigricans and carotenemia, may also accompany certain disorders, but their significance is unproven. Chronic nutritional insufficiency may lead to dyspigmentation — increased pigmentation in some areas and decreased pigmentation in others.

Typically asymptomatic and chronic, hyperpigmentation is a common problem that can have distressing psychological and social implications. It varies in location and intensity and may fade over time.

History and physical examination

Hyperpigmentation isn't an acute process, but an end result of another process, which should be the main target of your examination. Begin with a detailed patient history. Do any other family members have the same problem? Was the patient's hyperpigmentation present at birth? Did other signs or symptoms, such as a rash, accompany or precede it? Obtain a history of medical disorders (especially endocrine) as well as contact with or ingestion of chemicals, metals, plants, vegetables, citrus fruits, or perfumes. Is the hyperpigmentation related to exposure to sunlight or a change of season? Is the patient pregnant or taking prescription or over-the-counter drugs?

Explore other signs and symptoms too. Ask about fatigue, weakness, muscle aches, chills, irritability, fainting, and itching. Does the patient have any cardiopulmonary signs or symptoms, such as cough, shortness of breath, or swelling of the ankles, hands, or other areas? Any GI complaints, such as anorexia, nausea, vomiting, weight loss, abdominal pain, diarrhea, constipation, or epigastric fullness? Also, ask about genitourinary signs and symptoms, such as dark or pink urine, increased or decreased urination, menstrual irregularities, and loss of libido.

Next, examine the patient's skin. Note the color of hyperpigmented areas: Brown suggests excess melanin in the epidermis; slate gray or a bluish tone suggests excess pigment in the dermis. Inspect for other changes too — thickening and leatherlike texture as well as changes in hair distribution. Check the patient's skin and sclera for jaundice, and note any spider angiomas, palmar erythema, or purpura.

Take the patient's vital signs, noting fever, hypotension, or pulse irregularities. Evaluate his general appearance. Does he have exophthalmos or an enlarged jaw, an enlarged nose, or enlarged hands? Palpate for an enlarged thyroid, and auscultate for a bruit over the gland. Palpate muscles for atrophy and joints for swelling and tenderness. Assess the abdomen for ascites and edema, and palpate and percuss the liver and spleen to evaluate their size and position. Check the male patient for testicular atrophy and gynecomastia.

PEDIATRIC POINTERS

- *Most moles that are found in children are junctional nevi — flat, well demarcated, brown to black — that can appear anywhere on the skin. Although these lesions are considered benign, recent evidence suggests that some of them may become malignant later in life.*
- *Bizarre arrangements of linear or streaky hyperpigmented lesions on a child's sun-exposed lower legs suggest phytophotodermatitis.*
- *Congenital hyperpigmented lesions include mongolian spots (which are benign) and sharply defined or diffuse lesions occurring in such disorders as neurofibromatosis xeroderma pigmentosum; Gaucher's, Niemann-Pick, Wilson's diseases; Albright's, Fanconi's, Peutz-Jeghers syndromes; and phenylketonuria.*

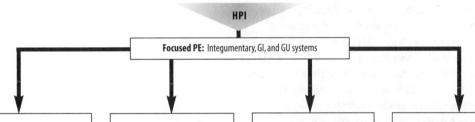

HPI

Focused PE: Integumentary, GI, and GU systems

ADRENOCORTICAL INSUFFICIENCY
Signs and symptoms
- Diffuse tan, brown, or bronze-to-black hyperpigmentation of the face, knees, knuckles, elbows, beltline, palmar creases, lips, gums, tongue, and buccal mucosa
- Hyperpigmentation of scars and moles
- Loss of axillary and pubic hair
- Possible vitiligo
- Slowly progressive fatigue
- Mental sluggishness
- Postural hypotension
- Weakness
- Anorexia
- Nausea and vomiting
- Weight loss
- Abdominal pain
- Orthostatic hypotension
- Irritability
- Diarrhea or constipation
- Decreased libido
- Amenorrhea
- Syncope
- Weak, irregular pulse
- Enhanced sense of taste, smell, and hearing (possibly)

DX: Labs (CBC, BUN, creatinine, electrolytes, cortisol levels, serum calcium, thyroid studies, ACTH stimulation test), imaging studies (CXR, CT scan), ECG
TX: Ventilatory and circulatory support, medication (glucocorticoid and mineral corticoid hormone replacement therapy), fluid and electrolyte replacement, treatment of underlying condition
F/U: Referral to endocrinologist

HEMOCHROMATOSIS, HEREDITARY
Signs and symptoms
- Early and progressive hyperpigmentation
- Generalized bronzing and metallic gray areas over sun-exposed areas, genitalia, and scars
- Weakness
- Lassitude
- Weight loss
- Abdominal pain
- Peripheral neuritis
- Arthritis
- Testicular atrophy
- Loss of libido
- Liver and cardiac involvement (late sign)

SIGNS OF DIABETES
- Polydipsia
- Polyuria

DX: Labs (iron level, ferritin level, CBC with differential), liver biopsy
TX: Weekly phlebotomy
F/U: Reevaluation every 3 months, referrals to hepatologist and hematologist

MALIGNANT MELANOMA
Signs and symptoms
- Hyperpigmented lesions of the skin (commonly moles) that are usually asymmetrical with border irregularity, color variation, and a diameter > 6 mm
- Inflamed, itchy, ulcerated, and bleeding lesions

DX: Skin examination, biopsy
TX: Surgery, sun exposure protection
F/U: Referrals to dermatologist and oncologist

CUSHING'S DISEASE
Signs and symptoms
- Increased hair growth on the face, abdomen, breasts, chest, or upper thighs
- Truncal obesity
- Buffalo hump
- Moonface
- Thin skin, purple striae
- Ecchymosis
- Petechiae
- Muscle wasting and weakness

DX: Labs (dexamethasone suppression test, cortisol levels, urine creatinine, ACTH), imaging studies (CT scan, MRI)
TX: Treatment of underlying cause, surgery if indicated
F/U: As needed (dependent on underlying cause), reevaluation of cortisol levels, referral to endocrinologist

---

Additional differential diagnoses: acromegaly ▪ biliary cirrhosis ▪ Laënnec's cirrhosis ▪ porphyria cutanea tarda ▪ scleroderma ▪ thyrotoxicosis ▪ tinea versicolor

---

Other causes: arsenic poisoning ▪ barbiturates ▪ phenolphthalein ▪ salicylates ▪ chemotherapeutic drugs, such as busulfan, cyclophosphamide, procarbazine, and nitrogen mustard ▪ chlorpromazine ▪ antimalarial drugs such as hydroxychloroquine ▪ hydantoin ▪ minocycline ▪ metals, such as silver and gold ▪ corticotropin ▪ phenothiazines

Hypopigmentation

Hypopigmentation (hypomelanosis) is a decrease in normal skin, hair, mucous membrane, or nail color resulting from deficiency, absence, or abnormal degradation of the pigment melanin. This sign may be congenital or acquired, asymptomatic or associated with other findings. Its causes include genetic disorders, nutritional deficiency, chemicals and drugs, inflammation, infection, and physical trauma. Typically chronic, hypopigmentation can be difficult to identify if the patient is light-skinned or has only slightly decreased coloring.

History and physical examination

Begin with a detailed patient history. Ask if any other family member has the same problem and if it was present from birth or developed after skin lesions or a rash. Were the lesions painful? Does the patient have any medical problems or a history of burns, physical injury, or physical contact with chemicals? Is he taking prescription or over-the-counter drugs? Find out if he has noticed other skin changes — such as erythema, scaling, ulceration, or hyperpigmentation — or if sun exposure causes unusually severe burning.

Next, examine the patient's skin, noting any erythema, scaling, ulceration, areas of hyperpigmentation, and other findings.

PEDIATRIC POINTERS

- In children, hypopigmentation results from genetic or acquired disorders, including albinism, phenylketonuria, and tuberous sclerosis.
- In neonates, hypopigmentation may indicate a metabolic or nervous system disorder.

ELDER CARE CUE

In elderly people, hypopigmentation is usually the result of cumulative exposure to ultraviolet light.

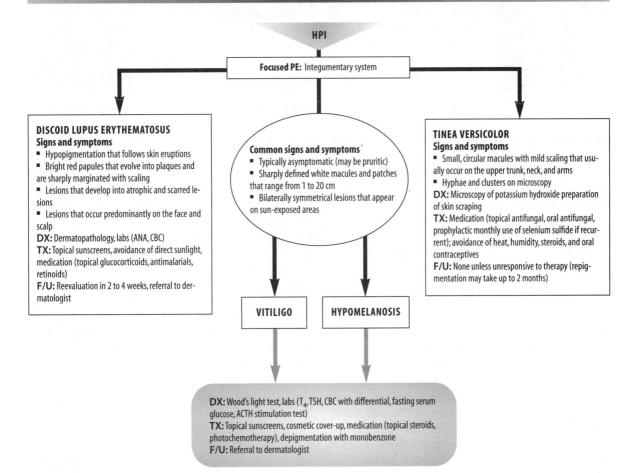

HPI

Focused PE: Integumentary system

DISCOID LUPUS ERYTHEMATOSUS
Signs and symptoms
- Hypopigmentation that follows skin eruptions
- Bright red papules that evolve into plaques and are sharply marginated with scaling
- Lesions that develop into atrophic and scarred lesions
- Lesions that occur predominantly on the face and scalp
DX: Dermatopathology, labs (ANA, CBC)
TX: Topical sunscreens, avoidance of direct sunlight, medication (topical glucocorticoids, antimalarials, retinoids)
F/U: Reevaluation in 2 to 4 weeks, referral to dermatologist

Common signs and symptoms
- Typically asymptomatic (may be pruritic)
- Sharply defined white macules and patches that range from 1 to 20 cm
- Bilaterally symmetrical lesions that appear on sun-exposed areas

TINEA VERSICOLOR
Signs and symptoms
- Small, circular macules with mild scaling that usually occur on the upper trunk, neck, and arms
- Hyphae and clusters on microscopy
DX: Microscopy of potassium hydroxide preparation of skin scraping
TX: Medication (topical antifungal, oral antifungal, prophylactic monthly use of selenium sulfide if recurrent); avoidance of heat, humidity, steroids, and oral contraceptives
F/U: None unless unresponsive to therapy (repigmentation may take up to 2 months)

VITILIGO

HYPOMELANOSIS

DX: Wood's light test, labs (T_4, TSH, CBC with differential, fasting serum glucose, ACTH stimulation test)
TX: Topical sunscreens, cosmetic cover-up, medication (topical steroids, photochemotherapy), depigmentation with monobenzone
F/U: Referral to dermatologist

Additional differential diagnoses: burns ▪ inflammatory and infectious disorders ▪ tuberculoid leprosy

Other causes: phenolic compounds (paratertiary butylphenol) ▪ germicides ▪ topical or intralesional administration of corticosteroids ▪ chloroquine

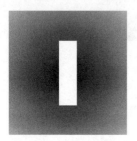

Impotence

Impotence is the inability to achieve and maintain penile erection sufficient to complete satisfactory intercourse; ejaculation may or may not be affected. Impotence varies from occasional and minimal to permanent and complete. Occasional impotence occurs in about one-half of adult men in the United States, whereas chronic impotence affects about 1 in 8 million men in the United States.

Impotence can be classified as primary or secondary. A man with *primary impotence* has never been potent with a partner but may achieve normal erections in other situations. This uncommon condition is difficult to treat. *Secondary impotence* carries a more favorable prognosis because, despite present erectile dysfunction, the patient has succeeded in completing intercourse in the past.

Penile erection involves increased arterial blood flow secondary to psychological, tactile, and other sensory stimulation. Trapping of blood within the penis produces increased length, circumference, and rigidity. Impotence results when any component of this process — psychological, vascular, neurologic, or hormonal — malfunctions.

Organic causes of impotence include vascular disease, diabetes mellitus, hypogonadism, a spinal cord lesion, alcohol and drug abuse, and surgical complications. (The incidence of organic impotence associated with other medical problems increases after age 50.) Psychogenic causes range from performance anxiety and marital discord to moral or religious conflicts.

History and physical examination

If the patient complains of impotence or of a condition that may be causing it, let him describe his problem without interruption. Then begin your examination in a systematic way, moving from less sensitive to more sensitive matters. Begin with a psychosocial history. Is the patient married, single, or widowed? How long has he been married or had a sexual relationship? What's the age and health status of his sexual partner? If you can do so discreetly, ask about sexual activity outside marriage or his primary sexual relationship. Also ask about his job history, his typical daily activities, and his living situation. How well does he get along with others in his household?

Focus your medical history on the causes of erectile dysfunction. Does the patient have type II diabetes mellitus, hypertension, or heart disease? If so, ask about its onset and treatment. Also ask about neurologic diseases such as multiple sclerosis. Obtain a surgical history, emphasizing neurologic, vascular, and urologic surgery. If trauma may be causing the patient's impotence, find out the date of the injury as well as its severity, associated effects, and treatment. Ask about intake of alcohol, drug use or abuse, smoking, diet, and exercise. Obtain a urologic history, including voiding problems and any past injury.

Next, ask the patient when his impotence began. How did it progress? What's its current status? Make your questions specific, but remember that many patients have difficulty discussing sexual problems, and many don't understand the physiology involved. The following sample questions may yield helpful data: When was the first time you remember not being able to initiate or maintain an erection? How often do you wake in the morning or at night with an erection? Do you have wet dreams? Has your sexual drive changed? How often do you try to have intercourse with your partner? How often would you *like* to? Can you ejaculate with or without an erection? Do you experience orgasm with ejaculation?

Ask the patient to rate the quality of a typical erection on a scale of 0 to 10, with 0 being completely flaccid and 10 being completely erect. Using the same scale, also ask him to rate his ability to ejaculate during sexual activity, with 0 being never and 10 being always.

Next, perform a brief physical examination. Inspect and palpate the genitalia and prostate for structural abnormalities. Assess the patient's sensory function, concentrating on the perineal area. Next, test motor strength and deep tendon reflexes in all extremities, and note other neurologic deficits. Take the patient's vital signs and palpate his pulses for quality. Note any signs of peripheral vascular disease, such as cyanosis and cool extremities. Auscultate for abdominal aortic, femoral, carotid, or iliac bruits, and palpate for thyroid gland enlargement.

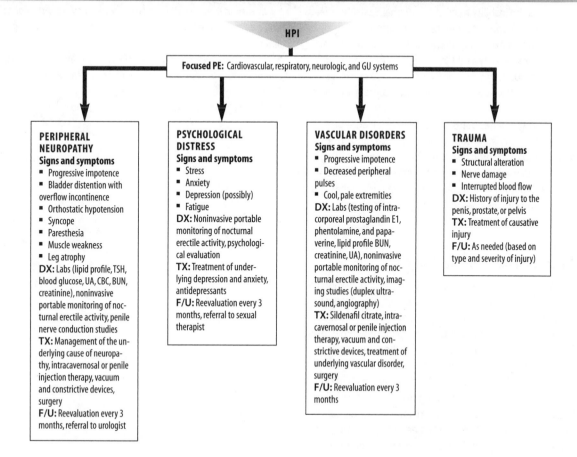

HPI

Focused PE: Cardiovascular, respiratory, neurologic, and GU systems

PERIPHERAL NEUROPATHY

Signs and symptoms
- Progressive impotence
- Bladder distention with overflow incontinence
- Orthostatic hypotension
- Syncope
- Paresthesia
- Muscle weakness
- Leg atrophy

DX: Labs (lipid profile, TSH, blood glucose, UA, CBC, BUN, creatinine), noninvasive portable monitoring of nocturnal erectile activity, penile nerve conduction studies

TX: Management of the underlying cause of neuropathy, intracavernosal or penile injection therapy, vacuum and constrictive devices, surgery

F/U: Reevaluation every 3 months, referral to urologist

PSYCHOLOGICAL DISTRESS

Signs and symptoms
- Stress
- Anxiety
- Depression (possibly)
- Fatigue

DX: Noninvasive portable monitoring of nocturnal erectile activity, psychological evaluation

TX: Treatment of underlying depression and anxiety, antidepressants

F/U: Reevaluation every 3 months, referral to sexual therapist

VASCULAR DISORDERS

Signs and symptoms
- Progressive impotence
- Decreased peripheral pulses
- Cool, pale extremities

DX: Labs (testing of intracorporeal prostaglandin E1, phentolamine, and papaverine, lipid profile BUN, creatinine, UA), noninvasive portable monitoring of nocturnal erectile activity, imaging studies (duplex ultrasound, angiography)

TX: Sildenafil citrate, intracavernosal or penile injection therapy, vacuum and constrictive devices, treatment of underlying vascular disorder, surgery

F/U: Reevaluation every 3 months

TRAUMA

Signs and symptoms
- Structural alteration
- Nerve damage
- Interrupted blood flow

DX: History of injury to the penis, prostate, or pelvis

TX: Treatment of causative injury

F/U: As needed (based on type and severity of injury)

Additional differential diagnoses: CNS disorders such as stroke ▪ endocrine disorders such as diabetes mellitus ▪ liver disease

Other causes: alcohol abuse ▪ antihypertensives ▪ drug abuse ▪ surgery ▪ urologic procedures such as prostatectomy ▪ radiation therapy ▪ various drugs

Insomnia

Insomnia is the inability to fall asleep, remain asleep, or feel refreshed by sleep. Acute and transient during periods of stress, insomnia may become chronic, causing constant fatigue, extreme anxiety as bedtime approaches, and even psychiatric disorders. This common complaint is experienced occasionally by about 25% of Americans, chronically by another 10%.

Physiologic causes of insomnia include jet lag, arguing, and lack of exercise. Pathophysiologic causes range from medical and psychiatric disorders to pain, drug adverse effects, and idiopathic factors. Complaints of insomnia are subjective and require close investigation; the patient may mistakenly attribute his insomnia to fatigue from an organic cause such as anemia.

History and physical examination

Take a thorough sleep and health history. Find out when the patient's insomnia began and the attending circumstances. Is the patient trying to stop using sedatives? Does he use central nervous system stimulants, such as amphetamines, pseudoephedrine, theophylline derivatives, phenylpropanolamine, cocaine, and caffeine-containing drugs and beverages?

Find out if the patient has a chronic or acute condition with effects that may be disturbing his sleep, particularly a cardiac or respiratory disease or a painful or pruritic condition. What about an endocrine or a neurologic disorder or a history of drug or alcohol abuse? Is he a frequent traveler who suffers from jet lag? Does he use his legs a lot during the day, then feel restless at night? Ask about daytime fatigue and regular exercise. Also ask if he experiences periods of gasping for air or apnea and frequent body repositioning. If possible, consult the patient's spouse or sleep partner because the patient may not be aware of his own behavior.

Assess the patient's emotional status, and try to estimate his level of self-esteem. Ask about personal and professional problems and psychological stress. Also ask if he has had hallucinations, and note behavior that may indicate alcohol withdrawal. After reviewing any complaints that suggest an undiagnosed disorder, perform a physical examination.

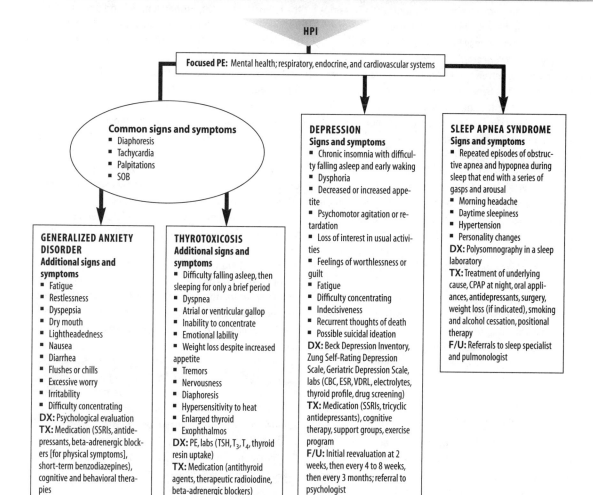

HPI

Focused PE: Mental health; respiratory, endocrine, and cardiovascular systems

Common signs and symptoms
- Diaphoresis
- Tachycardia
- Palpitations
- SOB

GENERALIZED ANXIETY DISORDER
Additional signs and symptoms
- Fatigue
- Restlessness
- Dyspepsia
- Dry mouth
- Lightheadedness
- Nausea
- Diarrhea
- Flushes or chills
- Excessive worry
- Irritability
- Difficulty concentrating

DX: Psychological evaluation
TX: Medication (SSRIs, antidepressants, beta-adrenergic blockers [for physical symptoms], short-term benzodiazepines), cognitive and behavioral therapies
F/U: Reevaluation every 2 to 3 weeks until stabilized on medication

THYROTOXICOSIS
Additional signs and symptoms
- Difficulty falling asleep, then sleeping for only a brief period
- Dyspnea
- Atrial or ventricular gallop
- Inability to concentrate
- Emotional lability
- Weight loss despite increased appetite
- Tremors
- Nervousness
- Diaphoresis
- Hypersensitivity to heat
- Enlarged thyroid
- Exophthalmos

DX: PE, labs (TSH, T_3, T_4, thyroid resin uptake)
TX: Medication (antithyroid agents, therapeutic radioiodine, beta-adrenergic blockers)
F/U: Reevaluation of thyroid function every 6 months; reevaluation at 6 weeks and 12 weeks, and then every 6 months, if undergoing radionuclide therapy

DEPRESSION
Signs and symptoms
- Chronic insomnia with difficulty falling asleep and early waking
- Dysphoria
- Decreased or increased appetite
- Psychomotor agitation or retardation
- Loss of interest in usual activities
- Feelings of worthlessness or guilt
- Fatigue
- Difficulty concentrating
- Indecisiveness
- Recurrent thoughts of death
- Possible suicidal ideation

DX: Beck Depression Inventory, Zung Self-Rating Depression Scale, Geriatric Depression Scale, labs (CBC, ESR, VDRL, electrolytes, thyroid profile, drug screening)
TX: Medication (SSRIs, tricyclic antidepressants), cognitive therapy, support groups, exercise program
F/U: Initial reevaluation at 2 weeks, then every 4 to 8 weeks, then every 3 months; referral to psychologist

SLEEP APNEA SYNDROME
Signs and symptoms
- Repeated episodes of obstructive apnea and hypopnea during sleep that end with a series of gasps and arousal
- Morning headache
- Daytime sleepiness
- Hypertension
- Personality changes

DX: Polysomnography in a sleep laboratory
TX: Treatment of underlying cause, CPAP at night, oral appliances, antidepressants, surgery, weight loss (if indicated), smoking and alcohol cessation, positional therapy
F/U: Referrals to sleep specialist and pulmonologist

Additional differential diagnoses: alcohol withdrawal syndrome ▪ mood (affective) disorders ▪ nocturnal myoclonus ▪ pain ▪ pheochromocytoma ▪ pruritus

---

Other causes: amphetamines ▪ caffeine-containing beverages ▪ cocaine ▪ ginseng ▪ green tea ▪ phenylpropanolamine ▪ pseudoephedrine ▪ theophylline derivatives ▪ withdrawal from sedatives or hypnotics

Intermittent claudication

Most common in the legs, intermittent claudication is cramping limb pain brought on by exercise and relieved by 1 or 2 minutes of rest. This pain may be acute or chronic; when acute, it may signal acute arterial occlusion. Intermittent claudication occurs most often in men ages 50 to 60 with a history of diabetes mellitus, hyperlipidemia, hypertension, or tobacco use. Without treatment, it may progress to pain at rest. In chronic arterial occlusion, limb loss is uncommon because collateral circulation usually develops.

In occlusive artery disease, intermittent claudication results from an inadequate blood supply. Pain in the calf (the most common area) or foot indicates disease of the femoral or popliteal arteries; pain in the buttocks and upper thigh, disease of the aortoiliac arteries. During exercise, the pain typically results from the release of lactic acid due to anaerobic metabolism in the ischemic segment, secondary to obstruction. When exercise stops, the lactic acid clears and the pain subsides.

Intermittent claudication may also have a neurologic cause: narrowing of the vertebral column at the level of the cauda equina. This condition creates pressure on the nerve roots to the lower extremities. Walking stimulates circulation to the cauda equina, causing increased pressure on those nerves and resultant pain.

History and physical examination

If the patient has sudden intermittent claudication with severe or aching leg pain at rest, check the leg's temperature and color and palpate pulses. Ask about numbness and tingling. Don't elevate the leg. Protect it and let nothing press on it. Arrange for an immediate surgical consult.

If the patient has chronic intermittent claudication, gather history data first. Ask how far he can walk before pain occurs and how long he must rest before it subsides. Can he walk less far now than before, or does he need to rest longer? Does the pain-rest pattern vary? Has this symptom affected his lifestyle?

Get a history of risk factors for atherosclerosis, such as smoking, diabetes, hypertension, and hyperlipidemia. Next, ask about associated signs and symptoms, such as paresthesia in the affected limb and visible changes in the color of the fingers (white to blue to pink) when he's smoking, exposed to cold, or under stress. If the patient is male, does he experience impotence?

Focus the physical examination on the cardiovascular system. Palpate for femoral, popliteal, dorsalis pedis, and posterior tibial pulses. Note character, amplitude, and bilateral equality. Diminished or absent popliteal and pedal pulses with the femoral pulse present may indicate atherosclerotic disease of the femoral artery. Diminished femoral and distal pulses may indicate disease of the terminal aorta or iliac branches. Absent pedal pulses with normal femoral and popliteal pulses may indicate Buerger's disease.

Listen for bruits over the major arteries. Note color and temperature differences between the legs or compared with the arms; also note the leg level where changes in temperature and color occur. Elevate the affected leg for 2 minutes; if it becomes pale or white, blood flow is severely decreased. When the leg hangs down, how long does it take for color to return? (Thirty seconds or longer indicates severe disease.) Check the patient's deep tendon reflexes after exercise; note if they're diminished in his lower extremities.

Examine the feet, toes, and fingers for ulceration, and inspect the hands and lower legs for small, tender nodules and erythema along blood vessels.

In the patient with arm pain, inspect the arms for a change in color (to white) on elevation. Next, palpate for changes in temperature, for muscle wasting, and for a pulsating mass in the subclavian area. Palpate and compare the radial, ulnar, brachial, axillary, and subclavian pulses to identify obstructed areas.

PEDIATRIC POINTERS

- *Intermittent claudication rarely occurs in children. Although it sometimes develops in coarctation of the aorta, extensive compensatory collateral circulation typically prevents manifestation of this sign.*
- *Muscle cramps from exercise and growing pains may be mistaken for intermittent claudication in children.*

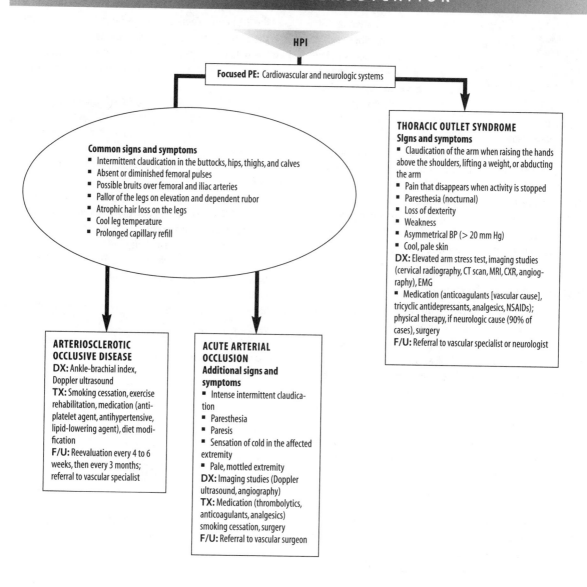

HPI

Focused PE: Cardiovascular and neurologic systems

Common signs and symptoms
- Intermittent claudication in the buttocks, hips, thighs, and calves
- Absent or diminished femoral pulses
- Possible bruits over femoral and iliac arteries
- Pallor of the legs on elevation and dependent rubor
- Atrophic hair loss on the legs
- Cool leg temperature
- Prolonged capillary refill

THORACIC OUTLET SYNDROME
Signs and symptoms
- Claudication of the arm when raising the hands above the shoulders, lifting a weight, or abducting the arm
- Pain that disappears when activity is stopped
- Paresthesia (nocturnal)
- Loss of dexterity
- Weakness
- Asymmetrical BP (> 20 mm Hg)
- Cool, pale skin

DX: Elevated arm stress test, imaging studies (cervical radiography, CT scan, MRI, CXR, angiography), EMG
- Medication (anticoagulants [vascular cause], tricyclic antidepressants, analgesics, NSAIDs); physical therapy, if neurologic cause (90% of cases), surgery

F/U: Referral to vascular specialist or neurologist

ARTERIOSCLEROTIC OCCLUSIVE DISEASE
DX: Ankle-brachial index, Doppler ultrasound
TX: Smoking cessation, exercise rehabilitation, medication (antiplatelet agent, antihypertensive, lipid-lowering agent), diet modification
F/U: Reevaluation every 4 to 6 weeks, then every 3 months; referral to vascular specialist

ACUTE ARTERIAL OCCLUSION
Additional signs and symptoms
- Intense intermittent claudication
- Paresthesia
- Paresis
- Sensation of cold in the affected extremity
- Pale, mottled extremity
DX: Imaging studies (Doppler ultrasound, angiography)
TX: Medication (thrombolytics, anticoagulants, analgesics) smoking cessation, surgery
F/U: Referral to vascular surgeon

Additional differential diagnoses: arteriosclerosis obliterans ▪ Buerger's disease ▪ Leriche's syndrome ▪ neurogenic claudication

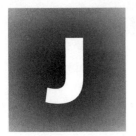

Jaundice

The yellow discoloration of the skin or mucous membranes, jaundice indicates excessive levels of conjugated or unconjugated bilirubin in the blood. In fair-skinned patients, it's most noticeable on the face, trunk, and sclerae; in dark-skinned patients, on the hard palate, sclerae, and conjunctivae.

Jaundice is most apparent in natural sunlight. In fact, it may be undetectable in artificial or poor light. It's commonly accompanied by pruritus (because bile pigment damages sensory nerves), dark urine, and clay-colored stools.

Jaundice may result from any of three pathophysiologic processes. It may be the only warning sign of certain disorders such as pancreatic cancer. (See *Classifying jaundice*.)

History and physical examination

Documenting a history of the patient's jaundice is critical in determining its cause. Begin by asking the patient when he first noted the jaundice. Does he also have pruritus, clay-colored stools, or dark urine? Ask about past episodes or a family history of jaundice. Does he have nonspecific signs or symptoms, such as fatigue, fever, or chills; GI signs or symptoms, such as anorexia, abdominal pain, nausea, or vomiting; or cardiopulmonary symptoms, such as shortness of breath or palpitations? Ask about alcohol use and a history of cancer or liver or gallbladder disease. Has the patient lost weight recently? Also, obtain a drug history.

Perform the physical examination in a room with natural light. Inspect the skin for texture and dryness and for hyperpigmentation and xanthomas. Look for spider angiomas or petechiae, clubbed fingers, and gynecomastia. If the patient has heart failure, auscultate for arrhythmias, murmurs, and gallops. For all patients, auscultate for crackles and abnormal bowel sounds. Palpate the lymph nodes for swelling and the abdomen for tenderness, pain, and swelling. Palpate and percuss the liver and spleen for enlargement, and test for ascites with the shifting dullness and fluid wave techniques. Obtain baseline data on the patient's mental status: Slight changes in sensorium may be an early sign of deteriorating hepatic function.

Classifying jaundice

Jaundice occurs in three forms: prehepatic, hepatic, and posthepatic. In all three, bilirubin levels in the blood increase due to impaired metabolism.

In *prehepatic jaundice,* certain conditions and disorders, such as transfusion reactions and sickle cell anemia, cause massive hemolysis. Red blood cells rupture faster than the liver can conjugate bilirubin, so large amounts of unconjugated bilirubin pass into the blood, causing increased intestinal conversion of this bilirubin to water-soluble urobilinogen for excretion in urine and stools. (Unconjugated bilirubin is insoluble in water, so it can't be directly excreted in urine.)

Hepatic jaundice results from the liver's inability to conjugate or excrete bilirubin, leading to increased blood levels of conjugated and unconjugated bilirubin. This occurs in such disorders as hepatitis, cirrhosis, and metastatic cancer and during prolonged use of drugs metabolized by the liver.

In *posthepatic jaundice,* which occurs in biliary and pancreatic disorders, bilirubin forms at its normal rate, but inflammation, scar tissue, a tumor, or gallstones block the flow of bile into the intestine. This causes an accumulation of conjugated bilirubin in the blood. Water-soluble, conjugated bilirubin is excreted in the urine.

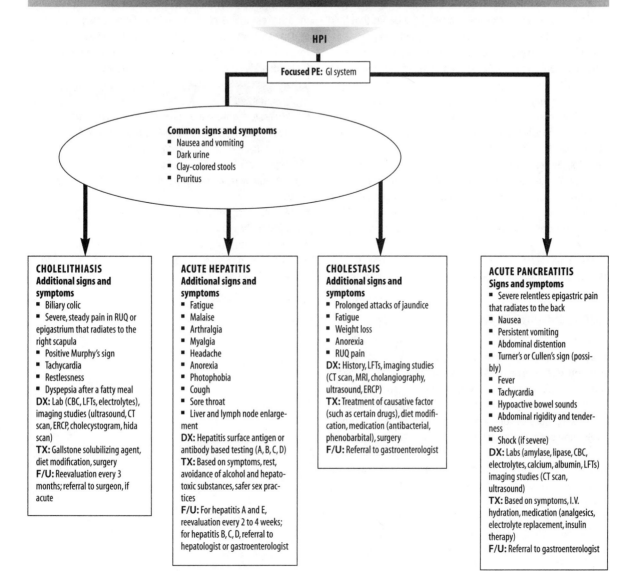

HPI

Focused PE: GI system

Common signs and symptoms
- Nausea and vomiting
- Dark urine
- Clay-colored stools
- Pruritus

CHOLELITHIASIS
Additional signs and symptoms
- Biliary colic
- Severe, steady pain in RUQ or epigastrium that radiates to the right scapula
- Positive Murphy's sign
- Tachycardia
- Restlessness
- Dyspepsia after a fatty meal

DX: Lab (CBC, LFTs, electrolytes), imaging studies (ultrasound, CT scan, ERCP, cholecystogram, hida scan)
TX: Gallstone solubilizing agent, diet modification, surgery
F/U: Reevaluation every 3 months; referral to surgeon, if acute

ACUTE HEPATITIS
Additional signs and symptoms
- Fatigue
- Malaise
- Arthralgia
- Myalgia
- Headache
- Anorexia
- Photophobia
- Cough
- Sore throat
- Liver and lymph node enlargement

DX: Hepatitis surface antigen or antibody based testing (A, B, C, D)
TX: Based on symptoms, rest, avoidance of alcohol and hepatotoxic substances, safer sex practices
F/U: For hepatitis A and E, reevaluation every 2 to 4 weeks; for hepatitis B, C, D, referral to hepatologist or gastroenterologist

CHOLESTASIS
Additional signs and symptoms
- Prolonged attacks of jaundice
- Fatigue
- Weight loss
- Anorexia
- RUQ pain

DX: History, LFTs, imaging studies (CT scan, MRI, cholangiography, ultrasound, ERCP)
TX: Treatment of causative factor (such as certain drugs), diet modification, medication (antibacterial, phenobarbital), surgery
F/U: Referral to gastroenterologist

ACUTE PANCREATITIS
Signs and symptoms
- Severe relentless epigastric pain that radiates to the back
- Nausea
- Persistent vomiting
- Abdominal distention
- Turner's or Cullen's sign (possibly)
- Fever
- Tachycardia
- Hypoactive bowel sounds
- Abdominal rigidity and tenderness
- Shock (if severe)

DX: Labs (amylase, lipase, CBC, electrolytes, calcium, albumin, LFTs) imaging studies (CT scan, ultrasound)
TX: Based on symptoms, I.V. hydration, medication (analgesics, electrolyte replacement, insulin therapy)
F/U: Referral to gastroenterologist

Additional differential diagnoses: agnogenic ▪ cholangitis ▪ cholecystitis ▪ cirrhosis ▪ Dubin-Johnson syndrome ▪ glucose-6-phosphate dehydrogenase deficiency ▪ hemolytic anemia (acquired) ▪ hepatic abscess ▪ hepatic cancer ▪ leptospirosis ▪ myeloid metaplasia ▪ pancreatic cancer ▪ sickle cell anemia ▪ Zieve syndrome

Other causes: androgenic steroids ▪ erythromycin estolate ▪ HMG-CoA reductase inhibitors ▪ I.V. tetracycline ▪ isoniazid ▪ mercaptopurine ▪ niacin ▪ oral contraceptives ▪ phenothiazines ▪ phenylbutazone ▪ portocaval shunt ▪ sulfonamides ▪ troleandomycin ▪ upper abdominal surgery

Jaw pain

Jaw pain may arise from either or both of the bones that hold the teeth in the jaw — the maxilla (upper jaw) and the mandible (lower jaw). Jaw pain also includes pain in the temporomandibular joint (TMJ), where the mandible meets the temporal bone.

Jaw pain may develop gradually or abruptly and may range from barely noticeable to excruciating, depending on its cause. It usually results from disorders of the teeth, soft tissue, or glands of the mouth or throat, or from local trauma or infection. Systemic causes include musculoskeletal, neurologic, cardiovascular, endocrine, immunologic, metabolic, or infectious disorders. Life-threatening disorders, such as myocardial infarction (MI) and tetany, also produce jaw pain, as do drugs (especially phenothiazines) and dental or surgical procedures.

Jaw pain is seldom a primary indicator of any one disorder; however, some of its causes are medical emergencies.

History and physical examination

Begin the patient history by asking the patient to describe the pain's character, intensity, and frequency. When did he first notice the jaw pain? Did it arise suddenly or gradually? Is it more severe or frequent now than when it first occurred? Sudden severe jaw pain, especially when associated with chest pain, shortness of breath, or arm pain, requires prompt evaluation because it may herald a life-threatening disorder. Where on the jaw does he feel pain? Does the pain radiate to other areas? Sharp or burning pain arises from the skin or subcutaneous tissues. Causalgia, an intense burning sensation, usually results from damage to the fifth cranial or trigeminal nerve. This type of superficial pain is easily localized, unlike dull, aching, boring, or throbbing pain, which originates in muscle, bone, or joints. Also, ask about aggravating or alleviating factors.

Ask about associated signs and symptoms, such as joint or chest pain, fatigue, headache, malaise, anorexia, weight loss, intermittent claudication, diplopia, and hearing loss. (Keep in mind that jaw pain may accompany more characteristic signs and symptoms of life-threatening disorders, such as chest pain in MI.)

Focus your physical examination on the jaw. Inspect the painful area for redness, and palpate for edema or warmth. Facing the patient directly, look for facial asymmetry indicating swelling. Check the TMJs by placing your fingertips just anterior to the external auditory meatus and asking the patient to open and close and to thrust out and retract his jaw. Note the presence of crepitus, an abnormal scraping or grinding sensation in the joint. (Clicks heard when the jaw is widely spread apart are normal.) How wide can the patient open his mouth? Less than 3 cm or more than 6 cm between upper and lower teeth is abnormal. Next, palpate the parotid area for pain and swelling, and inspect and palpate the oral cavity for lesions, elevation of the tongue, or masses.

JAW PAIN

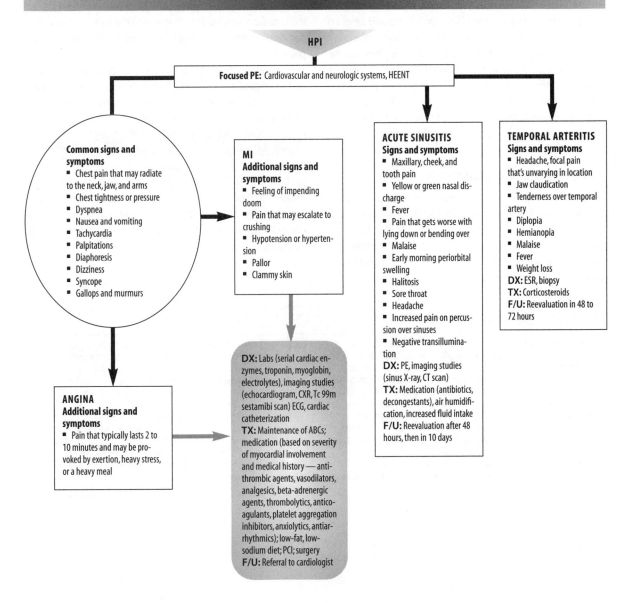

HPI

Focused PE: Cardiovascular and neurologic systems, HEENT

Common signs and symptoms
- Chest pain that may radiate to the neck, jaw, and arms
- Chest tightness or pressure
- Dyspnea
- Nausea and vomiting
- Tachycardia
- Palpitations
- Diaphoresis
- Dizziness
- Syncope
- Gallops and murmurs

MI
Additional signs and symptoms
- Feeling of impending doom
- Pain that may escalate to crushing
- Hypotension or hypertension
- Pallor
- Clammy skin

ACUTE SINUSITIS
Signs and symptoms
- Maxillary, cheek, and tooth pain
- Yellow or green nasal discharge
- Fever
- Pain that gets worse with lying down or bending over
- Malaise
- Early morning periorbital swelling
- Halitosis
- Sore throat
- Headache
- Increased pain on percussion over sinuses
- Negative transillumination
DX: PE, imaging studies (sinus X-ray, CT scan)
TX: Medication (antibiotics, decongestants), air humidification, increased fluid intake
F/U: Reevaluation after 48 hours, then in 10 days

TEMPORAL ARTERITIS
Signs and symptoms
- Headache, focal pain that's unvarying in location
- Jaw claudication
- Tenderness over temporal artery
- Diplopia
- Hemianopia
- Malaise
- Fever
- Weight loss
DX: ESR, biopsy
TX: Corticosteroids
F/U: Reevaluation in 48 to 72 hours

ANGINA
Additional signs and symptoms
- Pain that typically lasts 2 to 10 minutes and may be provoked by exertion, heavy stress, or a heavy meal

DX: Labs (serial cardiac enzymes, troponin, myoglobin, electrolytes), imaging studies (echocardiogram, CXR, Tc 99m sestamibi scan) ECG, cardiac catheterization
TX: Maintenance of ABCs; medication (based on severity of myocardial involvement and medical history — antithrombic agents, vasodilators, analgesics, beta-adrenergic agents, thrombolytics, anticoagulants, platelet aggregation inhibitors, anxiolytics, antiarrhythmics); low-fat, low-sodium diet; PCI; surgery
F/U: Referral to cardiologist

Additional differential diagnoses: arthritis ▪ head and neck cancer ▪ hypocalcemic tetany ▪ Ludwig's angina ▪ osteomyelitis ▪ sialolithiasis ▪ suppurative parotitis ▪ tetanus ▪ TMJ syndrome ▪ trauma ▪ trigeminal neuralgia

---

Other causes: phenothiazines ▪ drugs that reduce calcium

Jugular vein distention

Jugular vein distention is the abnormal fullness and height of the pulse waves in the internal or external jugular veins. When a supine patient's head is elevated 45 degrees, a pulse wave height greater than 4 cm above the angle of Louis indicates distention. Engorged, distended veins reflect increased venous pressure in the right side of the heart. This common sign characteristically occurs in heart failure and other cardiovascular disorders. (See *Evaluating jugular vein distention*.)

History and physical examination

If the patient isn't in severe distress, obtain a personal history. Has he gained weight recently? Does he have difficulty putting on shoes? Are his ankles swollen? Ask about chest pain, shortness of breath, paroxysmal nocturnal dyspnea, anorexia, nausea or vomiting, and a history of cancer or heart, pulmonary, or renal disease.

Next, perform a physical examination, beginning with vital signs. Tachycardia, tachypnea, and increased blood pressure indicate fluid overload that's stressing the heart. Inspect and palpate the extremities and face for edema. Then weigh the patient.

Auscultate the lungs for crackles and the heart for gallops and a pericardial friction rub. Inspect the abdomen for distention, and palpate and percuss for an enlarged liver. Finally, ask about any decrease in urine output.

PEDIATRIC POINTER

Jugular vein distention is difficult (sometimes impossible) to evaluate in most infants and toddlers because of their short, thick necks. Even in school-age children, measurement of jugular vein distention can be unreliable because the sternal angle may not be the same distance (5 to 7 cm) above the right atrium as it is in adults.

Evaluating jugular vein distention

To evaluate jugular vein distention, first place the patient in the supine position so that you can visualize pulsations reflected from the right atrium. Then elevate the head of the bed 45 to 90 degrees. (Normally, veins distend only when a patient lies flat.) Next, locate the angle of Louis (sternal notch) — the reference point for measuring venous pressure. To do so, palpate the clavicles where they join the sternum (the suprasternal notch). Place your first two fingers on the suprasternal notch. Then, without lifting them from the skin, slide them down the sternum until you feel a bony protuberance — this is the angle of Louis.

Find the internal jugular vein (which indicates venous pressure more reliably than the external jugular vein). Shine a flashlight across the patient's neck to create shadows that highlight his venous pulse. Be sure to distinguish jugular venous pulsations from carotid arterial pulsations. One way to do this is to palpate the vessel: Arterial pulsations continue, whereas venous pulsations disappear with light finger pressure. Also, venous pulsations increase or decrease with changes in body position, but arterial pulsations remain constant.

Next, locate the highest point along the vein where you can see pulsations. Using a centimeter ruler, measure the distance between that high point and the sternal notch. Record this finding as well as the angle at which the patient was lying. A finding greater than 4 cm above the sternal notch, with the head of the bed at a 45-degree angle, indicates jugular vein distention.

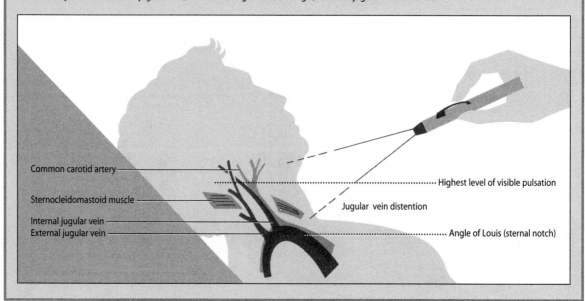

Common carotid artery

Sternocleidomastoid muscle

Internal jugular vein
External jugular vein

Highest level of visible pulsation

Jugular vein distention

Angle of Louis (sternal notch)

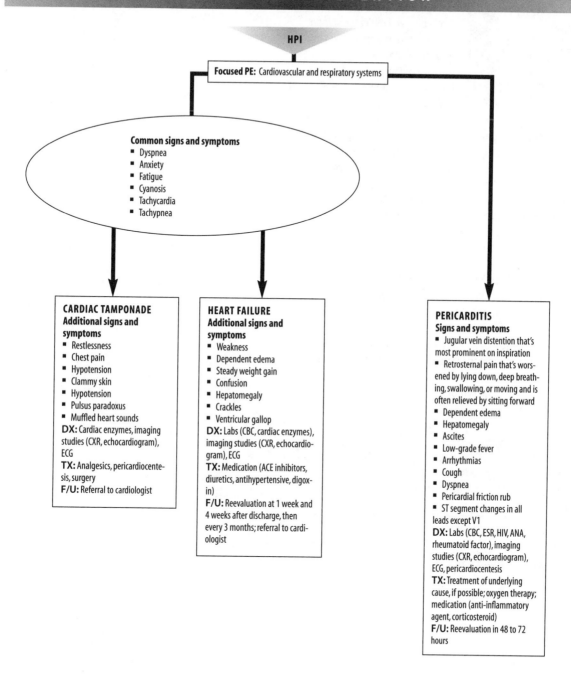

HPI

Focused PE: Cardiovascular and respiratory systems

Common signs and symptoms
- Dyspnea
- Anxiety
- Fatigue
- Cyanosis
- Tachycardia
- Tachypnea

CARDIAC TAMPONADE
Additional signs and symptoms
- Restlessness
- Chest pain
- Hypotension
- Clammy skin
- Hypotension
- Pulsus paradoxus
- Muffled heart sounds

DX: Cardiac enzymes, imaging studies (CXR, echocardiogram), ECG
TX: Analgesics, pericardiocentesis, surgery
F/U: Referral to cardiologist

HEART FAILURE
Additional signs and symptoms
- Weakness
- Dependent edema
- Steady weight gain
- Confusion
- Hepatomegaly
- Crackles
- Ventricular gallop

DX: Labs (CBC, cardiac enzymes), imaging studies (CXR, echocardiogram), ECG
TX: Medication (ACE inhibitors, diuretics, antihypertensive, digoxin)
F/U: Reevaluation at 1 week and 4 weeks after discharge, then every 3 months; referral to cardiologist

PERICARDITIS
Signs and symptoms
- Jugular vein distention that's most prominent on inspiration
- Retrosternal pain that's worsened by lying down, deep breathing, swallowing, or moving and is often relieved by sitting forward
- Dependent edema
- Hepatomegaly
- Ascites
- Low-grade fever
- Arrhythmias
- Cough
- Dyspnea
- Pericardial friction rub
- ST segment changes in all leads except V1

DX: Labs (CBC, ESR, HIV, ANA, rheumatoid factor), imaging studies (CXR, echocardiogram), ECG, pericardiocentesis
TX: Treatment of underlying cause, if possible; oxygen therapy; medication (anti-inflammatory agent, corticosteroid)
F/U: Reevaluation in 48 to 72 hours

Additional differential diagnoses: hypervolemia ▪ leiomyosarcoma ▪ superior vena cava obstruction

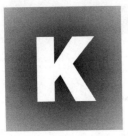

Kernig's sign

A reliable early indicator of meningeal irritation, Kernig's sign elicits both resistance and hamstring muscle pain when the examiner attempts to extend the knee while the hip and knee are both flexed 90 degrees. (See *Eliciting Kernig's sign.*) This sign is usually elicited in meningitis or subarachnoid hemorrhage. In these potentially life-threatening disorders, hamstring muscle resistance results from stretching the blood- or exudate-irritated meninges surrounding spinal nerve roots.

Kernig's sign can also indicate herniated disk and spinal tumor. In these disorders, sciatic pain results from disk or tumor pressure on spinal nerve roots.

History and physical examination

If you elicit a positive Kernig's sign and suspect life-threatening meningitis or subarachnoid hemorrhage, immediately prepare for emergency intervention.

If you don't suspect meningeal irritation, ask the patient if he feels any back pain that radiates down one or both legs. Does he also feel leg numbness, tingling, or weakness? Ask about other signs and symptoms, and find out if he has a history of cancer or back injury. Then perform a physical examination, concentrating on motor and sensory function.

> ### PEDIATRIC POINTER
>
> *Kernig's sign is considered ominous in children because of their greater potential for rapid deterioration.*

Eliciting Kernig's sign

To elicit Kernig's sign, place the patient in a supine position. Flex her leg at the hip and knee, as shown here. Then try to extend the leg while you keep the hip flexed. If the patient experiences pain and possibly spasm in the hamstring muscle and resists further extension, you can assume that meningeal irritation has occurred.

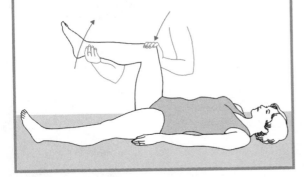

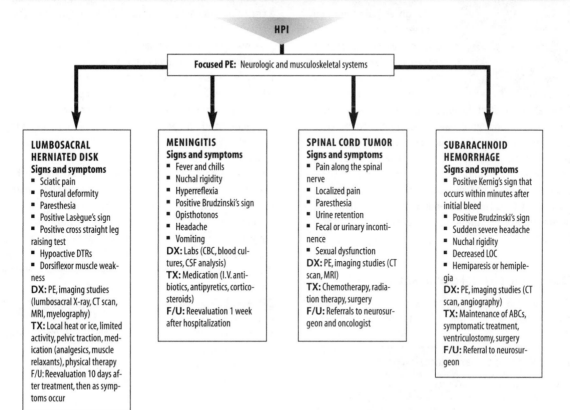

HPI

Focused PE: Neurologic and musculoskeletal systems

LUMBOSACRAL HERNIATED DISK
Signs and symptoms
- Sciatic pain
- Postural deformity
- Paresthesia
- Positive Lasègue's sign
- Positive cross straight leg raising test
- Hypoactive DTRs
- Dorsiflexor muscle weakness

DX: PE, imaging studies (lumbosacral X-ray, CT scan, MRI, myelography)
TX: Local heat or ice, limited activity, pelvic traction, medication (analgesics, muscle relaxants), physical therapy
F/U: Reevaluation 10 days after treatment, then as symptoms occur

MENINGITIS
Signs and symptoms
- Fever and chills
- Nuchal rigidity
- Hyperreflexia
- Positive Brudzinski's sign
- Opisthotonos
- Headache
- Vomiting

DX: Labs (CBC, blood cultures, CSF analysis)
TX: Medication (I.V. antibiotics, antipyretics, corticosteroids)
F/U: Reevaluation 1 week after hospitalization

SPINAL CORD TUMOR
Signs and symptoms
- Pain along the spinal nerve
- Localized pain
- Paresthesia
- Urine retention
- Fecal or urinary incontinence
- Sexual dysfunction

DX: PE, imaging studies (CT scan, MRI)
TX: Chemotherapy, radiation therapy, surgery
F/U: Referrals to neurosurgeon and oncologist

SUBARACHNOID HEMORRHAGE
Signs and symptoms
- Positive Kernig's sign that occurs within minutes after initial bleed
- Positive Brudzinski's sign
- Sudden severe headache
- Nuchal rigidity
- Decreased LOC
- Hemiparesis or hemiplegia

DX: PE, imaging studies (CT scan, angiography)
TX: Maintenance of ABCs, symptomatic treatment, ventriculostomy, surgery
F/U: Referral to neurosurgeon

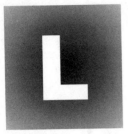

Leg pain

Although leg pain commonly signifies a musculoskeletal disorder, it can also result from more serious vascular or neurologic disorders. The pain may arise suddenly or gradually and may be localized or affect the entire leg. Constant or intermittent, it may feel dull, burning, sharp, shooting, or tingling. Leg pain often affects locomotion, limiting weight bearing. Severe leg pain that follows cast application for a fracture may signal limb-threatening compartment syndrome. Sudden onset of severe leg pain in a patient with underlying vascular insufficiency may signal acute deterioration, possibly requiring an arterial graft or amputation. (See *Highlighting causes of local leg pain*.)

History and physical examination

If the patient's condition permits, ask him when the pain began and have him describe its intensity, character, and pattern. Is the pain worse in the morning, at night, or with movement? If it doesn't prevent him from walking, must he rely on a crutch or other assistive device? Also, ask him about the presence of other signs and symptoms.

Find out if the patient has a history of leg injury or surgery, and if he or a family member has a history of joint, vascular, or back problems. Also, ask what medications he's taking and whether they've helped to relieve his leg pain.

Begin the physical examination by watching the patient walk, if his condition permits. Observe how he holds his leg while standing and sitting. Palpate the legs, buttocks, and lower back to determine the extent of pain and tenderness. If fracture has been ruled out, test range of motion in the hip and knee. Also, check reflexes with the patient's leg straightened and raised, noting any action that causes pain. Then compare both legs for symmetry, movement, and active range of motion. Also, assess pulses, color, sensation and strength. If the patient wears a leg cast, splint, or restrictive dressing, carefully check distal circulation, sensation, and mobility, and stretch his toes to elicit any associated pain.

PEDIATRIC POINTERS

- *Common pediatric causes of leg pain include fracture, osteomyelitis, and bone cancer.*
- *If parents fail to give an adequate explanation for a leg fracture, consider the possibility of child abuse.*

Highlighting causes of local leg pain

Various disorders cause ankle, foot, hip, or knee pain, which may radiate to surrounding tissues and be reported as leg pain. Local pain is commonly accompanied by tenderness, swelling, and deformity in the affected area.

ANKLE PAIN
Achilles tendon contracture
Arthritis
Dislocation
Fracture
Sprain
Tenosynovitis

FOOT PAIN
Arthritis
Bunion
Callus or corn
Dislocation
Flatfoot
Fracture
Gout
Hallux rigidus
Hammer toe
Ingrown toenail
Köhler's disease
Morton's neuroma
Occlusive vascular disease
Plantar fasciitis
Plantar wart
Radiculopathy
Tabes dorsalis
Tarsal tunnel syndrome

HIP PAIN
Arthritis
Avascular necrosis
Bursitis
Dislocation
Fracture
Sepsis
Tumor

KNEE PAIN
Arthritis
Bursitis
Chondromalacia
Contusion
Cruciate ligament injury
Dislocation
Fracture
Meniscal injury
Osteochondritis dissecans
Phlebitis
Popliteal cyst
Radiculopathy
Ruptured extensor mechanism
Sprain

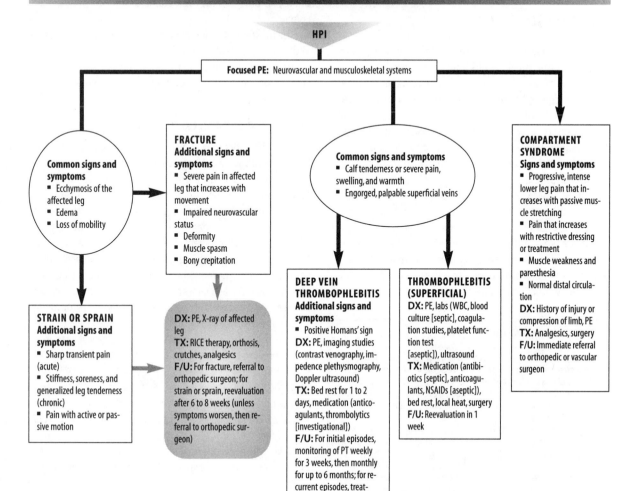

HPI

Focused PE: Neurovascular and musculoskeletal systems

Common signs and symptoms
- Ecchymosis of the affected leg
- Edema
- Loss of mobility

FRACTURE
Additional signs and symptoms
- Severe pain in affected leg that increases with movement
- Impaired neurovascular status
- Deformity
- Muscle spasm
- Bony crepitation

Common signs and symptoms
- Calf tenderness or severe pain, swelling, and warmth
- Engorged, palpable superficial veins

COMPARTMENT SYNDROME
Signs and symptoms
- Progressive, intense lower leg pain that increases with passive muscle stretching
- Pain that increases with restrictive dressing or treatment
- Muscle weakness and paresthesia
- Normal distal circulation
DX: History of injury or compression of limb, PE
TX: Analgesics, surgery
F/U: Immediate referral to orthopedic or vascular surgeon

STRAIN OR SPRAIN
Additional signs and symptoms
- Sharp transient pain (acute)
- Stiffness, soreness, and generalized leg tenderness (chronic)
- Pain with active or passive motion

DX: PE, X-ray of affected leg
TX: RICE therapy, orthosis, crutches, analgesics
F/U: For fracture, referral to orthopedic surgeon; for strain or sprain, reevaluation after 6 to 8 weeks (unless symptoms worsen, then referral to orthopedic surgeon)

DEEP VEIN THROMBOPHLEBITIS
Additional signs and symptoms
- Positive Homans' sign
DX: PE, imaging studies (contrast venography, impedence plethysmography, Doppler ultrasound)
TX: Bed rest for 1 to 2 days, medication (anticoagulants, thrombolytics [investigational])
F/U: For initial episodes, monitoring of PT weekly for 3 weeks, then monthly for up to 6 months; for recurrent episodes, treatment and monitoring once per year

THROMBOPHLEBITIS (SUPERFICIAL)
DX: PE, labs (WBC, blood culture [septic], coagulation studies, platelet function test [aseptic]), ultrasound
TX: Medication (antibiotics [septic], anticoagulants, NSAIDs [aseptic]), bed rest, local heat, surgery
F/U: Reevaluation in 1 week

Additional differential diagnoses: bone cancer ▪ infection ▪ occlusive vascular disease ▪ sciatica ▪ varicose veins ▪ venous stasis ulcers

Level of consciousness decrease

A decrease in level of consciousness (LOC), from lethargy to stupor to coma, usually results from neurologic disorders and often signals life-threatening complications of hemorrhage, trauma, or cerebral edema. However, this sign can also result from metabolic, GI, musculoskeletal, urologic, and cardiopulmonary disorders; severe nutritional deficiency; the effects of toxins; and drug use. LOC can deteriorate suddenly or gradually and can remain altered temporarily or permanently.

Consciousness is affected by the reticular activating system (RAS), an intricate network of neurons whose axons extend from the brain stem, thalamus, and hypothalamus to the cerebral cortex. A disturbance in any part of this integrated system prevents the intercommunication that makes consciousness possible. Loss of consciousness can result from a bilateral cerebral disturbance, an RAS disturbance, or both. Cerebral dysfunction characteristically produces the least dramatic decrease in a patient's LOC. In contrast, dysfunction of the RAS produces the most dramatic decrease in LOC — coma.

The most sensitive indicator of decreased LOC is a change in the patient's mental status. The Glasgow Coma Scale, which measures ability to respond to verbal, sensory, and motor stimulation, can be used to quickly evaluate a patient's LOC.

History and physical examination

Evaluate the patient's LOC by using the Glasgow Coma Scale. If the patient's score is 13 or less, the patient should be emergently evaluated for a life-threatening occurrence. Try to obtain history information from the patient if he's lucid and from his family. Did the patient complain of headache, dizziness, nausea, visual or hearing disturbances, weakness, fatigue, or any other problems before his LOC decreased? Has his family noticed any changes in the patient's behavior, personality, memory, or temperament? Also, ask about a history of neurologic disease, cancer, or recent trauma; drug and alcohol use; and the development of other signs and symptoms.

Because decreased LOC can result from disorders that affect virtually every body system, tailor the physical examination according to the patient's associated symptoms.

Glasgow Coma Scale

You've probably heard such terms as *lethargic, obtunded,* and *stuporous* used to describe progressive decrease in a patient's level of consciousness (LOC). However, the Glasgow Coma Scale provides a more accurate, less subjective method of recording such changes, grading consciousness in relation to eye opening and motor and verbal responses.

To use the Glasgow Coma Scale, test the patient's ability to respond to verbal, motor, and sensory stimulation. The scoring system doesn't determine exact LOC, but it does provide an easy way to describe the patient's basic status and helps to detect and interpret changes from baseline findings. A decreased reaction score in one or more categories may signal an impending neurologic crisis. A score of 7 or less indicates severe neurologic damage.

TEST	REACTION	SCORE
Eyes	Open spontaneously	4
	Open to verbal command	3
	Open to pain	2
	No response	1
Best motor response	Obeys verbal command	6
	Localizes painful stimulus	5
	Flexion — withdrawal	4
	Flexion — abnormal (decorticate rigidity)	3
	Extension (decerebrate rigidity)	2
	No response	1
	Oriented and converses	5
	Disoriented and converses	4
Best verbal response	Inappropriate words	3
	Incomprehensible sounds	2
	No response	1
Total		3 to 15

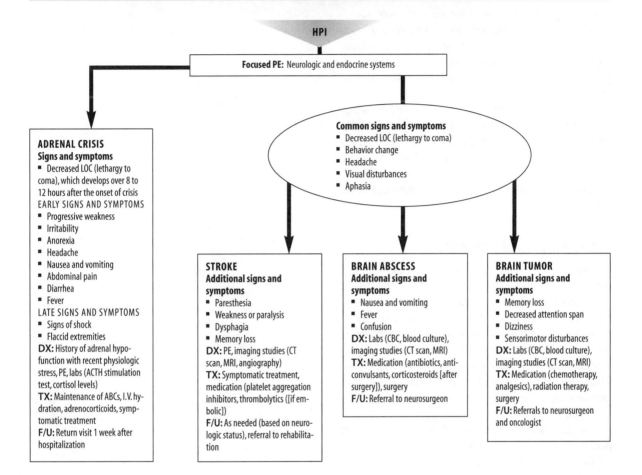

HPI

Focused PE: Neurologic and endocrine systems

ADRENAL CRISIS
Signs and symptoms
- Decreased LOC (lethargy to coma), which develops over 8 to 12 hours after the onset of crisis
EARLY SIGNS AND SYMPTOMS
- Progressive weakness
- Irritability
- Anorexia
- Headache
- Nausea and vomiting
- Abdominal pain
- Diarrhea
- Fever
LATE SIGNS AND SYMPTOMS
- Signs of shock
- Flaccid extremities
DX: History of adrenal hypofunction with recent physiologic stress, PE, labs (ACTH stimulation test, cortisol levels)
TX: Maintenance of ABCs, I.V. hydration, adrenocorticoids, symptomatic treatment
F/U: Return visit 1 week after hospitalization

Common signs and symptoms
- Decreased LOC (lethargy to coma)
- Behavior change
- Headache
- Visual disturbances
- Aphasia

STROKE
Additional signs and symptoms
- Paresthesia
- Weakness or paralysis
- Dysphagia
- Memory loss
DX: PE, imaging studies (CT scan, MRI, angiography)
TX: Symptomatic treatment, medication (platelet aggregation inhibitors, thrombolytics ([if embolic])
F/U: As needed (based on neurologic status), referral to rehabilitation

BRAIN ABSCESS
Additional signs and symptoms
- Nausea and vomiting
- Fever
- Confusion
DX: Labs (CBC, blood culture), imaging studies (CT scan, MRI)
TX: Medication (antibiotics, anticonvulsants, corticosteroids [after surgery]), surgery
F/U: Referral to neurosurgeon

BRAIN TUMOR
Additional signs and symptoms
- Memory loss
- Decreased attention span
- Dizziness
- Sensorimotor disturbances
DX: Labs (CBC, blood culture), imaging studies (CT scan, MRI)
TX: Medication (chemotherapy, analgesics), radiation therapy, surgery
F/U: Referrals to neurosurgeon and oncologist

Additional differential diagnoses: cerebral aneurysm (ruptured) ▪ cerebral contusion ▪ diabetic ketoacidosis ▪ encephalitis ▪ encephalomyelitis (postvaccinal) ▪ encephalopathy ▪ epidural hemorrhage (acute) ▪ heatstroke ▪ hypercapnia with pulmonary disease ▪ hyperglycemic hyperosmolar nonketotic coma ▪ hypernatremia ▪ hyperventilation syndrome ▪ hypokalemia ▪ hyponatremia ▪ hypothermia ▪ intracerebral hemorrhage ▪ meningitis ▪ myxedema crisis ▪ poisoning ▪ pontine hemorrhage ▪ seizure disorders ▪ shock ▪ subdural hematoma (chronic) ▪ subdural hemorrhage (acute) ▪ thyroid storm ▪ TIA ▪ West Nile encephalitis

Other causes: alcohol ▪ barbiturate overdose ▪ central nervous system depressants ▪ aspirin

Light flashes

A cardinal symptom of vision-threatening retinal detachment, light flashes (photopsias) can occur locally or throughout the visual field. The patient usually reports seeing spots, stars, or lightning-type streaks. Flashes can occur suddenly or gradually and can indicate temporary or permanent vision impairment.

In most cases, light flashes signal the splitting of the posterior vitreous membrane into two layers; the inner layer detaches from the retina and the outer layer remains fixed. The sensation of light flashes may result from vitreous traction on the retina, hemorrhage caused by a tear in the retinal capillary, or strands of solid vitreous floating in a local pool of liquid vitreous.

History and physical examination

Ask the patient when the light flashes began. Can he pinpoint their location or do they occur throughout the visual field? If the patient is experiencing eye pain or headache, have him describe it. Also, ask if the patient wears or has ever worn corrective lenses and if he or a family member has a history of eye or vision problems. Also ask if the patient has any other medical problems — especially hypertension or diabetes mellitus, which can cause retinopathy and possibly retinal detachment. Obtain an occupational history because light flashes may be related to job stress or eye strain.

Next, perform a complete eye and vision examination, especially if trauma is apparent or suspected. Begin by inspecting the external eye, lids, lashes, and tear puncta for any abnormalities and the iris and sclera for signs of bleeding. Observe pupil size and shape. Also, check for reaction to light, accommodation, and consensual light response. Then test visual acuity in each eye. Also test visual fields; document any light flashes the patient reports during this test.

PEDIATRIC POINTER

Children may experience light flashes after minor head trauma.

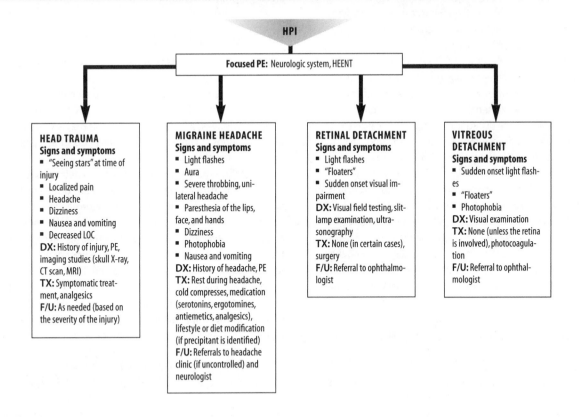

HPI

Focused PE: Neurologic system, HEENT

HEAD TRAUMA
Signs and symptoms
- "Seeing stars" at time of injury
- Localized pain
- Headache
- Dizziness
- Nausea and vomiting
- Decreased LOC

DX: History of injury, PE, imaging studies (skull X-ray, CT scan, MRI)
TX: Symptomatic treatment, analgesics
F/U: As needed (based on the severity of the injury)

MIGRAINE HEADACHE
Signs and symptoms
- Light flashes
- Aura
- Severe throbbing, unilateral headache
- Paresthesia of the lips, face, and hands
- Dizziness
- Photophobia
- Nausea and vomiting

DX: History of headache, PE
TX: Rest during headache, cold compresses, medication (serotonins, ergotomines, antiemetics, analgesics), lifestyle or diet modification (if precipitant is identified)
F/U: Referrals to headache clinic (if uncontrolled) and neurologist

---

RETINAL DETACHMENT
Signs and symptoms
- Light flashes
- "Floaters"
- Sudden onset visual impairment

DX: Visual field testing, slit-lamp examination, ultrasonography
TX: None (in certain cases), surgery
F/U: Referral to ophthalmologist

VITREOUS DETACHMENT
Signs and symptoms
- Sudden onset light flashes
- "Floaters"
- Photophobia

DX: Visual examination
TX: None (unless the retina is involved), photocoagulation
F/U: Referral to ophthalmologist

Additional differential diagnoses: CNS disorders such as stroke ▪ endocrine disorders such as diabetes mellitus ▪ liver disease

Other causes: alcohol abuse ▪ antihypertensives ▪ drug abuse ▪ surgery ▪ urologic procedures such as prostatectomy ▪ radiation therapy

Lymphadenopathy

Lymphadenopathy — enlargement of one or more lymph nodes — may result from increased production of lymphocytes or reticuloendothelial cells or from infiltration of cells that aren't normally present. This sign may be generalized (involving three or more node groups) or localized. Generalized lymphadenopathy may be caused by an inflammatory process, such as bacterial or viral infection; connective tissue disease; endocrine disorder; or neoplasm. Localized lymphadenopathy most commonly results from infection or trauma affecting the drained area. (See *Causes of localized lymphadenopathy.*)

Normally, lymph nodes range from 0.5 to 2.5 cm in diameter and are discrete, mobile, nontender and, except in children, nonpalpable. (However, palpable nodes may be normal in adults.) Nodes that exceed 3 cm in diameter are cause for concern. They may be tender and the skin overlying the lymph node may be erythematous, suggesting a draining lesion. Or they may be hard and fixed, tender or nontender, suggesting a malignant tumor. Assess for unilateral versus bilateral area lymphadenopathy.

History and physical examination

Ask the patient when he first noticed the swelling and if it's located on one side of his body or both. Are the swollen areas sore, hard, or red? Ask the patient if he has recently had an infection or any other health problems. Also ask if a biopsy has ever been done on any nodes because this may reveal a previously diagnosed cancer. Find out if the patient has a family history of cancer.

Palpate the entire lymph node system to determine the extent of lymphadenopathy and to detect any other areas of local enlargement. Use the pads of your index and middle fingers to move the skin over underlying tissues at the nodal area. If you detect enlarged nodes, note their size in centimeters and whether they're fixed or mobile, tender or nontender, and erythematous or not. Also note their texture: Is the node discrete or does the area feel matted? If you detect tender, erythematous lymph nodes, check the area drained by that part of the lymph system for signs of infection, such as erythema and swelling. Also, palpate for and percuss the spleen.

PEDIATRIC POINTER

Infection is the most common cause of lymphadenopathy in children. The condition is commonly associated with otitis media and pharyngitis.

Causes of localized lymphadenopathy

A variety of disorders can cause localized lymphadenopathy, but this sign usually results from infection or trauma affecting the drained area. Here you'll find some common causes of lymphadenopathy listed according to the areas affected.

OCCIPITAL
- Roseola
- Scalp infection
- Seborrheic dermatitis
- Tick bite
- Tinea capitis

AURICULAR
- Erysipelas
- Herpes zoster ophthalmicus
- Infection
- Rubella
- Squamous cell carcinoma
- Styes or chalazion
- Tularemia

CERVICAL
- Cat-scratch fever
- Facial or oral cancer
- Infection
- Mononucleosis
- Mucocutaneous lymph node syndrome
- Rubella
- Rubeola
- Thyrotoxicosis
- Tonsillitis
- Tuberculosis
- Varicella

SUBMAXILLARY AND SUBMENTAL
- Cystic fibrosis
- Dental infection
- Gingivitis
- Glossitis

SUPRACLAVICULAR
- Neoplastic disease

AXILLARY
- Breast cancer
- Lymphoma
- Mastitis

INGUINAL AND FEMORAL
- Carcinoma
- Chancroid
- Lymphogranuloma venereum
- Syphilis

POPLITEAL
- Infection

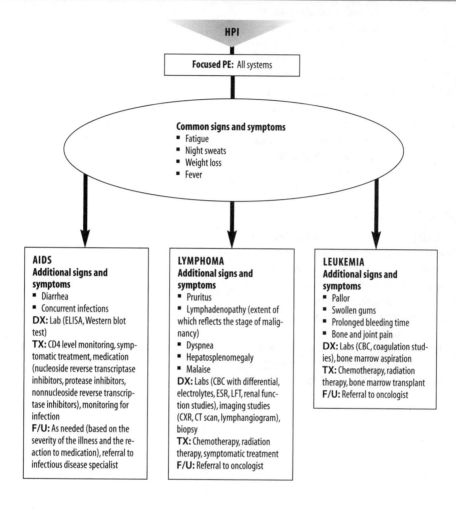

HPI

Focused PE: All systems

Common signs and symptoms
- Fatigue
- Night sweats
- Weight loss
- Fever

AIDS
Additional signs and symptoms
- Diarrhea
- Concurrent infections

DX: Lab (ELISA, Western blot test)

TX: CD4 level monitoring, symptomatic treatment, medication (nucleoside reverse transcriptase inhibitors, protease inhibitors, nonnucleoside reverse transcriptase inhibitors), monitoring for infection

F/U: As needed (based on the severity of the illness and the reaction to medication), referral to infectious disease specialist

LYMPHOMA
Additional signs and symptoms
- Pruritus
- Lymphadenopathy (extent of which reflects the stage of malignancy)
- Dyspnea
- Hepatosplenomegaly
- Malaise

DX: Labs (CBC with differential, electrolytes, ESR, LFT, renal function studies), imaging studies (CXR, CT scan, lymphangiogram), biopsy

TX: Chemotherapy, radiation therapy, symptomatic treatment

F/U: Referral to oncologist

LEUKEMIA
Additional signs and symptoms
- Pallor
- Swollen gums
- Prolonged bleeding time
- Bone and joint pain

DX: Labs (CBC, coagulation studies), bone marrow aspiration

TX: Chemotherapy, radiation therapy, bone marrow transplant

F/U: Referral to oncologist

Additional differential diagnoses: brucellosis ▪ chronic fatigue syndrome ▪ cytomegalovirus infection ▪ leptospirosis ▪ Lyme disease ▪ mononucleosis (infectious) ▪ mycosis fungoides ▪ rheumatoid arthritis ▪ sarcoidosis ▪ Sjögren's syndrome ▪ syphilis (secondary) ▪ SLE ▪ tuberculous lymphadenitis ▪ Waldenström's macroglobulinemia

Other causes: phenytoin ▪ immunizations such as typhoid vaccination

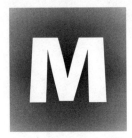

Masklike facies

A total loss of facial expression, masklike facies results from bradykinesia usually due to extrapyramidal damage. Even the rate of eye blinking is reduced — to 1 to 4 blinks per minute, producing a characteristic "reptilian" stare. Although a neurologic disorder is the most common cause, masklike facies can also result from certain systemic diseases and the effects of drugs and toxins. The sign often develops insidiously, at first mistaken by the observer for depression or apathy.

History and physical examination

Ask the patient and his family or friends when they first noticed the masklike facial expression and any other signs or symptoms. Find out what medications the patient is taking, if any, and ask about any changes in dosage or schedule. Determine the degree of facial muscle weakness by asking the patient to smile and to wrinkle his forehead. Typically, the patient's responses are slowed.

PEDIATRIC POINTER

Masklike facies occurs in the juvenile form of Parkinson's disease.

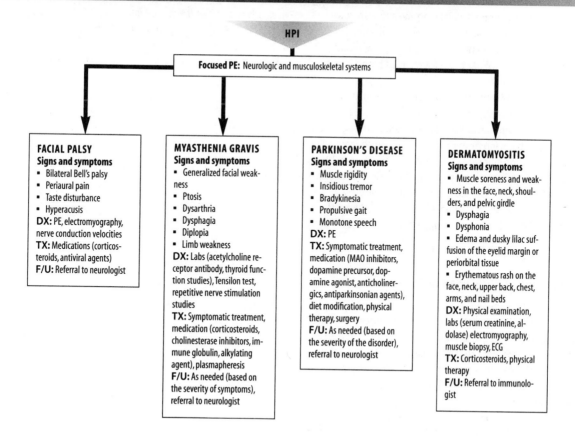

HPI

Focused PE: Neurologic and musculoskeletal systems

FACIAL PALSY
Signs and symptoms
- Bilateral Bell's palsy
- Periaural pain
- Taste disturbance
- Hyperacusis

DX: PE, electromyography, nerve conduction velocities
TX: Medications (corticosteroids, antiviral agents)
F/U: Referral to neurologist

MYASTHENIA GRAVIS
Signs and symptoms
- Generalized facial weakness
- Ptosis
- Dysarthria
- Dysphagia
- Diplopia
- Limb weakness

DX: Labs (acetylcholine receptor antibody, thyroid function studies), Tensilon test, repetitive nerve stimulation studies
TX: Symptomatic treatment, medication (corticosteroids, cholinesterase inhibitors, immune globulin, alkylating agent), plasmapheresis
F/U: As needed (based on the severity of symptoms), referral to neurologist

PARKINSON'S DISEASE
Signs and symptoms
- Muscle rigidity
- Insidious tremor
- Bradykinesia
- Propulsive gait
- Monotone speech

DX: PE
TX: Symptomatic treatment, medication (MAO inhibitors, dopamine precursor, dopamine agonist, anticholinergics, antiparkinsonian agents), diet modification, physical therapy, surgery
F/U: As needed (based on the severity of the disorder), referral to neurologist

DERMATOMYOSITIS
Signs and symptoms
- Muscle soreness and weakness in the face, neck, shoulders, and pelvic girdle
- Dysphagia
- Dysphonia
- Edema and dusky lilac suffusion of the eyelid margin or periorbital tissue
- Erythematous rash on the face, neck, upper back, chest, arms, and nail beds

DX: Physical examination, labs (serum creatinine, aldolase) electromyography, muscle biopsy, ECG
TX: Corticosteroids, physical therapy
F/U: Referral to immunologist

Additional differential diagnoses: Guillain-Barré syndrome ▪ scleroderma

Other causes: antipsychotics ▪ carbon monoxide poisoning ▪ manganese poisoning (chronic) ▪ metoclopramide ▪ metyrosine ▪ phenothiazines (particularly piperazine derivatives)

Melena

A common sign of upper GI bleeding, melena is the passage of black, tarry stools. Characteristic color results from bacterial degradation and hydrochloric acid acting on the blood as it travels through the GI tract. At least 60 ml of blood is needed to produce this sign.

Severe melena can signal acute bleeding and life-threatening hypovolemic shock. Usually, melena indicates bleeding from the esophagus, stomach, or duodenum, although it can also indicate bleeding from the jejunum, ileum, or ascending colon. In addition, this sign can result from swallowing blood, as in epistaxis; from certain drugs; and from alcohol. Because false melena may be caused by ingestion of lead, iron, bismuth, or licorice (which produces black stools without the presence of blood), all black stools should be tested for occult blood.

History and physical examination

If the patient is experiencing severe melena, quickly take orthostatic vital signs to detect hypovolemic shock. A decline of 10 mm Hg or more in systolic pressure or an increase of 10 beats or more in pulse rate indicates volume depletion. Quickly look for other signs of shock, such as tachycardia, tachypnea, and cool, clammy skin. Institute emergency measures, if necessary.

If the patient's condition permits, ask when he discovered his stools were black and tarry. Ask about the frequency and quantity of bowel movements. Has he had melena before? Ask about other signs and symptoms, notably hematemesis or hematochezia, and about use of anti-inflammatory drugs, alcohol, and other GI irritants. Also, find out if he has a history of GI lesions.

Next, inspect the patient's mouth and nasopharynx for evidence of bleeding. Perform an abdominal examination that includes inspection, auscultation, palpation, and percussion.

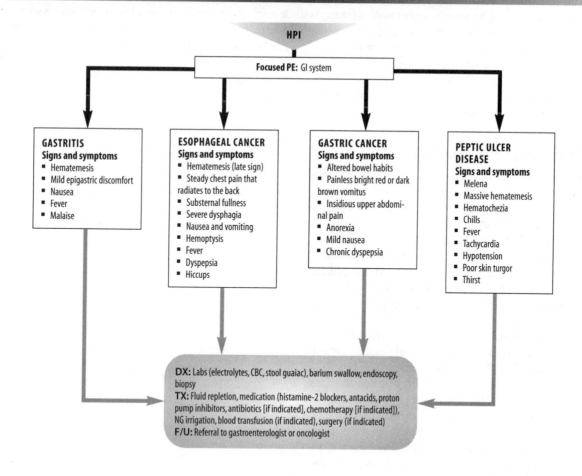

HPI

Focused PE: GI system

GASTRITIS
Signs and symptoms
- Hematemesis
- Mild epigastric discomfort
- Nausea
- Fever
- Malaise

ESOPHAGEAL CANCER
Signs and symptoms
- Hematemesis (late sign)
- Steady chest pain that radiates to the back
- Substernal fullness
- Severe dysphagia
- Nausea and vomiting
- Hemoptysis
- Fever
- Dyspepsia
- Hiccups

GASTRIC CANCER
Signs and symptoms
- Altered bowel habits
- Painless bright red or dark brown vomitus
- Insidious upper abdominal pain
- Anorexia
- Mild nausea
- Chronic dyspepsia

PEPTIC ULCER DISEASE
Signs and symptoms
- Melena
- Massive hematemesis
- Hematochezia
- Chills
- Fever
- Tachycardia
- Hypotension
- Poor skin turgor
- Thirst

DX: Labs (electrolytes, CBC, stool guaiac), barium swallow, endoscopy, biopsy
TX: Fluid repletion, medication (histamine-2 blockers, antacids, proton pump inhibitors, antibiotics [if indicated], chemotherapy [if indicated]), NG irrigation, blood transfusion (if indicated), surgery (if indicated)
F/U: Referral to gastroenterologist or oncologist

Additional differential diagnoses: colon cancer ▪ Ebola virus ▪ esophageal varices (ruptured) ▪ Mallory-Weiss syndrome ▪ small bowel tumors ▪ thrombocytopenia ▪ typhoid fever ▪ yellow fever

Other causes: alcohol ▪ aspirin ▪ NSAIDs

Menorrhagia

Heavy, or significantly heavier menstrual bleeding, menorrhagia may occur as a single episode or a chronic sign. In menorrhagia, bleeding is heavier than the patient's normal menstrual flow; menstrual blood loss is 80 ml or more per monthly period. A form of dysfunctional uterine bleeding, menorrhagia can result from endocrine and hematologic disorders, stress, and certain drugs and procedures.

History and physical examination

If the patient's condition permits, obtain a history. Determine her age at menarche, the duration of menstrual periods, and the interval between them. Establish the date of the patient's last menses and ask about any recent changes in her normal menstrual pattern. Have the patient describe the character and amount of bleeding. For example, how many pads or tampons does the patient use? Has she noted clots or tissue in the blood? Further, ask about the development of other signs and symptoms prior to and during the menstrual period.

Next, ask if the patient is sexually active. Does she use a method of birth control? If so, what kind? Could the patient be pregnant? Be sure to note the number of pregnancies, the outcome of each, and any pregnancy-related complications. Find out the dates of her most recent pelvic examination and Papanicolaou test and the details of previous gynecologic infections or neoplasms. In addition, be sure to ask about previous episodes of abnormal bleeding and the outcome of any treatment. If possible, obtain a pregnancy history of the patient's mother and determine if the patient was exposed to diethylstilbestrol in utero.

Be sure to ask the patient about her general health and medical history. Note particularly if the patient or her family has a history of thyroid, adrenal, or hepatic disease, blood dyscrasias, or tuberculosis because these may predispose her to menorrhagia. Also, ask about the patient's past surgical procedures and recent emotional stress. In addition, find out if the patient has undergone X-ray or other radiation therapy, as this may indicate prior treatment for menorrhagia. Then proceed with the physical examination, focusing on the pelvic examination, if appropriate.

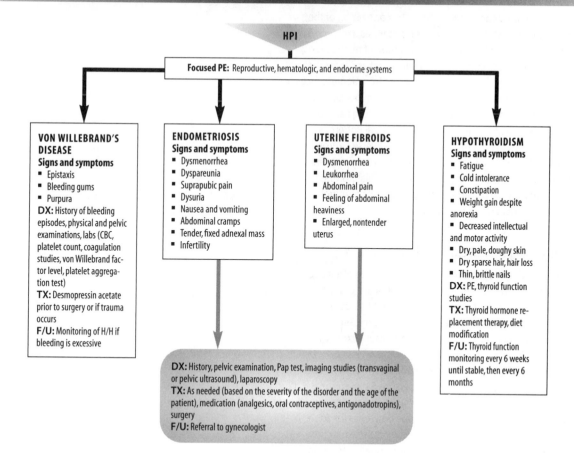

HPI

Focused PE: Reproductive, hematologic, and endocrine systems

VON WILLEBRAND'S DISEASE
Signs and symptoms
- Epistaxis
- Bleeding gums
- Purpura

DX: History of bleeding episodes, physical and pelvic examinations, labs (CBC, platelet count, coagulation studies, von Willebrand factor level, platelet aggregation test)
TX: Desmopressin acetate prior to surgery or if trauma occurs
F/U: Monitoring of H/H if bleeding is excessive

ENDOMETRIOSIS
Signs and symptoms
- Dysmenorrhea
- Dyspareunia
- Suprapubic pain
- Dysuria
- Nausea and vomiting
- Abdominal cramps
- Tender, fixed adnexal mass
- Infertility

UTERINE FIBROIDS
Signs and symptoms
- Dysmenorrhea
- Leukorrhea
- Abdominal pain
- Feeling of abdominal heaviness
- Enlarged, nontender uterus

HYPOTHYROIDISM
Signs and symptoms
- Fatigue
- Cold intolerance
- Constipation
- Weight gain despite anorexia
- Decreased intellectual and motor activity
- Dry, pale, doughy skin
- Dry sparse hair, hair loss
- Thin, brittle nails

DX: PE, thyroid function studies
TX: Thyroid hormone replacement therapy, diet modification
F/U: Thyroid function monitoring every 6 weeks until stable, then every 6 months

DX: History, pelvic examination, Pap test, imaging studies (transvaginal or pelvic ultrasound), laparoscopy
TX: As needed (based on the severity of the disorder and the age of the patient), medication (analgesics, oral contraceptives, antigonadotropins), surgery
F/U: Referral to gynecologist

Other causes: anticoagulants ▪ ginseng ▪ oral contraceptives ▪ injectable or implanted contraceptives ▪ intrauterine contraceptive devices

Miosis

Miosis — pupillary constriction caused by contraction of the sphincter muscle in the iris — occurs normally as a response to fatigue, increased light, and administration of miotic drugs; as part of the eye's accommodation reflex; and as part of the aging process (pupil size steadily decreases from adolescence to about age 60). However, it can also stem from ocular and neurologic disorders, trauma, use of systemic drugs, and contact lens overuse. A rare form of miosis — Argyll Robertson pupils — can stem from tabes dorsalis and diverse neurologic disorders. Occurring bilaterally, these miotic (often pinpoint), unequal, and irregularly shaped pupils don't dilate properly with mydriatic drug use and fail to react to light, although they do constrict on accommodation.

History and physical examination

Begin by asking the patient if he has experienced other ocular symptoms, and have him describe their onset, duration, and intensity. Does he wear contact lenses? While obtaining the patient's history, be sure to ask about trauma, serious systemic disease, and the use of topical and systemic medications.

Next, perform a thorough eye examination. Examine and compare both pupils for size (many persons have a normal discrepancy), color, shape, reaction to light, accommodation, and consensual light response. Examine both eyes for additional signs, and then evaluate extraocular muscle function by assessing the six cardinal fields of gaze. Finally, test visual acuity in each eye, with and without correction, paying particular attention to blurred or decreased vision in the miotic eye.

PEDIATRIC POINTERS

- *Miosis occurs frequently in the neonate because he's asleep or sleepy most of the time.*
- *Bilateral miosis occurs in congenital microcoria.*

HPI

Focused PE: Neurologic system, HEENT

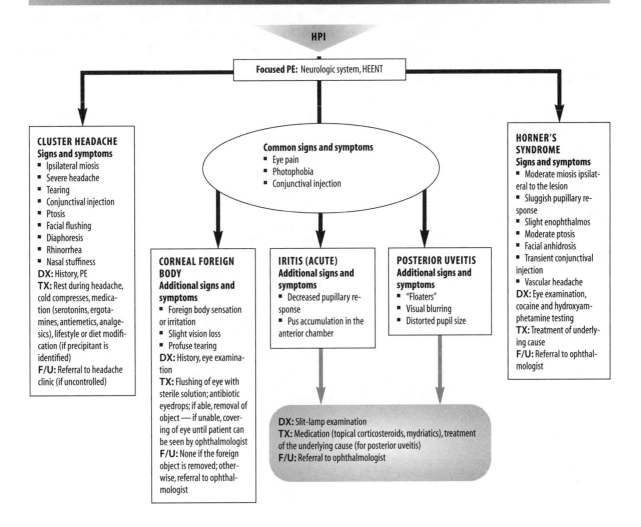

CLUSTER HEADACHE
Signs and symptoms
- Ipsilateral miosis
- Severe headache
- Tearing
- Conjunctival injection
- Ptosis
- Facial flushing
- Diaphoresis
- Rhinorrhea
- Nasal stuffiness

DX: History, PE
TX: Rest during headache, cold compresses, medication (serotonins, ergotamines, antiemetics, analgesics), lifestyle or diet modification (if precipitant is identified)
F/U: Referral to headache clinic (if uncontrolled)

Common signs and symptoms
- Eye pain
- Photophobia
- Conjunctival injection

CORNEAL FOREIGN BODY
Additional signs and symptoms
- Foreign body sensation or irritation
- Slight vision loss
- Profuse tearing

DX: History, eye examination
TX: Flushing of eye with sterile solution; antibiotic eyedrops; if able, removal of object — if unable, covering of eye until patient can be seen by ophthalmologist
F/U: None if the foreign object is removed; otherwise, referral to ophthalmologist

IRITIS (ACUTE)
Additional signs and symptoms
- Decreased pupillary response
- Pus accumulation in the anterior chamber

POSTERIOR UVEITIS
Additional signs and symptoms
- "Floaters"
- Visual blurring
- Distorted pupil size

DX: Slit-lamp examination
TX: Medication (topical corticosteroids, mydriatics), treatment of the underlying cause (for posterior uveitis)
F/U: Referral to ophthalmologist

HORNER'S SYNDROME
Signs and symptoms
- Moderate miosis ipsilateral to the lesion
- Sluggish pupillary response
- Slight enophthalmos
- Moderate ptosis
- Facial anhidrosis
- Transient conjunctival injection
- Vascular headache

DX: Eye examination, cocaine and hydroxyamphetamine testing
TX: Treatment of underlying cause
F/U: Referral to ophthalmologist

Additional differential diagnoses: cerebrovascular arteriosclerosis ▪ corneal ulcer ▪ hyphema ▪ neuropathy ▪ Parry-Romberg syndrome ▪ pontine hemorrhage ▪ tabes dorsalis

Other causes: chemical burns ▪ contact lens overuse ▪ deep anesthesia ▪ systemic drugs (barbiturates, cholinergics, cholinesterase inhibitors, clonidine [overdose], guanethidine, opiates, reserpine) ▪ topical drugs (acetylcholine, carbachol, demecarium bromide, echothiophate iodide, pilocarpine) ▪ trauma

Mouth lesions

Mouth lesions include ulcers (the most common type), cysts, firm nodules, hemorrhagic lesions, papules, vesicles, bullae, and erythematous lesions. They may occur anywhere on the lips, cheeks, hard and soft palate, salivary glands, tongue, gingivae, or mucous membranes. Many are painful and can be readily detected. Some, however, are asymptomatic; when these occur deep in the mouth, they may be discovered only through a complete oral examination. (See *Common mouth lesions*.)

Mouth lesions can result from trauma, infection, systemic disease, drugs, and radiation therapy.

History and physical examination

Begin your evaluation with a thorough history. Ask the patient when the lesions appeared and whether he has noticed any pain, odor, or drainage. Also ask about associated complaints, particularly skin lesions. Obtain a complete medication history, including drug allergies, and a complete medical history. Note especially any malignancy, sexually transmitted disease, I.V. drug use, recent infection, or trauma. Ask about his dental history, including oral hygiene habits, frequency of dental examinations, and the date of his most recent dental visit.

Next, perform a complete oral examination, noting lesion sites and character. Examine the patient's lips for color and texture. Inspect and palpate the buccal mucosa and tongue for color, texture, and contour; note especially any painless ulcers on the sides or base of the tongue. Hold the tongue with a piece of gauze, lift it, and examine its underside and the floor of the mouth. Depress the tongue with a tongue blade and examine the oropharynx. Inspect teeth and gums, noting missing, broken, or discolored teeth; dental caries; excessive debris; and bleeding, inflamed, swollen, or discolored gums.

Palpate the neck for adenopathy, especially in patients older than age 45 who smoke tobacco or use alcohol excessively.

PEDIATRIC POINTERS

- *In neonates, mouth ulcers can result from candidiasis or congenital syphilis.*
- *Causes of mouth ulcers in children include chicken pox, measles, scarlet fever, diphtheria, and hand-foot-and-mouth disease.*

Common mouth lesions

SQUAMOUS CELL CARCINOMA

LICHEN PLANUS

ULCERATION FROM TONGUE BITING

GINGIVAL HYPERPLASIA

RECURRENT APHTHOUS STOMATITIS

SYPHILITIC CHANCRE (RARE)

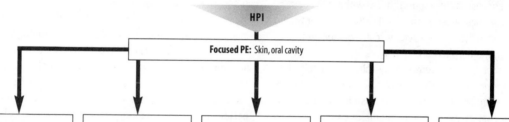

HPI

Focused PE: Skin, oral cavity

DISCOID LUPUS ERYTHEMATOSUS
Signs and symptoms
- Oral lesions on the tongue, buccal mucosa, and palate
- Erythematous areas with white spots and radiating white striae
- Lesions on the face, neck, ears, and scalp

DX: Immunofluorescent staining of skin biopsy
TX: Avoidance of sun exposure, excessive heat, cold, or trauma; medication (topical corticosteroid, antimalarials [if widespread])
F/U: Reevaluation 1 to 2 times per month

ERYTHEMA MULTIFORME
Signs and symptoms
- Sudden onset of vesicles and bullae on the lips and buccal mucosa
- Erythematous macules and papules on the hands, arms, feet, legs, face and neck
- Lymphadenopathy
- Fever
- Malaise
- Throat and chest pain

DX: PE, Nikolsky's sign
TX: Treatment of underlying cause, moist compresses to skin lesions, medications (analgesics, antipyretics, I.V. corticosteroids [in severe cases])
F/U: Referral to dermatologist

HERPES SIMPLEX
Signs and symptoms
- Prodromal tingling and itching
- Fever
- Pharyngitis
- Vesicles on the oral mucosa that form an erythematous base and then rupture, leaving a painful ulcer that's followed by a yellowish crust
- Submaxillary lymphadenopathy

DX: PE, labs (culture of lesion, Tzanck smear)
TX: Gentle cleansing, anesthetic mouthwash, antiviral agent
F/U: None unless lesions don't heal

SQUAMOUS CELL CANCER
Signs and symptoms
- Ulcer with an elevated indurated border (most commonly on the lower lip)
- Painless lesion

DX: History of smoking and alcohol use, oral examination, biopsy
TX: Surgery
F/U: Referrals to oncologist and surgeon

STOMATITIS
Signs and symptoms
- Recurrent painful ulcerations of the oral mucosa that are usually located on the dorsum of the tongue, gingivae, and hard palate
- Ulcers that are covered by a gray membrane and surrounded by a red halo

DX: Oral examination
TX: Mouth rinses, medication (topical or oral corticosteroids; OTC topical canker medication; for large, nonhealing ulcers, antibiotics)
F/U: None unless the condition continues

Additional differential diagnoses: actinomycosis (cervicofacial) ▪ AIDS ▪ Behçet's syndrome ▪ candidiasis ▪ epulis (giant cell) ▪ gingivitis (acute necrotizing ulcerative) ▪ gonorrhea ▪ herpes zoster ▪ inflammatory fibrous hyperplasia ▪ leukoplakia or erythroplakia ▪ lichen planus ▪ mucous duct obstruction ▪ pemphigus ▪ pyogenic granuloma ▪ syphilis ▪ SLE ▪ tuberculosis (oral mucosal)

Other causes: chemotherapeutic agents ▪ allergic reactions to penicillin, sulfonamides, gold, quinine, streptomycin, phenytoin, aspirin, and barbiturates ▪ radiation therapy ▪ trauma

Murmur

Murmurs are auscultatory sounds heard within the heart chambers or major arteries. They're classified by their timing and duration in the cardiac cycle, auscultatory location, loudness, configuration, pitch, and quality.

Timing can be characterized as systolic, holosystolic (continuous throughout systole), diastolic, or continuous throughout systole and diastole; systolic and diastolic murmurs can be further characterized as early, middle, or late. Location refers to the area of maximum loudness, such as the apex, the lower left sternal border, or an intercostal space. Loudness is graded on a scale of 1 to 6, with 1 signifying the faintest audible murmur. Configuration, or shape, refers to the nature of loudness — crescendo, decrescendo, crescendo-decrescendo, decrescendo-crescendo, plateau (even), or variable (uneven).

The murmur's pitch may be high or low. Its quality may be described as harsh, rumbling, blowing, scratching, buzzing, musical, or squeaking.

Murmurs can reflect accelerated blood flow through normal or abnormal valves; forward blood flow through a narrowed or irregular valve or into a dilated vessel; blood backflow through an incompetent valve, septal defect, or patent ductus arteriosus; or decreased blood viscosity. Often the result of organic heart disease, murmurs occasionally may signal an emergency situation — for example, a loud holosystolic murmur after acute myocardial infarction may signal papillary muscle rupture or ventricular septal defect. Murmurs may also result from surgical implantation of a prosthetic valve.

Some murmurs are innocent, or functional. An innocent systolic murmur is generally soft, medium-pitched, and loudest along the left sternal border at the second or third intercostal space. It's exacerbated by physical activity, excitement, fever, pregnancy, anemia, or thyrotoxicosis. Examples include Still's murmur in children and mammary souffle, often heard over either breast during late pregnancy and early post partum.

History and physical examination

If you discover a murmur, try to determine its type through careful auscultation. (See *Identifying common murmurs.*) Use the bell of your stethoscope for low-pitched murmurs; the diaphragm for high-pitched murmurs.

Next, obtain a patient history. Ask if the murmur is a new discovery or if it has been known since birth or childhood. Find out if the patient has experienced any associated symptoms, particularly palpitations, dizziness, syncope, chest pain, dyspnea, and fatigue. Explore the patient's medical history, noting especially any incidence of rheumatic fever, heart disease, or heart surgery, particularly prosthetic valve replacement.

Perform a systematic physical examination. Note especially the presence of cardiac arrhythmias, jugular vein distention, and such pulmonary signs as dyspnea, orthopnea, and crackles. Is the patient's liver tender or palpable? Does he have peripheral edema?

Identifying common murmurs

The timing and configuration of a murmur can help you identify its underlying cause. Learn to recognize the characteristics of these common murmurs.

AORTIC REGURGITATION (CHRONIC)

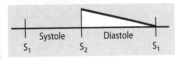

Thickened valve leaflets fail to close correctly, permitting backflow of blood into the left ventricle.

AORTIC STENOSIS

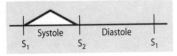

Thickened, scarred, or calcified valve leaflets impede ventricular systolic ejection.

MITRAL PROLAPSE

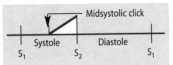

Incompetent mitral valve bulges into the left atrium because of an enlarged posterior leaflet and elongated chordae tendineae.

MITRAL REGURGITATION (CHRONIC)

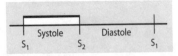

Incomplete mitral valve closure permits backflow of blood into the left atrium.

MITRAL STENOSIS

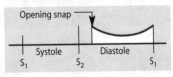

Thickened or scarred valve leaflets cause valve stenosis and restrict blood flow.

> ### PEDIATRIC POINTERS
>
> - *Pathognomonic heart murmurs in infants and young children usually result from congenital heart disease, such as atrial and ventricular septal defects.*
> - *Innocent murmurs, such as Still's murmur, are frequently heard in young children and often disappear in puberty.*
> - *Other murmurs can be acquired, as with rheumatic heart disease.*

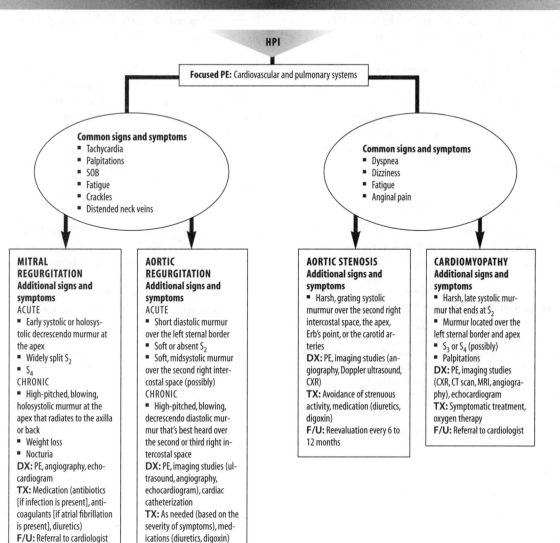

HPI

Focused PE: Cardiovascular and pulmonary systems

Common signs and symptoms
- Tachycardia
- Palpitations
- SOB
- Fatigue
- Crackles
- Distended neck veins

Common signs and symptoms
- Dyspnea
- Dizziness
- Fatigue
- Anginal pain

MITRAL REGURGITATION
Additional signs and symptoms
ACUTE
- Early systolic or holosystolic decrescendo murmur at the apex
- Widely split S_2
- S_4
CHRONIC
- High-pitched, blowing, holosystolic murmur at the apex that radiates to the axilla or back
- Weight loss
- Nocturia
DX: PE, angiography, echocardiogram
TX: Medication (antibiotics [if infection is present], anticoagulants [if atrial fibrillation is present], diuretics)
F/U: Referral to cardiologist

AORTIC REGURGITATION
Additional signs and symptoms
ACUTE
- Short diastolic murmur over the left sternal border
- Soft or absent S_2
- Soft, midsystolic murmur over the second right intercostal space (possibly)
CHRONIC
- High-pitched, blowing, decrescendo diastolic murmur that's best heard over the second or third right intercostal space
DX: PE, imaging studies (ultrasound, angiography, echocardiogram), cardiac catheterization
TX: As needed (based on the severity of symptoms), medications (diuretics, digoxin)
F/U: Referral to cardiologist

AORTIC STENOSIS
Additional signs and symptoms
- Harsh, grating systolic murmur over the second right intercostal space, the apex, Erb's point, or the carotid arteries
DX: PE, imaging studies (angiography, Doppler ultrasound, CXR)
TX: Avoidance of strenuous activity, medication (diuretics, digoxin)
F/U: Reevaluation every 6 to 12 months

CARDIOMYOPATHY
Additional signs and symptoms
- Harsh, late systolic murmur that ends at S_2
- Murmur located over the left sternal border and apex
- S_3 or S_4 (possibly)
- Palpitations
DX: PE, imaging studies (CXR, CT scan, MRI, angiography), echocardiogram
TX: Symptomatic treatment, oxygen therapy
F/U: Referral to cardiologist

Additional differential diagnoses: mitral prolapse ▪ mitral stenosis ▪ myxomas ▪ papillary muscle rupture ▪ tricuspid regurgitation ▪ tricuspid stenosis

Other causes: prosthetic valve replacement

Muscle atrophy

Muscle atrophy (muscle wasting) results from denervation or prolonged muscle disuse. When deprived of regular exercise, muscle fibers lose both bulk and length, producing a visible loss of muscle size and contour and apparent emaciation or deformity in the affected area. Even slight atrophy usually causes some loss of motion or power.

Atrophy usually results from neuromuscular disease or injury. However, it may also stem from certain metabolic and endocrine disorders and prolonged immobility. Some muscle atrophy also occurs with aging.

History and physical examination

Ask the patient when and where he first noticed the muscle wasting and how it has progressed. Also ask about any associated signs and symptoms, such as weakness, pain, loss of sensation, and recent weight loss. Review the patient's medical history for chronic illnesses; musculoskeletal or neurologic disorders, including trauma; and endocrine and metabolic disorders. Ask about his use of alcohol and drugs, particularly steroids.

Begin the physical examination by determining the location and extent of atrophy. Visually evaluate small and large muscles. Check all major muscle groups for size, tonicity, and strength. Measure the circumference of all limbs, comparing sides. (See *Measuring limb circumference.*) Check for muscle contractures in all limbs by fully extending joints and noting any pain or resistance. Complete the examination by palpating peripheral pulses for quality and rate, assessing sensory function in and around the atrophied area, and testing deep tendon reflexes.

Measuring limb circumference

To ensure accurate and consistent limb circumference measurements, use a consistent reference point each time and measure with the limb in full extension. The diagram here shows the correct reference points for arm and leg measurements.

ARM

Biceps circumference

Olecranon process

Forearm circumference

LEG

Quadriceps circumference

Patella

Calf circumference

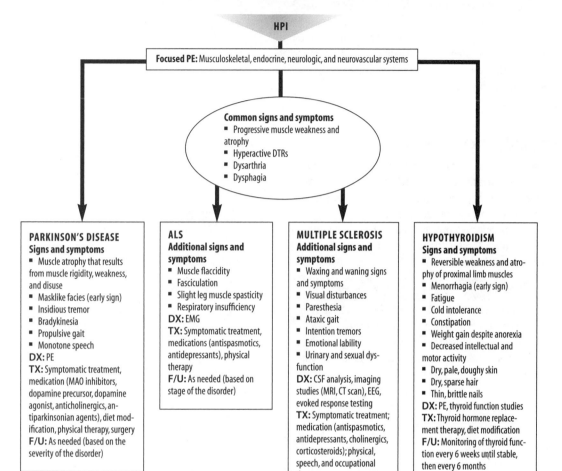

HPI

Focused PE: Musculoskeletal, endocrine, neurologic, and neurovascular systems

Common signs and symptoms
- Progressive muscle weakness and atrophy
- Hyperactive DTRs
- Dysarthria
- Dysphagia

PARKINSON'S DISEASE
Signs and symptoms
- Muscle atrophy that results from muscle rigidity, weakness, and disuse
- Masklike facies (early sign)
- Insidious tremor
- Bradykinesia
- Propulsive gait
- Monotone speech
DX: PE
TX: Symptomatic treatment, medication (MAO inhibitors, dopamine precursor, dopamine agonist, anticholinergics, antiparkinsonian agents), diet modification, physical therapy, surgery
F/U: As needed (based on the severity of the disorder)

ALS
Additional signs and symptoms
- Muscle flaccidity
- Fasciculation
- Slight leg muscle spasticity
- Respiratory insufficiency
DX: EMG
TX: Symptomatic treatment, medications (antispasmotics, antidepressants), physical therapy
F/U: As needed (based on stage of the disorder)

MULTIPLE SCLEROSIS
Additional signs and symptoms
- Waxing and waning signs and symptoms
- Visual disturbances
- Paresthesia
- Ataxic gait
- Intention tremors
- Emotional lability
- Urinary and sexual dysfunction
DX: CSF analysis, imaging studies (MRI, CT scan), EEG, evoked response testing
TX: Symptomatic treatment; medication (antispasmotics, antidepressants, cholinergics, corticosteroids); physical, speech, and occupational therapy
F/U: Referral to neurologist

HYPOTHYROIDISM
Signs and symptoms
- Reversible weakness and atrophy of proximal limb muscles
- Menorrhagia (early sign)
- Fatigue
- Cold intolerance
- Constipation
- Weight gain despite anorexia
- Decreased intellectual and motor activity
- Dry, pale, doughy skin
- Dry, sparse hair
- Thin, brittle nails
DX: PE, thyroid function studies
TX: Thyroid hormone replacement therapy, diet modification
F/U: Monitoring of thyroid function every 6 weeks until stable, then every 6 months

Additional differential diagnoses: burns ▪ compartment syndrome and Volkmann's ischemic contracture ▪ herniated disk ▪ hypercortisolism ▪ meniscal tear ▪ osteoarthritis ▪ peripheral nerve trauma ▪ peripheral neuropathy ▪ protein deficiency ▪ radiculopathy ▪ rheumatoid arthritis ▪ spinal cord injury ▪ stroke ▪ thyrotoxicosis

Other causes: prolonged steroid therapy ▪ immobility

Muscle flaccidity

Flaccid muscles (muscle hypotonicity) are profoundly weak and soft, with decreased resistance to movement, increased mobility, and greater than normal range of motion. The result of disrupted muscle innervation, flaccidity can be localized to a limb or muscle group or generalized over the entire body. Its onset may be acute, as in trauma, or chronic, as in neurologic disease.

History and physical examination

If the patient isn't in distress, ask about the onset and duration of muscle flaccidity and any precipitating factors. Ask about associated symptoms, notably weakness, other muscle changes, and sensory loss or paresthesia.

Examine the affected muscles for atrophy, which indicates a chronic problem. Test muscle strength and check deep tendon reflexes in all limbs.

PEDIATRIC POINTERS

- *An infant or young child with generalized flaccidity may lie in a froglike position, with his hips and knees abducted.*
- *Pediatric causes of muscle flaccidity include myelomeningocele, Lowe's disease, Werdnig-Hoffmann disease, and muscular dystrophy.*

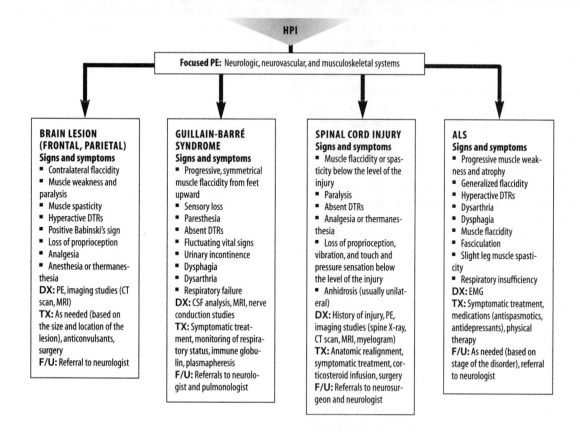

HPI

Focused PE: Neurologic, neurovascular, and musculoskeletal systems

BRAIN LESION (FRONTAL, PARIETAL)
Signs and symptoms
- Contralateral flaccidity
- Muscle weakness and paralysis
- Muscle spasticity
- Hyperactive DTRs
- Positive Babinski's sign
- Loss of proprioception
- Analgesia
- Anesthesia or thermanesthesia

DX: PE, imaging studies (CT scan, MRI)
TX: As needed (based on the size and location of the lesion), anticonvulsants, surgery
F/U: Referral to neurologist

GUILLAIN-BARRÉ SYNDROME
Signs and symptoms
- Progressive, symmetrical muscle flaccidity from feet upward
- Sensory loss
- Paresthesia
- Absent DTRs
- Fluctuating vital signs
- Urinary incontinence
- Dysphagia
- Dysarthria
- Respiratory failure

DX: CSF analysis, MRI, nerve conduction studies
TX: Symptomatic treatment, monitoring of respiratory status, immune globulin, plasmapheresis
F/U: Referrals to neurologist and pulmonologist

SPINAL CORD INJURY
Signs and symptoms
- Muscle flaccidity or spasticity below the level of the injury
- Paralysis
- Absent DTRs
- Analgesia or thermanesthesia
- Loss of proprioception, vibration, and touch and pressure sensation below the level of the injury
- Anhidrosis (usually unilateral)

DX: History of injury, PE, imaging studies (spine X-ray, CT scan, MRI, myelogram)
TX: Anatomic realignment, symptomatic treatment, corticosteroid infusion, surgery
F/U: Referrals to neurosurgeon and neurologist

ALS
Signs and symptoms
- Progressive muscle weakness and atrophy
- Generalized flaccidity
- Hyperactive DTRs
- Dysarthria
- Dysphagia
- Muscle flaccidity
- Fasciculation
- Slight leg muscle spasticity
- Respiratory insufficiency

DX: EMG
TX: Symptomatic treatment, medications (antispasmotics, antidepressants), physical therapy
F/U: As needed (based on stage of the disorder), referral to neurologist

Additional differential diagnoses: cerebellar disease ▪ Huntington's disease ▪ muscle disease ▪ peripheral nerve trauma ▪ peripheral neuropathy ▪ poliomyelitis ▪ seizure disorder

Muscle spasms and spasticity

Muscle spasms, also known as muscle cramps or muscle hypertonicity, are strong, painful contractions. They can occur in virtually any muscle but are most common in the calf and foot. Muscle spasms typically occur from simple muscle fatigue, after exercise, and during pregnancy. However, they may also develop in electrolyte imbalances and neuromuscular disorders, or as the result of certain drugs. They're often precipitated by movement and can usually be relieved by slow stretching.

Spasticity is a state of excessive muscle tone manifested by increased resistance to stretching and heightened reflexes. It's commonly detected by evaluating a muscle's response to passive movement; a spastic muscle offers more resistance when the passive movement is performed quickly. Caused by an upper-motor-neuron lesion, spasticity usually occurs in the arm and leg muscles. Long-term spasticity results in muscle fibrosis and contractures.

History and physical examination

If the patient isn't in distress, ask when the spasms began. How long did they last? How painful were they? Did anything worsen or lessen the pain? Ask about other symptoms, such as weakness, sensory loss, or paresthesia.

Evaluate muscle strength and tone. Then, check all major muscle groups, and note whether any movements precipitate spasms. Test the presence and quality of all peripheral pulses, and examine the limbs for color and temperature changes. Test capillary refill time and inspect for edema, especially in the involved area. Finally, test reflexes and sensory function in all extremities.

If you detect spasticity, ask the patient about its onset, duration, and progression. What, if any, events precipitate onset? Has he experienced other muscular changes or related symptoms? Does his medical history reveal any incidence of trauma or degenerative or vascular disease?

Take the patient's vital signs and perform a complete neurologic examination. Test reflexes and evaluate motor and sensory function in all limbs. Evaluate muscles for wasting and contractures.

During your examination, keep in mind that generalized spasticity and trismus in a patient with a recent skin puncture or laceration indicates tetanus. If you suspect this rare disorder, look for signs of respiratory distress. If necessary, provide ventilatory support and monitor the patient closely.

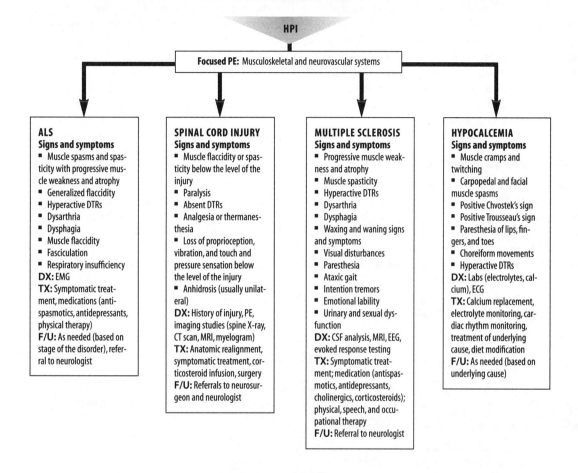

HPI

Focused PE: Musculoskeletal and neurovascular systems

ALS
Signs and symptoms
- Muscle spasms and spasticity with progressive muscle weakness and atrophy
- Generalized flaccidity
- Hyperactive DTRs
- Dysarthria
- Dysphagia
- Muscle flaccidity
- Fasciculation
- Respiratory insufficiency

DX: EMG
TX: Symptomatic treatment, medications (antispasmotics, antidepressants, physical therapy)
F/U: As needed (based on stage of the disorder), referral to neurologist

SPINAL CORD INJURY
Signs and symptoms
- Muscle flaccidity or spasticity below the level of the injury
- Paralysis
- Absent DTRs
- Analgesia or thermanesthesia
- Loss of proprioception, vibration, and touch and pressure sensation below the level of the injury
- Anhidrosis (usually unilateral)

DX: History of injury, PE, imaging studies (spine X-ray, CT scan, MRI, myelogram)
TX: Anatomic realignment, symptomatic treatment, corticosteroid infusion, surgery
F/U: Referrals to neurosurgeon and neurologist

MULTIPLE SCLEROSIS
Signs and symptoms
- Progressive muscle weakness and atrophy
- Muscle spasticity
- Hyperactive DTRs
- Dysarthria
- Dysphagia
- Waxing and waning signs and symptoms
- Visual disturbances
- Paresthesia
- Ataxic gait
- Intention tremors
- Emotional lability
- Urinary and sexual dysfunction

DX: CSF analysis, MRI, EEG, evoked response testing
TX: Symptomatic treatment; medication (antispasmotics, antidepressants, cholinergics, corticosteroids); physical, speech, and occupational therapy
F/U: Referral to neurologist

HYPOCALCEMIA
Signs and symptoms
- Muscle cramps and twitching
- Carpopedal and facial muscle spasms
- Positive Chvostek's sign
- Positive Trousseau's sign
- Paresthesia of lips, fingers, and toes
- Choreiform movements
- Hyperactive DTRs

DX: Labs (electrolytes, calcium), ECG
TX: Calcium replacement, electrolyte monitoring, cardiac rhythm monitoring, treatment of underlying cause, diet modification
F/U: As needed (based on underlying cause)

Additional differential diagnoses for muscle spasms: arterial occlusive disease ▪ dehydration ▪ fracture ▪ hypothyroidism ▪ respiratory alkalosis

Additional differential diagnoses for muscle spasticity: epidural hemorrhage ▪ stroke ▪ tetanus

Other causes for muscle spasm: diuretics ▪ corticosteroids ▪ estrogens

Muscle weakness

Muscle weakness is detected by observing and measuring the strength of an individual muscle or muscle group. It can result from a malfunction in the cerebral hemispheres, brain stem, spinal cord, nerve roots, peripheral nerves, or myoneural junctions and within the muscle itself. Muscle weakness occurs in certain neurologic, musculoskeletal, metabolic, endocrine, and cardiovascular disorders; as a response to certain drugs; and after prolonged immobilization.

History and physical examination

Begin by determining the location of the patient's muscle weakness. Ask if he has difficulty with any specific movements, such as rising from a chair. Find out when he first noticed the weakness; ask him whether it worsens with exercise or as the day progresses. Also ask about related symptoms, especially muscle or joint pain, altered sensory function, and fatigue.

Obtain a medical history, noting especially chronic disease such as hyperthyroidism; musculoskeletal or neurologic problems, including recent trauma; family history of chronic muscle weakness, especially in males; and alcohol and drug use.

Focus your physical examination on evaluating muscle strength. Test all major muscles bilaterally. (See *Testing muscle strength*.) When testing, be sure the patient's effort is constant; if it isn't, suspect pain or other reluctance to make the effort. If the patient complains of pain, ease or discontinue testing and have him try the movements again. Remember that the patient's dominant arm, hand, and leg are somewhat stronger than his nondominant counterparts. In addition to testing individual muscle strength, test for range of motion at all major joints (shoulder, elbow, wrist, hip, knee, ankle). Also test sensory function in the involved areas, and test deep tendon reflexes bilaterally.

PEDIATRIC POINTER

Muscular dystrophy, usually the Duchenne type, is a major cause of muscle weakness in children.

Testing muscle strength

Obtain an overall picture of your patient's motor function by testing muscle strength in ten selected muscle groups. Ask the patient to attempt normal range-of-motion movements against your resistance. If the muscle group is weak, vary the amount of resistance as necessary to permit accurate assessment. If necessary, position the patient so that his limbs don't have to resist gravity, and repeat the test.

Use the following scale to help you rate muscle strength.

0 = Total paralysis
1 = Visible or palpable contraction but no movement
2 = Full muscle movement with force of gravity eliminated
3 = Full muscle movement against gravity, but no movement against resistance

4 = Full muscle movement against gravity; partial movement against resistance
5 = Full muscle movement against both gravity and resistance — normal strength

ARM MUSCLES

Biceps
With your hand on the patient's hand, ask him to flex his forearm against your resistance; observe for biceps contraction.

Deltoid muscle
With the patient's arm fully extended, place one hand over his deltoid muscle and the other on his wrist. Ask him to abduct his arm to a horizontal position against your resistance; as he does so, palpate for deltoid contraction.

Triceps
Ask the patient to abduct and hold his arm midway between flexion and extension. Hold and support his arm at the wrist, and ask him to extend it against your resistance. Observe for triceps contraction.

Dorsal interossei
Ask the patient to extend and spread his fingers, and tell him to try to resist your attempt to squeeze them together.

Forearm and hand (grip)
Ask the patient to grasp your middle and index fingers and squeeze as hard as he can.

LEG MUSCLES

Anterior tibial
With the patient's leg extended, place your hand on his foot and ask him to dorsiflex his ankle against your resistance.

Psoas
While you support his leg, ask the patient to raise his knee and then flex his hip against your resistance. Observe for psoas muscle contraction.

Extensor hallucis longus
With your finger on the patient's great toe, ask him to dorsiflex the toe against your resistance. Palpate for extensor hallucis contraction.

Quadriceps
Ask the patient to bend his knee slightly while you support his lower leg. Then ask him to extend the knee against your resistance; as he's doing so, palpate for quadriceps contraction.

Gastrocnemius
With the patient on his side, support his foot and ask him to plantarflex his ankle against your resistance. Palpate for gastrocnemius contraction.

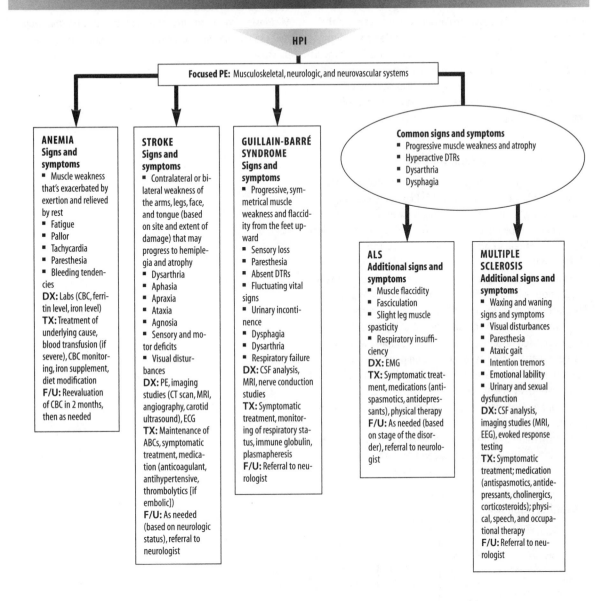

HPI

Focused PE: Musculoskeletal, neurologic, and neurovascular systems

ANEMIA
Signs and symptoms
- Muscle weakness that's exacerbated by exertion and relieved by rest
- Fatigue
- Pallor
- Tachycardia
- Paresthesia
- Bleeding tendencies

DX: Labs (CBC, ferritin level, iron level)
TX: Treatment of underlying cause, blood transfusion (if severe), CBC monitoring, iron supplement, diet modification
F/U: Reevaluation of CBC in 2 months, then as needed

STROKE
Signs and symptoms
- Contralateral or bilateral weakness of the arms, legs, face, and tongue (based on site and extent of damage) that may progress to hemiplegia and atrophy
- Dysarthria
- Aphasia
- Apraxia
- Ataxia
- Agnosia
- Sensory and motor deficits
- Visual disturbances

DX: PE, imaging studies (CT scan, MRI, angiography, carotid ultrasound), ECG
TX: Maintenance of ABCs, symptomatic treatment, medication (anticoagulant, antihypertensive, thrombolytics [if embolic])
F/U: As needed (based on neurologic status), referral to neurologist

GUILLAIN-BARRÉ SYNDROME
Signs and symptoms
- Progressive, symmetrical muscle weakness and flaccidity from the feet upward
- Sensory loss
- Paresthesia
- Absent DTRs
- Fluctuating vital signs
- Urinary incontinence
- Dysphagia
- Dysarthria
- Respiratory failure

DX: CSF analysis, MRI, nerve conduction studies
TX: Symptomatic treatment, monitoring of respiratory status, immune globulin, plasmapheresis
F/U: Referral to neurologist

Common signs and symptoms
- Progressive muscle weakness and atrophy
- Hyperactive DTRs
- Dysarthria
- Dysphagia

ALS
Additional signs and symptoms
- Muscle flaccidity
- Fasciculation
- Slight leg muscle spasticity
- Respiratory insufficiency

DX: EMG
TX: Symptomatic treatment, medications (antispasmotics, antidepressants), physical therapy
F/U: As needed (based on stage of the disorder), referral to neurologist

MULTIPLE SCLEROSIS
Additional signs and symptoms
- Waxing and waning signs and symptoms
- Visual disturbances
- Paresthesia
- Ataxic gait
- Intention tremors
- Emotional lability
- Urinary and sexual dysfunction

DX: CSF analysis, imaging studies (MRI, EEG), evoked response testing
TX: Symptomatic treatment; medication (antispasmotics, antidepressants, cholinergics, corticosteroids); physical, speech, and occupational therapy
F/U: Referral to neurologist

Additional differential diagnoses: brain tumor ▪ head trauma ▪ herniated disk ▪ Hodgkin's disease ▪ hypercortisolism ▪ hypothyroidism ▪ myasthenia gravis ▪ osteoarthritis ▪ Paget's disease ▪ Parkinson's disease ▪ peripheral nerve trauma ▪ peripheral neuropathy ▪ poliomyelitis ▪ polymyositis ▪ potassium imbalance ▪ protein deficiency ▪ rheumatoid arthritis ▪ seizure disorder ▪ spinal trauma and disease ▪ thyrotoxicosis

Other causes: prolonged corticosteroid use ▪ digitalis toxicity ▪ excessive doses of dantrolene ▪ aminoglycoside antibiotics (may worsen weakness in patients with myasthenia gravis) ▪ immobility ▪ prolonged bed rest ▪ inactivity

Mydriasis

Mydriasis — pupillary dilation caused by contraction of the dilator of the iris — is a normal response to decreased light, strong emotional stimuli, and topical administration of mydriatic and cycloplegic drugs. It can also result from ocular and neurologic disorders, eye trauma, and disorders that decrease level of consciousness. Mydriasis may be an adverse effect of antihistamines or other drugs.

History and physical examination

Begin by asking the patient about other eye problems, such as pain, blurring, diplopia, or visual field defects. Obtain a health history, focusing on eye or head trauma, glaucoma and other ocular problems, and neurologic and vascular disorders. In addition, obtain a complete medication history.

Next, perform a thorough eye and pupil examination. Inspect and compare the pupils' size, color, and shape — many people normally have unequal pupils. (See *Grading pupil size*.) Also, test each pupil for light reflex, consensual response, and accommodation. Perform a swinging flashlight test to evaluate a decreased response to direct light coupled with a normal consensual response (Marcus Gunn pupil). Be sure to check the eyes for ptosis, swelling, and ecchymosis. Test visual acuity in both eyes with and without correction. Evaluate extraocular muscle function by checking the six cardinal fields of gaze.

Keep in mind that mydriasis appears in two ocular emergencies: acute angle-closure glaucoma and traumatic iridoplegia.

Mydriasis occurs in children as a result of ocular trauma, drugs, Adie's syndrome and, most frequently, increased intracranial pressure.

Grading pupil size

To ensure accurate evaluation of pupillary size, compare your patient's pupils with the scale at right. Keep in mind that maximum constriction may be less than 1 mm and maximum dilation greater than 9 mm.

1 mm	2 mm	3 mm
4 mm	5 mm	6 mm
7 mm	8 mm	9 mm

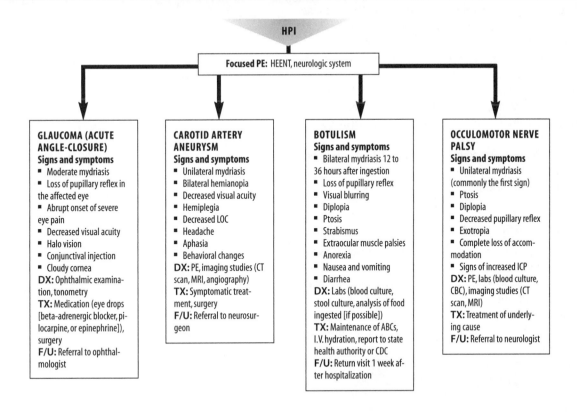

HPI

Focused PE: HEENT, neurologic system

GLAUCOMA (ACUTE ANGLE-CLOSURE)
Signs and symptoms
- Moderate mydriasis
- Loss of pupillary reflex in the affected eye
- Abrupt onset of severe eye pain
- Decreased visual acuity
- Halo vision
- Conjunctival injection
- Cloudy cornea

DX: Ophthalmic examination, tonometry
TX: Medication (eye drops [beta-adrenergic blocker, pilocarpine, or epinephrine]), surgery
F/U: Referral to ophthalmologist

CAROTID ARTERY ANEURYSM
Signs and symptoms
- Unilateral mydriasis
- Bilateral hemianopia
- Decreased visual acuity
- Hemiplegia
- Decreased LOC
- Headache
- Aphasia
- Behavioral changes

DX: PE, imaging studies (CT scan, MRI, angiography)
TX: Symptomatic treatment, surgery
F/U: Referral to neurosurgeon

BOTULISM
Signs and symptoms
- Bilateral mydriasis 12 to 36 hours after ingestion
- Loss of pupillary reflex
- Visual blurring
- Diplopia
- Ptosis
- Strabismus
- Extraocular muscle palsies
- Anorexia
- Nausea and vomiting
- Diarrhea

DX: Labs (blood culture, stool culture, analysis of food ingested [if possible])
TX: Maintenance of ABCs, I.V. hydration, report to state health authority or CDC
F/U: Return visit 1 week after hospitalization

OCCULOMOTOR NERVE PALSY
Signs and symptoms
- Unilateral mydriasis (commonly the first sign)
- Ptosis
- Diplopia
- Decreased pupillary reflex
- Exotropia
- Complete loss of accommodation
- Signs of increased ICP

DX: PE, labs (blood culture, CBC), imaging studies (CT scan, MRI)
TX: Treatment of underlying cause
F/U: Referral to neurologist

Additional differential diagnoses: Adie's syndrome ▪ aortic arch syndrome ▪ brain stem infarction ▪ traumatic iridoplegia

---

Other causes: anticholinergics ▪ antihistamines ▪ sympathomimetics ▪ barbiturate overdose ▪ estrogens ▪ tricyclic antidepressants ▪ anesthesia induction ▪ topical mydriatics and cycloplegics ▪ ocular surgery

Myoclonus

Myoclonus — sudden, shocklike contractions of a single muscle or muscle group — occurs in various neurologic disorders and often heralds onset of a seizure. These contractions may be isolated or repetitive, rhythmic or arrhythmic, symmetrical or asymmetrical, synchronous or asynchronous, and generalized or focal. They may be precipitated by bright flickering lights, a loud sound, or unexpected physical contact. One type, *intention myoclonus*, is evoked by intentional muscle movement.

Myoclonus occurs normally just before falling asleep and as a part of the natural startle reaction. It also occurs with some poisonings and, rarely, as a complication of hemodialysis.

History and physical examination

If the patient is stable, evaluate his level of consciousness and mental status. Ask about the frequency, severity, location, and circumstances of the myoclonus. Has he ever had a seizure? If so, did myoclonus precede it? Is the myoclonus ever precipitated by a sensory stimulus? During the physical examination, check for muscle rigidity and wasting, and test deep tendon reflexes.

PEDIATRIC POINTER

Although myoclonus is relatively uncommon in infants and children, it can result from subacute sclerosing panencephalitis, severe meningitis, progressive poliodystrophy, childhood myoclonic epilepsy, and encephalopathies, such as Reye's syndrome.

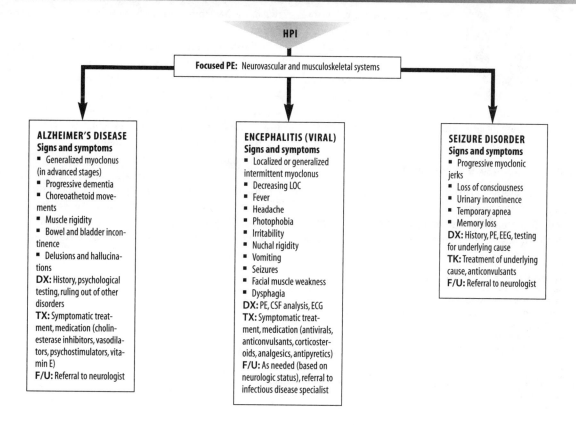

HPI

Focused PE: Neurovascular and musculoskeletal systems

ALZHEIMER'S DISEASE
Signs and symptoms
- Generalized myoclonus (in advanced stages)
- Progressive dementia
- Choreoathetoid movements
- Muscle rigidity
- Bowel and bladder incontinence
- Delusions and hallucinations

DX: History, psychological testing, ruling out of other disorders
TX: Symptomatic treatment, medication (cholinesterase inhibitors, vasodilators, psychostimulators, vitamin E)
F/U: Referral to neurologist

ENCEPHALITIS (VIRAL)
Signs and symptoms
- Localized or generalized intermittent myoclonus
- Decreasing LOC
- Fever
- Headache
- Photophobia
- Irritability
- Nuchal rigidity
- Vomiting
- Seizures
- Facial muscle weakness
- Dysphagia

DX: PE, CSF analysis, ECG
TX: Symptomatic treatment, medication (antivirals, anticonvulsants, corticosteroids, analgesics, antipyretics)
F/U: As needed (based on neurologic status), referral to infectious disease specialist

SEIZURE DISORDER
Signs and symptoms
- Progressive myoclonic jerks
- Loss of consciousness
- Urinary incontinence
- Temporary apnea
- Memory loss

DX: History, PE, EEG, testing for underlying cause
TK: Treatment of underlying cause, anticonvulsants
F/U: Referral to neurologist

Additional differential diagnoses: Creutzfeldt-Jakob disease ▪ encephalopathy

---

Other causes: drug withdrawal ▪ delirium tremens ▪ poisoning

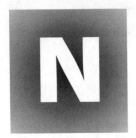

Nasal flaring

Nasal flaring is abnormal dilatation of the nostrils. It usually occurs during inspiration, although nasal flaring may occasionally occur during expiration or throughout the respiratory cycle. It indicates respiratory dysfunction, ranging from mild difficulty to potentially life-threatening respiratory distress.

History and physical examination

If you note nasal flaring in the patient, quickly evaluate his respiratory status. Inspiratory chest movement, absent breath sounds, cyanosis, diaphoresis, and tachycardia point to complete airway obstruction. As necessary, deliver back blows or abdominal thrusts (Heimlich maneuver) to relieve the obstruction. If these don't clear the airway, emergency intubation or tracheostomy and mechanical ventilation may be necessary.

If the patient displays breathing difficulty without an obstructed airway, give oxygen by nasal cannula or face mask. Intubation and mechanical ventilation may be necessary. After the patient is stabilized, obtain a pertinent history. Ask about cardiac and pulmonary disorders such as asthma. Does the patient have allergies? Has he experienced a recent illness (such as a respiratory infection) or trauma?

PEDIATRIC POINTERS

- *Nasal flaring is an important sign of respiratory distress in infants and very young children who can't verbalize their discomfort. (See Recognizing respiratory distress in infants.)*
- *Common causes include airway obstruction, hyaline membrane disease, croup, and acute epiglottiditis.*

Recognizing respiratory distress in infants

Because infants can't verbalize their symptoms, you'll need to teach parents how to recognize the signs of infant respiratory distress. Using these illustrations, show them how to evaluate nasal flaring. This sign, along with retractions and grunting on expiration, is graded to measure the severity of respiratory distress.

GRADE 0
The infant breathes normally, with no nasal flaring.

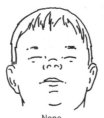

None

GRADE 1
The infant shows some signs of respiratory distress, including slightly flared nostrils and a slightly visible rib cage on inspiration. Instruct the parents to watch the infant closely and to begin measures to help him breathe more easily.

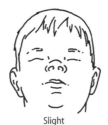

Slight

GRADE 2
The infant has pronounced respiratory distress. His nostrils flare widely, his rib cage is quite visible on exhalation, and he grunts as he exhales. Tell the parents to call the health care provider immediately and to continue measures to make breathing easier.

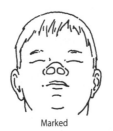

Marked

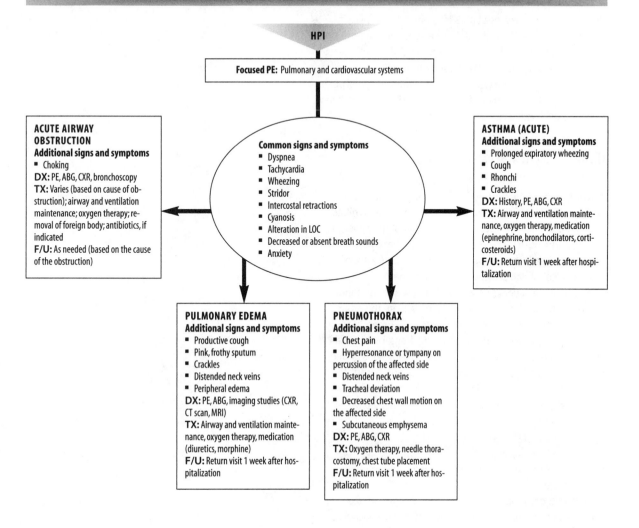

HPI

Focused PE: Pulmonary and cardiovascular systems

Common signs and symptoms
- Dyspnea
- Tachycardia
- Wheezing
- Stridor
- Intercostal retractions
- Cyanosis
- Alteration in LOC
- Decreased or absent breath sounds
- Anxiety

ACUTE AIRWAY OBSTRUCTION
Additional signs and symptoms
- Choking

DX: PE, ABG, CXR, bronchoscopy
TX: Varies (based on cause of obstruction); airway and ventilation maintenance; oxygen therapy; removal of foreign body; antibiotics, if indicated
F/U: As needed (based on the cause of the obstruction)

ASTHMA (ACUTE)
Additional signs and symptoms
- Prolonged expiratory wheezing
- Cough
- Rhonchi
- Crackles

DX: History, PE, ABG, CXR
TX: Airway and ventilation maintenance, oxygen therapy, medication (epinephrine, bronchodilators, corticosteroids)
F/U: Return visit 1 week after hospitalization

PULMONARY EDEMA
Additional signs and symptoms
- Productive cough
- Pink, frothy sputum
- Crackles
- Distended neck veins
- Peripheral edema

DX: PE, ABG, imaging studies (CXR, CT scan, MRI)
TX: Airway and ventilation maintenance, oxygen therapy, medication (diuretics, morphine)
F/U: Return visit 1 week after hospitalization

PNEUMOTHORAX
Additional signs and symptoms
- Chest pain
- Hyperresonance or tympany on percussion of the affected side
- Distended neck veins
- Tracheal deviation
- Decreased chest wall motion on the affected side
- Subcutaneous emphysema

DX: PE, ABG, CXR
TX: Oxygen therapy, needle thoracostomy, chest tube placement
F/U: Return visit 1 week after hospitalization

Additional differential diagnoses: anaphylaxis ▪ ARDS ▪ COPD ▪ pneumonia (bacterial) ▪ pulmonary embolus

Other causes: PFT such as vital capacity testing ▪ deep breathing

Nasal obstruction

Nasal obstruction may result from inflammatory, neoplastic, endocrine, and metabolic disorders as well as structural abnormalities and traumatic injuries. It may cause discomfort, alter a person's sense of taste and smell, and cause voice changes. Although a frequent and typically benign symptom, nasal obstruction may herald certain life-threatening disorders, such as a basilar skull fracture or malignant tumors.

History and physical examination

Begin the history by asking the patient about the duration and frequency of the obstruction. Did it begin suddenly or gradually? Is it intermittent or persistent? Unilateral or bilateral? Inquire about the presence and character of drainage. Is it watery, purulent, or bloody? Does the patient have nasal or sinus pain or headaches? Ask about recent travel, the use of drugs or alcohol, and previous trauma or surgery.

Examine the patient's nose; assess airflow and the condition of the turbinates and nasal septum. Evaluate the orbits for any evidence of dystopia, decreased vision, excess tearing, or abnormal appearance. Palpate over the frontal and maxillary sinuses for tenderness. Examine the ears for signs of middle ear effusions. Inspect the oral cavity, pharynx, nasopharynx, and larynx to detect inflammation, ulceration, excessive mucosal dryness, and neurologic deficits. Finally, palpate the neck for adenopathy.

PEDIATRIC POINTERS

- *Acute nasal obstruction in children often results from the common cold.*
- *In infants and children, especially between ages 3 and 6, chronic nasal obstruction typically results from large adenoids.*
- *In neonates, choanal atresia is the most common congenital cause of nasal obstruction, and it may be unilateral or bilateral.*
- *Cystic fibrosis may cause nasal polyps in children, resulting in nasal obstruction. However, if the child has unilateral nasal obstruction and rhinorrhea, you should assume a foreign body in the nose until proven otherwise.*

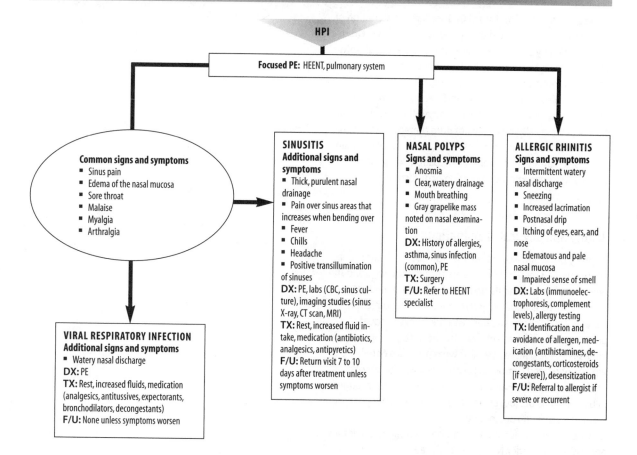

HPI

Focused PE: HEENT, pulmonary system

Common signs and symptoms
- Sinus pain
- Edema of the nasal mucosa
- Sore throat
- Malaise
- Myalgia
- Arthralgia

VIRAL RESPIRATORY INFECTION
Additional signs and symptoms
- Watery nasal discharge
DX: PE
TX: Rest, increased fluids, medication (analgesics, antitussives, expectorants, bronchodilators, decongestants)
F/U: None unless symptoms worsen

SINUSITIS
Additional signs and symptoms
- Thick, purulent nasal drainage
- Pain over sinus areas that increases when bending over
- Fever
- Chills
- Headache
- Positive transillumination of sinuses
DX: PE, labs (CBC, sinus culture), imaging studies (sinus X-ray, CT scan, MRI)
TX: Rest, increased fluid intake, medication (antibiotics, analgesics, antipyretics)
F/U: Return visit 7 to 10 days after treatment unless symptoms worsen

NASAL POLYPS
Signs and symptoms
- Anosmia
- Clear, watery drainage
- Mouth breathing
- Gray grapelike mass noted on nasal examination
DX: History of allergies, asthma, sinus infection (common), PE
TX: Surgery
F/U: Refer to HEENT specialist

ALLERGIC RHINITIS
Signs and symptoms
- Intermittent watery nasal discharge
- Sneezing
- Increased lacrimation
- Postnasal drip
- Itching of eyes, ears, and nose
- Edematous and pale nasal mucosa
- Impaired sense of smell
DX: Labs (immunoelectrophoresis, complement levels), allergy testing
TX: Identification and avoidance of allergen, medication (antihistamines, decongestants, corticosteroids [if severe]), desensitization
F/U: Referral to allergist if severe or recurrent

Additional differential diagnoses: basilar skull fracture ▪ hypothyroidism ▪ nasal deformities ▪ nasal fracture ▪ nasal tumors ▪ nasopharyngeal tumors ▪ sarcoidosis ▪ Wegener's granulomatosis

Other causes: topical nasal vasoconstrictors ▪ antihypertensives ▪ sinus or cranial surgery ▪ rhinoplasty

Nausea

Nausea, a common symptom of GI disorders, is a sensation of profound revulsion to food or of impending vomiting. Often accompanied by such autonomic signs as hypersalivation, diaphoresis, tachycardia, pallor, and tachypnea, it's closely associated with both anorexia and vomiting.

Nausea also occurs with fluid and electrolyte imbalance, infection, and metabolic, endocrine, labyrinthine, and cardiac disorders. It may also be a result of drug therapy, surgery, and radiation. Often present during the first trimester of pregnancy, nausea may also arise from severe pain, anxiety, alcohol intoxication, overeating, or ingestion of distasteful food or liquids.

History and physical examination

Begin by obtaining a complete medical history. Focus on GI, endocrine, and metabolic disorders; recent infections; and the presence of cancer and its treatment. Ask about medication use, alcohol consumption, and recent diet. If the patient is a female of childbearing age, ask whether she is or could be pregnant. Have the patient describe the onset, duration, and intensity of the nausea as well as what provokes or relieves it. Ask about related complaints, particularly vomiting (color, amount), abdominal pain, anorexia and weight loss, changes in bowel habits or stool character, excessive belching or flatus, and a sensation of bloating.

Inspect the skin for jaundice, bruises, and spider angiomas, and assess skin turgor. Next, inspect the abdomen for distention, auscultate for bowel sounds and bruits, palpate for rigidity and tenderness, and test for rebound tenderness. Palpate and percuss the liver for enlargement. Assess other body systems as appropriate.

PEDIATRIC POINTERS

- *Nausea, frequently described as stomachache, is one of the most common childhood complaints.*
- *Commonly the result of overeating, it can also occur as part of diverse disorders, ranging from acute infections to a conversion reaction caused by fear.*

ELDER CARE CUE

Elderly patients have increased dental caries; more frequent tooth loss; decreased salivary gland function, which causes mouth dryness; reduced gastric acid output and motility; and decreased senses of taste and smell. All of these may be factors contributing to nonpathologic nausea.

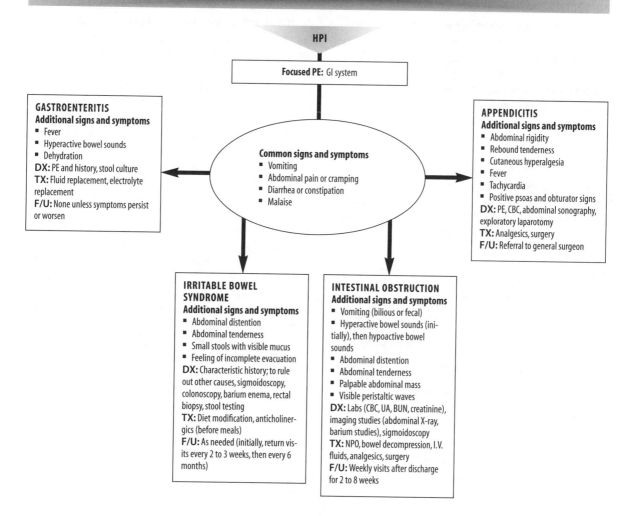

HPI

Focused PE: GI system

Common signs and symptoms
- Vomiting
- Abdominal pain or cramping
- Diarrhea or constipation
- Malaise

GASTROENTERITIS
Additional signs and symptoms
- Fever
- Hyperactive bowel sounds
- Dehydration

DX: PE and history, stool culture
TX: Fluid replacement, electrolyte replacement
F/U: None unless symptoms persist or worsen

APPENDICITIS
Additional signs and symptoms
- Abdominal rigidity
- Rebound tenderness
- Cutaneous hyperalgesia
- Fever
- Tachycardia
- Positive psoas and obturator signs

DX: PE, CBC, abdominal sonography, exploratory laparotomy
TX: Analgesics, surgery
F/U: Referral to general surgeon

IRRITABLE BOWEL SYNDROME
Additional signs and symptoms
- Abdominal distention
- Abdominal tenderness
- Small stools with visible mucus
- Feeling of incomplete evacuation

DX: Characteristic history; to rule out other causes, sigmoidoscopy, colonoscopy, barium enema, rectal biopsy, stool testing
TX: Diet modification, anticholinergics (before meals)
F/U: As needed (initially, return visits every 2 to 3 weeks, then every 6 months)

INTESTINAL OBSTRUCTION
Additional signs and symptoms
- Vomiting (bilious or fecal)
- Hyperactive bowel sounds (initially), then hypoactive bowel sounds
- Abdominal distention
- Abdominal tenderness
- Palpable abdominal mass
- Visible peristaltic waves

DX: Labs (CBC, UA, BUN, creatinine), imaging studies (abdominal X-ray, barium studies), sigmoidoscopy
TX: NPO, bowel decompression, I.V. fluids, analgesics, surgery
F/U: Weekly visits after discharge for 2 to 8 weeks

Additional differential diagnoses: adrenal insufficiency ▪ cholecystitis (acute) ▪ cholelithiasis ▪ diverticulitis ▪ ectopic pregnancy ▪ electrolyte imbalances ▪ gastric cancer ▪ gastritis ▪ hepatitis ▪ hyperemesis gravidarum ▪ infection ▪ inflammatory bowel disease ▪ labyrinthitis ▪ Ménière's disease ▪ mesenteric artery ischemia ▪ mesenteric venous thrombosis ▪ metabolic acidosis ▪ migraine headache ▪ motion sickness ▪ MI ▪ pancreatitis (acute) ▪ peptic ulcer ▪ peritonitis ▪ preeclampsia ▪ renal and urologic disorders ▪ thyrotoxicosis

Other causes: antineoplastics ▪ opiates ▪ ferrous sulfate ▪ levodopa ▪ oral potassium chloride replacements ▪ estrogens ▪ sulfasalazine ▪ antibiotics ▪ quinidine ▪ anesthetic agents ▪ digitalis or theophylline overdose ▪ ginkgo biloba ▪ St. John's wort ▪ radiation therapy ▪ abdominal surgery

Neck pain

Neck pain may originate from any neck structure, ranging from the meninges and cervical vertebrae to its blood vessels, muscles, and lymphatic tissue. This symptom can also be referred from other areas of the body. Its location, onset, and pattern help determine its origin and underlying causes. Neck pain usually results from trauma and degenerative, congenital, inflammatory, metabolic, and neoplastic disorders.

History and physical examination

If the patient's neck pain is due to trauma, first ensure proper cervical spine immobilization, preferably with a long backboard and a hard cervical collar. (See *Applying a Philadelphia collar.*) Then take vital signs, and perform a quick neurologic evaluation. If he shows signs of respiratory distress, give oxygen. Intubation and mechanical ventilation may be necessary. Ask the patient (or his companion, if the patient can't answer) how the injury occurred. Then examine the neck for abrasions, swelling, lacerations, erythema, and ecchymoses.

If the patient hasn't sustained trauma, find out the severity and onset of his neck pain. Where in the neck does he feel pain? Does anything relieve or worsen the pain? Also, ask about the development of other symptoms such as headaches. Next, focus on the patient's current and past illnesses and injuries, diet, medication use, and family health history.

Thoroughly inspect the patient's neck, shoulders, and cervical spine for swelling, masses, erythema, and ecchymoses. Palpate the cervical spine and paracervical area, checking for muscle spasm. Assess active range of motion in his neck by having him perform selection, extension, rotation, and lateral side bending. Note the degree of pain produced by these movements. Examine posture, and test muscle strength. Check the sensation in his arms, and assess his hand grasp and arm reflexes. Attempt to elicit Brudzinski's and Kernig's signs, and palpate the cervical lymph nodes for enlargement.

PEDIATRIC POINTERS

- *The most common causes of neck pain in children are meningitis and trauma.*
- *A rare cause of neck pain is congenital torticollis.*

Applying a Philadelphia collar

A lightweight molded polyethylene collar designed to hold the neck straight with the chin slightly elevated and tucked in, the Philadelphia cervical collar immobilizes the cervical spine, decreases muscle spasms, and relieves some pain. It also prevents further injury and promotes healing.

When applying the collar, fit it snugly around the patient's neck and attach the Velcro fasteners or buckles at the back. Be sure to check the patient's airway and his neurovascular status to ensure that the collar isn't too tight. Also, make sure that the collar isn't placed too high in front, which can hyperextend the neck. In a patient with a neck sprain, hyperextension may cause the ligaments to heal in a shortened position; in a patient with a cervical spine fracture, it could cause serious neurologic damage.

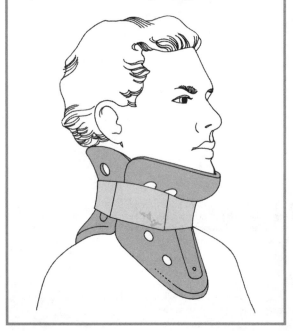

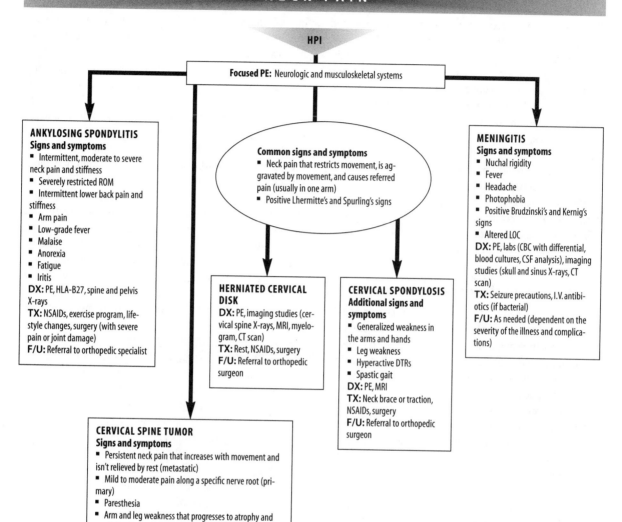

HPI

Focused PE: Neurologic and musculoskeletal systems

ANKYLOSING SPONDYLITIS
Signs and symptoms
- Intermittent, moderate to severe neck pain and stiffness
- Severely restricted ROM
- Intermittent lower back pain and stiffness
- Arm pain
- Low-grade fever
- Malaise
- Anorexia
- Fatigue
- Iritis

DX: PE, HLA-B27, spine and pelvis X-rays
TX: NSAIDs, exercise program, lifestyle changes, surgery (with severe pain or joint damage)
F/U: Referral to orthopedic specialist

Common signs and symptoms
- Neck pain that restricts movement, is aggravated by movement, and causes referred pain (usually in one arm)
- Positive Lhermitte's and Spurling's signs

HERNIATED CERVICAL DISK
DX: PE, imaging studies (cervical spine X-rays, MRI, myelogram, CT scan)
TX: Rest, NSAIDs, surgery
F/U: Referral to orthopedic surgeon

CERVICAL SPONDYLOSIS
Additional signs and symptoms
- Generalized weakness in the arms and hands
- Leg weakness
- Hyperactive DTRs
- Spastic gait

DX: PE, MRI
TX: Neck brace or traction, NSAIDs, surgery
F/U: Referral to orthopedic surgeon

MENINGITIS
Signs and symptoms
- Nuchal rigidity
- Fever
- Headache
- Photophobia
- Positive Brudzinski's and Kernig's signs
- Altered LOC

DX: PE, labs (CBC with differential, blood cultures, CSF analysis), imaging studies (skull and sinus X-rays, CT scan)
TX: Seizure precautions, I.V. antibiotics (if bacterial)
F/U: As needed (dependent on the severity of the illness and complications)

CERVICAL SPINE TUMOR
Signs and symptoms
- Persistent neck pain that increases with movement and isn't relieved by rest (metastatic)
- Mild to moderate pain along a specific nerve root (primary)
- Paresthesia
- Arm and leg weakness that progresses to atrophy and paralysis

DX: PE, imaging studies (cervical spine X-ray, CT scan, MRI)
TX: Medication (analgesics, chemotherapy), radiation therapy, surgery
F/U: Referrals to neurosurgeon and oncologist

Additional differential diagnoses: cervical extension injury ▪ cervical fibrositis ▪ cervical spine fracture ▪ cervical spine infection (acute) ▪ cervical stenosis ▪ esophageal trauma ▪ Hodgkin's lymphoma ▪ laryngeal cancer ▪ lymphadenitis ▪ neck sprain ▪ osteoporosis ▪ Paget's disease ▪ rheumatoid arthritis ▪ spinous process fracture ▪ subarachnoid hemorrhage ▪ thyroid trauma ▪ torticollis ▪ tracheal trauma

Nipple discharge

Nipple discharge can occur spontaneously or can be elicited by nipple stimulation. It's characterized by duration (intermittent or constant), extent (unilateral or bilateral), color, consistency, and composition. Its incidence increases with age and parity. This sign rarely occurs (but is more likely to be pathologic) in men and in nulligravid, regularly menstruating women. It's relatively common and often normal in parous women. A thick, grayish discharge — benign epithelial debris from inactive ducts — can often be elicited in middle-aged, parous women. Colostrum (a thin, yellowish or milky discharge) often occurs in the last weeks of pregnancy.

Nipple discharge can signal serious underlying disease, particularly when accompanied by other breast changes. Significant causes include endocrine disorders, cancer, certain drugs, and blocked lactiferous ducts.

History and physical examination

Ask the patient when she first noticed the discharge, and determine its duration, extent, quantity, color, and consistency. Has she had other nipple and breast changes, such as pain, tenderness, itching, warmth, changes in contour, and lumps? If she reports a lump, question her about its onset, location, size, and consistency.

Obtain a complete gynecologic and obstetric history, and determine her normal menstrual cycle and the date of her last menses. Ask whether she experiences breast swelling and tenderness, bloating, irritability, headaches, abdominal cramping, nausea, or diarrhea before or during menses. Note the number, date, and outcome of her pregnancies and, if she breast-fed, the approximate time of her last lactation. Also, check for any risk factors of breast cancer, such as family history, previous or current malignancies, nulliparity or first pregnancy after age 30, early menarche, or late menopause.

Start your physical examination by characterizing the discharge. If the discharge isn't frank, try to elicit it. (See *Eliciting nipple discharge.*) Then examine the nipples and breasts with the patient in four different positions: sitting with her arms at her sides, sitting with her arms overhead, sitting with her hands pressing on her hips, and leaning forward so her breasts are suspended. Check for nipple deviation, flattening, retraction, redness, asymmetry, thickening, excoriation, erosion, and cracking. Inspect her breasts for asymmetry, irregular contours, dimpling, erythema, and peau d'orange. With the patient supine, palpate the breasts and axilla for lumps, giving special attention to the areolae. Note the size, location, delineation, consistency, and mobility of any lump you find.

Is the patient taking hormones (oral contraceptive pills or hormone replacement therapy)? Is the discharge spontaneous, or does it have to be expressed? Is the discharge bloody?

Eliciting nipple discharge

If your patient has a history or evidence of nipple discharge, you can attempt to elicit it during your examination. Position the patient supine, and gently squeeze her nipple between your thumb and index finger; note any discharge through the nipple. Then place your fingers on the areola, as shown, and palpate the entire areolar surface, watching for any discharge through areolar ducts.

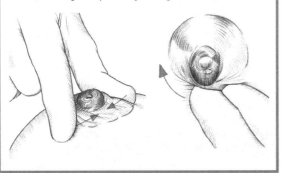

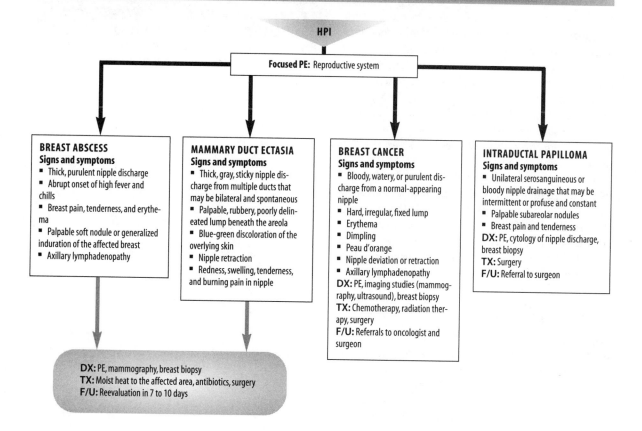

HPI

Focused PE: Reproductive system

BREAST ABSCESS
Signs and symptoms
- Thick, purulent nipple discharge
- Abrupt onset of high fever and chills
- Breast pain, tenderness, and erythema
- Palpable soft nodule or generalized induration of the affected breast
- Axillary lymphadenopathy

MAMMARY DUCT ECTASIA
Signs and symptoms
- Thick, gray, sticky nipple discharge from multiple ducts that may be bilateral and spontaneous
- Palpable, rubbery, poorly delineated lump beneath the areola
- Blue-green discoloration of the overlying skin
- Nipple retraction
- Redness, swelling, tenderness, and burning pain in nipple

BREAST CANCER
Signs and symptoms
- Bloody, watery, or purulent discharge from a normal-appearing nipple
- Hard, irregular, fixed lump
- Erythema
- Dimpling
- Peau d'orange
- Nipple deviation or retraction
- Axillary lymphadenopathy
DX: PE, imaging studies (mammography, ultrasound), breast biopsy
TX: Chemotherapy, radiation therapy, surgery
F/U: Referrals to oncologist and surgeon

INTRADUCTAL PAPILLOMA
Signs and symptoms
- Unilateral serosanguineous or bloody nipple drainage that may be intermittent or profuse and constant
- Palpable subareolar nodules
- Breast pain and tenderness
DX: PE, cytology of nipple discharge, breast biopsy
TX: Surgery
F/U: Referral to surgeon

DX: PE, mammography, breast biopsy
TX: Moist heat to the affected area, antibiotics, surgery
F/U: Reevaluation in 7 to 10 days

Additional differential diagnoses: choriocarcinoma ▪ herpes zoster ▪ hypothyroidism ▪ prolactin-secreting pituitary tumor ▪ proliferative (fibrocystic) breast disease ▪ trauma

Other causes: psychotropic agents (particularly phenothiazines and tricyclic antidepressants) ▪ antihypertensives (reserpine, methyldopa) ▪ oral contraceptives ▪ cimetidine ▪ metoclopramide ▪ verapamil ▪ chest wall surgery

Nocturia

Nocturia — excessive urination at night — may result from disruption of the normal diurnal pattern of urine concentration or from overstimulation of the nerves and muscles that control urination. Normally, more urine is concentrated during the night than during the day. As a result, most persons excrete three to four times more urine during the day and can sleep for 6 to 8 hours during the night without being awakened. In nocturia, the patient may awaken one or more times during the night to empty his bladder and may excrete 700 ml or more of urine.

Although nocturia usually results from renal and lower urinary tract disorders, it may also result from certain cardiovascular, endocrine, and metabolic disorders. This common sign may also result from drugs that induce diuresis — particularly when they're taken at night — and from the ingestion of large quantities of fluids, especially caffeinated beverages or alcohol, at bedtime.

History and physical examination

Begin by exploring the history of the patient's nocturia. When did it begin? How often does it occur? Can the patient identify a specific pattern or precipitating factors? Also, note the volume of urine voided. Ask the patient about any change in the color, odor, or consistency of his urine. Has the patient changed his usual pattern or volume of fluid intake? Next, explore associated symptoms. Ask about pain or burning on urination, difficulty initiating a urine stream, costovertebral angle tenderness, and flank, upper abdominal, or suprapubic pain.

Determine whether the patient or his family has a history of renal or urinary tract disorders or endocrine and metabolic diseases, particularly diabetes. Is the patient taking drugs that increase urine output, such as diuretics, cardiac glycosides, and antihypertensives?

Focus your physical examination on palpating and percussing the kidneys, the costovertebral angle, and the bladder. Carefully inspect the urinary meatus. Inspect a urine specimen for color, odor, and the presence of sediment.

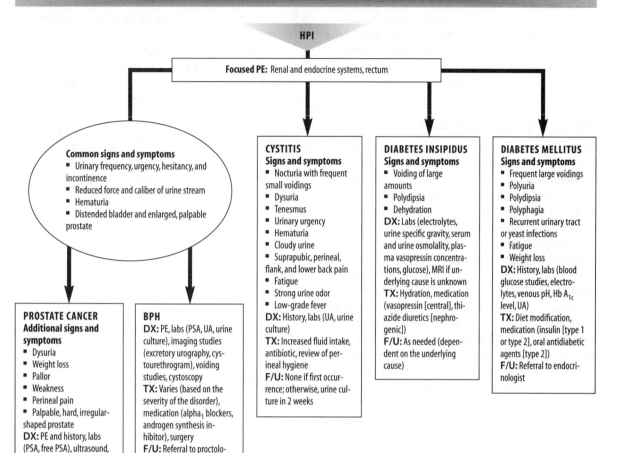

HPI

Focused PE: Renal and endocrine systems, rectum

Common signs and symptoms
- Urinary frequency, urgency, hesitancy, and incontinence
- Reduced force and caliber of urine stream
- Hematuria
- Distended bladder and enlarged, palpable prostate

PROSTATE CANCER
Additional signs and symptoms
- Dysuria
- Weight loss
- Pallor
- Weakness
- Perineal pain
- Palpable, hard, irregular-shaped prostate

DX: PE and history, labs (PSA, free PSA), ultrasound, biopsy
TX: Antineoplastic medication, surgery
F/U: Referrals to urologist and oncologist

BPH
DX: PE, labs (PSA, UA, urine culture), imaging studies (excretory urography, cystourethrogram), voiding studies, cystoscopy
TX: Varies (based on the severity of the disorder), medication (alpha$_1$ blockers, androgen synthesis inhibitor), surgery
F/U: Referral to proctologist

CYSTITIS
Signs and symptoms
- Nocturia with frequent small voidings
- Dysuria
- Tenesmus
- Urinary urgency
- Hematuria
- Cloudy urine
- Suprapubic, perineal, flank, and lower back pain
- Fatigue
- Strong urine odor
- Low-grade fever

DX: History, labs (UA, urine culture)
TX: Increased fluid intake, antibiotic, review of perineal hygiene
F/U: None if first occurrence; otherwise, urine culture in 2 weeks

DIABETES INSIPIDUS
Signs and symptoms
- Voiding of large amounts
- Polydipsia
- Dehydration

DX: Labs (electrolytes, urine specific gravity, serum and urine osmolality, plasma vasopressin concentrations, glucose), MRI if underlying cause is unknown
TX: Hydration, medication (vasopressin [central], thiazide diuretics [nephrogenic])
F/U: As needed (dependent on the underlying cause)

DIABETES MELLITUS
Signs and symptoms
- Frequent large voidings
- Polyuria
- Polydipsia
- Polyphagia
- Recurrent urinary tract or yeast infections
- Fatigue
- Weight loss

DX: History, labs (blood glucose studies, electrolytes, venous pH, Hb A$_{1c}$ level, UA)
TX: Diet modification, medication (insulin [type 1 or type 2], oral antidiabetic agents [type 2])
F/U: Referral to endocrinologist

Additional differential diagnoses: bladder neoplasm ▪ heart failure ▪ hypercalcemic nephropathy ▪ hypokalemic nephropathy ▪ pyelonephritis (acute) ▪ renal failure (chronic)

Other causes: drugs that mobilize edematous fluid or produce diuresis, such as diuretics and cardiac glycosides

Nuchal rigidity

Commonly an early sign of meningeal irritation, nuchal rigidity refers to stiffness of the neck that prevents flexion. Nuchal rigidity may herald life-threatening subarachnoid hemorrhage or meningitis. It may also be a late sign of cervical arthritis, in which joint mobility is gradually lost.

History and physical examination

Obtain a patient history; rely on family members for information if an altered level of consciousness prevents the patient from responding. Ask about the onset and duration of neck stiffness. Were there any precipitating factors? Also ask about associated symptoms, such as headache, fever, nausea and vomiting, and motor and sensory changes. Check for a history of hypertension, head trauma, cerebral aneurysm or arteriovenous malformation, endocarditis, recent infection (such as sinusitis or pneumonia), or recent dental work. Then obtain a complete drug history.

To elicit nuchal rigidity, attempt to passively flex the patient's neck and touch his chin to his chest. (See *Testing for nuchal rigidity*.) If nuchal rigidity is present, this maneuver triggers pain and muscle spasms. (Make sure that no cervical spinal misalignment, such as a fracture or dislocation, exists before testing for nuchal rigidity. Severe spinal cord damage could result.) The patient may also notice nuchal rigidity when he attempts to flex his neck during daily activities.

After eliciting nuchal rigidity, attempt to elicit Kernig's and Brudzinski's signs and evaluate level of consciousness. If signs of increased intracranial pressure are found, institute emergency treatment.

If the patient has no other signs of meningeal irritation, ask about a history of arthritis or neck trauma. Can the patient recall pulling a muscle in his neck? Inspect the patient's hands for swollen, tender joints, and palpate the neck for pain or tenderness.

PEDIATRIC POINTER

Nuchal rigidity reliably indicates meningeal irritation in children, unless they are paralyzed or comatose.

Testing for nuchal rigidity

To test for nuchal rigidity, place your hands behind the patient's neck and touch her chin to her chest, as shown here. Pain and muscle spasm will result if nuchal rigidity is present.

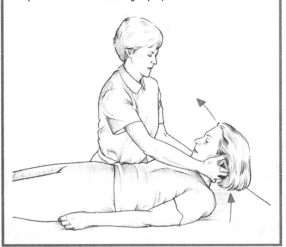

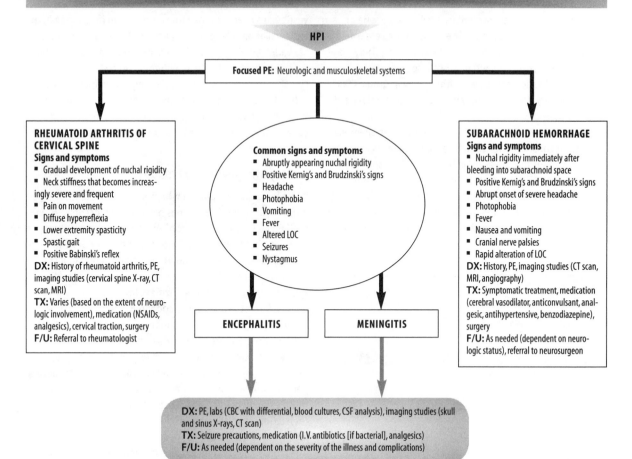

HPI

Focused PE: Neurologic and musculoskeletal systems

RHEUMATOID ARTHRITIS OF CERVICAL SPINE
Signs and symptoms
- Gradual development of nuchal rigidity
- Neck stiffness that becomes increasingly severe and frequent
- Pain on movement
- Diffuse hyperreflexia
- Lower extremity spasticity
- Spastic gait
- Positive Babinski's reflex

DX: History of rheumatoid arthritis, PE, imaging studies (cervical spine X-ray, CT scan, MRI)
TX: Varies (based on the extent of neurologic involvement), medication (NSAIDs, analgesics), cervical traction, surgery
F/U: Referral to rheumatologist

Common signs and symptoms
- Abruptly appearing nuchal rigidity
- Positive Kernig's and Brudzinski's signs
- Headache
- Photophobia
- Vomiting
- Fever
- Altered LOC
- Seizures
- Nystagmus

ENCEPHALITIS

MENINGITIS

SUBARACHNOID HEMORRHAGE
Signs and symptoms
- Nuchal rigidity immediately after bleeding into subarachnoid space
- Positive Kernig's and Brudzinski's signs
- Abrupt onset of severe headache
- Photophobia
- Fever
- Nausea and vomiting
- Cranial nerve palsies
- Rapid alteration of LOC

DX: History, PE, imaging studies (CT scan, MRI, angiography)
TX: Symptomatic treatment, medication (cerebral vasodilator, anticonvulsant, analgesic, antihypertensive, benzodiazepine), surgery
F/U: As needed (dependent on neurologic status), referral to neurosurgeon

DX: PE, labs (CBC with differential, blood cultures, CSF analysis), imaging studies (skull and sinus X-rays, CT scan)
TX: Seizure precautions, medication (I.V. antibiotics [if bacterial], analgesics)
F/U: As needed (dependent on the severity of the illness and complications)

Nystagmus

Nystagmus refers to the involuntary oscillations of one or, more commonly, both eyeballs. These oscillations are usually rhythmic and may be horizontal, vertical, or rotary. They may be transient or sustained and may occur spontaneously or on deviation or fixation of the eyes. Although nystagmus is fairly easy to identify, the patient may be unaware of it unless it affects his vision.

Nystagmus may be classified as pendular or jerk. Pendular nystagmus consists of horizontal (pendular) or vertical (seesaw) oscillations that are equal in both directions and resemble the movements of a clock's pendulum. Jerk nystagmus (convergence-retraction, downbeat, and vestibular) has a fast component and then a slow, perhaps unequal, corrective component in the opposite direction. (See *Classifying nystagmus.*)

Nystagmus is considered a supranuclear ocular palsy — that is, it results from pathology in the visual perceptual area, vestibular system, cerebellum, or brain stem rather than in the extraocular muscles or cranial nerves III, IV, and VI. Its causes are varied and include brain stem or cerebellar lesions, multiple sclerosis, encephalitis, labyrinthine disease, and drug toxicity. Occasionally, nystagmus is entirely normal; it's also considered a normal response in the unconscious patient during the doll's eye test (oculocephalic stimulation) or the cold caloric water test (oculovestibular stimulation).

History and physical examination

Begin by asking the patient whether he's aware of his nystagmus and, if so, how long he has had it. Does it occur intermittently? Does it affect his vision? Ask about recent infection, especially of the ear or respiratory tract, and about head trauma and cancer. Does the patient or anyone in his family have a history of stroke? Then assess for associated signs and symptoms, such as vertigo, dizziness, tinnitus, nausea or vomiting, numbness, weakness, bladder dysfunction, and fever.

Begin the physical examination by assessing the patient's level of consciousness and vital signs. Be alert for signs of increased intracranial pressure, such as pupillary changes, drowsiness, elevated systolic pressure, and altered respiratory pattern. Next, assess nystagmus fully by testing extraocular muscle function. Ask the patient to focus straight ahead and then to follow your finger up, down, and in an "X" across his face. Note when nystagmus occurs, as well as its velocity and direction. Finally, test reflexes, motor and sensory function, and the cranial nerves.

PEDIATRIC POINTER

In children, pendular nystagmus may be idiopathic or it may sometimes result from early impaired vision associated with such disorders as optic atrophy, albinism, congenital cataracts, and severe astigmatism.

Classifying nystagmus

JERK NYSTAGMUS

Convergence-retraction nystagmus refers to the irregular jerking of the eyes back into the orbit during upward gaze. It can indicate midbrain tegmental damage.

Downbeat nystagmus refers to the irregular downward jerking of the eyes during downward gaze. It can signal lower medullary damage.

Vestibular nystagmus, the horizontal or rotary movement of the eyes, suggests vestibular disease or cochlear dysfunction.

PENDULAR NYSTAGMUS

Horizontal, or pendular, nystagmus refers to oscillations of equal velocity around a center point. It can indicate congenital loss of visual acuity or multiple sclerosis.

Vertical, or seesaw, nystagmus, is the rapid seesaw movement of the eyes: one eye appears to rise while the other appears to fall. It suggests an optic chiasm lesion.

HPI

Focused PE: HEENT, neurologic system

BRAIN TUMOR
Signs and symptoms (dependent on size, type, and location of tumor)
- Insidious onset of jerk nystagmus (with tumors of the brain stem and cerebellum)
- Localized or general headache
- Intermittent deep pain that's more intense in the morning
- Associated personality changes
- Altered LOC
- Increased pain with Valsalva's maneuver
- Seizure
- Neurologic changes

DX: PE, imaging studies (CT scan, MRI, angiography), biopsy
TX: Symptomatic treatment, chemotherapy, radiation therapy, surgery
F/U: Referrals to neurosurgeon and oncologist

STROKE
Signs and symptoms
- Sudden horizontal or vertical jerk nystagmus that may be gaze dependent (with strokes involving the posterior inferior cerebellar artery)
- Dysphagia
- Dysarthria
- Sensory and motor loss
- Ipsilateral Horner's syndrome
- Ataxia
- Vertigo

DX: History, PE, imaging studies (CT scan, duplex carotid ultrasound, angiography)
TX: Maintenance of ABCs, symptomatic treatment, medication (platelet aggregation inhibitors, thrombolytics [if embolic])
F/U: As needed (dependent on neurologic status), referral to neurologist

ENCEPHALITIS
Signs and symptoms
- Abruptly appearing nuchal rigidity
- Jerk nystagmus
- Positive Kernig's and Brudzinski's signs
- Headache
- Photophobia
- Vomiting
- Fever
- Altered LOC
- Seizures

DX: PE, labs (CBC with differential, blood cultures, CSF analysis), imaging studies (skull and sinus X-rays, CT scan)
TX: Seizure precautions, medication (I.V. antibiotics [if bacterial], analgesics)
F/U: As needed (dependent on the severity of the illness and complications)

Common signs and symptoms
- Dizziness
- Vertigo
- Tinnitus
- Nausea and vomiting
- Gradual sensorineural hearing loss
- Positive Romberg's sign

LABYRINTHITIS (ACUTE)
Additional signs and symptoms
- Sudden onset of jerk nystagmus toward the unaffected ear

DX: CT scan, electronystagmography, calorie test, doll's eye test
TX: Treatment of the underlying cause, lying still in dark room during acute attack, medication (antivertigo agents, sedative-hypnotic)
F/U: Referral to otolaryngologist

MÉNIÈRE'S DISEASE
Additional signs and symptoms
- Acute attacks of jerk nystagmus that may last 10 minutes to several hours

DX: PE, otoscopy with air pressure applied to tympanic membrane, audiometry, caloric testing, MRI
TX: Medication (atropine, antiemetic-antivertigo agents, sedative-hypnotic)
F/U: Referral to otolaryngologist

Additional differential diagnoses: head trauma ▪ multiple sclerosis

Other causes: drugs (barbiturate, phenytoin, or carbamazepine toxicity) ▪ alcohol intoxication

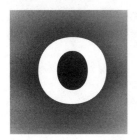

Ocular deviation

Ocular deviation refers to abnormal eye movement that may be conjugate (both eyes move together) or dysconjugate (one eye moves differently from the other). This common sign may result from ocular, neurologic, endocrine, and systemic disorders that interfere with the muscles, nerves, or brain centers governing eye movement. Occasionally, it signals a life-threatening disorder such as ruptured cerebral aneurysm. (See *Ocular deviation: Its characteristics and causes in cranial nerve damage.*)

Normally, eye movement is directly controlled by the extraocular muscles innervated by the oculomotor, trochlear, and abducens nerves (cranial nerves III, IV, and VI). Together, these muscles and nerves direct a visual stimulus to fall on corresponding parts of the retina. Dysconjugate ocular deviation may result from unequal muscle tone (nonparalytic strabismus) or from muscle paralysis associated with cranial nerve damage (paralytic strabismus). Conjugate ocular deviation may result from disorders that affect the centers in the cerebral cortex and brain stem responsible for conjugate eye movement. Typically, such disorders cause gaze palsy — difficulty moving the eyes in one or more directions.

Ocular deviation: Its characteristics and causes in cranial nerve damage

CHARACTERISTICS	CRANIAL NERVE AND EXTRAOCULAR MUSCLES INVOLVED	PROBABLE CAUSES
Inability to focus the eye upward, downward, inward, and outward; drooping eyelid; and, except in diabetes, a dilated pupil in the affected eye	Oculomotor nerve (III); medial rectus, superior rectus, inferior rectus, and inferior oblique muscles	Cerebral aneurysm, diabetes, temporal lobe herniation from increased intracranial pressure, brain tumor
Loss of downward and outward movement in the affected eye	Trochlear nerve (IV); superior oblique muscle	Head trauma
Loss of outward movement in the affected eye	Abducens nerve (VI); lateral rectus muscle	Brain tumor

History and physical examination

If the patient displays ocular deviation, quickly take his vital signs, and look for altered level of consciousness, pupil changes, motor or sensory dysfunction, and severe headache. If possible, ask the patient's family about behavioral changes. Is there a history of recent head trauma? Respiratory support may be necessary. Also, prepare the patient for emergency neurologic tests such as a computed tomography scan.

If the patient isn't in distress, find out how long he's had the ocular deviation. Is it accompanied by double vision, eye pain, or headache? Also ask whether he's noticed any associated motor or sensory changes or fever.

Check for a history of hypertension, diabetes, allergies, and thyroid, neurologic, or muscular disorders. Then obtain a thorough ocular history. Has the patient ever had extraocular muscle imbalance, eye or head trauma, or eye surgery?

During the physical examination, observe the patient for partial or complete ptosis. Does he spontaneously tilt his head or turn his face to compensate for ocular deviation? Check for eye redness or periorbital edema. Assess visual acuity; then evaluate extraocular muscle function by testing the six cardinal fields of gaze.

PEDIATRIC POINTERS

- *In children, the most common cause of ocular deviation is nonparalytic strabismus.*
- *Although severe strabismus is readily apparent, mild strabismus must be confirmed by tests for misalignment, such as the corneal light reflex test and the cover test. Testing is crucial — early corrective measures help preserve binocular vision and cosmetic appearance. Also, mild strabismus may indicate retinoblastoma, a tumor that may be asymptomatic before age 2, except for a characteristic whitish reflex in the pupil.*

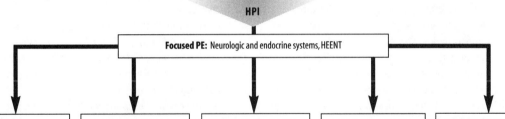

Focused PE: Neurologic and endocrine systems, HEENT

BRAIN TUMOR
Signs and symptoms
- Ocular deviation (dependent on site and extent of tumor)
- Localized or general headache
- Intermittent deep pain that's more intense in the morning
- Associated personality changes
- Changes in LOC
- Increased pain with Valsalva's maneuver

DX: PE, imaging studies (CT scan, MRI, arteriography)
TX: Medication (analgesics, anticonvulsants, osmotic diuretics, chemotherapy), radiation therapy, surgery
F/U: Referrals to neurosurgeon and oncologist

CEREBRAL ANEURYSM
Signs and symptoms
- Ocular deviation and diplopia (if aneurysm is near the internal carotid artery)
- Ptosis
- Dilated pupil on the affected side
- Severe unilateral frontal headache

DX: PE, imaging studies (CT scan, MRI, angiography)
TX: Medication (cerebral vasodilator, analgesics), surgery
F/U: Referral to neurosurgeon

MULTIPLE SCLEROSIS
Signs and symptoms
- Ocular deviation (early sign)
- Diplopia
- Blurred vision
- Sensory dysfunction
- Nystagmus
- Muscle weakness
- Hyperreflexia
- Intention tremor
- Gait ataxia

DX: PE, CSF analysis, MRI, EEG, evoked response studies
TX: Symptomatic treatment, medication (antispasmotics, antidepressants, corticosteroids)
F/U: Referral to neurologist

OPHTHALMOPLEGIC MIGRAINE
Signs and symptoms
- Ocular deviation and diplopia that persists for days after the headache subsides
- Unilateral headache
- Nausea and vomiting
- Temporary hemiplegia
- Sensory deficits

DX: PE and history
TX: Identification and avoidance of trigger, medication ($5-HT_1$ serotonin receptor agonist, ergotamines, barbiturates, analgesics, NSAIDs)
F/U: Referral to headache clinic if symptoms persist or worsen

ORBITAL CELLULITIS
Signs and symptoms
- Sudden onset of ocular deviation and diplopia
- Unilateral eye edema
- Fever
- Erythema
- Hyperemia
- Chemosis
- Extreme orbital pain
- Purulent eye discharge

DX: Labs (CBC, blood culture, throat and eye culture), imaging studies (orbit and sinus X-rays, CT scan)
TX: I.V. antibiotics, surgery
F/U: Referral to ophthalmologist

Additional differential diagnoses: cavernous sinus thrombosis ▪ diabetes mellitus ▪ encephalitis ▪ head trauma ▪ myasthenia gravis ▪ orbital blowout fracture ▪ orbital tumor ▪ stroke ▪ thyrotoxicosis

Oligomenorrhea

In most women, menstrual bleeding occurs every 28 days, plus or minus 4 days. Although some variation is normal, menstrual bleeding at intervals of greater than 36 days may indicate oligomenorrhea — abnormally infrequent menstrual bleeding characterized by three to six menstrual cycles per year. When menstrual bleeding does occur, it's usually profuse, prolonged (up to 10 days), and laden with clots and tissue. Occasionally, scant bleeding or spotting occurs between these heavy menses.

History and physical examination

After asking the patient how old she is, find out when menarche occurred. Has the patient ever experienced normal menstrual cycles? When did she begin having abnormal cycles? Ask her to describe the pattern of bleeding. How many days does the bleeding last, and how frequently does it occur? Are there clots and tissue fragments in her menstrual flow? Note when she last had menstrual bleeding.

Next, determine whether she's having symptoms of ovulatory bleeding. Does she experience mild, cramping abdominal pain 14 days before she bleeds? Is the bleeding accompanied by premenstrual symptoms, such as breast tenderness, irritability, bloating, weight gain, nausea, and diarrhea? Does she have cramping or pain with bleeding? Also, check for a history of infertility. Does the patient have any children? Is she trying to conceive? Ask whether she's currently using oral contraceptives or whether she's ever used them in the past. If she has, find out when she stopped taking them.

Then ask about previous gynecologic disorders such as ovarian cysts. If the patient is breast-feeding, has she experienced any problems with milk production? If she hasn't been breast-feeding recently, has she noticed milk leaking from her breasts? Ask about recent weight gain or loss. Is the patient less than 80% of her ideal weight? If so, does she claim that she's overweight? Ask whether she's exercising more vigorously than usual.

Screen for metabolic disorders by asking about excessive thirst, frequent urination, or fatigue. Has the patient been jittery or had palpitations? Ask about headache, dizziness, and impaired peripheral vision. Complete the history by finding out what drugs the patient is taking.

Begin the physical examination by taking the patient's vital signs and weighing her. Inspect for increased facial hair growth, sparse body hair, male distribution of fat and muscle, acne, and clitoral enlargement. Note if the skin is abnormally dry or moist, and check hair texture. Also, be alert for signs of psychological or physical stress.

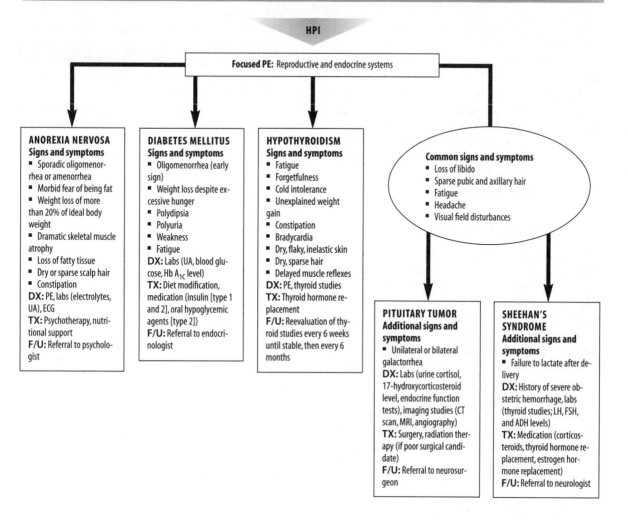

HPI

Focused PE: Reproductive and endocrine systems

ANOREXIA NERVOSA
Signs and symptoms
- Sporadic oligomenorrhea or amenorrhea
- Morbid fear of being fat
- Weight loss of more than 20% of ideal body weight
- Dramatic skeletal muscle atrophy
- Loss of fatty tissue
- Dry or sparse scalp hair
- Constipation
DX: PE, labs (electrolytes, UA), ECG
TX: Psychotherapy, nutritional support
F/U: Referral to psychologist

DIABETES MELLITUS
Signs and symptoms
- Oligomenorrhea (early sign)
- Weight loss despite excessive hunger
- Polydipsia
- Polyuria
- Weakness
- Fatigue
DX: Labs (UA, blood glucose, Hb A_{1C} level)
TX: Diet modification, medication (insulin [type 1 and 2], oral hypoglycemic agents [type 2])
F/U: Referral to endocrinologist

HYPOTHYROIDISM
Signs and symptoms
- Fatigue
- Forgetfulness
- Cold intolerance
- Unexplained weight gain
- Constipation
- Bradycardia
- Dry, flaky, inelastic skin
- Dry, sparse hair
- Delayed muscle reflexes
DX: PE, thyroid studies
TX: Thyroid hormone replacement
F/U: Reevaluation of thyroid studies every 6 weeks until stable, then every 6 months

Common signs and symptoms
- Loss of libido
- Sparse pubic and axillary hair
- Fatigue
- Headache
- Visual field disturbances

PITUITARY TUMOR
Additional signs and symptoms
- Unilateral or bilateral galactorrhea
DX: Labs (urine cortisol, 17-hydroxycorticosteroid level, endocrine function tests), imaging studies (CT scan, MRI, angiography)
TX: Surgery, radiation therapy (if poor surgical candidate)
F/U: Referral to neurosurgeon

SHEEHAN'S SYNDROME
Additional signs and symptoms
- Failure to lactate after delivery
DX: History of severe obstetric hemorrhage, labs (thyroid studies; LH, FSH, and ADH levels)
TX: Medication (corticosteroids, thyroid hormone replacement, estrogen hormone replacement)
F/U: Referral to neurologist

Additional differential diagnoses: adrenal hyperplasia ▪ hypothyroidism ▪ polycystic ovary disease ▪ thyrotoxicosis

Other causes: drugs that increase androgen levels (corticosteroids, corticotropin, anabolic steroids, danazol, injectable and implanted contraceptives) ▪ phenothiazine derivatives ▪ amphetamines ▪ antihypertensives

Oliguria

A cardinal sign of renal and urinary tract disorders, oliguria is clinically defined as urine output of less than 400 ml per 24 hours. Typically, this sign occurs abruptly and may herald serious — possibly life-threatening — hemodynamic instability. Its causes can be classified as prerenal (decreased renal blood flow), intrarenal (intrinsic renal damage), or postrenal (urinary tract obstruction); the pathophysiology differs for each classification. Oliguria associated with a prerenal or postrenal cause is usually promptly reversible with treatment, although it may lead to intrarenal damage if untreated. However, oliguria associated with an intrarenal cause is usually more persistent and may be irreversible.

History and physical examination

Begin by asking the patient about his usual daily voiding pattern, including frequency and amount. When did he first notice changes in this pattern and in the color, odor, or consistency of his urine? Ask about pain or burning on urination. Note his normal daily fluid intake. Has he recently been drinking more or less than usual? Has he had recent episodes of diarrhea or vomiting that might cause fluid loss? Next, explore associated complaints, especially fatigue, loss of appetite, thirst, dyspnea, chest pain, or recent weight gain.

Check for a history of renal, urinary tract, or cardiovascular disorders. Note recent traumatic injury or surgery associated with significant blood loss, as well as recent blood transfusions. Was the patient exposed to nephrotoxic agents, such as heavy metals, organic solvents, anesthetics, or radiographic contrast media? Next, obtain a drug history.

Begin the physical examination by taking the patient's vital signs and weighing him. Assess his overall appearance for edema. Palpate both kidneys for tenderness and enlargement, and percuss for costovertebral angle tenderness. Also, inspect the flank area for edema or erythema. Auscultate the heart and lungs for abnormal sounds and the flank area for renal artery bruits.

Obtain a urine sample and inspect for abnormal color, odor, or sediment. Use reagent strips to test for glucose, protein, and blood. Also, use a urinometer to measure specific gravity.

- In the neonate, oliguria may result from edema or dehydration. Major causes include congenital heart disease, respiratory distress syndrome, sepsis, congenital hydronephrosis, acute tubular necrosis, and renal vein thrombosis.

- Common causes of oliguria in children between ages 1 and 5 are acute poststreptococcal glomerulonephritis and hemolytic-uremic syndrome.

- After age 5, causes of oliguria are similar to those in adults.

- In elderly patients, oliguria may result from gradual progression of an underlying disorder.

- It may also result from overall poor muscle tone secondary to inactivity, poor fluid intake, and infrequent voiding attempts.

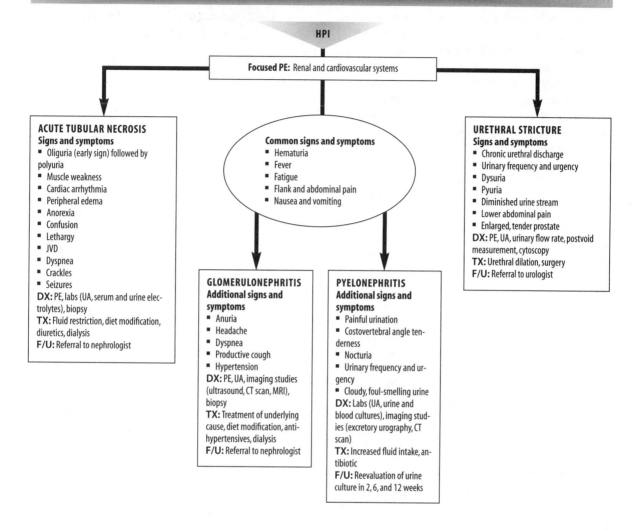

HPI

Focused PE: Renal and cardiovascular systems

ACUTE TUBULAR NECROSIS
Signs and symptoms
- Oliguria (early sign) followed by polyuria
- Muscle weakness
- Cardiac arrhythmia
- Peripheral edema
- Anorexia
- Confusion
- Lethargy
- JVD
- Dyspnea
- Crackles
- Seizures

DX: PE, labs (UA, serum and urine electrolytes), biopsy
TX: Fluid restriction, diet modification, diuretics, dialysis
F/U: Referral to nephrologist

Common signs and symptoms
- Hematuria
- Fever
- Fatigue
- Flank and abdominal pain
- Nausea and vomiting

URETHRAL STRICTURE
Signs and symptoms
- Chronic urethral discharge
- Urinary frequency and urgency
- Dysuria
- Pyuria
- Diminished urine stream
- Lower abdominal pain
- Enlarged, tender prostate

DX: PE, UA, urinary flow rate, postvoid measurement, cytoscopy
TX: Urethral dilation, surgery
F/U: Referral to urologist

GLOMERULONEPHRITIS
Additional signs and symptoms
- Anuria
- Headache
- Dyspnea
- Productive cough
- Hypertension

DX: PE, UA, imaging studies (ultrasound, CT scan, MRI), biopsy
TX: Treatment of underlying cause, diet modification, antihypertensives, dialysis
F/U: Referral to nephrologist

PYELONEPHRITIS
Additional signs and symptoms
- Painful urination
- Costovertebral angle tenderness
- Nocturia
- Urinary frequency and urgency
- Cloudy, foul-smelling urine

DX: Labs (UA, urine and blood cultures), imaging studies (excretory urography, CT scan)
TX: Increased fluid intake, antibiotic
F/U: Reevaluation of urine culture in 2, 6, and 12 weeks

Additional differential diagnoses: BPH ▪ bladder neoplasm ▪ calculi ▪ cirrhosis ▪ heart failure ▪ hypovolemia ▪ renal artery occlusion (bilateral) ▪ renal failure (chronic) ▪ renal vein occlusion (bilateral) ▪ retroperitoneal fibrosis ▪ sepsis ▪ toxemia of pregnancy

Other causes: contrast media ▪ drugs that cause decreased renal perfusion (diuretics), nephrotoxicity (most notably, aminoglycosides and chemotherapeutic agents), urine retention (adrenergic and anticholinergic agents), or urinary obstruction associated with precipitation of urinary crystals (sulfonamides and acyclovir)

Opisthotonos

A sign of severe meningeal irritation, opisthotonos is characterized by a strongly arched, rigid back; a hyperextended neck; heels that are bent back; and arms and hands that are flexed at the joints. Usually, this posture occurs spontaneously as well as continuously; however, it may be aggravated by movement. Because it immobilizes the spine, opisthotonos presumably represents a protective reflex that alleviates pain associated with meningeal irritation.

Usually caused by meningitis, opisthotonos may also result from subarachnoid hemorrhage, Arnold-Chiari syndrome, and tetanus. Occasionally, it occurs in achondroplastic dwarfism, although not necessarily as an indicator of meningeal irritation.

Opisthotonos is far more common in children — especially infants — than in adults. It's also more exaggerated in children because of nervous system immaturity. (See *Opisthotonos: Sign of meningeal irritation.*)

History and physical examination

If the patient's condition permits, obtain a history. Consult with a relative of the young child or infant. Ask about a history of cerebral aneurysm or arteriovenous malformation as well as hypertension. Note any recent infection that may have spread to the nervous system. Explore associated findings, such as headache, chills, and vomiting.

Focus the physical examination on the patient's neurologic status. Evaluate level of consciousness, and test sensorimotor and cranial nerve function. Then check for Brudzinski's and Kernig's signs as well as for nuchal rigidity.

Opisthotonos: Sign of meningeal irritation

In this characteristic posture, the back is severely arched with the neck hyperextended. The heels bend back on the legs, and the arms and hands flex rigidly at the joints, as shown.

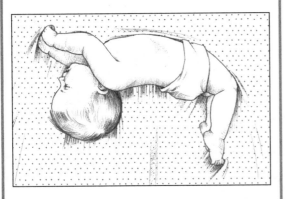

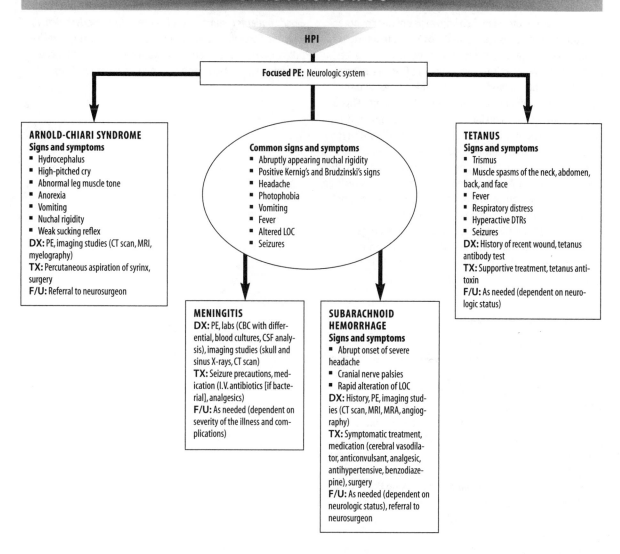

HPI

Focused PE: Neurologic system

ARNOLD-CHIARI SYNDROME
Signs and symptoms
- Hydrocephalus
- High-pitched cry
- Abnormal leg muscle tone
- Anorexia
- Vomiting
- Nuchal rigidity
- Weak sucking reflex

DX: PE, imaging studies (CT scan, MRI, myelography)
TX: Percutaneous aspiration of syrinx, surgery
F/U: Referral to neurosurgeon

Common signs and symptoms
- Abruptly appearing nuchal rigidity
- Positive Kernig's and Brudzinski's signs
- Headache
- Photophobia
- Vomiting
- Fever
- Altered LOC
- Seizures

TETANUS
Signs and symptoms
- Trismus
- Muscle spasms of the neck, abdomen, back, and face
- Fever
- Respiratory distress
- Hyperactive DTRs
- Seizures

DX: History of recent wound, tetanus antibody test
TX: Supportive treatment, tetanus anti-toxin
F/U: As needed (dependent on neurologic status)

MENINGITIS
DX: PE, labs (CBC with differential, blood cultures, CSF analysis), imaging studies (skull and sinus X-rays, CT scan)
TX: Seizure precautions, medication (I.V. antibiotics [if bacterial], analgesics)
F/U: As needed (dependent on severity of the illness and complications)

SUBARACHNOID HEMORRHAGE
Signs and symptoms
- Abrupt onset of severe headache
- Cranial nerve palsies
- Rapid alteration of LOC

DX: History, PE, imaging studies (CT scan, MRI, MRA, angiography)
TX: Symptomatic treatment, medication (cerebral vasodilator, anticonvulsant, analgesic, antihypertensive, benzodiazepine), surgery
F/U: As needed (dependent on neurologic status), referral to neurosurgeon

Other causes: antipsychotics such as phenothiazines

Orthostatic hypotension

In orthostatic hypotension, also known as postural hypotension, the patient's blood pressure drops 15 to 20 mm Hg or more — with or without an increase in the heart rate of at least 20 beats per minute — when he rises from a supine position to a sitting or standing position. (Blood pressure should be measured 5 minutes after the patient has changed his position.) This common sign indicates failure of compensatory vasomotor responses to adjust to position changes. It's typically associated with light-headedness, syncope, or blurred vision, and it may occur in a hypotensive, normotensive, or hypertensive patient. Although frequently a nonpathologic sign in elderly people, orthostatic hypotension may result from prolonged bed rest, fluid and electrolyte imbalance, endocrine or systemic disorders, and the effects of drugs.

To detect orthostatic hypotension, take and compare blood pressure readings with the patient supine, sitting, and standing.

History and physical examination

If you detect orthostatic hypotension, quickly check for tachycardia, altered level of consciousness, and pale, clammy skin. If these signs are present, suspect hypovolemic shock. If the patient is in no danger, obtain a history. Ask the patient whether he frequently experiences dizziness, weakness, or fainting when he stands. Also ask about associated symptoms, particularly fatigue, orthopnea, impotence, nausea, headache, abdominal or chest discomfort, and GI bleeding. Then obtain a complete drug history.

Begin the physical examination by checking the patient's skin turgor. Palpate peripheral pulses and auscultate the heart and lungs. Finally, test muscle strength and observe the patient's gait for unsteadiness.

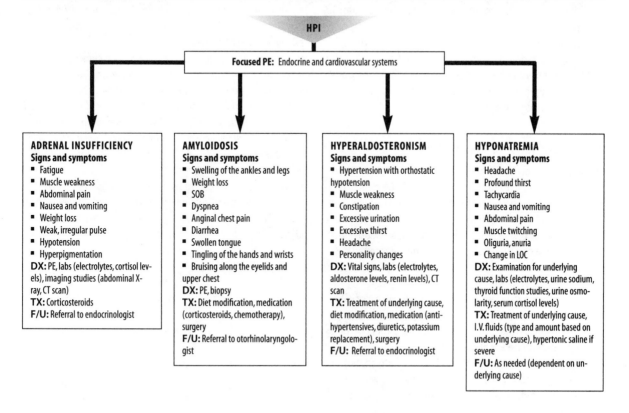

HPI

Focused PE: Endocrine and cardiovascular systems

ADRENAL INSUFFICIENCY
Signs and symptoms
- Fatigue
- Muscle weakness
- Abdominal pain
- Nausea and vomiting
- Weight loss
- Weak, irregular pulse
- Hypotension
- Hyperpigmentation

DX: PE, labs (electrolytes, cortisol levels), imaging studies (abdominal X-ray, CT scan)
TX: Corticosteroids
F/U: Referral to endocrinologist

AMYLOIDOSIS
Signs and symptoms
- Swelling of the ankles and legs
- Weight loss
- SOB
- Dyspnea
- Anginal chest pain
- Diarrhea
- Swollen tongue
- Tingling of the hands and wrists
- Bruising along the eyelids and upper chest

DX: PE, biopsy
TX: Diet modification, medication (corticosteroids, chemotherapy), surgery
F/U: Referral to otorhinolaryngologist

HYPERALDOSTERONISM
Signs and symptoms
- Hypertension with orthostatic hypotension
- Muscle weakness
- Constipation
- Excessive urination
- Excessive thirst
- Headache
- Personality changes

DX: Vital signs, labs (electrolytes, aldosterone levels, renin levels), CT scan
TX: Treatment of underlying cause, diet modification, medication (antihypertensives, diuretics, potassium replacement), surgery
F/U: Referral to endocrinologist

HYPONATREMIA
Signs and symptoms
- Headache
- Profound thirst
- Tachycardia
- Nausea and vomiting
- Abdominal pain
- Muscle twitching
- Oliguria, anuria
- Change in LOC

DX: Examination for underlying cause, labs (electrolytes, urine sodium, thyroid function studies, urine osmolarity, serum cortisol levels)
TX: Treatment of underlying cause, I.V. fluids (type and amount based on underlying cause), hypertonic saline if severe
F/U: As needed (dependent on underlying cause)

Additional differential diagnoses: alcoholism ▪ diabetic autonomic neuropathy ▪ hypovolemia ▪ pheochromocytoma ▪ Shy-Drager syndrome

Other causes: antihypertensives ▪ tricyclic antidepressants ▪ phenothiazines ▪ levodopa ▪ nitrates ▪ MAO inhibitors ▪ morphine ▪ spinal anesthesia ▪ large doses of diuretics ▪ prolonged bed rest (24 hours or longer) ▪ sympathectomy

Otorrhea

Otorrhea — drainage from the ear — may be bloody (otorrhagia), purulent, clear, or serosanguineous. Its onset, duration, and severity provide clues to the underlying cause. This sign may result from disorders that affect the external ear canal or the middle ear, including allergy, infection, neoplasms, trauma, and collagen diseases. Otorrhea may occur alone or with other symptoms such as ear pain.

History and physical examination

Begin your evaluation by asking the patient when the otorrhea began, noting how he recognized it. Did he clean the drainage from deep within the ear canal or did he wipe it from the auricle? Have him describe the color, consistency, and odor of the drainage. Is it clear, purulent, or bloody? Does it occur in one or both ears? Is it continuous or intermittent? If the patient wears cotton in his ear to absorb the drainage, ask how often he changes it.

Then explore associated otologic symptoms, especially pain. Is there tenderness on movement of the pinna or tragus? Ask about vertigo, which is absent in disorders of the external ear canal. Also ask about tinnitus.

Next, check the patient's medical history for recent upper respiratory infection or head trauma. Also, ask how he cleans his ears and whether he's an avid swimmer. Note a history of cancer, dermatitis, or immunosuppressive therapy.

Focus the physical examination on the patient's external ear, middle ear, and tympanic membrane. (If his symptoms are unilateral, examine the uninvolved ear first.) Inspect the external ear, and apply pressure on the tragus and mastoid area to elicit tenderness. Then insert an otoscope, using the largest speculum that will comfortably fit into the ear canal. If necessary, clean cerumen, pus, or other debris from the canal. Observe for edema, erythema, crusts, or polyps. Inspect the tympanic membrane, which should look like a shiny, pearl-gray cone. Note color changes, perforation, absence of the normal light reflex (a cone of light appearing toward the bottom of the drum), or a bulging membrane.

Next, test hearing acuity. Have the patient occlude one ear while you whisper some common two-syllable words toward the unoccluded ear. Stand behind him so he doesn't read your lips, and ask him to repeat what he heard. Perform the test on the other ear using different words. Then use a tuning fork to perform Weber's test and the Rinne test.

Complete your assessment by palpating the patient's neck and his preauricular, parotid, and postauricular (mastoid) areas for lymphadenopathy. Also, test the function of cranial nerves VII, IX, X, and XI.

PEDIATRIC POINTERS

- When you examine or clean a child's ear, remember that the auditory canal lies horizontally and that the pinna must be pulled downward and backward.
- Restrain a child during an ear procedure by having him sit on a parent's lap with the ear to be examined facing you. Have him put one arm around the parent's waist and the other arm down at his side and then ask the parent to hold the child in place. Or, if you're alone with the child, you can have him lie on his abdomen with his arms at his sides and his head turned so the affected ear faces the ceiling. Bend over him, restraining his upper body with your elbows and upper arms.
- Otitis media is the most common cause of otorrhea in infants and young children. Children are also likely to insert foreign bodies into their ears, resulting in infection, pain, and purulent discharge.

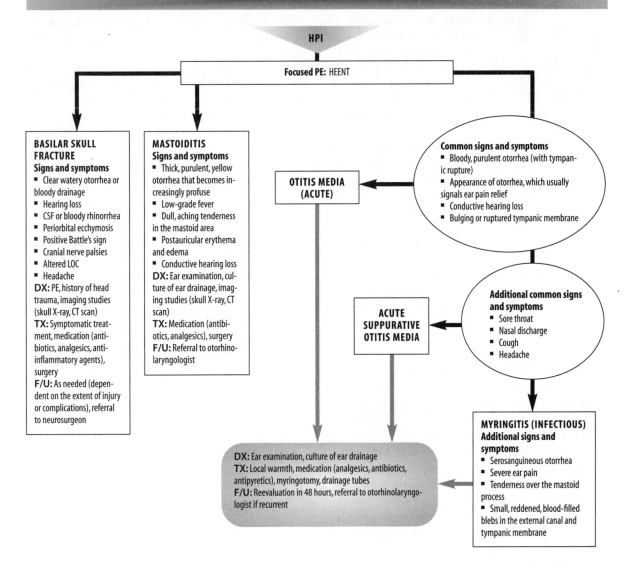

HPI

Focused PE: HEENT

BASILAR SKULL FRACTURE
Signs and symptoms
- Clear watery otorrhea or bloody drainage
- Hearing loss
- CSF or bloody rhinorrhea
- Periorbital ecchymosis
- Positive Battle's sign
- Cranial nerve palsies
- Altered LOC
- Headache

DX: PE, history of head trauma, imaging studies (skull X-ray, CT scan)
TX: Symptomatic treatment, medication (antibiotics, analgesics, anti-inflammatory agents), surgery
F/U: As needed (dependent on the extent of injury or complications), referral to neurosurgeon

MASTOIDITIS
Signs and symptoms
- Thick, purulent, yellow otorrhea that becomes increasingly profuse
- Low-grade fever
- Dull, aching tenderness in the mastoid area
- Postauricular erythema and edema
- Conductive hearing loss

DX: Ear examination, culture of ear drainage, imaging studies (skull X-ray, CT scan)
TX: Medication (antibiotics, analgesics), surgery
F/U: Referral to otorhinolaryngologist

OTITIS MEDIA (ACUTE)

Common signs and symptoms
- Bloody, purulent otorrhea (with tympanic rupture)
- Appearance of otorrhea, which usually signals ear pain relief
- Conductive hearing loss
- Bulging or ruptured tympanic membrane

ACUTE SUPPURATIVE OTITIS MEDIA

Additional common signs and symptoms
- Sore throat
- Nasal discharge
- Cough
- Headache

DX: Ear examination, culture of ear drainage
TX: Local warmth, medication (analgesics, antibiotics, antipyretics), myringotomy, drainage tubes
F/U: Reevaluation in 48 hours, referral to otorhinolaryngologist if recurrent

MYRINGITIS (INFECTIOUS)
Additional signs and symptoms
- Serosanguineous otorrhea
- Severe ear pain
- Tenderness over the mastoid process
- Small, reddened, blood-filled blebs in the external canal and tympanic membrane

Additional differential diagnoses: allergy ▪ aural polyps ▪ dermatitis of the external ear canal ▪ epidural abscess ▪ otitis externa ▪ perichondritis ▪ trauma ▪ tuberculosis ▪ tumor ▪ Wegener's granulomatosis

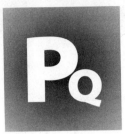

Pallor

Pallor is an abnormal paleness or loss of skin color, which may develop suddenly or gradually. Although generalized pallor affects the entire body, it's most apparent on the face, conjunctiva, oral mucosa, and nail beds. Localized pallor commonly affects a single limb.

How easily pallor is detected varies with skin color and the thickness and vascularity of underlying subcutaneous tissue. At times, it's merely a subtle lightening of skin color that may be difficult to detect in dark-skinned persons; sometimes, it's evident only on the conjunctiva and oral mucosa.

Pallor may result from decreased peripheral oxyhemoglobin or decreased total oxyhemoglobin. The former reflects diminished peripheral blood flow associated with peripheral vasoconstriction or arterial occlusion or with low cardiac output. (Transient peripheral vasoconstriction may occur with exposure to cold, causing nonpathologic pallor.) The latter usually results from anemia, the chief cause of pallor.

History and physical examination

If generalized pallor develops, look for signs of shock, such as tachycardia, hypotension, oliguria, and decreased level of consciousness. If the patient's condition permits, take a complete history. Does the patient or anyone in his family have a history of anemia? What about chronic disorders that might lead to pallor, such as renal failure, heart failure, ulcer disease, or diabetes? Ask about the patient's diet, particularly his intake of green vegetables.

Then explore the pallor more fully. Find out when the patient first noticed it. Is pallor constant or intermittent? Does it occur when he's exposed to the cold? Does it occur when he's under emotional stress? Explore associated signs and symptoms, such as dizziness, fainting, orthostasis, weakness and fatigue on exertion, chest pain, palpitations, menstrual irregularities, or loss of libido. Ask about the occurrence of melena or about any obvious signs of bleeding, such as epistaxis or hematemesis. If the pallor is confined to one or both legs, ask the patient whether walking is painful. Do his legs feel cold or numb? If the pallor is confined to his fingers, ask about tingling and numbness.

Start the physical examination by taking the patient's vital signs. Be sure to check for orthostatic hypotension. Auscultate the heart for gallops and murmurs and the lungs for crackles. Perform an abdominal exam, especially checking for tenderness. Check the patient's skin temperature — cold extremities commonly occur with vasoconstriction or arterial occlusion. Also, note skin ulceration. Finally, palpate peripheral pulses. An absent pulse in a pale extremity may indicate arterial occlusion, whereas a weak pulse may indicate low cardiac output.

HPI

Focused PE: Cardiovascular system

ANEMIA
Signs and symptoms
- Gradual pallor
- Sallow or gray skin
- Fatigue
- Dyspnea
- Tachycardia
- Bounding pulse

DX: Labs (CBC, serum ferritin level, serum iron, TIBC)

TX: Treatment of underlying cause (based on specific type of anemia)

F/U: As needed (dependent on the cause and severity of anemia)

SHOCK
Signs and symptoms
- Cool, pale, moist skin
- Tachycardia
- Tachypnea
- Fever
- Elevated or collapsed neck veins
- Crackles
- Arrhythmias, murmurs, or gallops
- Confusion
- Oliguria

DX: PE, labs (CBC, electrolytes, ABG, UA, blood cultures), CXR, ECG

TX: Varies (based on the specific type of shock), symptomatic treatment, I.V. fluids, cardiac monitoring, vasopressors

F/U: Referral to specialist as indicated by the type of shock

RAYNAUD'S PHENOMENON
Signs and symptoms
- Pallor of fingers on exposure to cold or stress (after which fingers become cyanotic and on rewarming become red and paresthetic)
- Ulceration
- Capillary nail fold abnormalities

TX: Avoidance of triggers to vasospasm, smoking cessation program, medication (calcium channel blockers, vasodilators, platelet aggregation inhibitor)

F/U: As needed (dependent on the severity of the phenomenon)

ARTERIAL OCCLUSION
Signs and symptoms
- Abrupt pallor of extremity
- Line of demarcation (with cool, cyanotic, mottled skin below and normal skin above)
- Severe pain
- Intense intermittent claudication
- Paresthesia
- Paresis
- Absent pulses and diminished capillary refill in the affected extremity

DX: PE, imaging studies (Doppler ultrasound, angiography)

TX: Medication (thrombolytics, anticoagulants, analgesics), surgery

F/U: Referral to vascular surgeon

ARTERIAL OCCLUSIVE DISEASE
Signs and symptoms
- Gradual pallor of extremity
- Increased pallor with elevation
- Intermittent claudication
- Weakness in the affected extremity
- Cool skin
- Diminished pulses in the affected extremity
- Ulceration or gangrene in the affected extremity

DX: History of arteriosclerosis, imaging studies (Doppler ultrasound, angiography)

TX: Smoking cessation program, diet modification, exercise program, medication (antiplatelet agents, vasodilators, analgesics), surgery

F/U: As needed (dependent on the severity of the disease)

Additional differential diagnoses: cardiac arrhythmias ▪ frostbite ▪ orthostatic hypotension ▪ shock ▪ vasopressor syncope

Palpitations

Defined as a conscious awareness of one's heartbeat, palpitations are usually felt over the precordium or in the throat or neck. The patient may describe them as pounding, jumping, turning, fluttering, or flopping or as missing or skipping beats. Palpitations may be regular or irregular, fast or slow, and paroxysmal or sustained.

Although frequently insignificant, this common symptom may result from cardiac and metabolic disorders as well as from the effects of certain drugs. Nonpathologic palpitations may occur with a newly implanted prosthetic valve because the valve's clicking sound heightens the patient's awareness of his heartbeat. Transient palpitations may accompany emotional stress, such as fright, anger, and anxiety, or physical stress, such as exercise and fever. They can also accompany use of stimulants, such as tobacco and caffeine.

To help characterize the palpitations, ask the patient to simulate their rhythm by tapping his finger on a hard surface. An irregular "skipped beat" rhythm points to premature ventricular contractions, whereas an episodic racing rhythm that ends abruptly suggests paroxysmal atrial tachycardia.

History and physical examination

If the patient complains of palpitations, ask him about dizziness and shortness of breath. Then inspect for pale, clammy skin. Assess vital signs for hypotension and irregular or abnormal pulse. If these signs are present, suspect cardiac arrhythmia. If the patient isn't in distress, perform a complete cardiac history and physical examination. Ask about cardiovascular or pulmonary disorders, which may produce arrhythmias. Does the patient have a history of hypertension or hypoglycemia? Be sure to obtain a drug history. Has the patient recently started digitalis glycoside therapy? In addition, ask about caffeine, tobacco, and alcohol consumption.

Then explore associated symptoms, such as weakness, fatigue, and anginal pain. Finally, auscultate for gallops, murmurs, and abnormal breath sounds.

PEDIATRIC POINTERS

- *Palpitations in children commonly result from fever and congenital heart defects, such as patent ductus arteriosus and septal defects.*
- *Because young children commonly can't describe this complaint, focus your attention on objective measurements, such as cardiac monitoring, physical examination, and laboratory tests.*

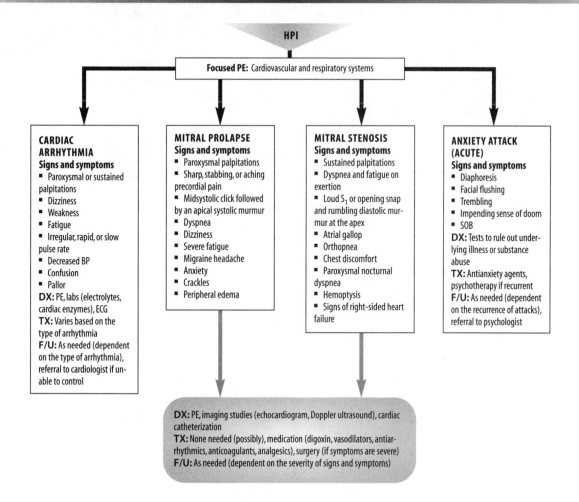

HPI

Focused PE: Cardiovascular and respiratory systems

CARDIAC ARRHYTHMIA
Signs and symptoms
- Paroxysmal or sustained palpitations
- Dizziness
- Weakness
- Fatigue
- Irregular, rapid, or slow pulse rate
- Decreased BP
- Confusion
- Pallor

DX: PE, labs (electrolytes, cardiac enzymes), ECG
TX: Varies based on the type of arrhythmia
F/U: As needed (dependent on the type of arrhythmia), referral to cardiologist if unable to control

MITRAL PROLAPSE
Signs and symptoms
- Paroxysmal palpitations
- Sharp, stabbing, or aching precordial pain
- Midsystolic click followed by an apical systolic murmur
- Dyspnea
- Dizziness
- Severe fatigue
- Migraine headache
- Anxiety
- Crackles
- Peripheral edema

MITRAL STENOSIS
Signs and symptoms
- Sustained palpitations
- Dyspnea and fatigue on exertion
- Loud S_1 or opening snap and rumbling diastolic murmur at the apex
- Atrial gallop
- Orthopnea
- Chest discomfort
- Paroxysmal nocturnal dyspnea
- Hemoptysis
- Signs of right-sided heart failure

ANXIETY ATTACK (ACUTE)
Signs and symptoms
- Diaphoresis
- Facial flushing
- Trembling
- Impending sense of doom
- SOB

DX: Tests to rule out underlying illness or substance abuse
TX: Antianxiety agents, psychotherapy if recurrent
F/U: As needed (dependent on the recurrence of attacks), referral to psychologist

DX: PE, imaging studies (echocardiogram, Doppler ultrasound), cardiac catheterization
TX: None needed (possibly), medication (digoxin, vasodilators, antiarrhythmics, anticoagulants, analgesics), surgery (if symptoms are severe)
F/U: As needed (dependent on the severity of signs and symptoms)

Additional differential diagnoses: anemia ▪ hypertension ▪ hypocalcemia ▪ hypoglycemia ▪ pheochromocytoma ▪ thyrotoxicosis

---

Other causes: herbal drugs, such as ginseng and ephedra ▪ drugs that precipitate cardiac arrhythmias or increase cardiac output (cardiac glycosides, sympathomimetics, cocaine, ganglionic blockers, atropine)

Papular rash

A papular rash consists of small, raised, circumscribed — and possibly discolored (red to purple) — lesions known as papules. It may erupt anywhere on the body in various configurations, and it may be acute or chronic. Papular rashes characterize many cutaneous disorders; they may also result from allergy and from infectious, neoplastic, and systemic disorders. (To compare papules with other skin lesions, see *Recognizing common skin lesions.*)

History and physical examination

Your first step is to evaluate the papular rash fully: Note its color, configuration, and location on the patient's body. Find out when it erupted. Has the patient noticed any changes in the rash? Is it itchy or burning? Painful or tender? Also, have him describe associated signs and symptoms, such as fever, headache, shortness of breath, and GI distress.

Next, obtain a medical history, including allergies, previous rashes or skin disorders, infections, childhood diseases, cancers, and sexual history, including any sexually transmitted diseases. Has the patient recently been bitten by an insect or rodent or exposed to anyone with an infectious disease? Ask about travel and food histories, pets, and environmental exposures. Finally, obtain a complete drug history.

PEDIATRIC POINTER

Common causes of papular rashes in children are infectious diseases, such as molluscum contagiosum and scarlet fever, scabies, insect bites, allergies and drug reactions, and miliaria, which occurs in three forms, depending on the depth of sweat gland involvement.

ELDER CARE CUE

In bedridden elderly patients, the first sign of pressure ulcers is often an erythematous area, sometimes with firm papules. If not properly managed, these lesions progress to deep ulcers and can lead to death.

Recognizing common skin lesions

MACULE

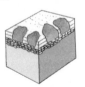

A small (usually less than 1 cm in diameter), flat blemish or discoloration that can be brown, tan, red, or white and has the same texture as the surrounding skin

VESICLE

A small (less than 0.5 cm in diameter), thin-walled, raised blister containing clear, serous, purulent, or bloody fluid

WHEAL

A slightly raised, firm lesion of variable size and shape that's surrounded by edema (skin may be red or pale)

PAPULE

A small, solid, raised lesion less than 1 cm in diameter with red to purple skin discoloration

BULLA

A raised, thin-walled blister that's greater than 0.5 cm in diameter and contains clear or serous fluid

PUSTULE

A circumscribed, pus- or lymph-filled, elevated lesion that varies in diameter and may be firm or soft and white or yellow

NODULE

A small, firm, circumscribed, elevated lesion approximately 1 to 2 cm in diameter with possible skin discoloration

TUMOR

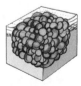

A solid, raised mass that's usually larger than 2 cm in diameter with possible skin discoloration

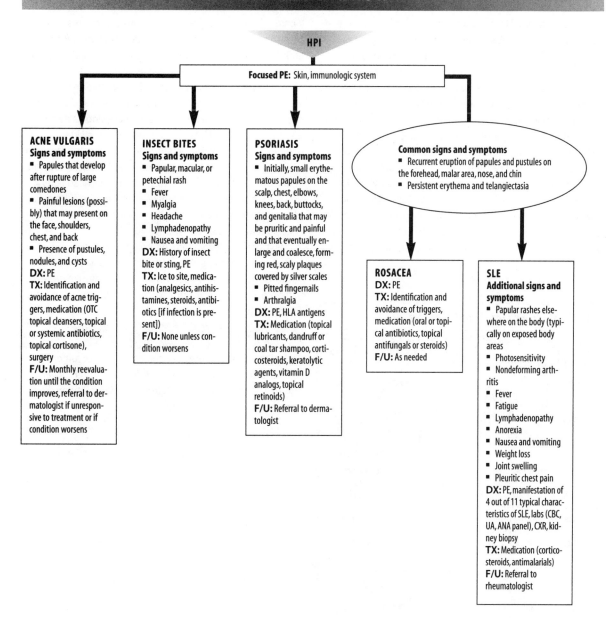

HPI

Focused PE: Skin, immunologic system

ACNE VULGARIS
Signs and symptoms
- Papules that develop after rupture of large comedones
- Painful lesions (possibly) that may present on the face, shoulders, chest, and back
- Presence of pustules, nodules, and cysts

DX: PE

TX: Identification and avoidance of acne triggers, medication (OTC topical cleansers, topical or systemic antibiotics, topical cortisone), surgery

F/U: Monthly reevaluation until the condition improves, referral to dermatologist if unresponsive to treatment or if condition worsens

INSECT BITES
Signs and symptoms
- Papular, macular, or petechial rash
- Fever
- Myalgia
- Headache
- Lymphadenopathy
- Nausea and vomiting

DX: History of insect bite or sting, PE

TX: Ice to site, medication (analgesics, antihistamines, steroids, antibiotics [if infection is present])

F/U: None unless condition worsens

PSORIASIS
Signs and symptoms
- Initially, small erythematous papules on the scalp, chest, elbows, knees, back, buttocks, and genitalia that may be pruritic and painful and that eventually enlarge and coalesce, forming red, scaly plaques covered by silver scales
- Pitted fingernails
- Arthralgia

DX: PE, HLA antigens

TX: Medication (topical lubricants, dandruff or coal tar shampoo, corticosteroids, keratolytic agents, vitamin D analogs, topical retinoids)

F/U: Referral to dermatologist

Common signs and symptoms
- Recurrent eruption of papules and pustules on the forehead, malar area, nose, and chin
- Persistent erythema and telangiectasia

ROSACEA

DX: PE

TX: Identification and avoidance of triggers, medication (oral or topical antibiotics, topical antifungals or steroids)

F/U: As needed

SLE
Additional signs and symptoms
- Papular rashes elsewhere on the body (typically on exposed body areas
- Photosensitivity
- Nondeforming arthritis
- Fever
- Fatigue
- Lymphadenopathy
- Anorexia
- Nausea and vomiting
- Weight loss
- Joint swelling
- Pleuritic chest pain

DX: PE, manifestation of 4 out of 11 typical characteristics of SLE, labs (CBC, UA, ANA panel), CXR, kidney biopsy

TX: Medication (corticosteroids, antimalarials)

F/U: Referral to rheumatologist

Additional differential diagnoses: dermatitis (perioral) ▪ dermatomyositis ▪ erythema chronicum migrans ▪ follicular mucinosis ▪ Fox-Fordyce disease ▪ gonococcemia ▪ granuloma annulare ▪ HIV infection ▪ leprosy ▪ lichen amyloidosis ▪ lichen planus ▪ mononucleosis (infectious) ▪ mycosis fungoides ▪ necrotizing vasculitis ▪ parapsoriasis (chronic) ▪ pityriasis rosea ▪ pityriasis rubra pilaris ▪ polymorphic light eruption ▪ rat bite fever ▪ sarcoidosis ▪ seborrheic keratosis ▪ syphilis ▪ syringoma

Other causes: antibiotics (tetracycline, ampicillin, cephalosporins, sulfonamides) ▪ benzodiazepines (diazepam) ▪ lithium ▪ phenylbutazone ▪ gold salts ▪ allopurino ▪ isoniazid ▪ salicylates

Paralysis

Paralysis — the total loss of voluntary motor function — results from severe cortical or pyramidal tract damage. It can occur in cerebrovascular disorders, degenerative neuromuscular disease, trauma, tumors, or central nervous system infection. Acute paralysis may be an early indicator of such life-threatening disorders as Guillain-Barré syndrome.

Paralysis can be local or widespread, symmetrical or asymmetrical, transient or permanent, and spastic or flaccid. It's often classified according to location and severity as paraplegia (sometimes transient paralysis of the legs), quadriplegia (permanent paralysis of the arms, legs, and body below the level of the spinal lesion), or hemiplegia (unilateral paralysis of varying severity and permanence). Incomplete paralysis with profound weakness (paresis) may precede total paralysis in some patients. (See *Understanding spinal cord syndromes*.)

History and physical examination

If paralysis has developed suddenly, suspect trauma or an acute vascular insult. Determine the level of consciousness and assess vital signs. If the patient is in no immediate danger, perform a complete neurologic assessment. Start with the history, relying on family members for information when necessary. Ask about the onset, duration, intensity, and progression of paralysis as well as the events preceding its development. Focus medical history questions on the incidence of degenerative neurologic or neuromuscular disease, recent infectious illness, sexually transmitted disease, cancer, or recent injury. Explore related symptoms, noting fever, headache, visual disturbances, dysphagia, nausea and vomiting, bowel or bladder dysfunction, muscle pain or weakness, and fatigue. Ask about any history of hypertension.

Next, perform a complete neurologic examination, testing cranial nerve, motor, and sensory function as well as deep tendon reflexes. Assess strength in all major muscle groups, and note any muscle atrophy. Document all findings to serve as a baseline.

PEDIATRIC POINTER

Besides the obvious causes — trauma, infection, or tumors — children may contract paralysis from hereditary and congenital disorders, such as Tay-Sachs disease, Werdnig-Hoffmann disease, spina bifida, and cerebral palsy.

Understanding spinal cord syndromes

When a patient's spinal cord is incompletely severed, he experiences partial motor and sensory loss. Most incomplete cord lesions fit into one of the syndromes described below.

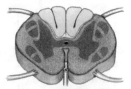

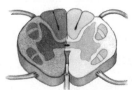

Anterior cord syndrome, usually resulting from a flexion injury, causes motor paralysis and loss of pain and temperature sensation below the level of injury. Touch, proprioception, and vibration sensation are usually preserved.

Brown-Séquard's syndrome can result from flexion, rotation, or penetration injury. It's characterized by unilateral motor paralysis ipsilateral to the injury and loss of pain and temperature sensation contralateral to the injury.

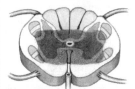

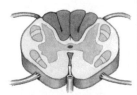

Central cord syndrome is caused by hyperextension or flexion injury. Motor loss is variable and greater in the arms than in the legs; sensory loss is usually slight.

Posterior cord syndrome, produced by a cervical hyperextension injury, causes only a loss of proprioception and light touch sensation. Motor function remains intact.

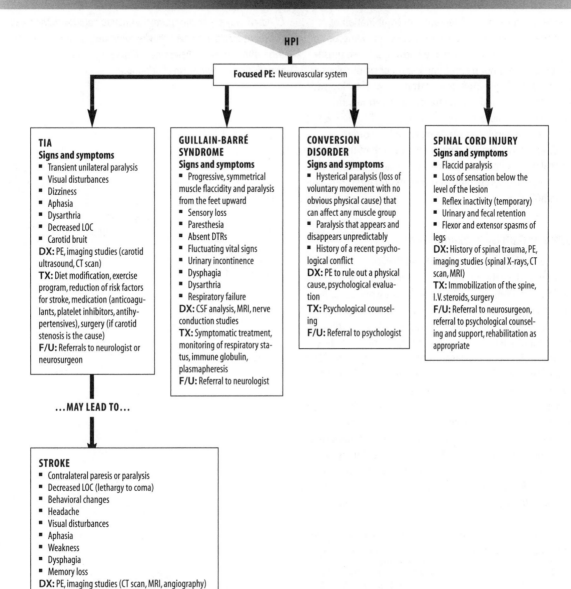

HPI

Focused PE: Neurovascular system

TIA
Signs and symptoms
- Transient unilateral paralysis
- Visual disturbances
- Dizziness
- Aphasia
- Dysarthria
- Decreased LOC
- Carotid bruit

DX: PE, imaging studies (carotid ultrasound, CT scan)

TX: Diet modification, exercise program, reduction of risk factors for stroke, medication (anticoagulants, platelet inhibitors, antihypertensives), surgery (if carotid stenosis is the cause)

F/U: Referrals to neurologist or neurosurgeon

GUILLAIN-BARRÉ SYNDROME
Signs and symptoms
- Progressive, symmetrical muscle flaccidity and paralysis from the feet upward
- Sensory loss
- Paresthesia
- Absent DTRs
- Fluctuating vital signs
- Urinary incontinence
- Dysphagia
- Dysarthria
- Respiratory failure

DX: CSF analysis, MRI, nerve conduction studies

TX: Symptomatic treatment, monitoring of respiratory status, immune globulin, plasmapheresis

F/U: Referral to neurologist

CONVERSION DISORDER
Signs and symptoms
- Hysterical paralysis (loss of voluntary movement with no obvious physical cause) that can affect any muscle group
- Paralysis that appears and disappears unpredictably
- History of a recent psychological conflict

DX: PE to rule out a physical cause, psychological evaluation

TX: Psychological counseling

F/U: Referral to psychologist

SPINAL CORD INJURY
Signs and symptoms
- Flaccid paralysis
- Loss of sensation below the level of the lesion
- Reflex inactivity (temporary)
- Urinary and fecal retention
- Flexor and extensor spasms of legs

DX: History of spinal trauma, PE, imaging studies (spinal X-rays, CT scan, MRI)

TX: Immobilization of the spine, I.V. steroids, surgery

F/U: Referral to neurosurgeon, referral to psychological counseling and support, rehabilitation as appropriate

...MAY LEAD TO...

STROKE
- Contralateral paresis or paralysis
- Decreased LOC (lethargy to coma)
- Behavioral changes
- Headache
- Visual disturbances
- Aphasia
- Weakness
- Dysphagia
- Memory loss

DX: PE, imaging studies (CT scan, MRI, angiography)

TX: Symptomatic treatment, medication (platelet aggregation inhibitors, thrombolytics [if embolic])

F/U: As needed (dependent on neurologic status), referral to rehabilitation program

Additional differential diagnoses: ALS ▪ Bell's palsy ▪ botulism ▪ brain abscess ▪ brain tumor ▪ encephalitis ▪ head trauma ▪ migraine headache ▪ multiple sclerosis ▪ myasthenia gravis ▪ neurosyphilis ▪ Parkinson's disease ▪ peripheral nerve trauma ▪ peripheral neuropathy ▪ poliomyelitis ▪ rabies ▪ seizure disorders ▪ spinal cord tumors ▪ subarachnoid hemorrhage ▪ syringomyelia ▪ thoracic aortic aneurysm ▪ West Nile encephalitis

Other causes: neuromuscular blocking agents (pancuronium, curare) ▪ electroconvulsive therapy

Paresthesia

Paresthesia is an abnormal sensation or combination of sensations — often described as numbness, prickling, or tingling — felt along peripheral nerve pathways. These sensations are generally not painful; unpleasant or painful sensations are termed dysesthesias. Paresthesia may develop suddenly or gradually and may be transient or permanent.

A common symptom of many neurologic disorders, paresthesia may also result from certain systemic disorders or drug effects. It may reflect damage or irritation of the parietal lobe, thalamus, spinothalamic tract, or spinal or peripheral nerves — the neural circuit that transmits and interprets sensory stimuli.

History and physical examination

First, explore the paresthesia. When did the abnormal sensations begin? Have the patient describe the character and distribution of the sensations. Also, ask about associated signs and symptoms, such as sensory loss and paresis or paralysis. Next, take a medical history, including neurologic, cardiovascular, metabolic, renal, and chronic inflammatory disorders, such as arthritis or lupus. Has the patient recently sustained a traumatic injury or had surgery or invasive procedures that may have damaged peripheral nerves?

Focus the physical examination on the patient's neurologic status. Assess his level of consciousness and cranial nerve function. Test muscle strength and deep tendon reflexes in limbs affected by paresthesia. Systematically evaluate light touch, pain, temperature, vibration, and position sensation. (See *Testing for analgesia*.) Also, note skin color and temperature, and palpate pulses.

Children may experience paresthesia associated with the same causes as adults. However, they're commonly unable to describe this symptom. Nevertheless, hereditary polyneuropathies are usually first recognized in childhood.

Testing for analgesia

By carefully and systematically testing your patient's sensitivity to pain, you can determine whether his nerve damage has a segmental or peripheral distribution and help locate the causative lesion.

Tell the patient to relax, and explain that you're going to lightly touch areas of his skin with a small pin. Have him close his eyes. Apply the pin firmly enough to produce pain without breaking the skin. (Practice on yourself first to learn how to apply the correct pressure.)

Starting with the patient's head and face, move down his body, pricking his skin on alternating sides. Have the patient report when he feels pain. Use the blunt end of the pin occasionally, and vary your test pattern to gauge the accuracy of his response.

Document your findings thoroughly, noting any areas of lost pain sensation either on a dermatome chart or on peripheral nerve diagrams (if available).

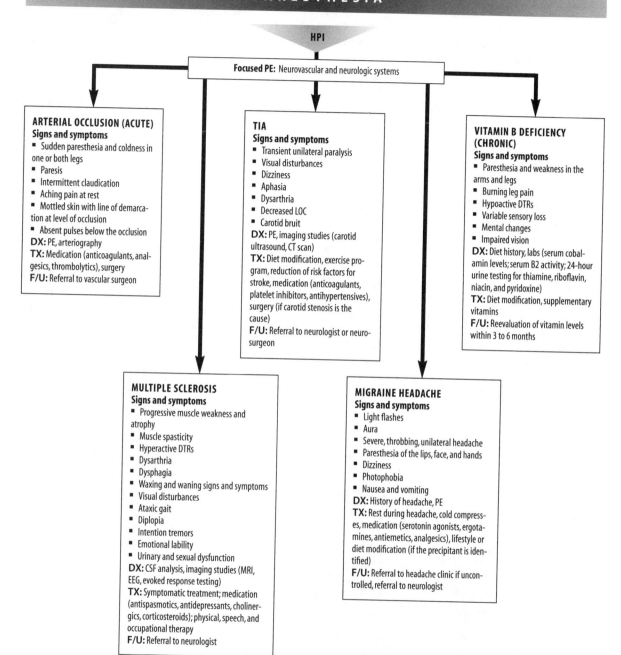

PARESTHESIA

HPI

Focused PE: Neurovascular and neurologic systems

ARTERIAL OCCLUSION (ACUTE)
Signs and symptoms
- Sudden paresthesia and coldness in one or both legs
- Paresis
- Intermittent claudication
- Aching pain at rest
- Mottled skin with line of demarcation at level of occlusion
- Absent pulses below the occlusion

DX: PE, arteriography
TX: Medication (anticoagulants, analgesics, thrombolytics), surgery
F/U: Referral to vascular surgeon

TIA
Signs and symptoms
- Transient unilateral paralysis
- Visual disturbances
- Dizziness
- Aphasia
- Dysarthria
- Decreased LOC
- Carotid bruit

DX: PE, imaging studies (carotid ultrasound, CT scan)
TX: Diet modification, exercise program, reduction of risk factors for stroke, medication (anticoagulants, platelet inhibitors, antihypertensives), surgery (if carotid stenosis is the cause)
F/U: Referral to neurologist or neurosurgeon

VITAMIN B DEFICIENCY (CHRONIC)
Signs and symptoms
- Paresthesia and weakness in the arms and legs
- Burning leg pain
- Hypoactive DTRs
- Variable sensory loss
- Mental changes
- Impaired vision

DX: Diet history, labs (serum cobalamin levels; serum B2 activity; 24-hour urine testing for thiamine, riboflavin, niacin, and pyridoxine)
TX: Diet modification, supplementary vitamins
F/U: Reevaluation of vitamin levels within 3 to 6 months

MULTIPLE SCLEROSIS
Signs and symptoms
- Progressive muscle weakness and atrophy
- Muscle spasticity
- Hyperactive DTRs
- Dysarthria
- Dysphagia
- Waxing and waning signs and symptoms
- Visual disturbances
- Ataxic gait
- Diplopia
- Intention tremors
- Emotional lability
- Urinary and sexual dysfunction

DX: CSF analysis, imaging studies (MRI, EEG, evoked response testing)
TX: Symptomatic treatment; medication (antispasmotics, antidepressants, cholinergics, corticosteroids); physical, speech, and occupational therapy
F/U: Referral to neurologist

MIGRAINE HEADACHE
Signs and symptoms
- Light flashes
- Aura
- Severe, throbbing, unilateral headache
- Paresthesia of the lips, face, and hands
- Dizziness
- Photophobia
- Nausea and vomiting

DX: History of headache, PE
TX: Rest during headache, cold compresses, medication (serotonin agonists, ergotamines, antiemetics, analgesics), lifestyle or diet modification (if the precipitant is identified)
F/U: Referral to headache clinic if uncontrolled, referral to neurologist

Additional differential diagnoses: arteriosclerosis obliterans ▪ arthritis ▪ brain tumor ▪ Buerger's disease ▪ diabetes mellitus ▪ Guillain-Barré syndrome ▪ head trauma ▪ heavy metal or solvent poisoning ▪ herniated disk ▪ herpes zoster ▪ hyperventilation syndrome ▪ hypocalcemia ▪ peripheral nerve trauma ▪ peripheral neuropathy ▪ rabies ▪ Raynaud's disease ▪ seizure disorders ▪ spinal cord injury ▪ spinal cord tumors ▪ SLE ▪ stroke ▪ tabes dorsalis ▪ thoracic outlet syndrome

Other causes: phenytoin ▪ chemotherapeutic agents (vincristine, vinblastine, procarbazine) ▪ isoniazid ▪ nitrofurantoin ▪ chloroquine ▪ parenteral gold therapy ▪ radiation therapy

Peau d'orange

Usually a late sign of breast cancer, peau d'orange (orange peel skin) is the edematous thickening and pitting of breast skin. This slowly developing sign can also occur with breast or axillary lymph node infection, erisypelas, and Graves' disease. Its striking orange peel appearance stems from lymphatic edema around deepened hair follicles. (See *Recognizing peau d'orange*.)

History and physical examination

Ask the patient when she first detected peau d'orange. Has she noticed any lumps, pain, or other breast changes? Does she have related symptoms, such as malaise, achiness, and weight loss? Is she lactating, or has she recently weaned her infant? Has she had previous axillary surgery that might have impaired lymphatic drainage of a breast?

In a well-lit examining room, observe the patient's breasts. Estimate the extent of the peau d'orange, and check for erythema. Assess the nipples for discharge, deviation, retraction, dimpling, and cracking. Gently palpate the area of peau d'orange, noting warmth or induration. Then palpate the entire breast, noting any fixed or mobile lumps, and the axillary lymph nodes, noting enlargement. Finally, take the patient's temperature.

Recognizing peau d'orange

In peau d'orange, the skin appears to be pitted (as shown at right). This condition usually indicates late-stage breast cancer.

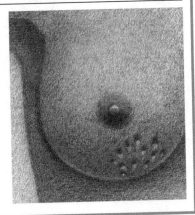

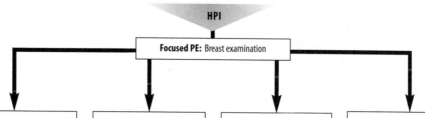

HPI

Focused PE: Breast examination

BREAST ABSCESS
Signs and symptoms
- Thick, purulent nipple discharge
- Abrupt onset of high fever and chills
- Breast pain, tenderness, and erythema
- Palpable soft nodule or generalized induration of the affected breast
- Axillary lymphadenopathy
DX: PE, mammography, breast biopsy
TX: Moist heat to the affected area, medication (antibiotics, analgesics), surgery
F/U: Reevaluation in 7 to 10 days

BREAST CANCER
Signs and symptoms
- Bloody, watery, or purulent discharge from a normal-appearing nipple
- Hard, irregular, fixed lump
- Erythema
- Dimpling
- Nipple deviation or retraction
- Axillary lymphadenopathy
DX: PE, imaging studies (mammography, ultrasound), breast biopsy
TX: Chemotherapy, radiation therapy, surgery
F/U: Referrals to oncologist and surgeon

ERYSIPELAS
Signs and symptoms
- Well-demarcated erythematous elevated area (commonly with peau d'orange texture)
- Pain
- Warmth
- Fever and chills
- Fatigue
DX: PE, labs (CBC, ESR, blood cultures), biopsy
TX: Warm, moist compresses; medication (analgesics, antipyretics, antibiotics)
F/U: Reevaluation in 48 to 72 hours, then in 7 to 10 days

GRAVES' DISEASE
Signs and symptoms
- Peau d'orange–like areas that coalesce
- Increasing appetite
- Weight loss
- Protruding eyes
- Restlessness
- Heat intolerance
- Increased swelling
- Fatigue
- Muscle cramps
- Tremor
- Frequent bowel movements
- Menstrual irregularities in women
- Goiter (possible)
DX: PE, labs (TSH, T_3, T_4, thyroid resin uptake, radioactive iodine uptake)
TX: Medication (antithyroid agents, radioactive iodine), surgery
F/U: Referral to endocrinologist

Photophobia

A common symptom, photophobia is an abnormal sensitivity to light. In many patients, photophobia simply indicates increased eye sensitivity without any underlying pathology. For example, it can stem from excessive wearing of contact lenses or use of poorly fitted lenses. In others, this symptom can result from systemic disorders, ocular disorders or trauma, or the use of certain drugs.

History and physical examination

If your patient reports photophobia, find out its onset and severity. Did it follow eye trauma, a chemical splash, or exposure to the rays of a sun lamp? If photophobia results from trauma, avoid eye manipulation. Ask the patient about eye pain, and have him describe its location, duration, and intensity. Does he have a sensation of a foreign body in his eye? Does he have any other signs and symptoms, such as increased tearing and vision changes?

Next, take the patient's vital signs and assess his neurologic status. Follow this with a careful eye examination, inspecting the eyes' external structures for any abnormalities. Examine the conjunctiva and sclera, noting especially their color. Characterize the amount and consistency of any discharge. Then check pupillary reaction to light. Evaluate extraocular muscle function by testing the six cardinal fields of gaze, and test visual acuity in both eyes.

During your assessment, keep in mind that photophobia can accompany life-threatening meningitis, although it isn't a cardinal sign of meningeal irritation.

PEDIATRIC POINTERS

- *Suspect photophobia in any child who squints, rubs his eyes frequently, or wears sunglasses indoors and outside.*
- *Congenital disorders (such as albinism) and childhood diseases (such as measles and rubella) can cause photophobia.*

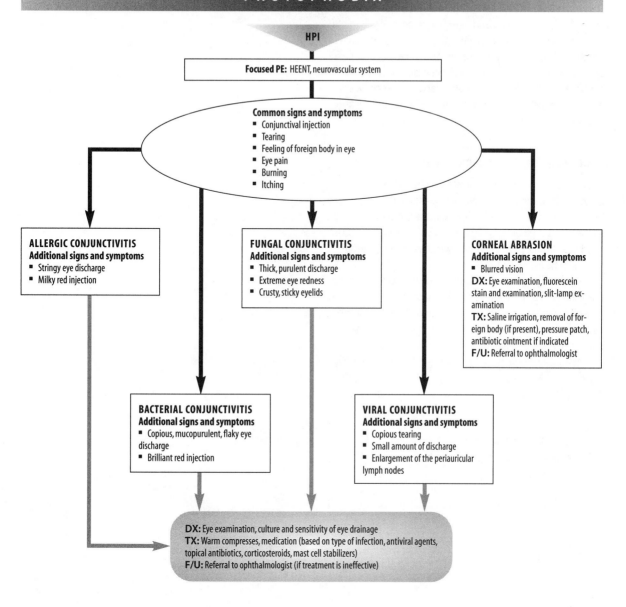

HPI

Focused PE: HEENT, neurovascular system

Common signs and symptoms
- Conjunctival injection
- Tearing
- Feeling of foreign body in eye
- Eye pain
- Burning
- Itching

ALLERGIC CONJUNCTIVITIS
Additional signs and symptoms
- Stringy eye discharge
- Milky red injection

FUNGAL CONJUNCTIVITIS
Additional signs and symptoms
- Thick, purulent discharge
- Extreme eye redness
- Crusty, sticky eyelids

CORNEAL ABRASION
Additional signs and symptoms
- Blurred vision

DX: Eye examination, fluorescein stain and examination, slit-lamp examination
TX: Saline irrigation, removal of foreign body (if present), pressure patch, antibiotic ointment if indicated
F/U: Referral to ophthalmologist

BACTERIAL CONJUNCTIVITIS
Additional signs and symptoms
- Copious, mucopurulent, flaky eye discharge
- Brilliant red injection

VIRAL CONJUNCTIVITIS
Additional signs and symptoms
- Copious tearing
- Small amount of discharge
- Enlargement of the periauricular lymph nodes

DX: Eye examination, culture and sensitivity of eye drainage
TX: Warm compresses, medication (based on type of infection, antiviral agents, topical antibiotics, corticosteroids, mast cell stabilizers)
F/U: Referral to ophthalmologist (if treatment is ineffective)

Additional differential diagnoses: burns ▪ corneal foreign body ▪ corneal ulcer ▪ dry eye syndrome ▪ iritis (acute) ▪ keratitis (interstitial) ▪ meningitis (acute bacterial) ▪ migraine headache ▪ scleritis ▪ sclerokeratitis ▪ trachoma ▪ uveitis

---

Other causes: mydriatics (phenylephrine, atropine, scopolamine, cyclopentolate, tropicamide) ▪ amphetamines ▪ cocaine ▪ ophthalmic antifungal drugs (trifluridine, vidarabine, idoxuridine)

Pica

Pica refers to the craving and ingestion of normally inedible substances, such as plaster, charcoal, clay, wool, ashes, paint, or dirt. In children, the most commonly affected group, pica typically results from nutritional deficiencies. However, in adults, pica may reflect a psychological disturbance. Depending on the substance eaten, pica can lead to poisoning and GI disorders.

History and physical examination

Begin by determining what substances the patient has been eating. If the patient has eaten toxic substances (such as lead), obtain a serum lead level. With a child, ask the parents to describe his eating habits and nutritional history. When did the child first display pica? Does he always crave the same substance? Is he listless or irritable?

Check the patient's vital signs, noting especially bradycardia, tachycardia, or hypotension. Then inspect the abdomen for visible peristaltic waves or other abnormalities. Also, observe the hair, skin, and mucous membranes for changes, such as dryness or pallor.

PEDIATRIC POINTER

Many older homes contain lead-based paints. Children who live in older homes may be at risk for lead poisoning from eating chipped paint or even from sucking their fingers if the lead paint has infiltrated house dust. Inner-city children and children in older homes should be monitored for serum lead levels.

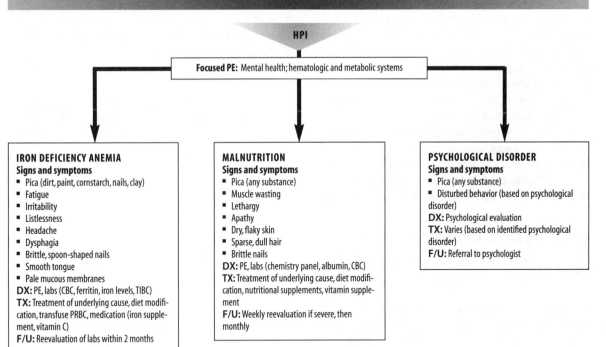

HPI

Focused PE: Mental health; hematologic and metabolic systems

IRON DEFICIENCY ANEMIA
Signs and symptoms
- Pica (dirt, paint, cornstarch, nails, clay)
- Fatigue
- Irritability
- Listlessness
- Headache
- Dysphagia
- Brittle, spoon-shaped nails
- Smooth tongue
- Pale mucous membranes

DX: PE, labs (CBC, ferritin, iron levels, TIBC)
TX: Treatment of underlying cause, diet modification, transfuse PRBC, medication (iron supplement, vitamin C)
F/U: Reevaluation of labs within 2 months

MALNUTRITION
Signs and symptoms
- Pica (any substance)
- Muscle wasting
- Lethargy
- Apathy
- Dry, flaky skin
- Sparse, dull hair
- Brittle nails

DX: PE, labs (chemistry panel, albumin, CBC)
TX: Treatment of underlying cause, diet modification, nutritional supplements, vitamin supplement
F/U: Weekly reevaluation if severe, then monthly

PSYCHOLOGICAL DISORDER
Signs and symptoms
- Pica (any substance)
- Disturbed behavior (based on psychological disorder)

DX: Psychological evaluation
TX: Varies (based on identified psychological disorder)
F/U: Referral to psychologist

Other causes: cultural beliefs (pica is an accepted practice in some cultures based on presumed nutritional or therapeutic properties or on religious or superstitious beliefs) ∎ pregnancy

Pleural friction rub

Commonly resulting from pulmonary disorders or trauma, this loud, coarse, and grating, creaking, or squeaking sound may be auscultated over one or both lungs during late inspiration or early expiration. It's heard best over the low axilla or the anterior, lateral, or posterior bases of the lung fields with the patient upright. Sometimes intermittent, it may resemble crackles or a pericardial friction rub.

A pleural friction rub indicates inflammation of the visceral and parietal pleural lining, which causes congestion and edema. The resultant fibrinous exudate covers both pleural surfaces, displacing the fluid that's normally between them and causing the surfaces to rub together.

History and physical examination

When you detect a pleural friction rub, quickly look for signs of respiratory distress. If the patient isn't in severe distress, explore related symptoms. Find out whether he has had chest pain. If so, ask him to describe its location and severity. How long does his chest pain last? Does it radiate to his shoulder, neck, or upper abdomen? Does the pain worsen with breathing, movement, coughing, or sneezing? Does it abate if he splints his chest, holds his breath, or exerts pressure or lies on the affected side? Has the patient experienced any fever?

Because pain is subjective and is exacerbated by anxiety, patients who are highly emotional may complain more readily of pleuritic pain than those who are habitually stoic about symptoms of illness.

Ask the patient about a history of rheumatoid arthritis, respiratory or cardiovascular disorders, recent trauma, asbestos exposure, or radiation therapy. If he smokes, obtain a history in pack-years.

Characterize the pleural friction rub by auscultating the lungs with the patient sitting upright and breathing deeply and slowly through his mouth. Is the friction rub unilateral or bilateral? Also, listen for absent or diminished breath sounds, noting their location and timing in the respiratory cycle. Do abnormal breath sounds clear with coughing? Observe for clubbing and pedal edema, which may indicate a chronic disorder. Then palpate for decreased chest motion and percuss for flatness or dullness.

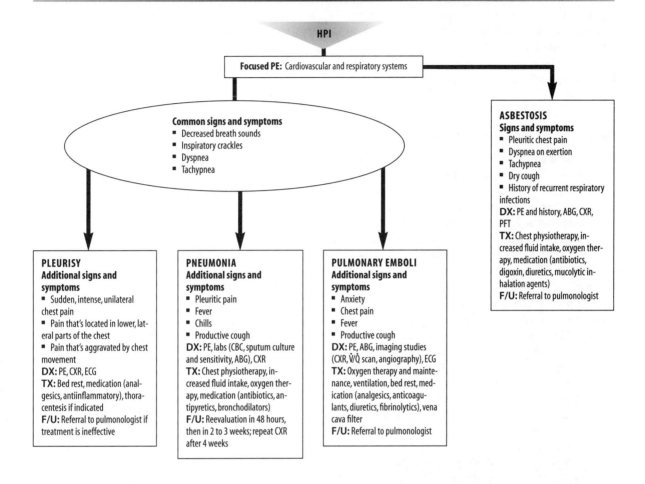

HPI

Focused PE: Cardiovascular and respiratory systems

Common signs and symptoms
- Decreased breath sounds
- Inspiratory crackles
- Dyspnea
- Tachypnea

ASBESTOSIS
Signs and symptoms
- Pleuritic chest pain
- Dyspnea on exertion
- Tachypnea
- Dry cough
- History of recurrent respiratory infections

DX: PE and history, ABG, CXR, PFT
TX: Chest physiotherapy, increased fluid intake, oxygen therapy, medication (antibiotics, digoxin, diuretics, mucolytic inhalation agents)
F/U: Referral to pulmonologist

PLEURISY
Additional signs and symptoms
- Sudden, intense, unilateral chest pain
- Pain that's located in lower, lateral parts of the chest
- Pain that's aggravated by chest movement

DX: PE, CXR, ECG
TX: Bed rest, medication (analgesics, antiinflammatory), thoracentesis if indicated
F/U: Referral to pulmonologist if treatment is ineffective

PNEUMONIA
Additional signs and symptoms
- Pleuritic pain
- Fever
- Chills
- Productive cough

DX: PE, labs (CBC, sputum culture and sensitivity, ABG), CXR
TX: Chest physiotherapy, increased fluid intake, oxygen therapy, medication (antibiotics, antipyretics, bronchodilators)
F/U: Reevaluation in 48 hours, then in 2 to 3 weeks; repeat CXR after 4 weeks

PULMONARY EMBOLI
Additional signs and symptoms
- Anxiety
- Chest pain
- Fever
- Productive cough

DX: PE, ABG, imaging studies (CXR, V̇/Q̇ scan, angiography), ECG
TX: Oxygen therapy and maintenance, ventilation, bed rest, medication (analgesics, anticoagulants, diuretics, fibrinolytics), vena cava filter
F/U: Referral to pulmonologist

Additional differential diagnoses: lung cancer ▪ rheumatoid arthritis ▪ SLE ▪ tuberculosis (pulmonary)

Other causes: thoracic surgery ▪ radiation therapy

Polydipsia

Polydipsia refers to excessive thirst, a common symptom associated with endocrine disorders and certain drugs. It may reflect decreased fluid intake, increased urine output, or excessive loss of water and salt. Polydipsia is also a common occurrence in psychiatric patients, especially those who are psychotic.

History and physical examination

Obtain a history. Ask when the increased thirst was first noticed. Find out how much fluid the patient drinks each day and at what time of the day the thirst occurs. How often and how much does he typically urinate? Does the need to urinate awaken him at night? Determine whether he or anyone in his family has diabetes or kidney disease. What medications does he use? Has his lifestyle changed recently? If so, have these changes upset him? Is there a history of a psychological disorder?

If the patient has polydipsia, take his blood pressure and pulse when he's in the supine and standing positions. A decrease of 10 mm Hg in systolic pressure and a pulse rate increase of 10 beats/minute from the supine to the standing position may indicate hypovolemia. Check for signs of dehydration, such as dry mucous membranes and decreased skin turgor. Check for signs of bleeding. Note any edema. Also, ask about recent weight loss or gain. Is there a history of recurrent infection? Review the patient's exercise and dietary habits. (See *Water intoxication*.)

PEDIATRIC POINTERS

- *In children, polydipsia usually stems from diabetes insipidus or diabetes mellitus.*
- *Rare causes include pheochromocytoma, neuroblastoma, and Prader-Willi syndrome.*
- *Some children develop habitual polydipsia that's unrelated to any disease.*

Water intoxication

Water intoxication, which can occur after ingestion of large amounts of water, causes cerebral swelling and fluid build-up in the lungs. Many athletes (such as marathon runners, cyclists, and hikers) consume large amounts of water to prevent dehydration. However, this over-consumption can cause blood plasma to increase, resulting in dilution of the sodium content of the blood. The athlete also loses sodium through sweat.

Water intoxication may also be a lethal consequence of ingestion of the street drug called "ecstasy," which induces syndrome of inappropriate antidiuretic hormone secretion.

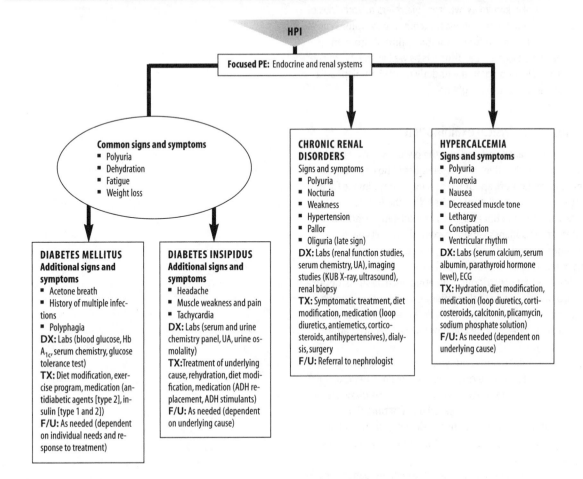

HPI

Focused PE: Endocrine and renal systems

Common signs and symptoms
- Polyuria
- Dehydration
- Fatigue
- Weight loss

DIABETES MELLITUS
Additional signs and symptoms
- Acetone breath
- History of multiple infections
- Polyphagia

DX: Labs (blood glucose, Hb A$_{1c}$, serum chemistry, glucose tolerance test)
TX: Diet modification, exercise program, medication (antidiabetic agents [type 2], insulin [type 1 and 2])
F/U: As needed (dependent on individual needs and response to treatment)

DIABETES INSIPIDUS
Additional signs and symptoms
- Headache
- Muscle weakness and pain
- Tachycardia

DX: Labs (serum and urine chemistry panel, UA, urine osmolality)
TX: Treatment of underlying cause, rehydration, diet modification, medication (ADH replacement, ADH stimulants)
F/U: As needed (dependent on underlying cause)

CHRONIC RENAL DISORDERS
Signs and symptoms
- Polyuria
- Nocturia
- Weakness
- Hypertension
- Pallor
- Oliguria (late sign)

DX: Labs (renal function studies, serum chemistry, UA), imaging studies (KUB X-ray, ultrasound), renal biopsy
TX: Symptomatic treatment, diet modification, medication (loop diuretics, antiemetics, corticosteroids, antihypertensives), dialysis, surgery
F/U: Referral to nephrologist

HYPERCALCEMIA
Signs and symptoms
- Polyuria
- Anorexia
- Nausea
- Decreased muscle tone
- Lethargy
- Constipation
- Ventricular rhythm

DX: Labs (serum calcium, serum albumin, parathyroid hormone level), ECG
TX: Hydration, diet modification, medication (loop diuretics, corticosteroids, calcitonin, plicamycin, sodium phosphate solution)
F/U: As needed (dependent on underlying cause)

Additional differential diagnoses: hypokalemia ▪ psychogenic polydipsia ▪ Sheehan's syndrome ▪ sickle cell anemia ▪ thyrotoxicosis

Other causes: diuretics ▪ demeclocycline ▪ phenothiazines ▪ anticholinergics

Polyphagia

Polyphagia, also known as hyperphagia, refers to voracious or excessive eating before satiety. This common symptom can be persistent or intermittent, resulting primarily from endocrine and psychological disorders as well as the use of certain drugs. Depending on the underlying cause, polyphagia may or may not cause weight gain.

History and physical examination

Begin your evaluation by asking the patient what he has had to eat and drink within the last 24 hours. (If he easily recalls this information, ask about the previous 2 days' intake for a broader view of his dietary habits.) Note the frequency of meals and the amount and types of food eaten. Find out whether the patient's eating or exercising habits have changed recently. Has he always had a large appetite? Does his overeating alternate with periods of anorexia? Ask about conditions that may trigger overeating, such as stress, depression, or menstruation (if the patient is female). Does the patient actually feel hungry or does he eat simply because food is available? Does he ever vomit or have a headache after overeating?

Explore related signs and symptoms. Has the patient recently gained or lost weight? Does he feel tired, nervous, or excitable? Has he experienced heat intolerance, dizziness, or palpitations? Diarrhea or increased thirst or urination? Ask about past medical history, such as diabetes or thyroid disease. Obtain a complete drug history, including use of laxatives or enemas.

During the physical examination, weigh the patient. Tell him his current weight, and watch for any expression of disbelief or anger. Inspect the skin to detect dryness or poor turgor. Palpate the thyroid for enlargement. Note any edema.

PEDIATRIC POINTERS

- *In children, polyphagia commonly results from juvenile diabetes.*
- *In infants ages 6 to 18 months, it can result from such malabsorptive disorders as celiac disease.*
- *Polyphagia may occur normally in a child who is experiencing a sudden growth spurt.*

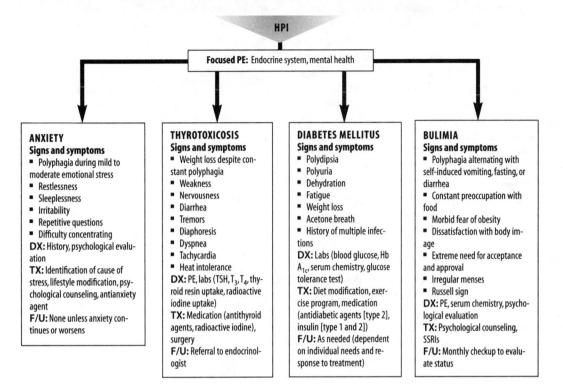

HPI

Focused PE: Endocrine system, mental health

ANXIETY
Signs and symptoms
- Polyphagia during mild to moderate emotional stress
- Restlessness
- Sleeplessness
- Irritability
- Repetitive questions
- Difficulty concentrating

DX: History, psychological evaluation

TX: Identification of cause of stress, lifestyle modification, psychological counseling, antianxiety agent

F/U: None unless anxiety continues or worsens

THYROTOXICOSIS
Signs and symptoms
- Weight loss despite constant polyphagia
- Weakness
- Nervousness
- Diarrhea
- Tremors
- Diaphoresis
- Dyspnea
- Tachycardia
- Heat intolerance

DX: PE, labs (TSH, T_3, T_4, thyroid resin uptake, radioactive iodine uptake)

TX: Medication (antithyroid agents, radioactive iodine), surgery

F/U: Referral to endocrinologist

DIABETES MELLITUS
Signs and symptoms
- Polydipsia
- Polyuria
- Dehydration
- Fatigue
- Weight loss
- Acetone breath
- History of multiple infections

DX: Labs (blood glucose, Hb A_{1c}, serum chemistry, glucose tolerance test)

TX: Diet modification, exercise program, medication (antidiabetic agents [type 2], insulin [type 1 and 2])

F/U: As needed (dependent on individual needs and response to treatment)

BULIMIA
Signs and symptoms
- Polyphagia alternating with self-induced vomiting, fasting, or diarrhea
- Constant preoccupation with food
- Morbid fear of obesity
- Dissatisfaction with body image
- Extreme need for acceptance and approval
- Irregular menses
- Russell sign

DX: PE, serum chemistry, psychological evaluation

TX: Psychological counseling, SSRIs

F/U: Monthly checkup to evaluate status

Additional differential diagnoses: migraine headache ▪ premenstrual syndrome

---

Other causes: corticosteroids ▪ cyproheptadine

Polyuria

A relatively common sign, polyuria is the daily production and excretion of more than 3,000 ml (3 L) of urine. It's usually reported by the patient as increased urination, especially when it occurs at night. Polyuria is aggravated by overhydration, consumption of caffeine or alcohol, and excessive ingestion of salt, glucose, or other hyperosmolar substances.

Polyuria most commonly results from the use of certain drugs (such as diuretics) and from psychological, neurologic, and renal disorders. It can reflect central nervous system dysfunction that diminishes or suppresses secretion of antidiuretic hormone (ADH), which regulates fluid balance. Or, when ADH levels are normal, it can reflect renal impairment. In both of these pathophysiologic mechanisms, the renal tubules fail to reabsorb sufficient water, causing polyuria.

History and physical examination

Because the patient with polyuria is at risk for developing hypovolemia, evaluate fluid status first. Take vital signs, noting especially increased body temperature, tachycardia, and orthostatic hypotension. Inspect for dry skin and mucous membranes, decreased skin turgor and elasticity, and reduced perspiration. Is the patient unusually tired or thirsty? Has he recently lost more than 5% of his body weight? If you detect these effects of hypovolemia, you'll need to infuse replacement fluids.

If the patient doesn't display signs of hypovolemia, explore the frequency and pattern of the polyuria. When did it begin? How long has it lasted? Was it precipitated by a certain event? Ask the patient to describe the pattern and amount of his daily fluid intake. Check for a history of visual deficits, headaches, or head trauma, which may precede diabetes insipidus. Also check for a history of urinary tract obstruction or infection, diabetes mellitus, renal disorders, chronic hypokalemia or hypercalcemia, and psychiatric disorders (both past and present). Find out the schedule and dosage of any drugs the patient is currently taking.

Perform a neurologic examination, noting especially any change in the patient's level of consciousness. Then palpate the bladder and inspect the urethral meatus. Obtain a urine specimen, and check its specific gravity.

- Because a child's fluid balance is more delicate than an adult's, check his urine specific gravity at each voiding and be alert for signs of dehydration. These include a decrease in body weight, decreased skin turgor, dry mucous membranes, decreased urine output, absence of tears when crying, and pale, mottled, or gray skin.

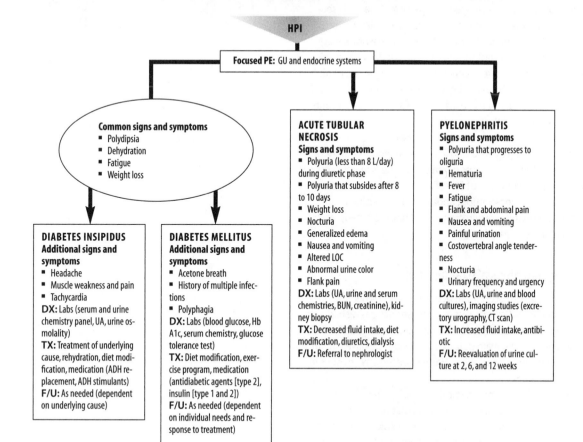

HPI

Focused PE: GU and endocrine systems

Common signs and symptoms
- Polydipsia
- Dehydration
- Fatigue
- Weight loss

DIABETES INSIPIDUS
Additional signs and symptoms
- Headache
- Muscle weakness and pain
- Tachycardia

DX: Labs (serum and urine chemistry panel, UA, urine osmolality)
TX: Treatment of underlying cause, rehydration, diet modification, medication (ADH replacement, ADH stimulants)
F/U: As needed (dependent on underlying cause)

DIABETES MELLITUS
Additional signs and symptoms
- Acetone breath
- History of multiple infections
- Polyphagia

DX: Labs (blood glucose, Hb A1c, serum chemistry, glucose tolerance test)
TX: Diet modification, exercise program, medication (antidiabetic agents [type 2], insulin [type 1 and 2])
F/U: As needed (dependent on individual needs and response to treatment)

ACUTE TUBULAR NECROSIS
Signs and symptoms
- Polyuria (less than 8 L/day) during diuretic phase
- Polyuria that subsides after 8 to 10 days
- Weight loss
- Nocturia
- Generalized edema
- Nausea and vomiting
- Altered LOC
- Abnormal urine color
- Flank pain

DX: Labs (UA, urine and serum chemistries, BUN, creatinine), kidney biopsy
TX: Decreased fluid intake, diet modification, diuretics, dialysis
F/U: Referral to nephrologist

PYELONEPHRITIS
Signs and symptoms
- Polyuria that progresses to oliguria
- Hematuria
- Fever
- Fatigue
- Flank and abdominal pain
- Nausea and vomiting
- Painful urination
- Costovertebral angle tenderness
- Nocturia
- Urinary frequency and urgency

DX: Labs (UA, urine and blood cultures), imaging studies (excretory urography, CT scan)
TX: Increased fluid intake, antibiotic
F/U: Reevaluation of urine culture at 2, 6, and 12 weeks

Additional differential diagnoses: hypercalcemia ▪ hypokalemia ▪ postobstructive uropathy ▪ psychogenic polydipsia ▪ Sheehan's syndrome ▪ sickle cell anemia

Other causes: contrast media ▪ diuretics ▪ cardiotonics ▪ vitamin D ▪ demeclocycline ▪ phenytoin ▪ lithium ▪ methoxyflurane ▪ propoxyphene

Priapism

A urologic emergency, priapism is a persistent, painful erection that's unrelated to sexual excitation. This relatively rare sign may begin during sleep and appear to be a normal erection; however, it may last for several hours or days. It's usually accompanied by a severe, constant, dull aching in the penis. Despite the pain, the patient may be too embarrassed to seek medical help and may try to achieve detumescence through continued sexual activity.

Priapism occurs when the veins of the corpora cavernosa fail to drain correctly, resulting in persistent engorgement of the tissues. Without prompt treatment, penile ischemia and thrombosis occur. In about half of all cases, priapism is idiopathic and develops without apparent predisposing factors. Secondary priapism results from blood disorders, neoplasms, trauma, and the use of certain drugs.

History and physical examination

When the patient's condition permits, ask him when the priapism began. Is it continuous or intermittent? Has he had a prolonged erection before? If so, what did he do to relieve it? How long did he remain detumescent? Does he have pain or tenderness when he urinates? Has he noticed any changes in sexual function?

Explore the patient's medical history. If he reports sickle cell anemia, find out about any factors that could precipitate a crisis, such as dehydration and infection. Ask whether he has recently suffered genital trauma, and obtain a thorough drug history.

Examine the patient's penis, noting its color and temperature. Check for any loss of sensation, and look for signs of infection, such as redness or drainage. Finally, take his vital signs, particularly noting fever.

PEDIATRIC POINTERS

- *In neonates, priapism can result from hypoxia but is usually resolved with oxygen therapy.*
- *Priapism is more likely to develop in children with sickle cell disease than in adults with the disease.*

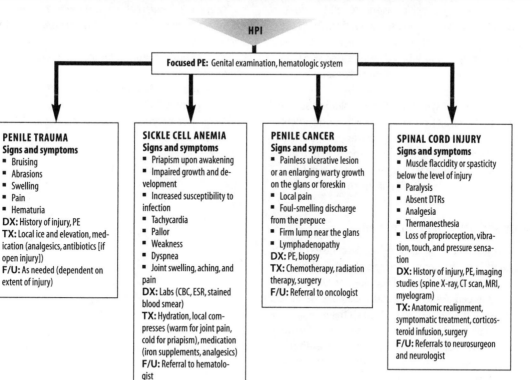

HPI

Focused PE: Genital examination, hematologic system

PENILE TRAUMA
Signs and symptoms
- Bruising
- Abrasions
- Swelling
- Pain
- Hematuria

DX: History of injury, PE
TX: Local ice and elevation, medication (analgesics, antibiotics [if open injury])
F/U: As needed (dependent on extent of injury)

SICKLE CELL ANEMIA
Signs and symptoms
- Priapism upon awakening
- Impaired growth and development
- Increased susceptibility to infection
- Tachycardia
- Pallor
- Weakness
- Dyspnea
- Joint swelling, aching, and pain

DX: Labs (CBC, ESR, stained blood smear)
TX: Hydration, local compresses (warm for joint pain, cold for priapism), medication (iron supplements, analgesics)
F/U: Referral to hematologist

PENILE CANCER
Signs and symptoms
- Painless ulcerative lesion or an enlarging warty growth on the glans or foreskin
- Local pain
- Foul-smelling discharge from the prepuce
- Firm lump near the glans
- Lymphadenopathy

DX: PE, biopsy
TX: Chemotherapy, radiation therapy, surgery
F/U: Referral to oncologist

SPINAL CORD INJURY
Signs and symptoms
- Muscle flaccidity or spasticity below the level of injury
- Paralysis
- Absent DTRs
- Analgesia
- Thermanesthesia
- Loss of proprioception, vibration, touch, and pressure sensation

DX: History of injury, PE, imaging studies (spine X-ray, CT scan, MRI, myelogram)
TX: Anatomic realignment, symptomatic treatment, corticosteroid infusion, surgery
F/U: Referrals to neurosurgeon and neurologist

Other causes: phenothiazines ▪ thioridazine ▪ trazodone ▪ androgenic steroids ▪ anticoagulants ▪ antihypertensives ▪ intracorporeal injection of papaverine

Pruritus

Commonly provoking scratching as an attempt to gain relief, pruritus is an unpleasant itching sensation that affects the skin, certain mucous membranes, and the eyes. Most severe at night, pruritus may be exacerbated by increased skin temperature, poor skin turgor, local vasodilation, dermatoses, and stress.

The most common symptom of dermatologic disorders, pruritus may also result from local and systemic disorders and from drug use. Physiologic pruritus (such as pruritic urticarial papules and plaques of pregnancy) may occur in primigravidas late in the third trimester. Pruritus can also stem from emotional upset or contact with skin irritants.

History and physical examination

If the patient reports pruritus, have him describe its onset, frequency, and intensity. If pruritus occurs at night, ask him whether it prevents him from falling asleep or awakens him after he falls asleep. (Generally, pruritus related to dermatoses prevents — but doesn't disturb — sleep.) Is the itching localized or generalized? When is it most severe? How long does it last? Is there a relationship to activities (physical exertion, bathing, applying makeup, or use of perfumes)? Has there been any recent change in soap, detergent, or medications? Locate the area of pruritis.

Ask the patient how he cleans his skin. In particular, look for excessive bathing, harsh soaps, contact allergy, and excessively hot water. Does he have occupational exposure to known skin irritants, such as fiberglass insulation or chemicals? Ask about the patient's general health and what medications he takes (new medications are suspect). Has he recently traveled abroad? Does he have any pets? Does anyone else in the house report itching? Does exercise, stress, fear, depression, or illness seem to aggravate the itching? Ask about contact with skin irritants, previous skin disorders, and related symptoms. Then obtain a complete drug history.

Examine the patient for signs of scratching, such as excoriation, purpura, scabs, scars, or lichenification. Look for primary lesions to help confirm dermatoses.

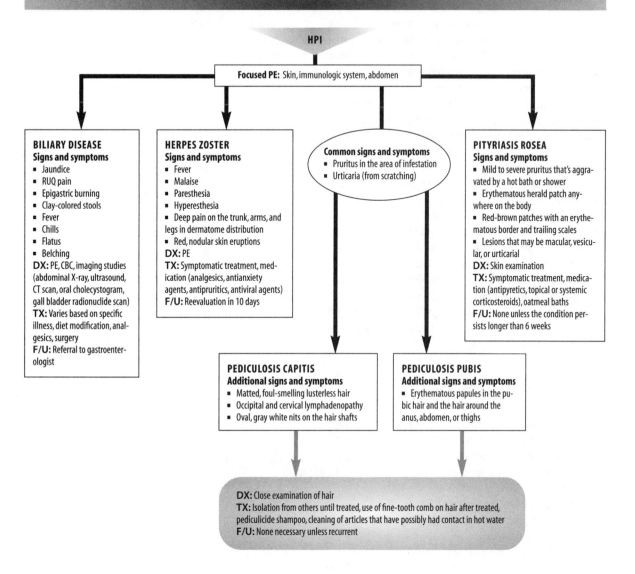

HPI

Focused PE: Skin, immunologic system, abdomen

BILIARY DISEASE
Signs and symptoms
- Jaundice
- RUQ pain
- Epigastric burning
- Clay-colored stools
- Fever
- Chills
- Flatus
- Belching

DX: PE, CBC, imaging studies (abdominal X-ray, ultrasound, CT scan, oral cholecystogram, gall bladder radionuclide scan)
TX: Varies based on specific illness, diet modification, analgesics, surgery
F/U: Referral to gastroenterologist

HERPES ZOSTER
Signs and symptoms
- Fever
- Malaise
- Paresthesia
- Hyperesthesia
- Deep pain on the trunk, arms, and legs in dermatome distribution
- Red, nodular skin eruptions

DX: PE
TX: Symptomatic treatment, medication (analgesics, antianxiety agents, antipruritics, antiviral agents)
F/U: Reevaluation in 10 days

Common signs and symptoms
- Pruritus in the area of infestation
- Urticaria (from scratching)

PITYRIASIS ROSEA
Signs and symptoms
- Mild to severe pruritus that's aggravated by a hot bath or shower
- Erythematous herald patch anywhere on the body
- Red-brown patches with an erythematous border and trailing scales
- Lesions that may be macular, vesicular, or urticarial

DX: Skin examination
TX: Symptomatic treatment, medication (antipyretics, topical or systemic corticosteroids), oatmeal baths
F/U: None unless the condition persists longer than 6 weeks

PEDICULOSIS CAPITIS
Additional signs and symptoms
- Matted, foul-smelling lusterless hair
- Occipital and cervical lymphadenopathy
- Oval, gray white nits on the hair shafts

PEDICULOSIS PUBIS
Additional signs and symptoms
- Erythematous papules in the pubic hair and the hair around the anus, abdomen, or thighs

DX: Close examination of hair
TX: Isolation from others until treated, use of fine-tooth comb on hair after treated, pediculicide shampoo, cleaning of articles that have possibly had contact in hot water
F/U: None necessary unless recurrent

Additional differential diagnoses: anemia (iron deficiency) ▪ conjunctivitis ▪ dermatitis ▪ enterobiasis ▪ hemorrhoids ▪ herpes zoster ▪ Hodgkin's disease ▪ leukemia (chronic lymphocytic) ▪ lichen planus ▪ lichen simplex chronicus ▪ liver failure ▪ mastocytosis ▪ multiple myeloma ▪ mycosis fungoides ▪ myringitis (chronic) ▪ polycythemia vera ▪ psoriasis ▪ psychogenic pruritus ▪ renal failure (chronic) ▪ scabies ▪ thyrotoxicosis ▪ tinea pedis ▪ urticaria ▪ vaginitis

Other causes: ingestion of fruit pulp from ginkgo tree ▪ bedbug bites ▪ drug hypersensitivity

Ptosis

Ptosis is the excessive drooping of one or both upper eyelids. This sign can be constant, progressive, or intermittent as well as unilateral or bilateral. When it's unilateral, it's easy to detect by comparing the eyelids' relative positions. When it's bilateral or mild, it's difficult to detect — the eyelids may be abnormally low, covering the upper part of the iris or even part of the pupil instead of overlapping the iris slightly. Other clues include a furrowed forehead or a tipped-back head — signs that the patient is compensating to see under his drooping lids. In severe ptosis, the patient may not be able to raise his eyelids voluntarily. Because ptosis can resemble enophthalmos, exophthalmometry may be required.

Ptosis can be classified as congenital or acquired. Classification is important for proper treatment. Congenital ptosis results from levator muscle underdevelopment or disorders of the third cranial (oculomotor) nerve. Acquired ptosis may result from trauma to or inflammation of these muscles and nerves or from certain drugs, systemic diseases, intracranial lesions, or life-threatening aneurysms. However, the most common cause is advanced age, which reduces muscle elasticity and produces senile ptosis.

History and physical examination

Ask the patient when he first noticed his drooping eyelid and whether it has worsened or improved. Find out whether he's suffered a traumatic eye injury recently. (If he has, avoid manipulating the eye to prevent further damage.) Ask about eye pain or headache, and determine its location and severity. Has the patient experienced any vision changes? If so, have him describe them. Does the patient wear corrective lenses or contact lenses? Obtain a drug history, noting especially any chemotherapeutic agents.

Assess the degree of ptosis, and check for eyelid edema, exophthalmos, deviation, and conjunctival injection. Evaluate extraocular muscle function by testing the six cardinal fields of gaze. Carefully examine the pupil's size, color, shape, and reaction to light, and test visual acuity. Is there any convergence, photosensitivity, or photophobia present?

Keep in mind that ptosis occasionally indicates a life-threatening condition. For example, sudden unilateral ptosis can herald a cerebral aneurysm.

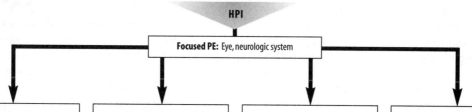

HPI

Focused PE: Eye, neurologic system

HORNER'S SYNDROME
Signs and symptoms
- Moderate unilateral ptosis that almost disappears when the eye is opened widely
- Unilateral miosis
- Ipsilateral anhidrosis of the face and neck
- Transient conjunctivitis
- Vascular headache on the affected side
- Vertigo

DX: Eye examination, pharmacologic testing of the pupil
TX: Treatment of underlying cause
F/U: As needed (dependent on underlying cause)

LACRIMAL GLAND TUMOR
Signs and symptoms
- Mild to severe ptosis (based on tumor size and location)
- Brow elevation
- Exophthalmos
- Eye deviation
- Eye pain

DX: Eye examination, imaging studies (CT scan, MRI)
TX: Radiation therapy, surgery
F/U: Referrals to ophthalmologist and oncologist

MYOTONIC DYSTROPHY
Signs and symptoms
- Mild to severe bilateral ptosis
- Distinctive cataracts with iridescent dots in the cortex
- Miosis
- Diplopia
- Decreased tearing
- Facial weakness
- Slack jaw
- Muscular and testicular atrophy

DX: History and PE, DNA analysis, EMG, ECG, muscle biopsy
TX: Symptomatic treatment, physical and speech therapy, diet modification, antiarrhythmics
F/U: As needed (dependent on the severity of symptoms)

PARRY-ROMBERG SYNDROME
Signs and symptoms
- Unilateral ptosis
- Facial hemiatrophy
- Miosis
- Sluggish pupil
- Enophthalmos
- Different colored irises
- Ocular muscle paralysis
- Nystagmus
- Muscle atrophy

DX: PE
TX: Symptomatic treatment, speech therapy, surgery
F/U: Referral to neurologist

Additional differential diagnoses: alcoholism ▪ botulism ▪ cerebral aneurysm ▪ multiple sclerosis ▪ dacryoadenitis ▪ hemangioma ▪ levator muscle maldevelopment ▪ myasthenia gravis ▪ ocular muscle dystrophy ▪ ocular trauma ▪ Parinaud's syndrome ▪ subdural hematoma (chronic)

Other causes: vinca alkaloids ▪ lead poisoning

Pulse, absent or weak

An absent or a weak pulse may be generalized or may affect only one extremity. When generalized, this sign is an important indicator of such life-threatening conditions as shock and arrhythmia. Localized loss or weakness of a pulse that's normally present and strong may indicate acute arterial occlusion, which could require emergency surgery. However, the pressure of palpation may temporarily diminish or obliterate superficial pulses, such as the posterior tibial or the dorsal pedal. Thus, bilateral weakness or absence of these pulses doesn't necessarily indicate underlying pathology. (See *Evaluating peripheral pulses.*)

History and physical examination

If a patient is unconscious and the pulse is absent, institute emergency measures. If you detect an absent or a weak pulse, quickly palpate the remaining arterial pulses to distinguish between localized or generalized loss or weakness. Then quickly check other vital signs, evaluate cardiopulmonary status, and obtain a brief history. Is there any history of claudication? Does the patient have pain? Is the pulse absent or weak in only one extremity? What is the color and temperature of the extremity? Check for capillary refill. Does the patient have an existing history of venous insufficiency? Perform an abdominal exam to evaluate the presence of an abdominal aortic aneurysm or renal stenosis through the detection of bruits. Based on your findings, proceed with interventions.

Evaluating peripheral pulses

The rate, amplitude, and symmetry of peripheral pulses provide important clues to cardiac function and the quality of peripheral perfusion. To gather these clues, palpate peripheral pulses lightly with the pads of your index, middle, and ring fingers, as space permits.

RATE
Count all pulses for at least 30 seconds (60 seconds when recording vital signs). The normal rate is between 60 and 100 beats/minute.

AMPLITUDE
Palpate the blood vessel during ventricular systole. Describe pulse amplitude by using a scale such as this:
    4+ = bounding
    3+ = normal
    2+ = difficult to palpate
    1+ = weak, thready
    0 = absent.
    Use a stick figure to easily document the location and amplitude of all pulses.

SYMMETRY
Simultaneously palpate pulses (except the carotid pulse) on both sides of the patient's body, and note inequality. Always assess peripheral pulses methodically, moving from the arms to the legs.

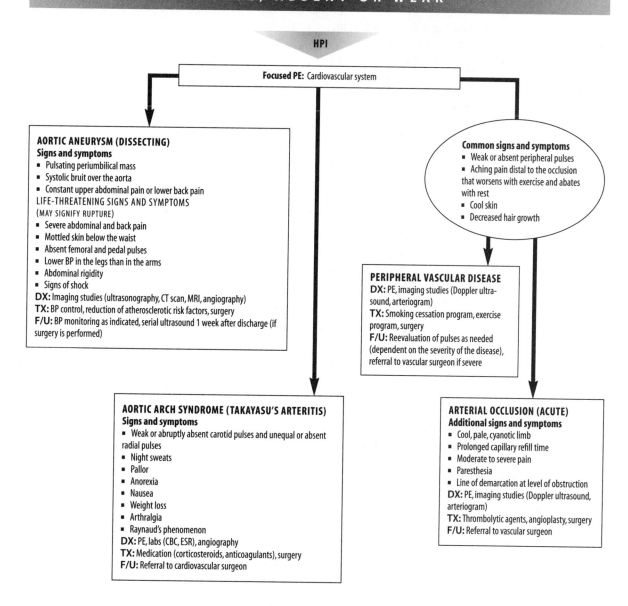

HPI

Focused PE: Cardiovascular system

AORTIC ANEURYSM (DISSECTING)
Signs and symptoms
- Pulsating periumbilical mass
- Systolic bruit over the aorta
- Constant upper abdominal pain or lower back pain
LIFE-THREATENING SIGNS AND SYMPTOMS
(MAY SIGNIFY RUPTURE)
- Severe abdominal and back pain
- Mottled skin below the waist
- Absent femoral and pedal pulses
- Lower BP in the legs than in the arms
- Abdominal rigidity
- Signs of shock
DX: Imaging studies (ultrasonography, CT scan, MRI, angiography)
TX: BP control, reduction of atherosclerotic risk factors, surgery
F/U: BP monitoring as indicated, serial ultrasound 1 week after discharge (if surgery is performed)

Common signs and symptoms
- Weak or absent peripheral pulses
- Aching pain distal to the occlusion that worsens with exercise and abates with rest
- Cool skin
- Decreased hair growth

PERIPHERAL VASCULAR DISEASE
DX: PE, imaging studies (Doppler ultrasound, arteriogram)
TX: Smoking cessation program, exercise program, surgery
F/U: Reevaluation of pulses as needed (dependent on the severity of the disease), referral to vascular surgeon if severe

AORTIC ARCH SYNDROME (TAKAYASU'S ARTERITIS)
Signs and symptoms
- Weak or abruptly absent carotid pulses and unequal or absent radial pulses
- Night sweats
- Pallor
- Anorexia
- Nausea
- Weight loss
- Arthralgia
- Raynaud's phenomenon
DX: PE, labs (CBC, ESR), angiography
TX: Medication (corticosteroids, anticoagulants), surgery
F/U: Referral to cardiovascular surgeon

ARTERIAL OCCLUSION (ACUTE)
Additional signs and symptoms
- Cool, pale, cyanotic limb
- Prolonged capillary refill time
- Moderate to severe pain
- Paresthesia
- Line of demarcation at level of obstruction
DX: PE, imaging studies (Doppler ultrasound, arteriogram)
TX: Thrombolytic agents, angioplasty, surgery
F/U: Referral to vascular surgeon

Additional differential diagnoses: aortic bifurcation occlusion (acute) ▪ aortic stenosis ▪ arrhythmias ▪ cardiac tamponade ▪ coarctation of the aorta ▪ pulmonary embolism ▪ shock ▪ thoracic outlet syndrome

Other causes: arteriovenous shunts for dialysis

Pulse, bounding

Produced by large waves of pressure as blood ejects from the left ventricle with each contraction, a bounding pulse is strong and easily palpable and may be visible over superficial peripheral arteries. It's characterized by regular, recurrent expansion and contraction of the arterial walls, and it isn't obliterated by the pressure of palpation. A healthy person develops a bounding pulse during exercise, pregnancy, and periods of anxiety. However, this sign also results from fever and certain endocrine, hematologic, and cardiovascular disorders that increase the basal metabolic rate.

History and physical examination

When taking the patient's history, ask if he noticed the bounding pulse. If he did, ask how long it has been present and ask if it's present continuously or intermittently. Ask him if he has noticed any palpitations? You should also ask about pregnancy (for a female patient), fever, and feelings of anxiety or stress. Also ask the patient whether he's noticed any weakness, fatigue, shortness of breath, or other health changes. Review his medical history for hyperthyroidism, anemia, or cardiovascular disorders, and ask about his use of alcohol. After you detect a bounding pulse, check other vital signs; then auscultate the heart and lungs for any abnormal sounds, rates, or rhythms.

PEDIATRIC POINTERS

- *A bounding pulse can be normal in infants or children because arteries lie close to the skin surface.*
- *It can also result from patent ductus arteriosus if the left-to-right shunt is large.*

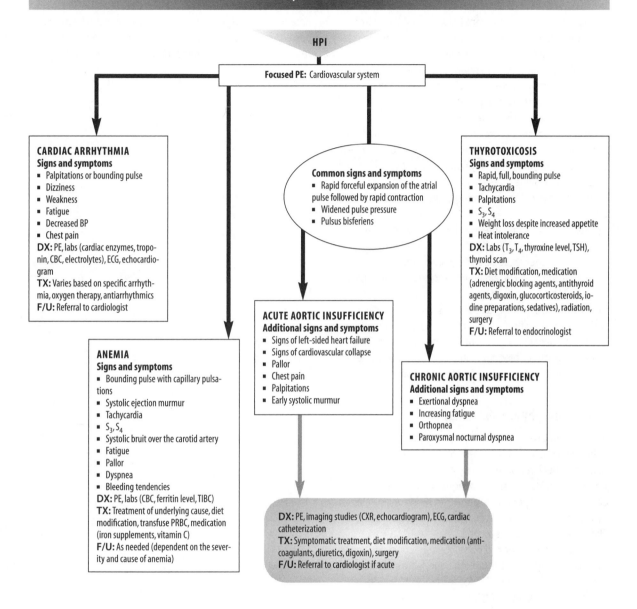

HPI

Focused PE: Cardiovascular system

CARDIAC ARRHYTHMIA
Signs and symptoms
- Palpitations or bounding pulse
- Dizziness
- Weakness
- Fatigue
- Decreased BP
- Chest pain

DX: PE, labs (cardiac enzymes, troponin, CBC, electrolytes), ECG, echocardiogram
TX: Varies based on specific arrhythmia, oxygen therapy, antiarrhythmics
F/U: Referral to cardiologist

Common signs and symptoms
- Rapid forceful expansion of the atrial pulse followed by rapid contraction
- Widened pulse pressure
- Pulsus bisferiens

THYROTOXICOSIS
Signs and symptoms
- Rapid, full, bounding pulse
- Tachycardia
- Palpitations
- S_3, S_4
- Weight loss despite increased appetite
- Heat intolerance

DX: Labs (T_3, T_4, thyroxine level, TSH), thyroid scan
TX: Diet modification, medication (adrenergic blocking agents, antithyroid agents, digoxin, glucocorticosteroids, iodine preparations, sedatives), radiation, surgery
F/U: Referral to endocrinologist

ANEMIA
Signs and symptoms
- Bounding pulse with capillary pulsations
- Systolic ejection murmur
- Tachycardia
- S_3, S_4
- Systolic bruit over the carotid artery
- Fatigue
- Pallor
- Dyspnea
- Bleeding tendencies

DX: PE, labs (CBC, ferritin level, TIBC)
TX: Treatment of underlying cause, diet modification, transfuse PRBC, medication (iron supplements, vitamin C)
F/U: As needed (dependent on the severity and cause of anemia)

ACUTE AORTIC INSUFFICIENCY
Additional signs and symptoms
- Signs of left-sided heart failure
- Signs of cardiovascular collapse
- Pallor
- Chest pain
- Palpitations
- Early systolic murmur

CHRONIC AORTIC INSUFFICIENCY
Additional signs and symptoms
- Exertional dyspnea
- Increasing fatigue
- Orthopnea
- Paroxysmal nocturnal dyspnea

DX: PE, imaging studies (CXR, echocardiogram), ECG, cardiac catheterization
TX: Symptomatic treatment, diet modification, medication (anticoagulants, diuretics, digoxin), surgery
F/U: Referral to cardiologist if acute

Additional differential diagnosis: febrile disorder

Pulse pressure, abnormal

Pulse pressure — the difference between systolic and diastolic blood pressures — is measured by sphygmomanometry or intra-arterial monitoring. Normally, systolic pressure exceeds diastolic pressure by about 40 mm Hg. Narrowed pressure — a difference of less than 30 mm Hg — occurs when peripheral vascular resistance increases, cardiac output declines, or intravascular volume markedly decreases.

In conditions that cause mechanical obstruction (such as aortic stenosis), pulse pressure is directly related to the severity of the underlying condition. Usually a late sign, narrowed pulse pressure alone doesn't signal an emergency, even though it commonly occurs in shock and other life-threatening disorders.

Widened pulse pressure — a difference of more than 50 mm Hg — commonly occurs as a physiologic response to fever, hot weather, exercise, anxiety, anemia, or pregnancy. It can also result from certain neurologic disorders — especially life-threatening increased intracranial pressure (ICP) — or from cardiovascular disorders such as aortic insufficiency, which causes backflow of blood into the heart with each contraction. Widened pulse pressure can be easily identified by monitoring arterial blood pressure and is commonly detected during routine sphygmomanometric recordings.

History and physical examination

If you detect a narrowed pulse pressure, check for other signs of heart failure, such as hypotension, tachycardia, dyspnea, distended neck veins, pulmonary crackles, and decreased urine output. Also check for changes in skin temperature or color, strength of peripheral pulses, and level of consciousness. Auscultate the heart for murmurs. Ask about a history of chest pain, dizziness, or syncope.

If you detect a widened pulse pressure, check for signs of increased ICP. Perform a thorough neurologic examination, which will serve as a baseline for subsequent changes. If you don't suspect increased ICP, ask about associated symptoms, such as chest pain, shortness of breath, weakness, fatigue, or syncope. Check for edema and auscultate for murmurs.

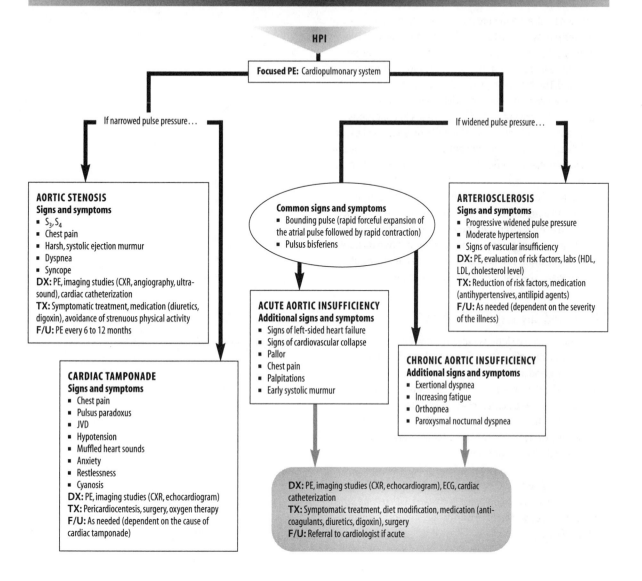

HPI

Focused PE: Cardiopulmonary system

If narrowed pulse pressure...

If widened pulse pressure...

AORTIC STENOSIS
Signs and symptoms
- S_3, S_4
- Chest pain
- Harsh, systolic ejection murmur
- Dyspnea
- Syncope
DX: PE, imaging studies (CXR, angiography, ultrasound), cardiac catheterization
TX: Symptomatic treatment, medication (diuretics, digoxin), avoidance of strenuous physical activity
F/U: PE every 6 to 12 months

Common signs and symptoms
- Bounding pulse (rapid forceful expansion of the atrial pulse followed by rapid contraction)
- Pulsus bisferiens

ARTERIOSCLEROSIS
Signs and symptoms
- Progressive widened pulse pressure
- Moderate hypertension
- Signs of vascular insufficiency
DX: PE, evaluation of risk factors, labs (HDL, LDL, cholesterol level)
TX: Reduction of risk factors, medication (antihypertensives, antilipid agents)
F/U: As needed (dependent on the severity of the illness)

ACUTE AORTIC INSUFFICIENCY
Additional signs and symptoms
- Signs of left-sided heart failure
- Signs of cardiovascular collapse
- Pallor
- Chest pain
- Palpitations
- Early systolic murmur

CHRONIC AORTIC INSUFFICIENCY
Additional signs and symptoms
- Exertional dyspnea
- Increasing fatigue
- Orthopnea
- Paroxysmal nocturnal dyspnea

CARDIAC TAMPONADE
Signs and symptoms
- Chest pain
- Pulsus paradoxus
- JVD
- Hypotension
- Muffled heart sounds
- Anxiety
- Restlessness
- Cyanosis
DX: PE, imaging studies (CXR, echocardiogram)
TX: Pericardiocentesis, surgery, oxygen therapy
F/U: As needed (dependent on the cause of cardiac tamponade)

DX: PE, imaging studies (CXR, echocardiogram), ECG, cardiac catheterization
TX: Symptomatic treatment, diet modification, medication (anticoagulants, diuretics, digoxin), surgery
F/U: Referral to cardiologist if acute

Additional differential diagnoses for narrowed pulse pressure: heart failure ▪ shock

Additional differential diagnoses for widened pulse pressure: febrile disorders ▪ increased ICP

Pulsus bisferiens

A bisferiens pulse is a hyperdynamic, double-beating pulse characterized by two systolic peaks separated by a midsystolic dip. Both peaks may be equal or either may be larger; however, the first peak is typically taller or more forceful than the second. The first peak (percussion wave) is believed to be the pulse pressure; the second (tidal wave), reverberation from the periphery. Pulsus bisferiens occurs in conditions such as aortic insufficiency, in which a large volume of blood is rapidly ejected from the left ventricle. The pulse can be palpated in peripheral arteries or observed on an arterial pressure wave recording.

To detect pulsus bisferiens, *lightly* palpate the carotid, brachial, radial, or femoral artery. (The pulse is easiest to palpate in the carotid artery.) At the same time, listen to the patient's heart sounds to determine whether the two palpable peaks occur during systole. If they do, you'll feel the double pulse between the first and second heart sounds.

History and physical examination

After you detect a bisferiens pulse, review the patient's history for cardiac disorders. Next, find out what medication he's taking, if any, and ask whether he has any other illnesses. Also, ask about the development of any associated signs and symptoms, such as dyspnea, chest pain, or fatigue. Find out how long he's had these symptoms and whether they change with activity or rest. Then take his vital signs and auscultate for abnormal heart or lung sounds.

PEDIATRIC POINTER

Pulsus bisferiens may be palpated in children with a large patent ductus arteriosus and in those with congenital aortic stenosis and insufficiency.

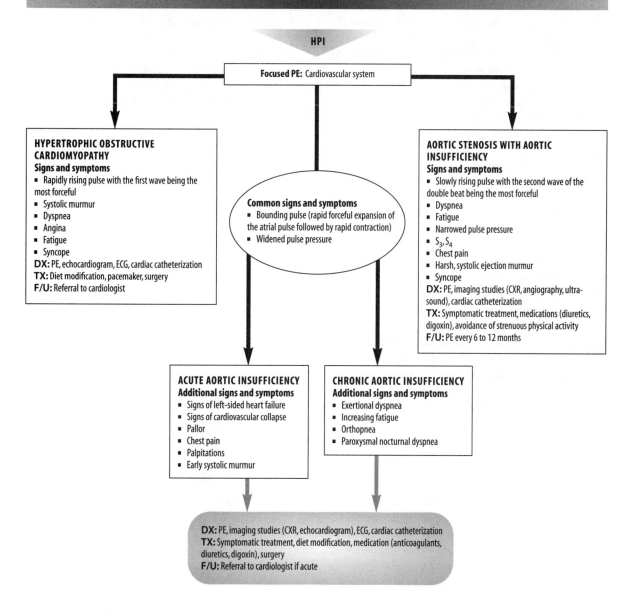

HPI

Focused PE: Cardiovascular system

HYPERTROPHIC OBSTRUCTIVE CARDIOMYOPATHY
Signs and symptoms
- Rapidly rising pulse with the first wave being the most forceful
- Systolic murmur
- Dyspnea
- Angina
- Fatigue
- Syncope

DX: PE, echocardiogram, ECG, cardiac catheterization
TX: Diet modification, pacemaker, surgery
F/U: Referral to cardiologist

Common signs and symptoms
- Bounding pulse (rapid forceful expansion of the atrial pulse followed by rapid contraction)
- Widened pulse pressure

AORTIC STENOSIS WITH AORTIC INSUFFICIENCY
Signs and symptoms
- Slowly rising pulse with the second wave of the double beat being the most forceful
- Dyspnea
- Fatigue
- Narrowed pulse pressure
- S_3, S_4
- Chest pain
- Harsh, systolic ejection murmur
- Syncope

DX: PE, imaging studies (CXR, angiography, ultrasound), cardiac catheterization
TX: Symptomatic treatment, medications (diuretics, digoxin), avoidance of strenuous physical activity
F/U: PE every 6 to 12 months

ACUTE AORTIC INSUFFICIENCY
Additional signs and symptoms
- Signs of left-sided heart failure
- Signs of cardiovascular collapse
- Pallor
- Chest pain
- Palpitations
- Early systolic murmur

CHRONIC AORTIC INSUFFICIENCY
Additional signs and symptoms
- Exertional dyspnea
- Increasing fatigue
- Orthopnea
- Paroxysmal nocturnal dyspnea

DX: PE, imaging studies (CXR, echocardiogram), ECG, cardiac catheterization
TX: Symptomatic treatment, diet modification, medication (anticoagulants, diuretics, digoxin), surgery
F/U: Referral to cardiologist if acute

Additional differential diagnoses: high cardiac output states (such as anemia, thyrotoxicosis, fever, and exercise)

Pulsus paradoxus

Pulsus paradoxus, or paradoxical pulse, is an exaggerated decline in blood pressure during inspiration. Normally, systolic pressure falls less than 10 mm Hg during inspiration. In pulsus paradoxus, however, it falls more than 10 mm Hg. When systolic pressure falls more than 20 mm Hg, the peripheral pulses may be barely palpable or may disappear during inspiration.

Pulsus paradoxus is thought to result from an exaggerated inspirational increase in negative intrathoracic pressure. Normally, systolic pressure drops during inspiration because of blood pooling in the pulmonary system. This, in turn, reduces left ventricular filling and stroke volume and transmits negative intrathoracic pressure to the aorta. Conditions associated with large intrapleural pressure swings, such as asthma, or those that reduce left-sided heart filling, such as pericardial tamponade, produce paradoxical pulse.

To accurately detect and measure paradoxical pulse, use a sphygmomanometer or an intra-arterial monitoring device. Inflate the blood pressure cuff 10 to 20 mm Hg beyond the peak systolic pressure. Then deflate the cuff at a rate of 2 mm Hg per second until you hear the first Korotkoff's sound during expiration. Note the systolic pressure. As you continue to slowly deflate the cuff, observe the patient's respiratory pattern. If a paradoxical pulse is present, the Korotkoff's sounds will disappear with inspiration and return with expiration. Continue to deflate the cuff until you hear Korotkoff's sounds during both inspiration and expiration and, again, note the systolic pressure. Subtract this reading from the first one to determine the degree of paradoxical pulse. A difference of more than 10 mm Hg is abnormal.

You can also detect paradoxical pulse by palpating the radial pulse over several cycles of slow inspiration and expiration. Marked pulse diminution during inspiration indicates paradoxical pulse. When you check for paradoxical pulse, remember that irregular heart rhythms and tachycardia cause variations in pulse amplitude and must be ruled out before a true paradoxical pulse can be identified.

History and physical examination

A paradoxical pulse may signal cardiac tamponade. When you detect paradoxical pulse, quickly assess all vital signs. Check for additional signs and symptoms of cardiac tamponade. If the patient doesn't have cardiac tamponade, find out whether he has a history of chronic cardiac or pulmonary disease. Ask about the development of associated signs and symptoms, such as cough or chest pain. Then auscultate for abnormal breath sounds.

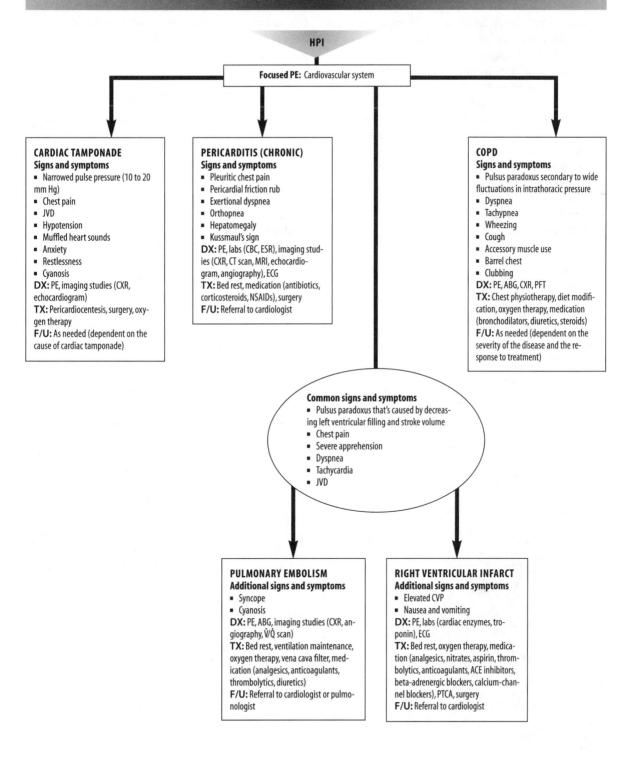

PULSUS PARADOXUS

HPI

Focused PE: Cardiovascular system

CARDIAC TAMPONADE
Signs and symptoms
- Narrowed pulse pressure (10 to 20 mm Hg)
- Chest pain
- JVD
- Hypotension
- Muffled heart sounds
- Anxiety
- Restlessness
- Cyanosis

DX: PE, imaging studies (CXR, echocardiogram)
TX: Pericardiocentesis, surgery, oxygen therapy
F/U: As needed (dependent on the cause of cardiac tamponade)

PERICARDITIS (CHRONIC)
Signs and symptoms
- Pleuritic chest pain
- Pericardial friction rub
- Exertional dyspnea
- Orthopnea
- Hepatomegaly
- Kussmaul's sign

DX: PE, labs (CBC, ESR), imaging studies (CXR, CT scan, MRI, echocardiogram, angiography), ECG
TX: Bed rest, medication (antibiotics, corticosteroids, NSAIDs), surgery
F/U: Referral to cardiologist

COPD
Signs and symptoms
- Pulsus paradoxus secondary to wide fluctuations in intrathoracic pressure
- Dyspnea
- Tachypnea
- Wheezing
- Cough
- Accessory muscle use
- Barrel chest
- Clubbing

DX: PE, ABG, CXR, PFT
TX: Chest physiotherapy, diet modification, oxygen therapy, medication (bronchodilators, diuretics, steroids)
F/U: As needed (dependent on the severity of the disease and the response to treatment)

Common signs and symptoms
- Pulsus paradoxus that's caused by decreasing left ventricular filling and stroke volume
- Chest pain
- Severe apprehension
- Dyspnea
- Tachycardia
- JVD

PULMONARY EMBOLISM
Additional signs and symptoms
- Syncope
- Cyanosis

DX: PE, ABG, imaging studies (CXR, angiography, V̇/Q̇ scan)
TX: Bed rest, ventilation maintenance, oxygen therapy, vena cava filter, medication (analgesics, anticoagulants, thrombolytics, diuretics)
F/U: Referral to cardiologist or pulmonologist

RIGHT VENTRICULAR INFARCT
Additional signs and symptoms
- Elevated CVP
- Nausea and vomiting

DX: PE, labs (cardiac enzymes, troponin), ECG
TX: Bed rest, oxygen therapy, medication (analgesics, nitrates, aspirin, thrombolytics, anticoagulants, ACE inhibitors, beta-adrenergic blockers, calcium-channel blockers), PTCA, surgery
F/U: Referral to cardiologist

Pupils, nonreactive

Nonreactive (fixed) pupils fail to constrict in response to light or fail to dilate when the light is removed. The development of a unilateral or bilateral nonreactive response indicates an important change in the patient's condition and may signal a life-threatening emergency and, possibly, brain death. It also occurs with use of certain optic drugs.

To evaluate pupillary reaction to light, first test the patient's direct light reflex. Darken the room, and cover one of the patient's eyes while you hold open the opposite eyelid. Using a bright penlight, bring the light toward the patient from the side and shine it directly into his opened eye. If normal, the pupil will promptly constrict. Next, test the consensual light reflex. Hold the patient's eyelids open and shine the light into one eye while watching the pupil of the opposite eye. If normal, both pupils will promptly constrict. Repeat both procedures in the opposite eye. A unilateral or bilateral nonreactive response indicates dysfunction of cranial nerves II and III, which mediate the pupillary light reflex. (See *Innervation of direct and consensual light reflexes*.)

History and physical examination

If the patient is unconscious and develops unilateral or bilateral nonreactive pupils, quickly assess all vital signs. Be alert for decerebrate or decorticate posture, bradycardia, elevated systolic blood pressure, and other untoward changes in the patient's condition. A unilateral dilated, nonreactive pupil may be a sign of uncal brain herniation.

If the patient is conscious, obtain a brief history. Ask him what type of eyedrops he's using, if any, and when they were last instilled. Also ask whether he's experiencing any pain and, if so, try to determine its location, intensity, and duration. Assess extraocular movement to evaluate cranial nerves III, IV and VI. Assess for photosensitivity and photophobia. Check the patient's visual acuity in both eyes. Then test the pupillary reaction to accommodation: Normally, both pupils constrict equally as the patient shifts his glance from a distant to a near object.

Next, hold a penlight at the side of each eye and examine the cornea and iris for any abnormalities. Estimate intraocular pressure (IOP) by placing your second and third fingers over the patient's closed eyelid. If the eyeball feels rock hard, suspect elevated IOP. Ophthalmoscopic and slit-lamp examinations of the eye will need to be performed. If the patient has experienced ocular trauma, don't manipulate the affected eye. After the examination, be sure to cover the affected eye with a protective metal shield but don't let the shield rest on the globe.

PEDIATRIC POINTERS

- *Children have nonreactive pupils for the same reasons as adults.*
- *The most common cause is oculomotor nerve palsy from increased intracranial pressure.*

Innervation of direct and consensual light reflexes

Two reactions — direct and consensual — constitute the pupillary light reflex. Normally, when a light is shined directly onto the retina of one eye, the parasympathetic nerves are stimulated to cause brisk constriction of that pupil — the *direct light reflex*. The pupil of the opposite eye also constricts — the *consensual light reflex*.

The optic nerve (CN II) mediates the afferent arc of this reflex from each eye, while the oculomotor nerve (CN III) mediates the efferent arc to both eyes. A nonreactive or sluggish response in one or both pupils indicates dysfunction of these cranial nerves, usually due to degenerative disease of the central nervous system.

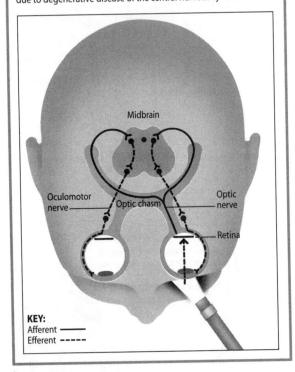

Midbrain

Oculomotor nerve

Optic chasm

Optic nerve

Retina

KEY:
Afferent ———
Efferent -----

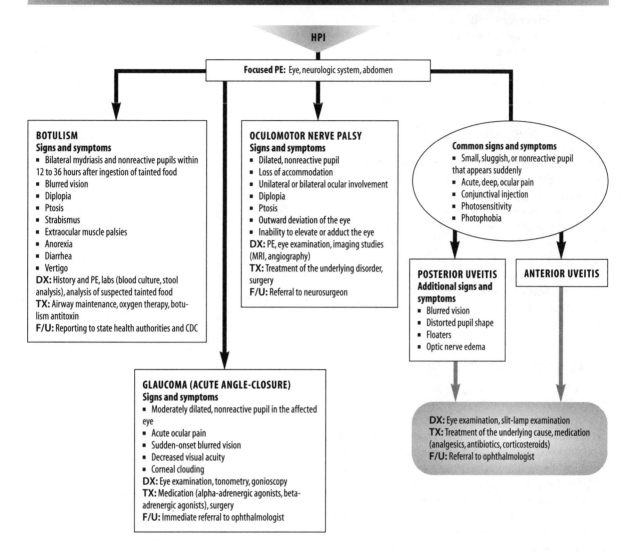

HPI

Focused PE: Eye, neurologic system, abdomen

BOTULISM
Signs and symptoms
- Bilateral mydriasis and nonreactive pupils within 12 to 36 hours after ingestion of tainted food
- Blurred vision
- Diplopia
- Ptosis
- Strabismus
- Extraocular muscle palsies
- Anorexia
- Diarrhea
- Vertigo

DX: History and PE, labs (blood culture, stool analysis), analysis of suspected tainted food
TX: Airway maintenance, oxygen therapy, botulism antitoxin
F/U: Reporting to state health authorities and CDC

OCULOMOTOR NERVE PALSY
Signs and symptoms
- Dilated, nonreactive pupil
- Loss of accommodation
- Unilateral or bilateral ocular involvement
- Diplopia
- Ptosis
- Outward deviation of the eye
- Inability to elevate or adduct the eye

DX: PE, eye examination, imaging studies (MRI, angiography)
TX: Treatment of the underlying disorder, surgery
F/U: Referral to neurosurgeon

Common signs and symptoms
- Small, sluggish, or nonreactive pupil that appears suddenly
- Acute, deep, ocular pain
- Conjunctival injection
- Photosensitivity
- Photophobia

POSTERIOR UVEITIS
Additional signs and symptoms
- Blurred vision
- Distorted pupil shape
- Floaters
- Optic nerve edema

ANTERIOR UVEITIS

GLAUCOMA (ACUTE ANGLE-CLOSURE)
Signs and symptoms
- Moderately dilated, nonreactive pupil in the affected eye
- Acute ocular pain
- Sudden-onset blurred vision
- Decreased visual acuity
- Corneal clouding

DX: Eye examination, tonometry, gonioscopy
TX: Medication (alpha-adrenergic agonists, beta-adrenergic agonists), surgery
F/U: Immediate referral to ophthalmologist

DX: Eye examination, slit-lamp examination
TX: Treatment of the underlying cause, medication (analgesics, antibiotics, corticosteroids)
F/U: Referral to ophthalmologist

Additional differential diagnoses: Adie's syndrome ▪ encephalitis ▪ familial amyloid polyneuropathy ▪ iris disease (degenerative or inflammatory) ▪ midbrain lesions ▪ ocular trauma ▪ Wernicke's disease

Other causes: topical mydriatics and cycloplegics ▪ opiates (heroin, morphine) ▪ atropine poisoning

Pupils, sluggish

A sluggish pupillary reaction is an abnormally slow pupillary response to light. It can occur in one pupil or both, unlike the normal reaction, which is always bilateral. A sluggish reaction accompanies degenerative disease of the central nervous system and diabetic neuropathy. It can occur normally in elderly people, whose pupils become smaller and less responsive with age.

To assess pupillary reaction to light, first test the patient's direct light reflex. Darken the room, and cover one of the patient's eyes while you hold open the opposite eyelid. Using a bright penlight, bring the light toward the patient from the side and shine it directly into his uncovered eye. If normal, the pupil will promptly constrict. Next, test the consensual light reflex. Hold both of the patient's eyelids open, and shine the light into one eye while watching the pupil of the opposite eye. If normal, both pupils will promptly constrict. Repeat both procedures to test light reflexes in the opposite eye. A sluggish reaction in one or both pupils indicates dysfunction of cranial nerves II and III, which mediate the pupillary light reflex.

History and physical examination

If you detect a sluggish pupillary reaction, determine the patient's visual function. Start by testing visual acuity in both eyes, using the Snellen chart. Assess extraocular movements. Determine whether the patient suffers from photosensitivity or photophobia. Then test the pupillary reaction to accommodation; the pupils should constrict equally as the patient shifts his glance from a distant to a near object.

Next, hold a penlight at the side of each eye and examine the cornea and iris for irregularities, scars, and foreign bodies. Estimate intraocular pressure (IOP) by placing your fingers over the patient's closed eyelid. If the eyeball feels rock hard, suspect elevated IOP. In addition, ophthalmoscopic and slit-lamp examinations of the eye will need to be performed.

PEDIATRIC POINTER

Children experience sluggish pupillary reactions for the same reasons as adults.

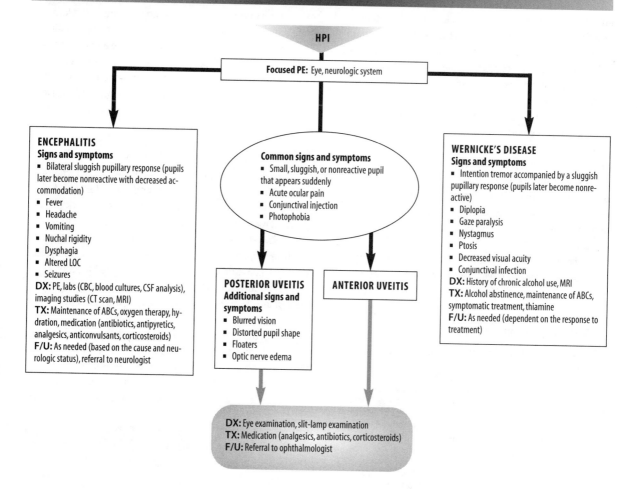

HPI

Focused PE: Eye, neurologic system

ENCEPHALITIS
Signs and symptoms
- Bilateral sluggish pupillary response (pupils later become nonreactive with decreased accommodation)
- Fever
- Headache
- Vomiting
- Nuchal rigidity
- Dysphagia
- Altered LOC
- Seizures

DX: PE, labs (CBC, blood cultures, CSF analysis), imaging studies (CT scan, MRI)
TX: Maintenance of ABCs, oxygen therapy, hydration, medication (antibiotics, antipyretics, analgesics, anticonvulsants, corticosteroids)
F/U: As needed (based on the cause and neurologic status), referral to neurologist

Common signs and symptoms
- Small, sluggish, or nonreactive pupil that appears suddenly
- Acute ocular pain
- Conjunctival injection
- Photophobia

POSTERIOR UVEITIS
Additional signs and symptoms
- Blurred vision
- Distorted pupil shape
- Floaters
- Optic nerve edema

ANTERIOR UVEITIS

WERNICKE'S DISEASE
Signs and symptoms
- Intention tremor accompanied by a sluggish pupillary response (pupils later become nonreactive)
- Diplopia
- Gaze paralysis
- Nystagmus
- Ptosis
- Decreased visual acuity
- Conjunctival infection

DX: History of chronic alcohol use, MRI
TX: Alcohol abstinence, maintenance of ABCs, symptomatic treatment, thiamine
F/U: As needed (dependent on the response to treatment)

DX: Eye examination, slit-lamp examination
TX: Medication (analgesics, antibiotics, corticosteroids)
F/U: Referral to ophthalmologist

Additional differential diagnoses: Adie's syndrome ■ diabetic neuropathy ■ familial amyloid polyneuropathy ■ herpes zoster ■ multiple sclerosis ■ myotonic dystrophy ■ tertiary syphilis

Purpura

Purpura is the extravasation of red blood cells from the blood vessels into the skin, subcutaneous tissue, or mucous membranes. It's characterized by discoloration — usually purplish or brownish red — that's easily visible through the epidermis. Purpuric lesions include petechiae, ecchymoses, and hematomas. (See *Identifying purpuric lesions*.) Purpura differs from erythema in that it doesn't blanch with pressure because it involves blood in the tissues, not just dilated vessels.

Purpura results from damage to the endothelium of small blood vessels, coagulation defects, ineffective perivascular support, capillary fragility and permeability, or a combination of these factors. These faulty hemostatic factors, in turn, can result from thrombocytopenia or other hematologic disorders, invasive procedures and, of course, the use of anticoagulant drugs.

Additional causes are nonpathologic. Purpura can be a consequence of aging, when loss of collagen decreases connective tissue support of upper skin blood vessels. In the elderly or cachectic person, skin atrophy and inelasticity and loss of subcutaneous fat increase susceptibility to minor trauma, causing purpura to appear along the veins of the forearms, hands, legs, and feet. Prolonged coughing or vomiting can produce crops of petechiae in loose face and neck tissue. Violent muscle contraction — for example, in seizures or weight lifting — sometimes results in localized ecchymoses from increased intraluminal pressure and rupture. High fever, which increases capillary fragility, can also produce purpura.

History and physical examination

Ask the patient when he first noticed the lesion and whether he has noticed other lesions on his body. Does he or his family have a history of bleeding disorders or easy bruising? Find out what medications he's taking, if any, and ask him to describe his diet. Ask about recent trauma or transfusions and the development of associated signs, such as epistaxis, bleeding gums, hematuria, vaginal bleeding, and hematochezia. Also ask about systemic complaints such as fever that may suggest infection. If the patient is female, ask about heavy menstrual flow.

Inspect the patient's entire skin surface to determine the type, size, location, distribution, and severity of purpuric lesions. Also inspect the mucous membranes. Remember that the same mechanisms that cause purpura can also cause internal hemorrhage, although purpura isn't a cardinal indicator of this condition.

Identifying purpuric lesions

Purpuric lesions fall into three categories: petechiae, ecchymoses, and hematomas.

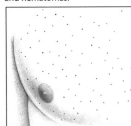

PETECHIAE

Petechiae are painless, round, pinpoint lesions, 1 to 3 mm in diameter. Caused by extravasation of red blood cells into cutaneous tissue, these red or brown lesions usually arise on dependent portions of the body. They appear and fade in crops and can group to form ecchymoses.

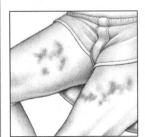

ECCHYMOSES

Ecchymoses, another form of blood extravasation, are larger than petechiae. These purple, blue, or yellow-green bruises vary in size and shape and can arise anywhere on the body as a result of trauma. Ecchymoses usually appear on the arms and legs of patients with bleeding disorders.

HEMATOMAS

Hematomas are palpable ecchymoses that are painful and swollen. Usually the result of trauma, superficial hematomas are red, whereas deep hematomas are blue. Hematomas often exceed 1 cm in diameter, but their size varies widely.

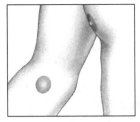

PEDIATRIC POINTERS

- *Neonates commonly exhibit petechiae, particularly on the head, neck, and shoulders, after vertex deliveries. Thought to result from the trauma of birth, these petechiae disappear within a few days.*
- *Other causes in infants include thrombocytopenia, vitamin K deficiency, and infantile scurvy.*
- *The most common type of purpura in children is allergic purpura.*
- *Other causes in children include trauma, hemophilia, autoimmune hemolytic anemia, Gaucher's disease, thrombasthenia, congenital factor deficiencies, Wiskott-Aldrich syndrome, acute idiopathic thrombocytopenic purpura, von Willebrand's disease, and the rare but life-threatening purpura fulminans, which most often follows bacterial or viral infection.*
- *When you assess a child with purpura, be alert for signs of possible child abuse: bruises in different stages of resolution, from repeated beatings; bruise patterns resembling a familiar object, such as a belt, hand, or thumb and finger; and bruises on areas unlikely to be injured accidentally, such as the face, buttocks, or genitalia.*

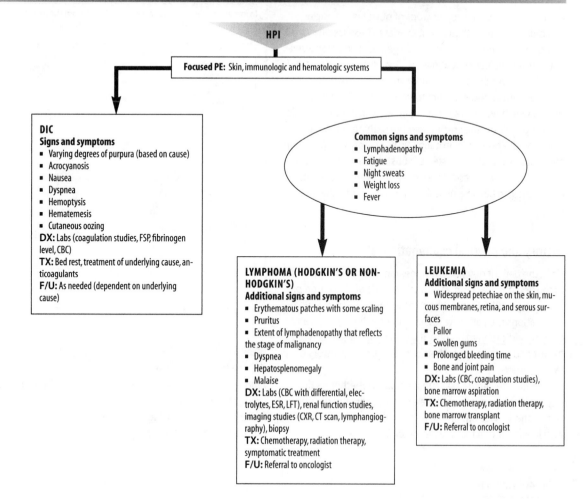

HPI

Focused PE: Skin, immunologic and hematologic systems

DIC
Signs and symptoms
- Varying degrees of purpura (based on cause)
- Acrocyanosis
- Nausea
- Dyspnea
- Hemoptysis
- Hematemesis
- Cutaneous oozing

DX: Labs (coagulation studies, FSP, fibrinogen level, CBC)
TX: Bed rest, treatment of underlying cause, anticoagulants
F/U: As needed (dependent on underlying cause)

Common signs and symptoms
- Lymphadenopathy
- Fatigue
- Night sweats
- Weight loss
- Fever

LYMPHOMA (HODGKIN'S OR NON-HODGKIN'S)
Additional signs and symptoms
- Erythematous patches with some scaling
- Pruritus
- Extent of lymphadenopathy that reflects the stage of malignancy
- Dyspnea
- Hepatosplenomegaly
- Malaise

DX: Labs (CBC with differential, electrolytes, ESR, LFT), renal function studies, imaging studies (CXR, CT scan, lymphangiography), biopsy
TX: Chemotherapy, radiation therapy, symptomatic treatment
F/U: Referral to oncologist

LEUKEMIA
Additional signs and symptoms
- Widespread petechiae on the skin, mucous membranes, retina, and serous surfaces
- Pallor
- Swollen gums
- Prolonged bleeding time
- Bone and joint pain

DX: Labs (CBC, coagulation studies), bone marrow aspiration
TX: Chemotherapy, radiation therapy, bone marrow transplant
F/U: Referral to oncologist

Additional differential diagnoses: amyloidosis ▪ autoerythrocyte sensitivity ▪ coagulopathy ▪ dermatoses (pigmented) ▪ dysproteinemias ▪ easy bruising syndrome ▪ Ehlers-Danlos syndrome ▪ liver disease ▪ myeloproliferative disorders ▪ nutritional deficiencies ▪ septicemia ▪ stasis ▪ SLE ▪ thrombotic thrombocytopenic purpura ▪ trauma

Other causes: invasive procedures (venipuncture, arterial catheterization) ▪ anticoagulants ▪ antiplatelet agents ▪ nonsteroidal anti-inflammatories ▪ procedures that disrupt circulation, coagulation, or platelet activity or production (pulmonary and cardiac surgery, radiation therapy, chemotherapy, hemodialysis, multiple blood transfusions with platelet-poor blood, use of plasma expanders)

Pustular rash

A pustular rash is made up of crops of pustules — vesicles and bullae that fill with purulent exudate. These lesions vary greatly in size and shape and can be generalized or localized to the hair follicles or sweat glands. (See *Identifying a pustule*.) Pustules can result from skin and systemic disorders, the use of certain drugs, and exposure to skin irritants. For example, people who have been swimming in salt water commonly develop a papulopustular rash under the bathing suit or elsewhere on the body from irritation by sea organisms. Although many pustular lesions are sterile, a pustular rash usually indicates infection. Any vesicular eruption, or even acute contact dermatitis, can become pustular if secondary infection occurs.

History and physical examination

Have the patient describe the appearance, location, and onset of the first pustular lesion. Did another type of skin lesion precede the pustule? Find out how the lesions spread. Ask what medications the patient takes and whether he's applied any topical medication to his rash. If so, what type and when did he last apply it? Find out whether he has a family history of skin disorders.

Examine the entire skin surface, noting whether it's dry, oily, moist, or greasy. Record the exact location and distribution of the skin lesions and their color, shape, and size. Is the rash linear? Does it follow a dermatome?

Recognizing impetigo

In impetigo, when vesicles break, crusts form from the exudate. This infection is especially contagious among young children.

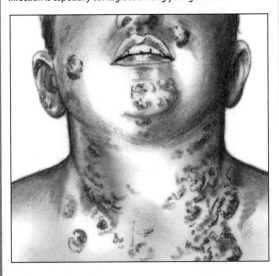

PEDIATRIC POINTER

Among the various disorders that produce pustular rash in children are varicella, erythema toxicum neonatorum, candidiasis, impetigo (see Recognizing impetigo*), infantile acropustulosis, and acrodermatitis enteropathica.*

Identifying a pustule

A pustule is a raised, circumscribed lesion that's usually less than ³/₈″ (1 cm) in diameter and contains purulent material, which makes it a yellow-white color.

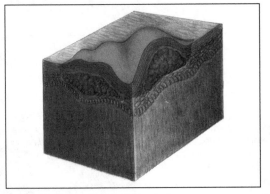

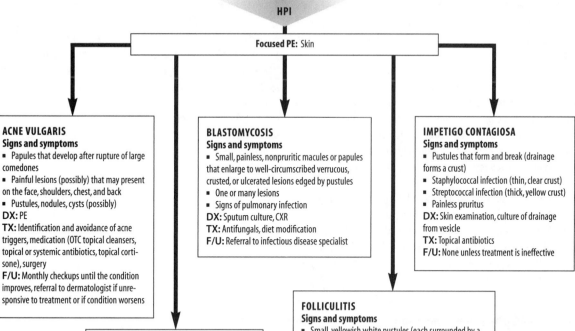

HPI

Focused PE: Skin

ACNE VULGARIS
Signs and symptoms
- Papules that develop after rupture of large comedones
- Painful lesions (possibly) that may present on the face, shoulders, chest, and back
- Pustules, nodules, cysts (possibly)
DX: PE
TX: Identification and avoidance of acne triggers, medication (OTC topical cleansers, topical or systemic antibiotics, topical cortisone), surgery
F/U: Monthly checkups until the condition improves, referral to dermatologist if unresponsive to treatment or if condition worsens

BLASTOMYCOSIS
Signs and symptoms
- Small, painless, nonpruritic macules or papules that enlarge to well-circumscribed verrucous, crusted, or ulcerated lesions edged by pustules
- One or many lesions
- Signs of pulmonary infection
DX: Sputum culture, CXR
TX: Antifungals, diet modification
F/U: Referral to infectious disease specialist

IMPETIGO CONTAGIOSA
Signs and symptoms
- Pustules that form and break (drainage forms a crust)
- Staphylococcal infection (thin, clear crust)
- Streptococcal infection (thick, yellow crust)
- Painless pruritus
DX: Skin examination, culture of drainage from vesicle
TX: Topical antibiotics
F/U: None unless treatment is ineffective

ROSACEA
Signs and symptoms
- Recurrent eruption of papules and pustules on the forehead, malar area, nose, and chin
- Persistent erythema and telangiectasia
DX: PE
TX: Identification and avoidance of triggers, medication (oral or topical antibiotics, topical antifungals or steroids)
F/U: As needed

FOLLICULITIS
Signs and symptoms
- Small, yellowish white pustules (each surrounded by a red ring and pierced by a hair)
- Blood-stained pus
- Pruritus
- "Hot tub" folliculitis (pustules on areas covered by a bathing suit)
DX: Skin or scalp examination, culture of pustule drainage
TX: Medication (topical or oral antibiotics or antifungal agents), diet modification
F/U: None unless treatment is ineffective, then referral to dermatologist

Additional differential diagnoses: furunculosis ▪ gonococcemia ▪ nummular or annular dermatitis ▪ pompholyx ▪ pustular miliaria ▪ pustular psoriasis ▪ scabies

Other causes: bromides ▪ iodides ▪ corticotropin ▪ corticosteroids ▪ dactinomycin ▪ trimethadione ▪ lithium ▪ phenytoin ▪ phenobarbital ▪ isoniazid ▪ oral contraceptives ▪ androgens ▪ anabolic steroids

Pyrosis

Caused by reflux of gastric contents into the esophagus, pyrosis (heartburn) is a substernal burning sensation that rises in the chest and may radiate to the neck or throat. It's frequently accompanied by regurgitation, which also results from gastric reflux. Because increased intra-abdominal pressure contributes to reflux, pyrosis commonly occurs with pregnancy, ascites, or obesity. It also accompanies various GI disorders, connective tissue disease, and the use of numerous drugs. Pyrosis usually develops after meals or when the patient lies down (especially on his right side), bends over, lifts heavy objects, or exercises vigorously. It typically worsens with swallowing and improves when the patient sits upright or takes antacids.

A patient experiencing a myocardial infarction (MI) may mistake chest pain for pyrosis. However, he'll probably develop other signs and symptoms — such as dyspnea, tachycardia, palpitations, nausea, and vomiting — that will help distinguish MI from pyrosis. And, of course, his chest pain won't be relieved by antacids.

History and physical examination

Ask the patient whether he's experienced heartburn before. Do certain foods or beverages trigger it? Does stress or fatigue aggravate his discomfort? Does movement, a certain body position, or ingestion of very hot or cold liquids worsen or help relieve the heartburn? Ask where the pain is located and whether it radiates to other areas. Also, find out whether the patient regurgitates sour- or bitter-tasting fluids. (See *Regurgitation: Mechanism and causes.*) Does the patient have

any associated signs and symptoms? Then perform a complete physical examination, focusing on the cardiovascular and GI systems.

PEDIATRIC POINTER

A child may have difficulty distinguishing esophageal pain from pyrosis. To gain information, help him describe the sensation.

ELDER CARE CUE

Elderly patients with peptic ulcer disease commonly present with nonspecific abdominal discomfort or weight loss. Older people are also at greater risk for complications due to esophageal sphincter weakness.

Regurgitation: Mechanism and causes

When gastric reflux moves up the esophagus and passes through the upper esophageal sphincter, regurgitation occurs. Unlike vomiting, regurgitation is effortless and unaccompanied by nausea. It usually happens when the patient is lying down or bending over and often accompanies pyrosis. Aspiration of regurgitated gastric contents can lead to recurrent pulmonary infections.

In adults, regurgitation usually results from esophageal disorders such as achalasia. However, it can also occur when the gag reflex is absent, as in bulbar palsy, or when the patient has an overfilled stomach or esophagus.

In infants, regurgitation can signal pyloric stenosis or dysphagia lusoria. Usually, however, infants "spit up" because their esophageal sphincters aren't fully developed during the first year of life. To help reduce regurgitation in an infant, teach the parents to handle the infant gently during feeding and to burp him frequently. After feeding, they should place the infant on his right side or on his stomach with his head slightly elevated to avoid gravitational regurgitation and to help prevent aspiration.

PYROSIS

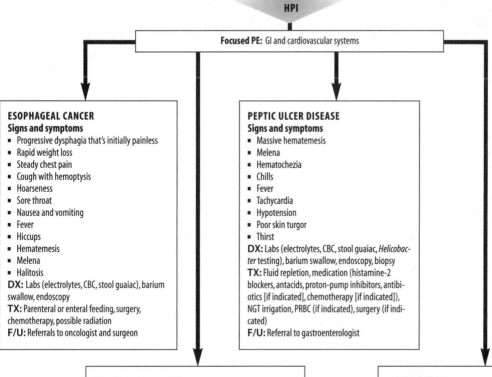

HPI

Focused PE: GI and cardiovascular systems

ESOPHAGEAL CANCER
Signs and symptoms
- Progressive dysphagia that's initially painless
- Rapid weight loss
- Steady chest pain
- Cough with hemoptysis
- Hoarseness
- Sore throat
- Nausea and vomiting
- Fever
- Hiccups
- Hematemesis
- Melena
- Halitosis

DX: Labs (electrolytes, CBC, stool guaiac), barium swallow, endoscopy
TX: Parenteral or enteral feeding, surgery, chemotherapy, possible radiation
F/U: Referrals to oncologist and surgeon

PEPTIC ULCER DISEASE
Signs and symptoms
- Massive hematemesis
- Melena
- Hematochezia
- Chills
- Fever
- Tachycardia
- Hypotension
- Poor skin turgor
- Thirst

DX: Labs (electrolytes, CBC, stool guaiac, *Helicobacter* testing), barium swallow, endoscopy, biopsy
TX: Fluid repletion, medication (histamine-2 blockers, antacids, proton-pump inhibitors, antibiotics [if indicated], chemotherapy [if indicated]), NGT irrigation, PRBC (if indicated), surgery (if indicated)
F/U: Referral to gastroenterologist

REFLUX ESOPHAGITIS
Signs and symptoms
- Dysphagia (late sign)
- Pyrosis that's aggravated by strenuous exercise, bending over, or lying down
- Frequent, effortless vomiting
- Dry, nocturnal cough
- Hypersalivation
- Substernal chest pain

DX: Labs (electrolytes, CBC, stool guaiac), barium swallow, ECG, endoscopy
TX: Dietary modification, medication (H_2 receptor antagonist, sucralfate, proton-pump inhibitor), smoking cessation program
F/U: Return visit within 2 weeks, then every 6 to 12 weeks

HIATAL HERNIA
Signs and symptoms
- Eructation after eating
- Pyrosis that worsens when lying down
- Regurgitation of sour-tasting fluid
- Abdominal distention
- Dull, substernal or epigastric pain
- Dysphagia
- Nausea
- Cough

DX: History, imaging studies (barium swallow, CT scan), endoscopy
TX: Diet modification, repositioning (sleeping with HOB elevated and avoiding lying down after meals), medication (antacids, histamine-2 blockers, GI stimulant)
F/U: None unless symptoms worsen

Additional differential diagnoses: esophageal diverticula or stenosis ▪ gastritis ▪ GERD ▪ obesity ▪ scleroderma

---

Other causes: acetohexamide ▪ tolbutamide ▪ lypressin ▪ aspirin ▪ anticholinergic agents ▪ NSAIDs ▪ drugs with anticholinergic effects

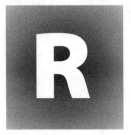

Rectal pain

A common symptom of anorectal disorders, rectal pain is discomfort that arises in the anal-rectal area. Although the anal canal is separated from the rest of the rectum by the internal sphincter, the patient may refer to all local pain as rectal pain.

Because the mucocutaneous border of the anal canal and the perianal skin contains somatic nerve fibers, lesions in this area are especially painful. This pain may result from or be aggravated by diarrhea, constipation, or passage of hardened stools. It may also be aggravated by intense pruritus and continued scratching associated with drainage of mucous, blood, or fecal matter that irritates the skin and nerve endings. Other possible causes of rectal pain include rectal trauma and presence of a foreign object.

History and physical examination

If your patient reports rectal pain, inspect for rectal bleeding; abnormal drainage such as pus; foreign objects; or protrusions, such as skin tags or thrombosed hemorrhoids. In addition, observe the patient for inflammation and other lesions. A rectal examination may be necessary.

After examination, proceed with your evaluation by taking the patient's history. Ask the patient to describe the pain. Is it sharp or dull, burning or knifelike? How often does it occur? Ask if the pain is worse during or immediately after defecation. Does the patient avoid having bowel movements because of anticipated pain? Is there a history of rectal trauma? In addition, find out what alleviates the pain.

Be sure to ask appropriate questions about the development of any associated signs and symptoms. For example, does the patient experience bleeding along with rectal pain? If so, find out how frequently this occurs and whether the blood appears on the toilet tissue, on the surface of the stool, or in the toilet bowl. Is the blood bright or dark red? Also, ask whether the patient has noticed other drainage, such as mucous or pus, and whether he's experiencing constipation or diarrhea.

PEDIATRIC POINTERS

- *Observe any child with rectal pain for associated bleeding, drainage, and signs and symptoms of infection (fever and irritability).*
- *Acute anal fissure is a common cause of rectal pain and bleeding in children, whose fear of provoking the pain may lead to constipation.*

- *Infants who seem to have pain on defecation should be evaluated for congenital anomalies of the rectum.*
- *Consider the possibility of sexual abuse in all children who complain of rectal pain.*

ELDER CARE CUE

Because elderly people typically underreport their symptoms and have an increased risk of neoplastic disorders, they should always be thoroughly evaluated.

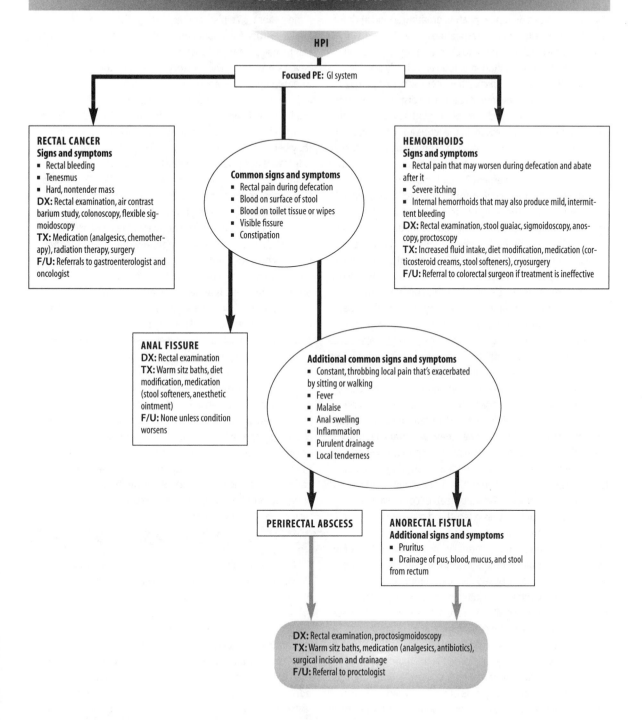

HPI

Focused PE: GI system

RECTAL CANCER
Signs and symptoms
- Rectal bleeding
- Tenesmus
- Hard, nontender mass

DX: Rectal examination, air contrast barium study, colonoscopy, flexible sigmoidoscopy
TX: Medication (analgesics, chemotherapy), radiation therapy, surgery
F/U: Referrals to gastroenterologist and oncologist

Common signs and symptoms
- Rectal pain during defecation
- Blood on surface of stool
- Blood on toilet tissue or wipes
- Visible fissure
- Constipation

HEMORRHOIDS
Signs and symptoms
- Rectal pain that may worsen during defecation and abate after it
- Severe itching
- Internal hemorrhoids that may also produce mild, intermittent bleeding

DX: Rectal examination, stool guaiac, sigmoidoscopy, anoscopy, proctoscopy
TX: Increased fluid intake, diet modification, medication (corticosteroid creams, stool softeners), cryosurgery
F/U: Referral to colorectal surgeon if treatment is ineffective

ANAL FISSURE
DX: Rectal examination
TX: Warm sitz baths, diet modification, medication (stool softeners, anesthetic ointment)
F/U: None unless condition worsens

Additional common signs and symptoms
- Constant, throbbing local pain that's exacerbated by sitting or walking
- Fever
- Malaise
- Anal swelling
- Inflammation
- Purulent drainage
- Local tenderness

PERIRECTAL ABSCESS

ANORECTAL FISTULA
Additional signs and symptoms
- Pruritus
- Drainage of pus, blood, mucus, and stool from rectum

DX: Rectal examination, proctosigmoidoscopy
TX: Warm sitz baths, medication (analgesics, antibiotics), surgical incision and drainage
F/U: Referral to proctologist

Additional differential diagnoses: cryptitis ▪ proctalgia fugax ▪ prostatic abscess ▪ rectal prolapse ▪ rectal ulcer

Respirations, abnormal

Characterized by a deep, low-pitched grunting sound at the end of each breath, grunting respirations are a chief sign of respiratory distress in infants and children. They may be soft and heard only on auscultation or loud and clearly audible without a stethoscope. Typically, the intensity of grunting respirations reflects the severity of respiratory distress. The grunting sound coincides with closure of the glottis, an effort to increase end-expiratory pressure in the lungs and prolong alveolar gas exchange, thereby enhancing ventilation and perfusion.

Grunting respirations indicate intrathoracic disease with lower respiratory involvement. Though most common in children, they sometimes occur in adults who are in severe respiratory distress. Whether they occur in children or adults, grunting respirations demand immediate medical attention.

Respirations are *shallow* when a diminished volume of air enters the lungs during inspiration. The patient with shallow respirations usually breathes at an accelerated rate. However, as he tires or as his muscles weaken, this compensatory increase in respirations diminishes, leading to inadequate gas exchange and such signs and symptoms as dyspnea, cyanosis, confusion, agitation, loss of consciousness, and tachycardia.

Shallow respirations may develop suddenly or gradually and may last briefly or become chronic. They're a key sign of respiratory distress and neurologic deterioration. Causes include inadequate central respiratory control over breathing, neuromuscular disorders, increased resistance to airflow into the lungs, respiratory muscle fatigue or weakness, voluntary alterations in breathing, and decreased activity from prolonged bed rest.

Characterized by a harsh, rattling, or snoring sound, *stertorous* respirations usually result from the vibration of relaxed oropharyngeal structures during sleep or coma, causing partial airway obstruction. Less often, these respirations result from retained mucus in the upper airway.

Stertorous respirations normally occur in about 10% of individuals, especially middle-aged, obese men. They may be aggravated by alcohol or sedative use before bed, which increases oropharyngeal flaccidity, and by sleeping in the supine position, which allows the relaxed tongue to slip back into the airway. The major pathologic causes of stertorous respirations are obstructive sleep apnea and life-threatening upper airway obstruction associated with an oropharyngeal tumor or with uvular or palatal edema. Obstruction may also occur during the postictal phase of a generalized seizure when mucous secretions or a relaxed tongue blocks the airway.

Occasionally, stertorous respirations are mistaken for stridor, which is another sign of upper airway obstruction. However, stridor indicates laryngeal or tracheal obstruction, whereas stertorous respirations signal higher airway obstruction.

History and physical examination

If the patient isn't in severe respiratory distress, begin by taking his history. Ask about chronic illness, surgery, and trauma. Has he had a tetanus booster in the past 10 years? Does he have asthma, allergies, a history of heart failure or vascular disease, chronic respiratory disorders or infections, or neurologic or neuromuscular disease? Does he smoke? Obtain a medication history and explore the possibility of drug abuse.

Ask about the patient's abnormal respirations: When did they begin? How long do they last? What makes them subside? What aggravates them? Ask about changes in appetite, weight, activity level, and behavior. If the patient is a premature infant, find out his gestational age. If the patient is a child, ask the parents if anyone in the home has had an upper respiratory infection (URI) recently. Has the child had signs of a URI, such as a runny nose, cough, low-grade fever, or anorexia? Does he have a history of frequent colds or URIs? Ask the parents to describe changes in the child's activity level to determine if the child is lethargic or less alert than usual.

Begin the physical examination by assessing the patient's level of consciousness and his orientation to time, person, and place. Observe spontaneous movements, and test muscle strength and deep tendon reflexes. Next, inspect the chest for deformities or abnormal movements such as intercostal retractions. Inspect the extremities for cyanosis and digital clubbing. Then palpate for expansion and diaphragmatic tactile fremitus and percuss for hyperresonance or dullness. Auscultate the lungs, especially the lower lobes. Note diminished or abnormal sounds, such as crackles or sibilant rhonchi, which may indicate mucus or fluid buildup. In addition, characterize the color, amount, and consistency of any discharge or sputum. Note any peripheral edema. Finally, examine the abdomen for distention, tenderness, or masses.

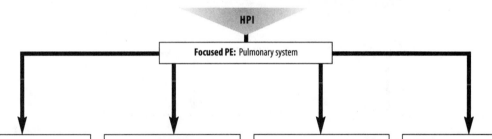

Focused PE: Pulmonary system

ASTHMA
Signs and symptoms
- Acute dyspneic attacks
- Audible or auscultated wheezing
- Dry cough
- Hyperpnea
- Chest tightness
- Accessory muscle use
- Nasal flaring
- Intercostal and supraclavicular retractions
- Tachypnea
- Tachycardia
- Diaphoresis
- Prolonged expiration
- Flushing or cyanosis
- Apprehension

DX: Labs (CBC, ABG, allergy skin testing), CXR, PFT
TX: Avoidance of allergens, tobacco, and beta-adrenergic blockers; medication (inhaled beta$_2$-agonists, inhaled corticosteroids [nedocromil or cromolyn if < age 12], leukotriene receptor agonist [possibly], corticosteroids during infections and exacerbations), peak expiratory flow monitoring
F/U: For acute exacerbation, return visit within 24 hours, then every 3 to 5 days, then every 1 to 3 months; referral to pulmonologist if treatment is ineffective

HEART FAILURE
Signs and symptoms
- Grunting respirations (late sign)
- Increasing pulmonary edema
- Productive cough
- Crackles
- Chest wall retractions

DX: Labs (CBC, cardiac enzymes), imaging studies (CXR, echocardiogram), ECG
TX: Medication (ACE inhibitors, diuretics, carvedilol [possibly], digoxin to improve ejection fraction and exercise tolerance [possibly])
DX: Imaging studies (echocardiography, CXR), ECG
F/U: Return visit within 1 week after discharge, at 4 weeks, and then every 3 months; referral to cardiologist if chronic

PNEUMONIA
Signs and symptoms
- High-grade fever
- Tachypnea
- Productive cough
- Anorexia
- Lethargy
- Decreased breath sounds
- Scattered crackles
- Sibilant rhonchi
- Severe dyspnea
- Substernal and subcostal retractions
- Nasal flaring
- Cyanosis

DX: PE, labs (sputum gram stain, CBC, ABG), CXR
TX: Medication (analgesics, antipyretics, antibiotics), oxygen therapy, chest physiotherapy
F/U: Reevaluation in 7 to 10 days unless the condition worsens

RESPIRATORY DISTRESS SYNDROME
Signs and symptoms
- Audible expiratory grunting
- Intercostal, subcostal, or substernal retractions
- Nasal flaring
- Tachycardia
- Tachypnea
- Signs of severe respiratory distress
- Harsh, diminished breath sounds
- Crackles

DX: ABG, CXR, PFT
TX: Oxygen therapy, treatment of underlying cause, symptomatic treatment, lung surfactant (infants)
F/U: Referral to pulmonologist

Other causes: abdominal pain ■ hiccups ■ tracheal obstruction or trauma

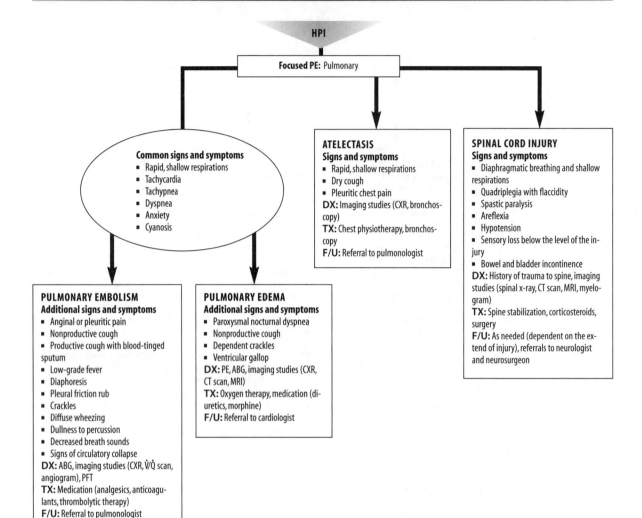

HPI

Focused PE: Pulmonary

Common signs and symptoms
- Rapid, shallow respirations
- Tachycardia
- Tachypnea
- Dyspnea
- Anxiety
- Cyanosis

ATELECTASIS
Signs and symptoms
- Rapid, shallow respirations
- Dry cough
- Pleuritic chest pain

DX: Imaging studies (CXR, bronchoscopy)
TX: Chest physiotherapy, bronchoscopy
F/U: Referral to pulmonologist

SPINAL CORD INJURY
Signs and symptoms
- Diaphragmatic breathing and shallow respirations
- Quadriplegia with flaccidity
- Spastic paralysis
- Areflexia
- Hypotension
- Sensory loss below the level of the injury
- Bowel and bladder incontinence

DX: History of trauma to spine, imaging studies (spinal x-ray, CT scan, MRI, myelogram)
TX: Spine stabilization, corticosteroids, surgery
F/U: As needed (dependent on the extend of injury), referrals to neurologist and neurosurgeon

PULMONARY EMBOLISM
Additional signs and symptoms
- Anginal or pleuritic pain
- Nonproductive cough
- Productive cough with blood-tinged sputum
- Low-grade fever
- Diaphoresis
- Pleural friction rub
- Crackles
- Diffuse wheezing
- Dullness to percussion
- Decreased breath sounds
- Signs of circulatory collapse

DX: ABG, imaging studies (CXR, V̇/Q̇ scan, angiogram), PFT
TX: Medication (analgesics, anticoagulants, thrombolytic therapy)
F/U: Referral to pulmonologist

PULMONARY EDEMA
Additional signs and symptoms
- Paroxysmal nocturnal dyspnea
- Nonproductive cough
- Dependent crackles
- Ventricular gallop

DX: PE, ABG, imaging studies (CXR, CT scan, MRI)
TX: Oxygen therapy, medication (diuretics, morphine)
F/U: Referral to cardiologist

Additional differential diagnoses: ARDS ▪ ALS ▪ asthma ▪ botulism ▪ bronchiectasis ▪ chronic bronchitis ▪ coma ▪ emphysema ▪ flail chest ▪ Guillain-Barré syndrome ▪ kyphoscoliosis ▪ multiple sclerosis ▪ muscular dystrophy ▪ myasthenia gravis ▪ obesity ▪ Parkinson's disease ▪ pleural effusion ▪ pneumonia ▪ pneumothorax ▪ tetanus ▪ upper airway obstruction

---

Other causes: drugs (narcotics, sedatives and hypnotics, tranquilizers, neuromuscular blockers, magnesium sulfate, anesthetics) ▪ abdominal or thoracic surgery (due to postoperative pain)

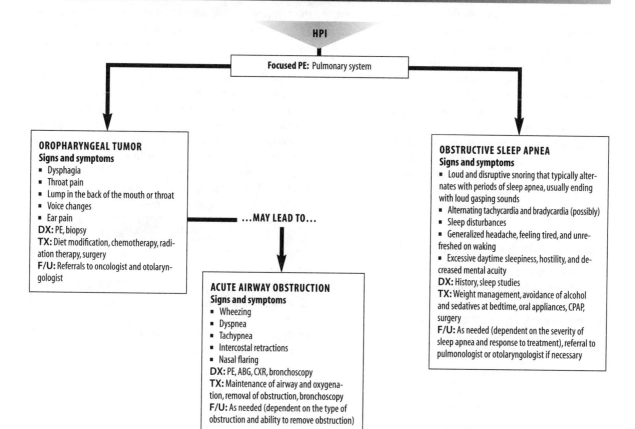

HPI

Focused PE: Pulmonary system

OROPHARYNGEAL TUMOR
Signs and symptoms
- Dysphagia
- Throat pain
- Lump in the back of the mouth or throat
- Voice changes
- Ear pain

DX: PE, biopsy
TX: Diet modification, chemotherapy, radiation therapy, surgery
F/U: Referrals to oncologist and otolaryngologist

...MAY LEAD TO...

ACUTE AIRWAY OBSTRUCTION
Signs and symptoms
- Wheezing
- Dyspnea
- Tachypnea
- Intercostal retractions
- Nasal flaring

DX: PE, ABG, CXR, bronchoscopy
TX: Maintenance of airway and oxygenation, removal of obstruction, bronchoscopy
F/U: As needed (dependent on the type of obstruction and ability to remove obstruction)

OBSTRUCTIVE SLEEP APNEA
Signs and symptoms
- Loud and disruptive snoring that typically alternates with periods of sleep apnea, usually ending with loud gasping sounds
- Alternating tachycardia and bradycardia (possibly)
- Sleep disturbances
- Generalized headache, feeling tired, and unrefreshed on waking
- Excessive daytime sleepiness, hostility, and decreased mental acuity

DX: History, sleep studies
TX: Weight management, avoidance of alcohol and sedatives at bedtime, oral appliances, CPAP, surgery
F/U: As needed (dependent on the severity of sleep apnea and response to treatment), referral to pulmonologist or otolaryngologist if necessary

Additional differential diagnoses: obstructive hypoventilation syndrome ▪ stroke

Other causes: endotracheal surgery, intubation, or suction

Retractions

A cardinal sign of respiratory distress in infants and children, costal and sternal retractions are visible indentations of the soft tissue covering the chest wall. They may be suprasternal (directly above the sternum and clavicles), intercostal (between the ribs), subcostal (below the lower costal margin of the rib cage), or substernal (just below the xiphoid process). Retractions may be mild or severe, producing barely visible to deep indentations.

Normally, infants and young children use abdominal muscles for breathing, unlike older children and adults, who use the diaphragm. When breathing requires extra effort, accessory muscles assist respiration, especially inspiration. Retractions typically accompany accessory muscle use.

History and physical examination

If you detect retractions in a child, check quickly for other signs of respiratory distress, such as cyanosis, tachypnea, and tachycardia. Observe the depth and location of retractions. Also, note the rate, depth, and quality of respirations. Look for accessory muscle use, nasal flaring during inspiration, or grunting during expiration. If the child has a cough, record the color, consistency, and odor of any sputum. Note whether the child appears restless or lethargic. Finally, auscultate the child's lungs to detect abnormal breath sounds. (See *Observing retractions*.)

If the child's condition permits, ask his parents about his medical history. Was he born prematurely? Was the delivery complicated? Ask about recent signs of an upper respiratory infection, such as a runny nose, cough, and a low-grade fever. How often has the child had respiratory problems during the past year? Has he been in contact with anyone who has had a cold, the flu, or other respiratory ailments? Did he aspirate any food, liquid, or foreign body? Inquire about any personal or family history of allergies or asthma.

PEDIATRIC POINTER

When examining a child for retractions, know that crying may accentuate the contractions.

ELDER CARE CUE

Although retractions may occur at any age, they're more difficult to assess in an older patient who is obese or in a patient who has chronic chest wall stiffness or deformity.

Observing retractions

When you observe retractions in infants and children, be sure to note their exact location — an important clue to the cause and severity of respiratory distress. For example, subcostal and substernal retractions usually result from lower respiratory tract disorders, whereas suprasternal retractions usually result from upper respiratory tract disorders.

Mild intercostal retractions alone may be normal. However, intercostal retractions accompanied by subcostal and substernal retractions may indicate moderate respiratory distress. Deep suprasternal retractions typically indicate severe distress.

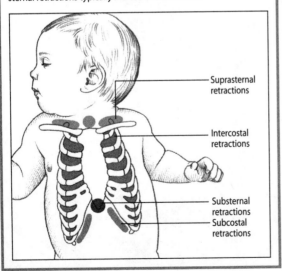

Suprasternal retractions

Intercostal retractions

Substernal retractions

Subcostal retractions

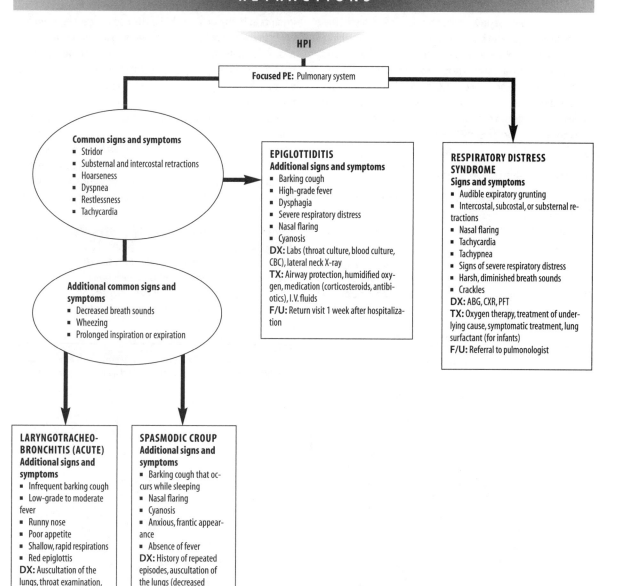

HPI

Focused PE: Pulmonary system

Common signs and symptoms
- Stridor
- Substernal and intercostal retractions
- Hoarseness
- Dyspnea
- Restlessness
- Tachycardia

Additional common signs and symptoms
- Decreased breath sounds
- Wheezing
- Prolonged inspiration or expiration

EPIGLOTTIDITIS
Additional signs and symptoms
- Barking cough
- High-grade fever
- Dysphagia
- Severe respiratory distress
- Nasal flaring
- Cyanosis

DX: Labs (throat culture, blood culture, CBC), lateral neck X-ray
TX: Airway protection, humidified oxygen, medication (corticosteroids, antibiotics), I.V. fluids
F/U: Return visit 1 week after hospitalization

RESPIRATORY DISTRESS SYNDROME
Signs and symptoms
- Audible expiratory grunting
- Intercostal, subcostal, or substernal retractions
- Nasal flaring
- Tachycardia
- Tachypnea
- Signs of severe respiratory distress
- Harsh, diminished breath sounds
- Crackles

DX: ABG, CXR, PFT
TX: Oxygen therapy, treatment of underlying cause, symptomatic treatment, lung surfactant (for infants)
F/U: Referral to pulmonologist

LARYNGOTRACHEO-BRONCHITIS (ACUTE)
Additional signs and symptoms
- Infrequent barking cough
- Low-grade to moderate fever
- Runny nose
- Poor appetite
- Shallow, rapid respirations
- Red epiglottis

DX: Auscultation of the lungs, throat examination, neck X-ray
TX: Warm or cool humidified air, oxygen therapy, antibiotics
F/U: Return visit 1 week after treatment is started (unless condition worsens) or 1 week after hospitalization

SPASMODIC CROUP
Additional signs and symptoms
- Barking cough that occurs while sleeping
- Nasal flaring
- Cyanosis
- Anxious, frantic appearance
- Absence of fever

DX: History of repeated episodes, auscultation of the lungs (decreased breath sounds, wheezing, prolonged inspiration or expiration), no signs of infection
TX: Oxygen therapy, humidified air
F/U: Referral to an allergist

Additional differential diagnoses: asthmatic attack ▪ bronchiolitis ▪ exacerbated COPD ▪ heart failure ▪ pneumonia (bacterial) ▪ rib fracture ▪ sepsis ▪ tracheal obstruction ▪ unstable sternum

Rhinorrhea

Common but rarely serious, rhinorrhea is the free discharge of thin nasal mucus. It can be self-limiting or chronic, resulting from nasal, sinus, or systemic disorders or from a basilar skull fracture. Rhinorrhea can also result from sinus or cranial surgery, excessive use of vasoconstricting nose drops or sprays, or inhalation of an irritant, such as tobacco smoke, dust, and fumes. Depending on the cause, the discharge may be clear, purulent, bloody, or serosanguineous.

History and physical examination

Begin the patient's history by asking him if the discharge runs from both nostrils. Is the discharge intermittent or persistent? Did it begin suddenly or gradually? Does the position of his head affect the discharge?

Next, ask the patient to characterize the discharge. Is it watery, bloody, purulent, or foul-smelling? Is it copious or scanty? Does the discharge worsen or improve with the time of day?

In addition, find out if the patient is using any medications, especially nose drops or sprays. Has he been exposed to nasal irritants at home or at work? Has he had a recent head injury?

Examine the patient's nose, checking airflow from each nostril. Evaluate the size, color, and condition of the turbinate mucosa (normally pale pink). Note if the mucosa is red, unusually pale, blue, or gray. Then examine the area beneath each turbinate. (See *Using a nasal speculum*.) Be sure to palpate over the frontal, ethmoid, and maxillary sinuses for tenderness.

To differentiate nasal mucus from cerebrospinal fluid (CSF), collect a small amount of drainage on a glucose test strip. If CSF (which contains glucose) is present, the test will be positive. Finally, using a nonirritating substance, be sure to test for anosmia.

PEDIATRIC POINTER

Be aware that rhinorrhea in children may stem from choanal atresia, allergic or chronic rhinitis, acute ethmoiditis, or congenital syphilis. Assume that unilateral rhinorrhea and nasal obstruction is caused by a foreign body in the nose until this is proven otherwise.

ELDER CARE CUE

Elderly patients may suffer increased adverse effects from medications used to treat rhinorrhea.

Using a nasal speculum

To visualize the interior of the nares, you'll need a nasal speculum and a good light source such as a penlight. Hold the speculum in the palm of one hand and the penlight in the other hand. Have the patient tilt her head back slightly and rest it against a wall or other firm support, if possible. Insert the speculum blades about ½ inch (1.3 cm) into the nasal vestibule, as shown.

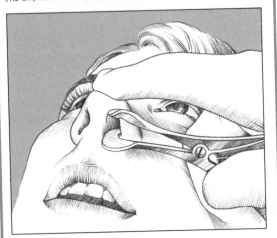

Place your index finger on the tip of the patient's nose for stability. Carefully open the speculum blades. Shine the light source in the direction of the nares. Now, inspect the nares, as shown. The mucosa should be deep pink. Note any discharge, masses, lesions, or mucosal swellings. Check the nasal septum for perforation, bleeding, or crusting. Bluish turbinates suggest allergy. A rounded, elongated projection suggests a polyp.

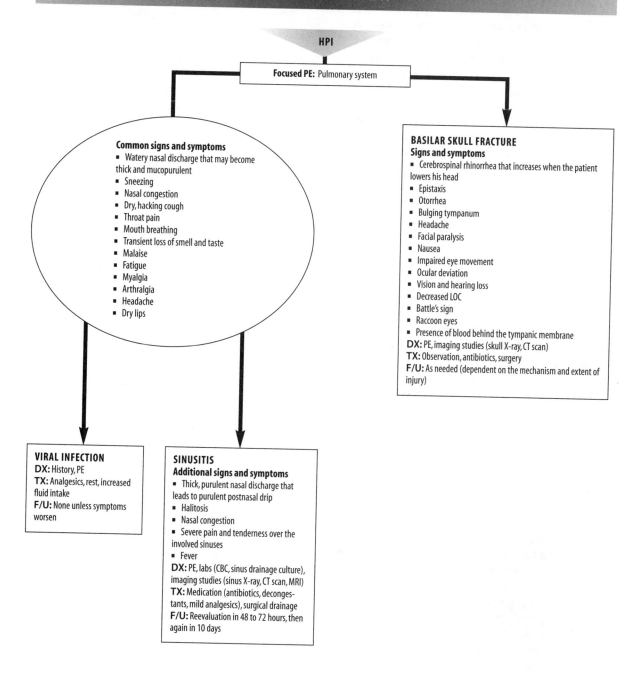

HPI

Focused PE: Pulmonary system

Common signs and symptoms
- Watery nasal discharge that may become thick and mucopurulent
- Sneezing
- Nasal congestion
- Dry, hacking cough
- Throat pain
- Mouth breathing
- Transient loss of smell and taste
- Malaise
- Fatigue
- Myalgia
- Arthralgia
- Headache
- Dry lips

BASILAR SKULL FRACTURE
Signs and symptoms
- Cerebrospinal rhinorrhea that increases when the patient lowers his head
- Epistaxis
- Otorrhea
- Bulging tympanum
- Headache
- Facial paralysis
- Nausea
- Impaired eye movement
- Ocular deviation
- Vision and hearing loss
- Decreased LOC
- Battle's sign
- Raccoon eyes
- Presence of blood behind the tympanic membrane

DX: PE, imaging studies (skull X-ray, CT scan)
TX: Observation, antibiotics, surgery
F/U: As needed (dependent on the mechanism and extent of injury)

VIRAL INFECTION
DX: History, PE
TX: Analgesics, rest, increased fluid intake
F/U: None unless symptoms worsen

SINUSITIS
Additional signs and symptoms
- Thick, purulent nasal discharge that leads to purulent postnasal drip
- Halitosis
- Nasal congestion
- Severe pain and tenderness over the involved sinuses
- Fever

DX: PE, labs (CBC, sinus drainage culture), imaging studies (sinus X-ray, CT scan, MRI)
TX: Medication (antibiotics, decongestants, mild analgesics), surgical drainage
F/U: Reevaluation in 48 to 72 hours, then again in 10 days

Additional differential diagnoses: headache (cluster) ▪ mucormycosis ▪ nasal or sinus tumors ▪ rhinitis ▪ rhinoscleroma ▪ Wegener's granulomatosis

Other causes: nasal sprays or drops containing vasoconstrictors ▪ sinus or cranial surgery

Rhonchi

Rhonchi are continuous adventitious breath sounds detected by auscultation. They're usually louder and lower-pitched than crackles — more like a hoarse moan or a deep snore — though they may be described as rattling, sonorous, bubbling, rumbling, or musical. However, sibilant rhonchi, or wheezes, are high-pitched.

Rhonchi are heard over large airways, such as the trachea. They occur in pulmonary disorders when air flows through passages that have been narrowed by secretions, a tumor or foreign body, bronchospasm, or mucosal thickening. The resulting vibration of airway walls produces the rhonchi.

History and physical examination

If you auscultate rhonchi, take the patient's vital signs and be alert for signs of respiratory distress. Characterize the patient's respirations as rapid or slow, shallow or deep, and regular or irregular. Inspect the chest, noting the use of accessory muscles. Is the patient audibly wheezing or gurgling? Auscultate for other abnormal breath sounds, such as crackles and a pleural friction rub. If you detect these sounds, note their location. Are breath sounds diminished or absent? Next, percuss the chest. If the patient has a cough, note its frequency and characterize its sound. If it's productive, examine the sputum for color, odor, consistency, and blood.

Ask related questions: Does the patient smoke? If so, obtain a history in pack-years. Has he recently lost weight or felt tired or weak? Does he have asthma or other pulmonary disorders? Is he currently taking any prescribed or over-the-counter drugs?

During the examination, keep in mind that thick or excessive secretions, bronchospasm, or inflammation of mucous membranes may lead to airway obstruction. If necessary, suction the patient and keep equipment available for inserting an airway. Keep bronchodilators available to treat bronchospasm.

PEDIATRIC POINTERS

- *Rhonchi in children can result from bacterial pneumonia, cystic fibrosis, and croup syndrome.*
- *Because a respiratory tract disorder may begin abruptly and progress rapidly in an infant or a child, observe closely for signs of airway obstruction.*

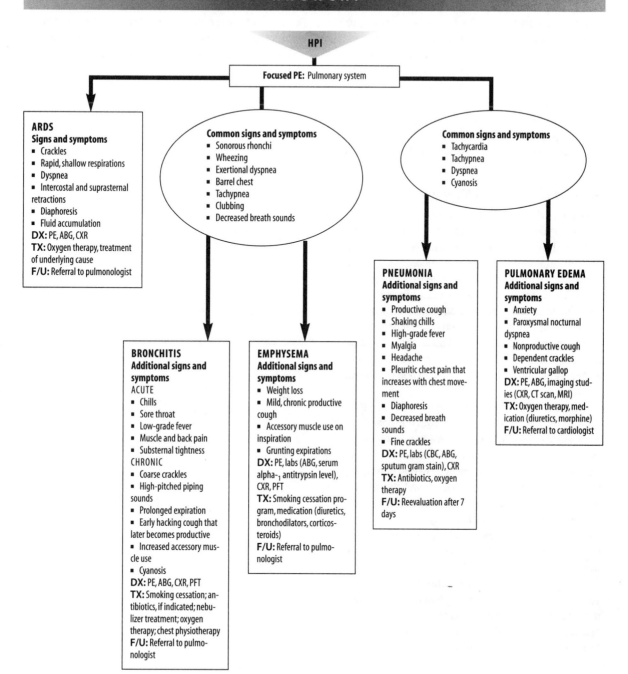

HPI

Focused PE: Pulmonary system

ARDS
Signs and symptoms
- Crackles
- Rapid, shallow respirations
- Dyspnea
- Intercostal and suprasternal retractions
- Diaphoresis
- Fluid accumulation

DX: PE, ABG, CXR
TX: Oxygen therapy, treatment of underlying cause
F/U: Referral to pulmonologist

Common signs and symptoms
- Sonorous rhonchi
- Wheezing
- Exertional dyspnea
- Barrel chest
- Tachypnea
- Clubbing
- Decreased breath sounds

Common signs and symptoms
- Tachycardia
- Tachypnea
- Dyspnea
- Cyanosis

PNEUMONIA
Additional signs and symptoms
- Productive cough
- Shaking chills
- High-grade fever
- Myalgia
- Headache
- Pleuritic chest pain that increases with chest movement
- Diaphoresis
- Decreased breath sounds
- Fine crackles

DX: PE, labs (CBC, ABG, sputum gram stain), CXR
TX: Antibiotics, oxygen therapy
F/U: Reevaluation after 7 days

PULMONARY EDEMA
Additional signs and symptoms
- Anxiety
- Paroxysmal nocturnal dyspnea
- Nonproductive cough
- Dependent crackles
- Ventricular gallop

DX: PE, ABG, imaging studies (CXR, CT scan, MRI)
TX: Oxygen therapy, medication (diuretics, morphine)
F/U: Referral to cardiologist

BRONCHITIS
Additional signs and symptoms
ACUTE
- Chills
- Sore throat
- Low-grade fever
- Muscle and back pain
- Substernal tightness
CHRONIC
- Coarse crackles
- High-pitched piping sounds
- Prolonged expiration
- Early hacking cough that later becomes productive
- Increased accessory muscle use
- Cyanosis

DX: PE, ABG, CXR, PFT
TX: Smoking cessation; antibiotics, if indicated; nebulizer treatment; oxygen therapy; chest physiotherapy
F/U: Referral to pulmonologist

EMPHYSEMA
Additional signs and symptoms
- Weight loss
- Mild, chronic productive cough
- Accessory muscle use on inspiration
- Grunting expirations

DX: PE, labs (ABG, serum alpha-$_1$ antitrypsin level), CXR, PFT
TX: Smoking cessation program, medication (diuretics, bronchodilators, corticosteroids)
F/U: Referral to pulmonologist

Additional differential diagnoses: asthma ▪ bronchiectasis ▪ pulmonary coccidioidomycosis

Other causes: PFTs ▪ bronchoscopy ▪ foreign body aspiration ▪ respiratory therapy

Romberg's sign

A positive Romberg's sign refers to a patient's inability to maintain balance when standing erect with his feet together and his eyes closed. It indicates a vestibular or proprioceptive disorder, or a disorder of the spinal tracts (the posterior columns) that carry proprioceptive information — the perception of one's position in space, of joint movements, and of pressure sensations — to the brain. Insufficient vestibular or proprioceptive information causes an inability to execute precise movements and maintain balance without visual cues.

History and physical examination

Once you've detected a positive Romberg's sign, perform other neurologic screening tests. A positive Romberg's sign only indicates the presence of a defect; it doesn't pinpoint its cause or location. First, test proprioception. If the patient can maintain his balance with his eyes open, ask him to hop on one foot and then on the other. Next, ask him to do a knee bend and to walk a straight line, placing heel to toe. Lastly, ask him to walk a short distance so you can evaluate his gait.

Test the patient's awareness of body part position by changing the position of one of his fingers, or any other joint, while his eyes are closed. Ask him to describe the change you've made.

Next, test the patient's direction of movement. Ask him to close his eyes and to touch his nose with the index finger of one hand and then with the other. Ask him to repeat this movement several times, gradually increasing his speed. Then test the accuracy of his movement by having him rapidly touch each finger of one hand to the thumb. Next, test sensation in all dermatomes, using a pin or cold object. Also test two-point discrimination by touching two pins (one in each hand) to his skin simultaneously. Does he feel one or two pinpricks? Finally, test and characterize the patient's deep tendon reflexes.

To test the patient's vibratory sense, ask him to close his eyes; then apply a mildly vibrating tuning fork to his feet. If the patient doesn't feel the stimulus initially, increase the vibration, and then test the knee or hip. This procedure can also be done to test the fingers, the elbow, and the shoulder.

Record all test results. Also, ask the patient if he has noticed sensory changes, such as numbness and tingling in his limbs. If so, when did they begin?

PEDIATRIC POINTER

Romberg's sign can't be tested in children until they can stand without support and follow commands. However, a positive sign in children commonly results from spinal cord disease.

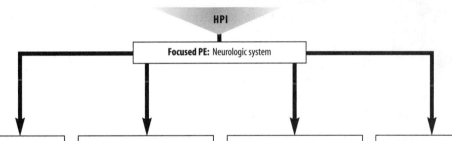

HPI

Focused PE: Neurologic system

MULTIPLE SCLEROSIS
Signs and symptoms
- Vision changes
- Diplopia
- Paresthesia
- Nystagmus
- Constipation
- Muscle weakness
- Spasticity
- Hyperreflexia
- Dysphagia
- Dysarthria
- Incontinence
- Urinary frequency and urgency
- Impotence
- Emotional instability

DX: PE, CSF analysis, MRI, EEG
TX: Medication (antispasmodics, cholinergics, antidepressants, amantadine, corticosteroids); physical, occupational, and speech therapy
F/U: Referral to neurologist

PERNICIOUS ANEMIA
Signs and symptoms
- Loss of proprioception in the lower limbs
- Gait changes
- Muscle weakness
- Impaired coordination
- Paresthesia
- Sensory loss
- Hypoactive or hyperactive DTRs
- Sore tongue
- Positive Babinski's reflex
- Fatigue
- Blurred vision
- Diplopia
- Light-headedness

DX: Labs (CBC, vitamin B_{12} level, Schilling test), bone marrow analysis
TX: Vitamin B_{12} injections
F/U: Referral to hematologist

PERIPHERAL NERVE DISEASE
Signs and symptoms
- Impotence
- Fatigue
- Paresthesia
- Hyperesthesia
- Anesthesia of the hands and feet
- Incoordination
- Ataxia
- Burning pain in the affected area
- Progressive muscle weakness and atrophy
- Loss of vibration sense
- Hypoactive DTRs (possibly)

DX: PE, EMG, nerve conduction tests, nerve biopsy
TX: Treatment of underlying cause, analgesics
F/U: Referral to neurologist

MÉNIÈRE'S DISEASE
Signs and symptoms
- Dizziness
- Vertigo
- Tinnitus
- Nausea and vomiting
- Gradual sensorineural hearing loss
- Acute attacks of jerk nystagmus that last 10 minutes to several hours

DX: PE (otoscopy with air pressure applied to the tympanic membrane), audiometry, caloric testing, MRI
TX: Medication (atropine, antiemetic-antivertigo agents), sedative-hypnotic
F/U: Referral to otolaryngologist

Additional differential diagnoses: head trauma ▪ spinal cerebellar degeneration ▪ spinal cord disease ▪ stroke ▪ tabes dorsalis ▪ vestibular disorders

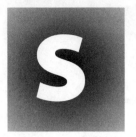

Scotoma

A scotoma is an area of partial or complete blindness within an otherwise normal or slightly impaired visual field. Usually located within the central 30° area, the defect ranges from absolute blindness to a barely detectable loss of visual acuity. Typically, the patient can pinpoint the scotoma's location in the visual field.

A scotoma can result from retinal, choroid, or optic nerve disorders. It can be classified as absolute, relative, or scintillating. An *absolute scotoma* refers to the total inability to see all sizes of test objects used in mapping the visual field. A *relative scotoma,* in contrast, refers to the ability to see only large test objects. A *scintillating scotoma* refers to the flashes or bursts of light commonly seen during a migraine headache.

History and physical examination

First, identify and characterize the scotoma, using such visual field tests as the tangent screen examination, the Goldmann perimeter test, and the automated perimetry test. Two other visual field tests — confrontation testing and the Amsler's grid — may also help in identifying a scotoma.

Next, test the patient's visual acuity and inspect his pupils for size, equality, and reaction to light. An ophthalmoscopic examination and measurement of intraocular pressure are necessary.

Explore the patient's history for eye disorders, vision problems, or chronic systemic disorders. Find out if he takes medications or uses eyedrops.

PEDIATRIC POINTER

In young children, visual field testing is difficult and requires patience. Confrontation testing is the method of choice.

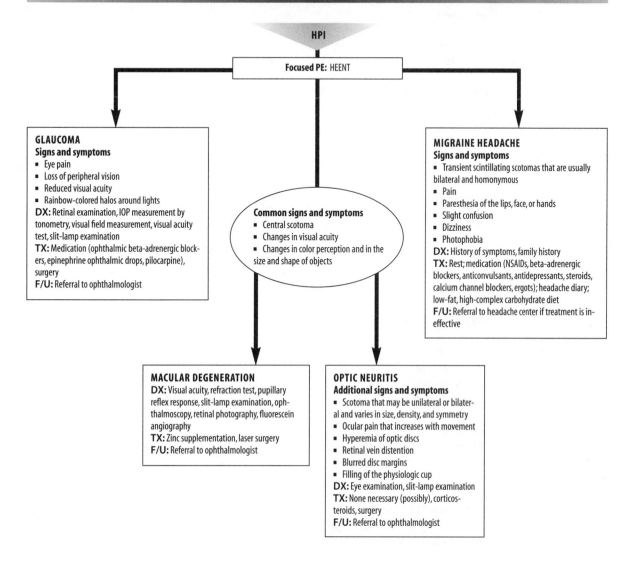

HPI

Focused PE: HEENT

GLAUCOMA
Signs and symptoms
- Eye pain
- Loss of peripheral vision
- Reduced visual acuity
- Rainbow-colored halos around lights

DX: Retinal examination, IOP measurement by tonometry, visual field measurement, visual acuity test, slit-lamp examination
TX: Medication (ophthalmic beta-adrenergic blockers, epinephrine ophthalmic drops, pilocarpine), surgery
F/U: Referral to ophthalmologist

Common signs and symptoms
- Central scotoma
- Changes in visual acuity
- Changes in color perception and in the size and shape of objects

MIGRAINE HEADACHE
Signs and symptoms
- Transient scintillating scotomas that are usually bilateral and homonymous
- Pain
- Paresthesia of the lips, face, or hands
- Slight confusion
- Dizziness
- Photophobia

DX: History of symptoms, family history
TX: Rest; medication (NSAIDs, beta-adrenergic blockers, anticonvulsants, antidepressants, steroids, calcium channel blockers, ergots); headache diary; low-fat, high-complex carbohydrate diet
F/U: Referral to headache center if treatment is ineffective

MACULAR DEGENERATION
DX: Visual acuity, refraction test, pupillary reflex response, slit-lamp examination, ophthalmoscopy, retinal photography, fluorescein angiography
TX: Zinc supplementation, laser surgery
F/U: Referral to ophthalmologist

OPTIC NEURITIS
Additional signs and symptoms
- Scotoma that may be unilateral or bilateral and varies in size, density, and symmetry
- Ocular pain that increases with movement
- Hyperemia of optic discs
- Retinal vein distention
- Blurred disc margins
- Filling of the physiologic cup

DX: Eye examination, slit-lamp examination
TX: None necessary (possibly), corticosteroids, surgery
F/U: Referral to ophthalmologist

Additional differential diagnoses: chorioretinitis ▪ retinal pigmentary degeneration

Other cause: direct visualization of eclipse

Scrotal swelling

Scrotal swelling occurs when a condition affecting the testicles, epididymis, or scrotal skin produces edema or a mass; the penis may or may not be involved. Scrotal swelling can affect males of any age. It can be unilateral or bilateral and painful or painless.

The sudden onset of painful scrotal swelling suggests torsion of a testicle or testicular appendages, especially in a prepubescent male. This emergency requires immediate surgery to untwist and stabilize the spermatic cord or to remove the appendage.

History and physical examination

If the patient isn't in distress, proceed with obtaining his history. Ask about injuries to the scrotum, urethral discharge, cloudy urine, increased urinary frequency, and dysuria. Is the patient sexually active? When was his last sexual contact? Find out about recent illnesses, particularly mumps. Does he have a history of prostate surgery or prolonged catheterization? Does changing his body position or level of activity affect the swelling?

Take the patient's vital signs, noting especially fever, and palpate his abdomen for tenderness. Then examine the entire genital area. Assess the scrotum with the patient supine and standing. Note its size and color. Is the swelling unilateral or bilateral? Do you see signs of trauma or bruising? Gently palpate the scrotum for a cyst or a lump. Note especially tenderness or increased firmness. Check the testicles' position in the scrotum. Finally, transilluminate the scrotum to distinguish a fluid-filled cyst from a solid mass. (A solid mass can't be transilluminated.)

PEDIATRIC POINTERS

- *A thorough physical assessment is especially important for children with scrotal swelling, who may be unable to provide history data.*
- *In children up to age 1, a hernia or hydrocele of the spermatic cord may stem from abnormal fetal development.*
- *In infants, scrotal swelling may stem from ammonia-related dermatitis, if diapers aren't changed often enough.*
- *In prepubescent males, it usually results from torsion of the spermatic cord.*
- *Other disorders that can produce scrotal swelling in children include epididymitis (rare before age 10), adherence of the foreskin to the penile head, traumatic orchitis from contact sports, and mumps, which occurs most commonly after puberty.*

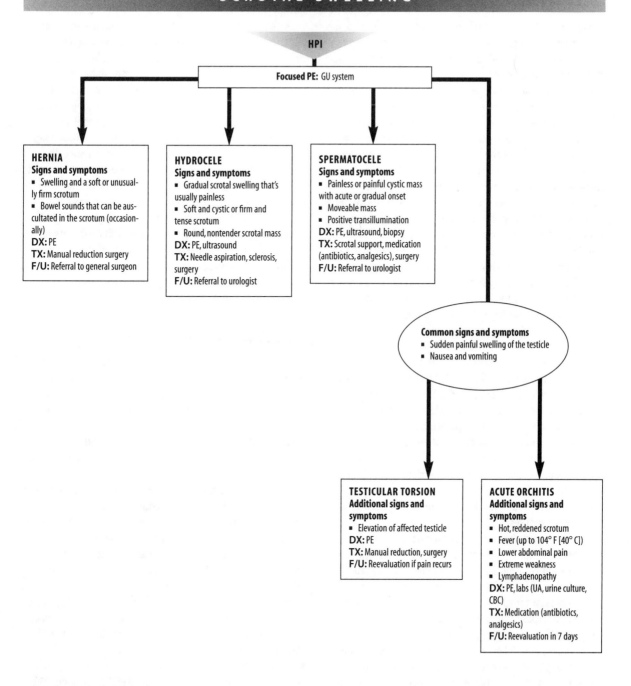

HPI

Focused PE: GU system

HERNIA
Signs and symptoms
- Swelling and a soft or unusually firm scrotum
- Bowel sounds that can be auscultated in the scrotum (occasionally)
DX: PE
TX: Manual reduction surgery
F/U: Referral to general surgeon

HYDROCELE
Signs and symptoms
- Gradual scrotal swelling that's usually painless
- Soft and cystic or firm and tense scrotum
- Round, nontender scrotal mass
DX: PE, ultrasound
TX: Needle aspiration, sclerosis, surgery
F/U: Referral to urologist

SPERMATOCELE
Signs and symptoms
- Painless or painful cystic mass with acute or gradual onset
- Moveable mass
- Positive transillumination
DX: PE, ultrasound, biopsy
TX: Scrotal support, medication (antibiotics, analgesics), surgery
F/U: Referral to urologist

Common signs and symptoms
- Sudden painful swelling of the testicle
- Nausea and vomiting

TESTICULAR TORSION
Additional signs and symptoms
- Elevation of affected testicle
DX: PE
TX: Manual reduction, surgery
F/U: Reevaluation if pain recurs

ACUTE ORCHITIS
Additional signs and symptoms
- Hot, reddened scrotum
- Fever (up to 104° F [40° C])
- Lower abdominal pain
- Extreme weakness
- Lymphadenopathy
DX: PE, labs (UA, urine culture, CBC)
TX: Medication (antibiotics, analgesics)
F/U: Reevaluation in 7 days

Additional differential diagnoses: elephantiasis of the scrotum ▪ epididymal cysts ▪ epididymal tuberculosis ▪ epididymitis ▪ fistula ▪ granuloma ▪ gumma ▪ idiopathic scrotal edema ▪ lymphoma ▪ scrotal burns ▪ scrotal trauma ▪ testicular tumor ▪ torsion of a hydatid of Morgagni

Other cause: surgery

Seizures

A *simple partial seizure* is also known as a *focal seizure* and may manifest in different areas of the body. A *focal motor seizure* is a series of unilateral clonic (muscle jerking) and tonic (muscle stiffening) movements of one part of the body. The patient's head and eyes characteristically turn away from the hemispheric focus — usually the frontal lobe near the motor strip. A tonic-clonic contraction of the trunk or extremities may follow.

A *jacksonian motor seizure* typically begins with a tonic contraction of a finger, the corner of the mouth, or one foot. Clonic movements follow, spreading to other muscles on the same side of the body, moving up the arm or leg and, eventually, involving the whole side. Alternatively, clonic movements may spread to the opposite side, becoming generalized and leading to a loss of consciousness. In the postictal phase, the patient may experience paralysis (Todd's paralysis) in the affected limbs, which usually resolves within 24 hours.

A *focal somatosensory seizure* affects a localized body area on one side. Usually, this type of seizure initially causes numbness, tingling, or crawling or "electric" sensations; occasionally, it causes pain or burning sensations in the lips, fingers, or toes. A *visual seizure* involves sensations of darkness or of stationary or moving lights or spots, usually red at first, then blue, green, and yellow. It can affect both visual fields or the visual field on the side opposite the lesion. The irritable focus is in the occipital lobe. In contrast, the irritable focus in an *auditory* or *olfactory seizure* is in the temporal lobe.

A *complex partial seizure* occurs when a focal seizure begins in the temporal lobe and causes a partial alteration of consciousness — usually confusion. Psychomotor seizures can occur at any age, but their incidence usually increases during adolescence and adulthood. Two-thirds of patients also have generalized seizures.

An aura — usually a complex hallucination or illusion — typically precedes a psychomotor seizure. The hallucination may be audiovisual (images with sounds), auditory (abnormal or normal sounds or voices from the patient's past), or olfactory (unpleasant smells, such as rotten eggs or burning materials). Other types of auras include sensations of déjà vu, unfamiliarity with surroundings, or depersonalization. Some patients become fearful or anxious, experience lip smacking, or have an unpleasant feeling in the epigastric region that rises toward the chest and throat. A period of unresponsiveness follows the aura. The patient may experience automatisms, appear dazed and wander aimlessly, perform inappropriate acts (such as undressing in public), be unresponsive, utter incoherent phrases, or (rarely) go into a rage or tantrum. After the seizure, the patient is confused, drowsy, and doesn't remember the seizure. Behavioral automatisms rarely last longer than 5 minutes, but postseizure confusion and amnesia may persist.

A *generalized tonic-clonic seizure* may begin with or without an aura. As seizure activity spreads to the subcortical structures, the patient loses consciousness, falls to the ground, and may utter a loud cry that's precipitated by air rushing from the lungs through the vocal cords. His body stiffens (tonic phase), then undergoes rapid, synchronous muscle jerking and hyperventilation (clonic phase). Tongue biting, incontinence, diaphoresis, profuse salivation, and signs of respiratory distress may also occur. The seizure usually stops after 2 to 5 minutes. The patient then regains consciousness but displays confusion. He may complain of headache, fatigue, muscle soreness, and arm and leg weakness.

Generalized tonic-clonic seizures usually occur singly. The patient may be asleep or awake and active. Life-threatening status epilepticus is marked by prolonged seizure activity or by rapidly recurring seizures with no intervening periods of recovery. It's most commonly triggered by abrupt discontinuation of anticonvulsant drugs.

History and physical examination

If you didn't witness the seizure, obtain a description from the patient's companion. Ask when the seizure started and how long it lasted. Did the patient report any unusual sensations before the seizure began? Did the seizure start in one area of the body and spread, or did it affect the entire body right away? Did the patient fall on a hard surface? Did his eyes or head turn? Did he turn blue? Did he lose bladder control? Did he have any other seizures before recovering?

Next, obtain a patient history. Has he ever had generalized or focal seizures before? If so, do they occur frequently? Do other family members also have them? Is the patient receiving drug therapy? Is he compliant? Also, ask about any sleep deprivation, or emotional or physical stress at the time the seizure occurred. Then perform a full neurologic assessment.

PEDIATRIC POINTERS

- *Complex partial seizures in children can result from birth injury, abuse, infection, or cancer. In about one-third of patients, their cause is unknown.*
- *Many children between the ages of 3 months and 3 years experience generalized seizures associated with fever. About 25% of febrile seizures may present as focal seizures.*

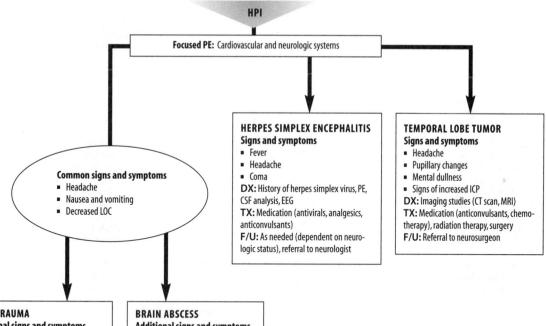

HPI

Focused PE: Cardiovascular and neurologic systems

Common signs and symptoms
- Headache
- Nausea and vomiting
- Decreased LOC

HERPES SIMPLEX ENCEPHALITIS
Signs and symptoms
- Fever
- Headache
- Coma

DX: History of herpes simplex virus, PE, CSF analysis, EEG

TX: Medication (antivirals, analgesics, anticonvulsants)

F/U: As needed (dependent on neurologic status), referral to neurologist

TEMPORAL LOBE TUMOR
Signs and symptoms
- Headache
- Pupillary changes
- Mental dullness
- Signs of increased ICP

DX: Imaging studies (CT scan, MRI)

TX: Medication (anticonvulsants, chemotherapy), radiation therapy, surgery

F/U: Referral to neurosurgeon

HEAD TRAUMA
Additional signs and symptoms
- Seizures that occur months or years after trauma
- Seizures that increase in frequency or eventually stop
- Behavior and personality changes
- Obvious wound

DX: History of trauma, PE, imaging studies (CT scan, MRI)

TX: Varies based on the extent of trauma, safety maintenance during seizure, medication (analgesics, anticonvulsants), surgery (if indicated)

F/U: As needed (dependent on the severity of trauma and neurologic status)

BRAIN ABSCESS
Additional signs and symptoms
- Central facial weakness
- Auditory receptive aphasia
- Hemiparesis
- Ocular disturbances

DX: Imaging studies (CT scan, MRI), EEG

TX: Medication (antibiotics, analgesics, anticonvulsants), surgery

F/U: Referral to neurosurgeon

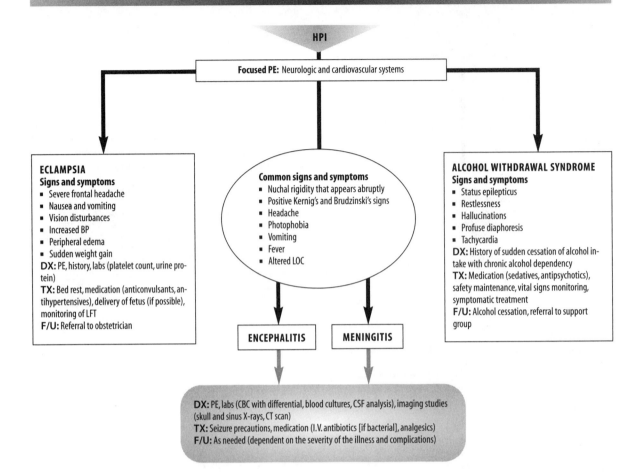

HPI

Focused PE: Neurologic and cardiovascular systems

ECLAMPSIA
Signs and symptoms
- Severe frontal headache
- Nausea and vomiting
- Vision disturbances
- Increased BP
- Peripheral edema
- Sudden weight gain

DX: PE, history, labs (platelet count, urine protein)
TX: Bed rest, medication (anticonvulsants, antihypertensives), delivery of fetus (if possible), monitoring of LFT
F/U: Referral to obstetrician

Common signs and symptoms
- Nuchal rigidity that appears abruptly
- Positive Kernig's and Brudzinski's signs
- Headache
- Photophobia
- Vomiting
- Fever
- Altered LOC

ALCOHOL WITHDRAWAL SYNDROME
Signs and symptoms
- Status epilepticus
- Restlessness
- Hallucinations
- Profuse diaphoresis
- Tachycardia

DX: History of sudden cessation of alcohol intake with chronic alcohol dependency
TX: Medication (sedatives, antipsychotics), safety maintenance, vital signs monitoring, symptomatic treatment
F/U: Alcohol cessation, referral to support group

ENCEPHALITIS

MENINGITIS

DX: PE, labs (CBC with differential, blood cultures, CSF analysis), imaging studies (skull and sinus X-rays, CT scan)
TX: Seizure precautions, medication (I.V. antibiotics [if bacterial], analgesics)
F/U: As needed (dependent on the severity of the illness and complications)

Additional differential diagnoses: brain abscess ▪ brain tumor ▪ cerebral aneurysm ▪ chronic renal failure ▪ epilepsy (idiopathic) ▪ head trauma ▪ hepatic encephalopathy ▪ hypertensive encephalopathy ▪ hypoglycemia ▪ hyponatremia ▪ hypoparathyroidism ▪ hypoxic encephalopathy ▪ multiple sclerosis ▪ neurofibromatosis ▪ porphyria (intermittent acute) ▪ sarcoidosis ▪ stroke

Other causes: arsenic poisoning ▪ barbiturate withdrawal ▪ contrast agents ▪ toxic levels of theophylline, lidocaine, meperidine, penicillin, or cimetidine ▪ phenothiazines ▪ tricyclic antidepressants ▪ amphetamines ▪ isoniazid ▪ vincristine (in patients with preexisting seizure disorders)

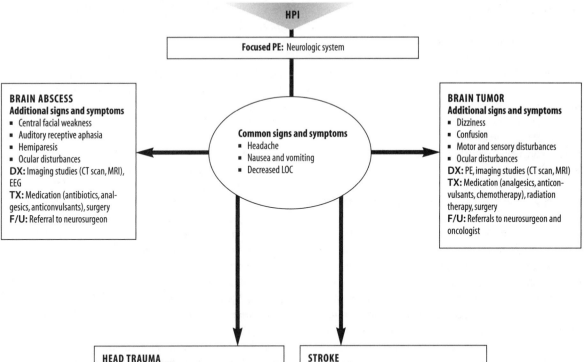

HPI

Focused PE: Neurologic system

Common signs and symptoms
- Headache
- Nausea and vomiting
- Decreased LOC

BRAIN ABSCESS
Additional signs and symptoms
- Central facial weakness
- Auditory receptive aphasia
- Hemiparesis
- Ocular disturbances

DX: Imaging studies (CT scan, MRI), EEG
TX: Medication (antibiotics, analgesics, anticonvulsants), surgery
F/U: Referral to neurosurgeon

BRAIN TUMOR
Additional signs and symptoms
- Dizziness
- Confusion
- Motor and sensory disturbances
- Ocular disturbances

DX: PE, imaging studies (CT scan, MRI)
TX: Medication (analgesics, anticonvulsants, chemotherapy), radiation therapy, surgery
F/U: Referrals to neurosurgeon and oncologist

HEAD TRAUMA
Additional signs and symptoms
- Seizures that occur months or years after trauma
- Seizures that increase in frequency or eventually stop
- Behavior and personality changes
- Obvious wound

DX: History of trauma, PE, imaging studies (CT scan, MRI)
TX: Varies based on the extent of trauma, safety maintenance during seizure, medication (analgesics, anticonvulsants), surgery (if indicated)
F/U: As needed (dependent on the severity of trauma and neurologic status)

STROKE
Additional signs and symptoms
- Seizures that may not occur until 6 months after onset
- Contralateral hemiplegia
- Dysarthria
- Dysphagia
- Ataxia
- Unilateral sensory loss
- Aphasia

DX: History of illness, imaging studies (skull X-ray, CT scan, MRI, angiography), EEG
TX: Airway stabilization, treatment of cause of injury, control of extension of injury, medication (for embolic stroke, thrombolytics; anticonvulsants; analgesics), surgery
F/U: Referral to neurologist or neurosurgeon, transfer to brain injury center

Additional differential diagnoses: multiple sclerosis ▪ neurofibromatosis ▪ sarcoidosis

Skin, abnormal

Clammy skin — moist, cool, and often pale — is a sympathetic response to stress, which triggers release of the hormones epinephrine and norepinephrine. These hormones cause cutaneous vasoconstriction and secretion of cold sweat from eccrine glands, particularly on the palms, forehead, and soles.

Clammy skin typically accompanies shock, acute hypoglycemia, anxiety reactions, arrhythmias, and heat exhaustion. It also occurs as a vasovagal reaction to severe pain associated with nausea, anorexia, epigastric distress, hyperpnea, tachypnea, weakness, confusion, tachycardia, and pupillary dilation or a combination of these findings. Marked bradycardia and syncope may follow.

Mottled skin is patchy discoloration indicating primary or secondary changes of the deep, middle, or superficial dermal blood vessels. It can result from hematologic, immune, or connective tissue disorders; chronic occlusive arterial disease; dysproteinemias; immobility; exposure to heat or cold; or shock. Mottled skin can be a normal reaction, such as the diffuse mottling that occurs when exposure to cold causes venous stasis in cutaneous blood vessels (cutis marmorata).

Scaly skin results when cells of the uppermost skin layer (stratum corneum) desiccate and shed, causing excessive accumulation of loosely adherent flakes of normal or abnormal keratin. Scaly skin varies in texture from fine and delicate to branny, coarse, or stratified. Scales are typically dry, brittle, and shiny, but they can be greasy and dull. Their color ranges from whitish gray, yellow, or brown to a silvery sheen.

History and physical examination

If you detect clammy skin, immediately ask about a history of insulin-dependent diabetes mellitus or cardiac disorders. Is the patient currently taking any medications, especially antiarrhythmics? Is he experiencing pain, chest pressure, nausea, or epigastric distress? Does he feel weak? Does he have a dry mouth? Does he have diarrhea or increased urination? Next, examine the pupils for dilation. Also, check for abdominal distention and increased muscle tension.

Mottled skin may indicate an emergency condition requiring rapid evaluation and intervention. However, if the patient isn't in distress, obtain a history. Ask if the mottling began suddenly or gradually. What precipitated it? How long has he had it? Does anything make it go away? Does the patient have other symptoms, such as pain, numbness, or tingling in an extremity? If so, do they disappear with temperature changes?

Observe the patient's skin color, and palpate his arms and legs for skin texture, swelling, and temperature differences between extremities. Palpate for the presence (or absence) of pulses and for their quality. Note breaks in the skin, muscle appearance, and hair distribution. Assess motor and sensory function.

If the patient has scaly skin, begin by asking how long the patient has had scaly skin and whether he has had it before. Where did it appear first? Did a lesion or skin eruption such as erythema precede it? Has the patient used a topical skin product recently? How often does he bathe? Has he had recent joint pain, illness, or malaise? Ask the patient about work exposure to chemicals, use of prescribed drugs, and a family history of skin disorders. Find out what kinds of soap, cosmetics, skin lotion, and hair preparations he uses.

Next, examine the entire skin surface. Is it dry, oily, moist, or greasy? Observe the general pattern of skin lesions, and record their location, color, shape, and size. Are they thick or fine? Do they itch? Does the patient have other lesions in addition to scaly skin?

PEDIATRIC POINTERS

- *A common cause of mottled skin in children is systemic vasoconstriction from shock.*
- *In children, scaly skin may stem from infantile eczema, pityriasis rosea, epidermolytic hyperkeratosis, psoriasis, various forms of ichthyosis, atopic dermatitis, a viral infection, or an acute transient dermatitis. Desquamation may follow a febrile illness.*

ELDER CARE CUE

Elderly patients develop clammy or mottled skin easily because of decreased tissue perfusion.

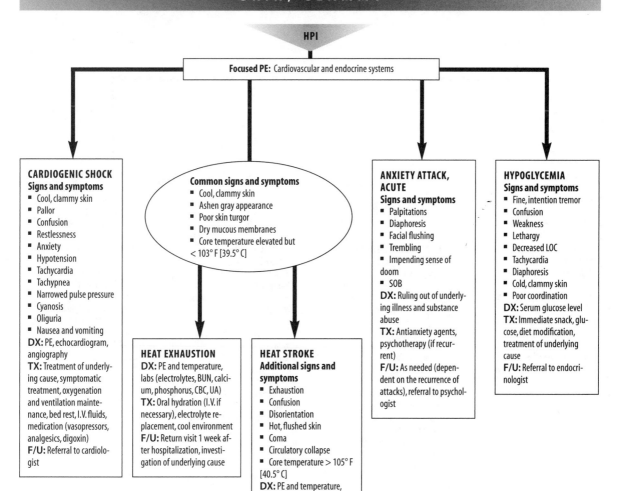

HPI

Focused PE: Cardiovascular and endocrine systems

CARDIOGENIC SHOCK
Signs and symptoms
- Cool, clammy skin
- Pallor
- Confusion
- Restlessness
- Anxiety
- Hypotension
- Tachycardia
- Tachypnea
- Narrowed pulse pressure
- Cyanosis
- Oliguria
- Nausea and vomiting

DX: PE, echocardiogram, angiography
TX: Treatment of underlying cause, symptomatic treatment, oxygenation and ventilation maintenance, bed rest, I.V. fluids, medication (vasopressors, analgesics, digoxin)
F/U: Referral to cardiologist

Common signs and symptoms
- Cool, clammy skin
- Ashen gray appearance
- Poor skin turgor
- Dry mucous membranes
- Core temperature elevated but < 103° F [39.5° C]

HEAT EXHAUSTION
DX: PE and temperature, labs (electrolytes, BUN, calcium, phosphorus, CBC, UA)
TX: Oral hydration (I.V. if necessary), electrolyte replacement, cool environment
F/U: Return visit 1 week after hospitalization, investigation of underlying cause

HEAT STROKE
Additional signs and symptoms
- Exhaustion
- Confusion
- Disorientation
- Hot, flushed skin
- Coma
- Circulatory collapse
- Core temperature > 105° F [40.5° C]

DX: PE and temperature, labs (electrolytes, BUN, creatinine)
TX: I.V. hydration, careful electrolyte monitoring, airway and ventilation maintenance, hemodynamic monitoring, rapid cooling with ice packs, cooling blanket
F/U: Return visit 1 week after hospitalization, investigation of underlying cause

ANXIETY ATTACK, ACUTE
Signs and symptoms
- Palpitations
- Diaphoresis
- Facial flushing
- Trembling
- Impending sense of doom
- SOB

DX: Ruling out of underlying illness and substance abuse
TX: Antianxiety agents, psychotherapy (if recurrent)
F/U: As needed (dependent on the recurrence of attacks), referral to psychologist

HYPOGLYCEMIA
Signs and symptoms
- Fine, intention tremor
- Confusion
- Weakness
- Lethargy
- Decreased LOC
- Tachycardia
- Diaphoresis
- Cold, clammy skin
- Poor coordination

DX: Serum glucose level
TX: Immediate snack, glucose, diet modification, treatment of underlying cause
F/U: Referral to endocrinologist

Additional differential diagnoses: arrhythmias ▪ hypovolemic shock ▪ septic shock

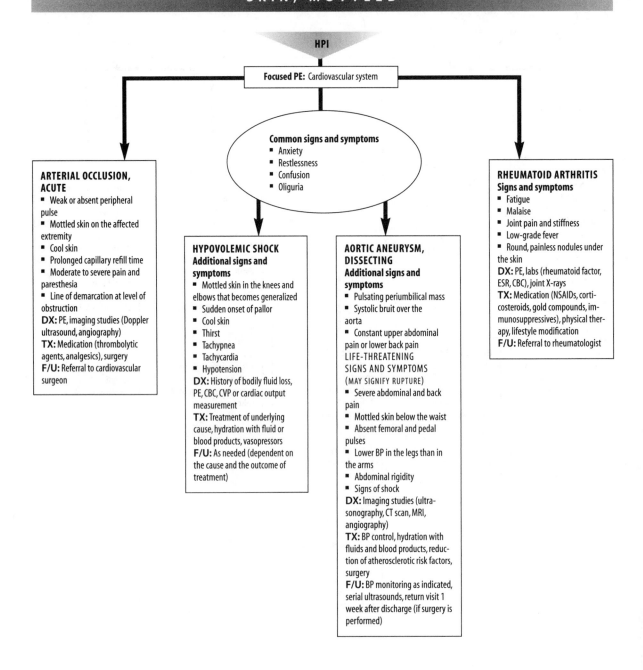

HPI

Focused PE: Cardiovascular system

Common signs and symptoms
- Anxiety
- Restlessness
- Confusion
- Oliguria

ARTERIAL OCCLUSION, ACUTE
- Weak or absent peripheral pulse
- Mottled skin on the affected extremity
- Cool skin
- Prolonged capillary refill time
- Moderate to severe pain and paresthesia
- Line of demarcation at level of obstruction

DX: PE, imaging studies (Doppler ultrasound, angiography)
TX: Medication (thrombolytic agents, analgesics), surgery
F/U: Referral to cardiovascular surgeon

HYPOVOLEMIC SHOCK
Additional signs and symptoms
- Mottled skin in the knees and elbows that becomes generalized
- Sudden onset of pallor
- Cool skin
- Thirst
- Tachypnea
- Tachycardia
- Hypotension

DX: History of bodily fluid loss, PE, CBC, CVP or cardiac output measurement
TX: Treatment of underlying cause, hydration with fluid or blood products, vasopressors
F/U: As needed (dependent on the cause and the outcome of treatment)

AORTIC ANEURYSM, DISSECTING
Additional signs and symptoms
- Pulsating periumbilical mass
- Systolic bruit over the aorta
- Constant upper abdominal pain or lower back pain
LIFE-THREATENING SIGNS AND SYMPTOMS
(MAY SIGNIFY RUPTURE)
- Severe abdominal and back pain
- Mottled skin below the waist
- Absent femoral and pedal pulses
- Lower BP in the legs than in the arms
- Abdominal rigidity
- Signs of shock

DX: Imaging studies (ultra-sonography, CT scan, MRI, angiography)
TX: BP control, hydration with fluids and blood products, reduction of atherosclerotic risk factors, surgery
F/U: BP monitoring as indicated, serial ultrasounds, return visit 1 week after discharge (if surgery is performed)

RHEUMATOID ARTHRITIS
Signs and symptoms
- Fatigue
- Malaise
- Joint pain and stiffness
- Low-grade fever
- Round, painless nodules under the skin

DX: PE, labs (rheumatoid factor, ESR, CBC), joint X-rays
TX: Medication (NSAIDs, corticosteroids, gold compounds, immunosuppressives), physical therapy, lifestyle modification
F/U: Referral to rheumatologist

Additional differential diagnoses: acrocyanosis ▪ arteriosclerosis obliterans ▪ Buerger's disease ▪ livedo reticularis (idiopathic or primary) ▪ periarteritis nodosa ▪ polycythemia vera ▪ SLE

Other causes: immobility ▪ thermal exposure

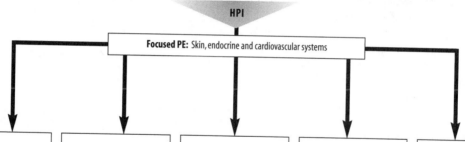

HPI

Focused PE: Skin, endocrine and cardiovascular systems

SEBORRHEIC DERMATITIS
Signs and symptoms
MILD
- Fine, dry, white or yellow scales on inflamed base
MODERATE
- Dull, red plaques with thick white or yellow scales in a diffuse distribution
- Pruritus
DX: Skin examination
TX: Medicated shampoo, medication (topical corticosteroids, ketoconazole, selenium)
F/U: None unless signs and symptoms worsen

NUMMULAR DERMATITIS
Signs and symptoms
- Round, pustular lesions
- Purulent exudate
- Encrustation and scaling
- Pruritus
DX: Skin examination, personal and family history
TX: Symptomatic treatment, medication (antipruritics, topical tar lotions, topical corticosteroids)
F/U: Referral to dermatologist

PITYRIASIS ROSEA
Signs and symptoms
- Mild to severe pruritus that's aggravated by a hot bath or shower
- Erythematous herald patch anywhere on the body
- Red-brown patches with erythematous borders and trailing scales
- Lesions that may be macular, vesicular, or urticarial
DX: Skin examination
TX: Symptomatic treatment, medication (antipyretics, antihistamines, topical or systemic corticosteroids), oatmeal baths
F/U: None unless the condition persists longer than 6 weeks

PSORIASIS
Signs and symptoms
- Initially small erythematous papules on the scalp, chest, elbows, knees, back, buttocks, and genitalia that may be pruritic and painful and eventually enlarge and coalesce, forming red, scaly plaques covered by silver scales
- Pitted fingernails
- Arthralgia
DX: PE, HLAs
TX: Medication (topical lubricants, dandruff or coal tar shampoo, corticosteroids, keratolytic agents, vitamin D analogs, topical retinoids)
F/U: Referral to dermatologist

TINEA VERSICOLOR
Signs and symptoms
- Macular, hyperpigmented, scaly patches of varying size and shapes
- Lesions that usually affect the upper trunk, arms, and lower abdomen
DX: Skin examination, potassium preparation of scales
TX: Tar preparation shampoo, topical antifungal
F/U: None unless treatment is ineffective

Additional differential diagnoses: Bowen's disease ▪ dermatophytosis ▪ discoid lupus erythematosus ▪ lichen planus ▪ lymphoma ▪ parapsoriasis (chronic) ▪ syphilis (secondary) ▪ SLE

Other causes: drugs, such as penicillins, sulfonamides, barbiturates, quinidine, diazepam, phenytoin, and isoniazid

Stools, clay-colored

Normally, bile pigments give the stool its characteristic brown color. However, hepatocellular degeneration or biliary obstruction may interfere with the formation or release of these pigments into the intestine, resulting in clay-colored stools. These stools are commonly associated with jaundice and dark urine. Pale, putty-colored stools usually result from hepatic, gallbladder, or pancreatic disorders.

History and physical examination

After documenting when the patient first noticed clay-colored stools, explore associated signs and symptoms, such as abdominal pain, nausea and vomiting, fatigue, anorexia, weight loss, and dark urine. Does the patient have trouble digesting fatty foods or heavy meals? Does he bruise easily?

Next, review the patient's medical history for gallbladder, hepatic, or pancreatic disorders. Has he ever had biliary surgery? Has he recently undergone barium studies? (Barium lightens stool color for several days.) Also, ask about antacid use because large amounts may lighten stool color. Note a history of alcoholism or exposure to other hepatotoxic substances.

After assessing the patient's general appearance, take his vital signs and check his skin and eyes for jaundice. Then examine the abdomen; inspect for distention and auscultate for hypoactive bowel sounds. Percuss and palpate for masses and rebound tenderness. Finally, obtain urine and stool specimens for laboratory analysis.

 PEDIATRIC POINTER

Clay-colored stools may occur in infants with biliary atresia.

 ELDER CARE CUE

Because elderly patients with cholelithiasis have a greater risk of developing complications if the condition isn't treated, surgery should be considered early on for treatment of persistent systems.

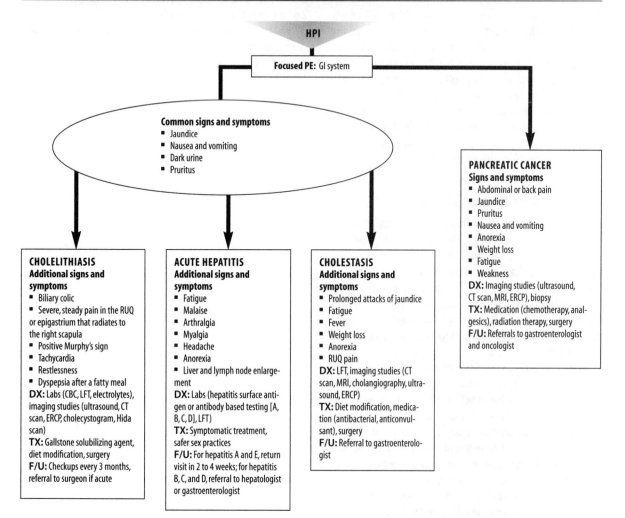

HPI

Focused PE: GI system

Common signs and symptoms
- Jaundice
- Nausea and vomiting
- Dark urine
- Pruritus

CHOLELITHIASIS
Additional signs and symptoms
- Biliary colic
- Severe, steady pain in the RUQ or epigastrium that radiates to the right scapula
- Positive Murphy's sign
- Tachycardia
- Restlessness
- Dyspepsia after a fatty meal

DX: Labs (CBC, LFT, electrolytes), imaging studies (ultrasound, CT scan, ERCP, cholecystogram, Hida scan)
TX: Gallstone solubilizing agent, diet modification, surgery
F/U: Checkups every 3 months, referral to surgeon if acute

ACUTE HEPATITIS
Additional signs and symptoms
- Fatigue
- Malaise
- Arthralgia
- Myalgia
- Headache
- Anorexia
- Liver and lymph node enlargement

DX: Labs (hepatitis surface antigen or antibody based testing [A, B, C, D], LFT)
TX: Symptomatic treatment, safer sex practices
F/U: For hepatitis A and E, return visit in 2 to 4 weeks; for hepatitis B, C, and D, referral to hepatologist or gastroenterologist

CHOLESTASIS
Additional signs and symptoms
- Prolonged attacks of jaundice
- Fatigue
- Fever
- Weight loss
- Anorexia
- RUQ pain

DX: LFT, imaging studies (CT scan, MRI, cholangiography, ultrasound, ERCP)
TX: Diet modification, medication (antibacterial, anticonvulsant), surgery
F/U: Referral to gastroenterologist

PANCREATIC CANCER
Signs and symptoms
- Abdominal or back pain
- Jaundice
- Pruritus
- Nausea and vomiting
- Anorexia
- Weight loss
- Fatigue
- Weakness

DX: Imaging studies (ultrasound, CT scan, MRI, ERCP), biopsy
TX: Medication (chemotherapy, analgesics), radiation therapy, surgery
F/U: Referrals to gastroenterologist and oncologist

Additional differential diagnoses: bile duct cancer ▪ biliary cirrhosis ▪ cholangitis (sclerosing) ▪ cholelithiasis ▪ hepatic cancer ▪ pancreatitis (acute)

Other cause: biliary surgery

Stridor

A loud, harsh, musical respiratory sound, stridor results from an obstruction in the trachea or larynx. Usually heard during inspiration, this sign may also occur during expiration in severe upper airway obstruction. It may begin as low-pitched "croaking" and progress to high-pitched "crowing" as respirations become more vigorous.

Life-threatening upper airway obstruction can stem from foreign-body aspiration, increased secretions, intraluminal tumor, localized edema or muscle spasms, and external compression by a tumor or aneurysm.

History and physical examination

If you hear stridor, quickly examine the patient for other signs of partial airway obstruction — choking or gagging, tachypnea, dyspnea, shallow respirations, intercostal retractions, nasal flaring, tachycardia, cyanosis, and diaphoresis. (Be aware that abrupt cessation of stridor signals complete obstruction in which the patient has inspiratory chest movement but absent breath sounds. Unable to talk, he quickly becomes lethargic and loses consciousness.) Emergency interventions may be necessary.

When the patient's condition permits, obtain a patient history from him or a family member. First, find out when the stridor began. Has he had it before? Does he have an upper respiratory infection? If so, how long has he had it?

Ask about a history of allergies, tumors, and respiratory and vascular disorders. Note recent exposure to smoke or noxious fumes or gases. Next, explore associated signs and symptoms. Does stridor occur with pain or a cough?

Then examine the patient's mouth for excessive secretions, foreign matter, inflammation, and swelling. Assess his neck for swelling, masses, subcutaneous crepitation, and scars. Observe the patient's chest for delayed, decreased, or asymmetrical chest expansion. Auscultate for wheezes, rhonchi, crackles, rubs, and other abnormal breath sounds. Percuss for dullness, tympany, or flatness. Finally, note any burns or signs of trauma, such as ecchymoses and lacerations.

PEDIATRIC POINTERS

■ *Stridor is a major sign of airway obstruction in children. When you hear this sign, you must intervene quickly to prevent total airway obstruction. This emergency can happen more rapidly in a child because his airway is narrower than an adult's.*

■ *Causes of stridor include foreign-body aspiration, croup syndrome, laryngeal diphtheria, pertussis, retropharyngeal abscess, and congenital abnormalities of the larynx.*

■ *Therapy for partial airway obstruction typically involves hot or cold steam in a mist tent or hood, parenteral fluids and electrolytes, and plenty of rest.*

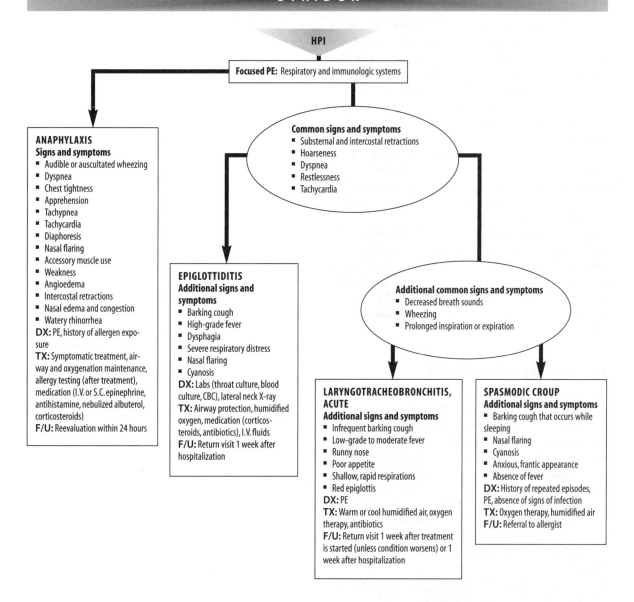

HPI

Focused PE: Respiratory and immunologic systems

ANAPHYLAXIS
Signs and symptoms
- Audible or auscultated wheezing
- Dyspnea
- Chest tightness
- Apprehension
- Tachypnea
- Tachycardia
- Diaphoresis
- Nasal flaring
- Accessory muscle use
- Weakness
- Angioedema
- Intercostal retractions
- Nasal edema and congestion
- Watery rhinorrhea

DX: PE, history of allergen exposure
TX: Symptomatic treatment, airway and oxygenation maintenance, allergy testing (after treatment), medication (I.V. or S.C. epinephrine, antihistamine, nebulized albuterol, corticosteroids)
F/U: Reevaluation within 24 hours

Common signs and symptoms
- Substernal and intercostal retractions
- Hoarseness
- Dyspnea
- Restlessness
- Tachycardia

EPIGLOTTIDITIS
Additional signs and symptoms
- Barking cough
- High-grade fever
- Dysphagia
- Severe respiratory distress
- Nasal flaring
- Cyanosis

DX: Labs (throat culture, blood culture, CBC), lateral neck X-ray
TX: Airway protection, humidified oxygen, medication (corticosteroids, antibiotics), I.V. fluids
F/U: Return visit 1 week after hospitalization

Additional common signs and symptoms
- Decreased breath sounds
- Wheezing
- Prolonged inspiration or expiration

LARYNGOTRACHEOBRONCHITIS, ACUTE
Additional signs and symptoms
- Infrequent barking cough
- Low-grade to moderate fever
- Runny nose
- Poor appetite
- Shallow, rapid respirations
- Red epiglottis

DX: PE
TX: Warm or cool humidified air, oxygen therapy, antibiotics
F/U: Return visit 1 week after treatment is started (unless condition worsens) or 1 week after hospitalization

SPASMODIC CROUP
Additional signs and symptoms
- Barking cough that occurs while sleeping
- Nasal flaring
- Cyanosis
- Anxious, frantic appearance
- Absence of fever

DX: History of repeated episodes, PE, absence of signs of infection
TX: Oxygen therapy, humidified air
F/U: Referral to allergist

Additional differential diagnoses: airway trauma ▪ hypocalcemia ▪ inhalation injury ▪ laryngeal tumor ▪ mediastinal tumor ▪ retrosternal thyroid ▪ thoracic aortic aneurysm

Other causes: bronchoscopy ▪ laryngoscopy ▪ prolonged intubation ▪ foreign body aspiration ▪ neck surgery

Syncope

A common neurologic sign, syncope (or fainting) refers to transient loss of consciousness associated with impaired cerebral blood supply. It usually occurs abruptly and lasts for seconds to minutes. Typically, the patient lies motionless with his skeletal muscles relaxed but sphincter muscles controlled. However, the depth of unconsciousness varies — some patients can hear voices or see blurred outlines; others are unaware of their surroundings.

In many ways, syncope simulates death: The patient is strikingly pale with a slow, weak pulse, hypotension, and almost imperceptible breathing. If severe hypotension lasts for 20 seconds or longer, the patient may also develop convulsive, tonic-clonic movements.

Syncope may result from cardiac and cerebrovascular disorders, hypoxemia, and postural changes in the presence of autonomic dysfunction. It may also follow vigorous coughing (tussive syncope) and emotional stress, injury, shock, or pain (vasovagal syncope, or common fainting). Hysterical syncope may also follow emotional stress but isn't accompanied by other vasodepressor effects.

History and physical examination

If you see a patient faint, ensure a patent airway and take vital signs. Be ready to begin cardiopulmonary resuscitation. If the patient reports a fainting episode, gather information about the episode from him and his family. Did he feel weak, lightheaded, nauseous, or sweaty just before he fainted? Did he get up quickly from a chair or from lying down? During the fainting episode, did he have muscle spasms or incontinence? How long was he unconscious? When he regained consciousness, was he alert or confused? Did he have a headache? Has he fainted before? If so, how often does it occur?

Examine him for any injuries that may have occurred during his fall.

PEDIATRIC POINTER

Syncope is much less common in children than in adults. It may result from cardiac or neurologic disorders, allergy, or emotional stress.

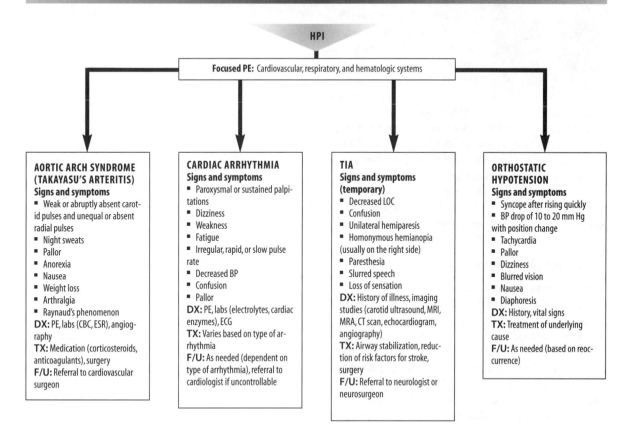

HPI

Focused PE: Cardiovascular, respiratory, and hematologic systems

AORTIC ARCH SYNDROME (TAKAYASU'S ARTERITIS)
Signs and symptoms
- Weak or abruptly absent carotid pulses and unequal or absent radial pulses
- Night sweats
- Pallor
- Anorexia
- Nausea
- Weight loss
- Arthralgia
- Raynaud's phenomenon
DX: PE, labs (CBC, ESR), angiography
TX: Medication (corticosteroids, anticoagulants), surgery
F/U: Referral to cardiovascular surgeon

CARDIAC ARRHYTHMIA
Signs and symptoms
- Paroxysmal or sustained palpitations
- Dizziness
- Weakness
- Fatigue
- Irregular, rapid, or slow pulse rate
- Decreased BP
- Confusion
- Pallor
DX: PE, labs (electrolytes, cardiac enzymes), ECG
TX: Varies based on type of arrhythmia
F/U: As needed (dependent on type of arrhythmia), referral to cardiologist if uncontrollable

TIA
Signs and symptoms (temporary)
- Decreased LOC
- Confusion
- Unilateral hemiparesis
- Homonymous hemianopia (usually on the right side)
- Paresthesia
- Slurred speech
- Loss of sensation
DX: History of illness, imaging studies (carotid ultrasound, MRI, MRA, CT scan, echocardiogram, angiography)
TX: Airway stabilization, reduction of risk factors for stroke, surgery
F/U: Referral to neurologist or neurosurgeon

ORTHOSTATIC HYPOTENSION
Signs and symptoms
- Syncope after rising quickly
- BP drop of 10 to 20 mm Hg with position change
- Tachycardia
- Pallor
- Dizziness
- Blurred vision
- Nausea
- Diaphoresis
DX: History, vital signs
TX: Treatment of underlying cause
F/U: As needed (based on reoccurrence)

Additional differential diagnoses: aortic stenosis ▪ carotid sinus hypersensitivity ▪ hypoxemia ▪ vagal glossopharyngeal neuralgia

Other causes: drugs, such as quinidine, prazosin, griseofulvin, levodopa, and indomethacin

Tachycardia

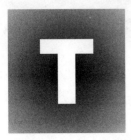

Easily detected by counting the apical, carotid, or radial pulse, tachycardia is a heart rate greater than 100 beats/minute. The patient with tachycardia usually complains of palpitations or of a "racing" heart. This common sign normally occurs in response to emotional or physical stress, such as excitement, exercise, pain, and fever. It may also result from the use of stimulants, such as caffeine and tobacco. However, tachycardia may be an early sign of a life-threatening disorder, such as cardiogenic, hypovolemic, or septic shock. It may also result from cardiovascular, respiratory, and metabolic disorders and from the effects of certain drugs, tests, and treatments.

History and physical examination

After detecting tachycardia, first perform electrocardiography to examine for reduced cardiac output, which may initiate or result from tachycardia. Take the patient's other vital signs and determine his level of consciousness. If the patient's condition permits, take a focused history. Find out if he has had palpitations before. If so, how were they treated? Explore associated symptoms. Is the patient dizzy or short of breath? Weak or fatigued? Is he experiencing chest pain? Next, ask about a history of trauma, diabetes, or cardiac, pulmonary, or thyroid disorders. Also, obtain a drug history.

Inspect the patient's skin for pallor or cyanosis. Assess pulses, noting peripheral edema. Finally, auscultate the heart and lungs for abnormal sounds or rhythms.

PEDIATRIC POINTERS

- *When examining a child for tachycardia, recognize that normal heart rates for children are higher than those for adults.*
- *In children, tachycardia may result from many of the adult causes described above.*

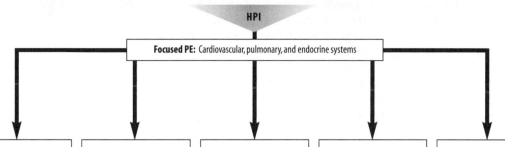

TACHYCARDIA

HPI

Focused PE: Cardiovascular, pulmonary, and endocrine systems

CARDIAC ARRHYTHMIA
Signs and symptoms
- Bradycardia
- Palpitations
- Hypotension
- Dizziness
- Weakness
- Fatigue

DX: PE, ECG, electrophysiology study, labs (serum chemistry, digoxin level, cardiac enzymes, troponin)
TX: Varies based on the type of arrhythmia and the underlying cause, antiarrhythmic if needed
F/U: Referral to cardiologist if treatment is ineffective

ANXIETY
Signs and symptoms
- Intermittent, sharp, stabbing pain behind the breast bone
- Precordial tenderness
- Palpitations
- Fatigue
- Headache
- Insomnia
- Nausea and vomiting
- Breathlessness
- Tachypnea
- Diarrhea
- Tremors

DX: Labs (CBC, UA, thyroid studies), psychological testing
TX: Medication (based on the type of anxiety disorder; benzodiazepines, SSRIs, azapirones, TCAs), psychological counseling, exercise program
F/U: Regular office visits, referral to psychologist

HHNS
Signs and symptoms
- Rapidly deteriorating LOC
- Hypotension
- Seizure disorder
- Oliguria
- Dehydration

DX: Labs (serum electrolytes, ABG)
TX: I.V. normal saline solution infusion, I.V. insulin, frequent blood glucose monitoring
F/U: Referral to endocrinologist

THYROTOXICOSIS
Signs and symptoms
- Ptosis
- Progressive exophthalmus
- Increased tearing
- Visual changes
- Lid edema
- Lid lag
- Photophobia
- Enlarged thyroid
- Nervousness
- Heat intolerance
- Weight loss
- Tremors
- Palpitation
- Dyspnea

DX: PE, thyroid function studies, thyroid scan
TX: Medication (antithyroid therapy, radioiodine, beta-adrenergic blockers)
F/U: Thyroid function testing 6 weeks after treatment is initiated, then biannually if at euthyroid state

ANEMIA
Signs and symptoms
- Fatigue
- Pallor
- Dyspnea
- Postural hypotension
- Atrial gallop

DX: PE, CBC
TX: Treatment of underlying cause, medication (iron supplements, PRBC if indicated), diet modification
F/U: Regular checkups

Additional differential diagnoses: adrenocortical insufficiency ▪ ARDS ▪ alcohol withdrawal syndrome ▪ anaphylactic shock ▪ aortic insufficiency ▪ aortic stenosis ▪ cardiac contusion ▪ cardiac tamponade ▪ cardiogenic shock ▪ COPD ▪ diabetic ketoacidosis ▪ febrile illness ▪ heart failure ▪ hypertensive crisis ▪ hypoglycemia ▪ hyponatremia ▪ hypovolemia ▪ hypovolemic shock ▪ hypoxemia ▪ MI ▪ myocardial ischemia ▪ neurogenic shock ▪ orthostatic hypotension ▪ pheochromocytoma ▪ pneumothorax ▪ pulmonary edema ▪ pulmonary embolism ▪ septic shock

Other causes: cardiac catheterization ▪ electrophysiologic studies ▪ drugs (sympathomimetics, phenothiazines, anticholinergics, thyroid drugs, vasodilators, acetylcholinesterase inhibitors, nitrates, alpha-adrenergic blockers) ▪ alcohol ▪ excessive caffeine intake ▪ cardiac surgery ▪ pacemaker malfunction

Tachypnea

A common sign of cardiopulmonary disorders, tachypnea is an abnormally fast respiratory rate — 20 breaths/minute or more. Tachypnea may reflect the need to increase minute volume — the amount of air breathed each minute. Under these circumstances, it may be accompanied by an increase in tidal volume — the volume of air inhaled or exhaled per breath — resulting in hyperventilation. Tachypnea, however, may also reflect stiff lungs or overloaded ventilatory muscles, in which case tidal volume may actually be reduced.

Tachypnea may result from reduced arterial oxygen tension or arterial oxygen content, decreased perfusion, or increased oxygen demand. Heightened oxygen demand, for example, may result from fever, exertion, anxiety, and pain. It may also occur as a compensatory response to metabolic acidosis or may result from pulmonary irritation, stretch receptor stimulation, or neurologic disorders that upset medullary respiratory control. Generally, respirations increase by 4 breaths/minute for every 1° F (0.6° C) increase in body temperature.

History and physical examination

After detecting tachypnea, quickly evaluate cardiopulmonary status; check for cyanosis, chest pain, dyspnea, tachycardia, and hypotension.

If the patient's condition permits, obtain a medical history. Find out when the tachypnea began. Did it follow activity? Has he had it before? Then have him describe associated signs and symptoms, such as diaphoresis and recent weight loss. Is he anxious about anything or does he have a history of anxiety attacks? Note whether he's taking any analgesics. If so, how effective are they?

Begin the physical examination by taking the patient's other vital signs, if you haven't already done so, and observing his overall behavior. Does he seem restless? Then auscultate the chest for abnormal heart and breath sounds. If the patient has a productive cough, record the color, amount, and consistency of sputum. Finally, check for jugular vein distention and examine the skin for pallor, cyanosis, edema, and warmth or coolness.

PEDIATRIC POINTERS

When assessing a child for tachypnea, be aware that the normal respiratory rate varies with the child's age. If you detect tachypnea, first rule out the causes listed above. Then consider these pediatric causes: congenital heart defects, meningitis, metabolic

acidosis, and cystic fibrosis. Keep in mind, though, that hunger and anxiety may also cause tachypnea.

ELDER CARE CUE

Tachypnea may have a variety of causes in elderly patients, and mild increases in respiratory rate may go unnoticed.

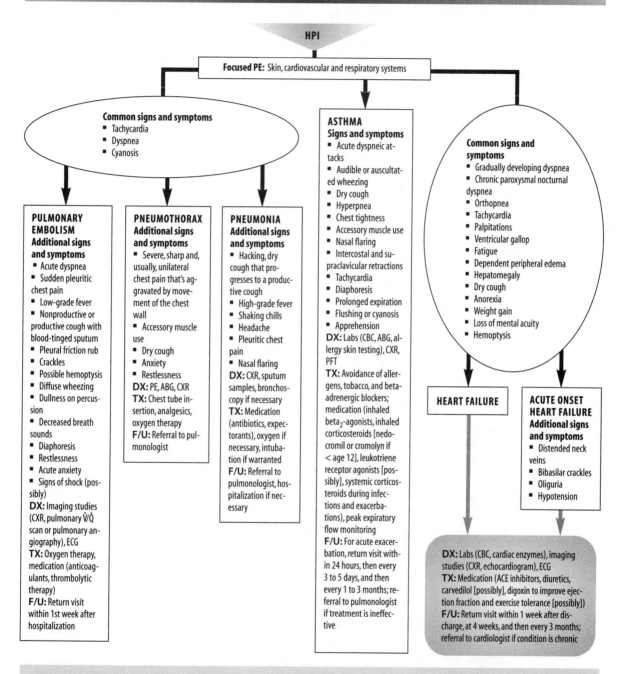

HPI

Focused PE: Skin, cardiovascular and respiratory systems

Common signs and symptoms
- Tachycardia
- Dyspnea
- Cyanosis

PULMONARY EMBOLISM
Additional signs and symptoms
- Acute dyspnea
- Sudden pleuritic chest pain
- Low-grade fever
- Nonproductive or productive cough with blood-tinged sputum
- Pleural friction rub
- Crackles
- Possible hemoptysis
- Diffuse wheezing
- Dullness on percussion
- Decreased breath sounds
- Diaphoresis
- Restlessness
- Acute anxiety
- Signs of shock (possibly)

DX: Imaging studies (CXR, pulmonary $\dot{V}/\dot{Q}$ scan or pulmonary angiography), ECG
TX: Oxygen therapy, medication (anticoagulants, thrombolytic therapy)
F/U: Return visit within 1st week after hospitalization

PNEUMOTHORAX
Additional signs and symptoms
- Severe, sharp and, usually, unilateral chest pain that's aggravated by movement of the chest wall
- Accessory muscle use
- Dry cough
- Anxiety
- Restlessness

DX: PE, ABG, CXR
TX: Chest tube insertion, analgesics, oxygen therapy
F/U: Referral to pulmonologist

PNEUMONIA
Additional signs and symptoms
- Hacking, dry cough that progresses to a productive cough
- High-grade fever
- Shaking chills
- Headache
- Pleuritic chest pain
- Nasal flaring

DX: CXR, sputum samples, bronchoscopy if necessary
TX: Medication (antibiotics, expectorants), oxygen if necessary, intubation if warranted
F/U: Referral to pulmonologist, hospitalization if necessary

ASTHMA
Signs and symptoms
- Acute dyspneic attacks
- Audible or auscultated wheezing
- Dry cough
- Hyperpnea
- Chest tightness
- Accessory muscle use
- Nasal flaring
- Intercostal and supraclavicular retractions
- Tachycardia
- Diaphoresis
- Prolonged expiration
- Flushing or cyanosis
- Apprehension

DX: Labs (CBC, ABG, allergy skin testing), CXR, PFT
TX: Avoidance of allergens, tobacco, and beta-adrenergic blockers; medication (inhaled beta$_2$-agonists, inhaled corticosteroids [nedocromil or cromolyn if < age 12], leukotriene receptor agonists [possibly], systemic corticosteroids during infections and exacerbations), peak expiratory flow monitoring
F/U: For acute exacerbation, return visit within 24 hours, then every 3 to 5 days, and then every 1 to 3 months; referral to pulmonologist if treatment is ineffective

Common signs and symptoms
- Gradually developing dyspnea
- Chronic paroxysmal nocturnal dyspnea
- Orthopnea
- Tachycardia
- Palpitations
- Ventricular gallop
- Fatigue
- Dependent peripheral edema
- Hepatomegaly
- Dry cough
- Anorexia
- Weight gain
- Loss of mental acuity
- Hemoptysis

HEART FAILURE

ACUTE ONSET HEART FAILURE
Additional signs and symptoms
- Distended neck veins
- Bibasilar crackles
- Oliguria
- Hypotension

DX: Labs (CBC, cardiac enzymes), imaging studies (CXR, echocardiogram), ECG
TX: Medication (ACE inhibitors, diuretics, carvedilol [possibly], digoxin to improve ejection fraction and exercise tolerance [possibly])
F/U: Return visit within 1 week after discharge, at 4 weeks, and then every 3 months; referral to cardiologist if condition is chronic

Additional differential diagnoses: abdominal pain ▪ anaphylactic shock ▪ anemia ▪ ARDS ▪ ascites ▪ bronchiectasis ▪ bronchitis (chronic) ▪ cardiac arrhythmias ▪ cardiac tamponade ▪ cardiogenic shock ▪ chest trauma ▪ COPD ▪ emphysema ▪ febrile illness ▪ flail chest ▪ foreign body aspiration ▪ head trauma ▪ hepatic failure ▪ HHNS ▪ hypovolemic shock ▪ hypoxia ▪ interstitial fibrosis ▪ lung abscess ▪ lung, pleural, or mediastinal tumor ▪ mesothelioma (malignant) ▪ neurogenic shock ▪ pancreatitis ▪ pleural effusion ▪ pulmonary edema ▪ pulmonary hypertension ▪ septic shock

Other cause: salicylates

Throat pain

Throat pain — commonly known as a sore throat — refers to discomfort in any part of the pharynx: the nasopharynx, the oropharynx, or the hypopharynx. This common symptom ranges from a sensation of scratchiness to severe pain. It's often accompanied by ear pain because cranial nerves IX and X innervate the pharynx as well as the middle and external ear.

Throat pain may result from infection, trauma, allergy, cancer, and certain systemic disorders. It may also follow surgery and endotracheal intubation. Nonpathologic causes include dry mucous membranes associated with mouth breathing and laryngeal irritation associated with alcohol consumption, inhaling smoke or chemicals such as ammonia, and vocal strain.

History and physical examination

Ask the patient when he first noticed the pain and have him describe it. Has he had throat pain before? Is it accompanied by fever, ear pain, or dysphagia? Review the patient's medical history for throat problems, allergies, and systemic disorders.

Next, carefully examine the pharynx, noting redness, exudate, or swelling. Examine the oropharynx, using a warmed metal spatula or tongue blade, and the nasopharynx, using a warmed laryngeal mirror or a fiber-optic nasopharyngoscope. Laryngoscopic examination of the hypopharynx may be required. (If necessary, spray the soft palate and pharyngeal wall with a local anesthetic to prevent gagging.)

Observe the tonsils for redness, swelling, or exudate. In addition, obtain an exudate specimen for culture. Then examine the nose, using a nasal speculum. Also, check the patient's ears, especially if he reports ear pain. Finally, palpate the patient's neck and oropharynx for nodules or lymph node enlargement.

PEDIATRIC POINTERS

- *Sore throat is a common complaint in children and may result from many of the same disorders that affect adults.*
- *Other pediatric causes of sore throat include acute epiglottitis, herpangina, scarlet fever, acute follicular tonsillitis, and retropharyngeal abscess.*

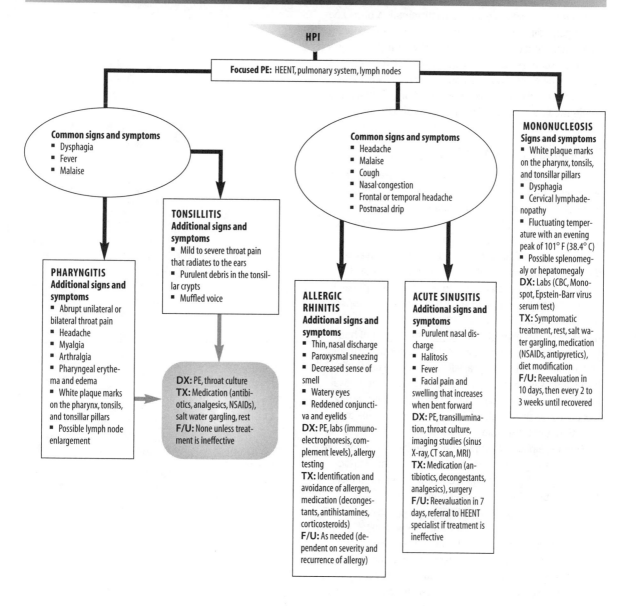

HPI

Focused PE: HEENT, pulmonary system, lymph nodes

Common signs and symptoms
- Dysphagia
- Fever
- Malaise

TONSILLITIS
Additional signs and symptoms
- Mild to severe throat pain that radiates to the ears
- Purulent debris in the tonsillar crypts
- Muffled voice

PHARYNGITIS
Additional signs and symptoms
- Abrupt unilateral or bilateral throat pain
- Headache
- Myalgia
- Arthralgia
- Pharyngeal erythema and edema
- White plaque marks on the pharynx, tonsils, and tonsillar pillars
- Possible lymph node enlargement

DX: PE, throat culture
TX: Medication (antibiotics, analgesics, NSAIDs), salt water gargling, rest
F/U: None unless treatment is ineffective

Common signs and symptoms
- Headache
- Malaise
- Cough
- Nasal congestion
- Frontal or temporal headache
- Postnasal drip

ALLERGIC RHINITIS
Additional signs and symptoms
- Thin, nasal discharge
- Paroxysmal sneezing
- Decreased sense of smell
- Watery eyes
- Reddened conjunctiva and eyelids

DX: PE, labs (immunoelectrophoresis, complement levels), allergy testing
TX: Identification and avoidance of allergen, medication (decongestants, antihistamines, corticosteroids)
F/U: As needed (dependent on severity and recurrence of allergy)

ACUTE SINUSITIS
Additional signs and symptoms
- Purulent nasal discharge
- Halitosis
- Fever
- Facial pain and swelling that increases when bent forward

DX: PE, transillumination, throat culture, imaging studies (sinus X-ray, CT scan, MRI)
TX: Medication (antibiotics, decongestants, analgesics), surgery
F/U: Reevaluation in 7 days, referral to HEENT specialist if treatment is ineffective

MONONUCLEOSIS
Signs and symptoms
- White plaque marks on the pharynx, tonsils, and tonsillar pillars
- Dysphagia
- Cervical lymphadenopathy
- Fluctuating temperature with an evening peak of 101° F (38.4° C)
- Possible splenomegaly or hepatomegaly
DX: Labs (CBC, Monospot, Epstein-Barr virus serum test)
TX: Symptomatic treatment, rest, salt water gargling, medication (NSAIDs, antipyretics), diet modification
F/U: Reevaluation in 10 days, then every 2 to 3 weeks until recovered

Additional differential diagnoses: agranulocytosis ▪ bronchitis (acute) ▪ chronic fatigue syndrome ▪ contact ulcers ▪ eagle's syndrome ▪ foreign body ▪ glossopharyngeal neuralgia ▪ herpes simplex virus ▪ influenza ▪ laryngeal cancer ▪ laryngitis (acute) ▪ necrotizing ulcerative gingivitis (acute) ▪ peritonsillar abscess ▪ pharyngomaxillary space abscess ▪ reflux laryngopharyngitis ▪ tongue cancer ▪ tonsillar cancer ▪ uvulitis ▪ viral infection

Other causes: endotracheal intubation ▪ local surgery (tonsillectomy, adenoidectomy)

Thyroid enlargement

An enlarged thyroid can result from inflammation, physiologic changes, iodine deficiency, and thyroid tumors. Depending on the medical cause, hyperfunction or hypofunction may occur with resulting excess or deficiency, respectively, of the hormone thyroxine. If no infection is present, enlargement is usually slow and progressive. An enlarged thyroid that causes visible swelling in the front of the neck is called a goiter.

History and physical examination

The patient's history commonly reveals the cause of thyroid enlargement. Important data include a family history of thyroid disease, when the thyroid enlargement began, any previous irradiation of the thyroid or the neck, recent infections, and the use of thyroid replacement drugs.

Begin the physical examination by inspecting the patient's trachea for midline deviation. Although you can frequently see an enlarged gland, you should always palpate it. To palpate the thyroid gland, you'll need to stand in front of or behind the patient. Give the patient a cup of water, and have him extend his neck slightly. Place the fingers of both hands on the patient's neck, just below the cricoid cartilage and just lateral to the trachea. Tell the patient to take a sip of water and swallow. The thyroid gland should rise as he swallows. Use your fingers to palpate laterally and downward to feel the whole thyroid gland. Palpate over the midline to feel the isthmus of the thyroid.

During palpation, be sure to note the size, shape, and consistency of the gland, and the presence or absence of nodules. Using the bell of a stethoscope, listen over the lateral lobes for a bruit. The bruit is often continuous.

PEDIATRIC POINTER

Congenital goiter, a syndrome of infantile myxedema or cretinism, is characterized by mental retardation, growth failure, and other signs and symptoms of hypothyroidism. Early treatment can prevent mental retardation. Genetic counseling is important, as subsequent children are at risk.

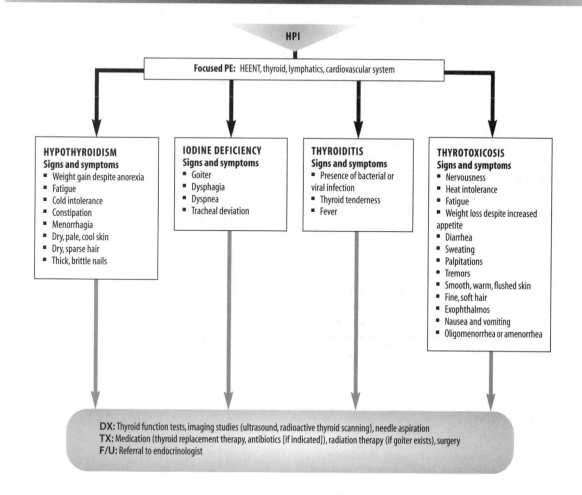

HPI

Focused PE: HEENT, thyroid, lymphatics, cardiovascular system

HYPOTHYROIDISM
Signs and symptoms
- Weight gain despite anorexia
- Fatigue
- Cold intolerance
- Constipation
- Menorrhagia
- Dry, pale, cool skin
- Dry, sparse hair
- Thick, brittle nails

IODINE DEFICIENCY
Signs and symptoms
- Goiter
- Dysphagia
- Dyspnea
- Tracheal deviation

THYROIDITIS
Signs and symptoms
- Presence of bacterial or viral infection
- Thyroid tenderness
- Fever

THYROTOXICOSIS
Signs and symptoms
- Nervousness
- Heat intolerance
- Fatigue
- Weight loss despite increased appetite
- Diarrhea
- Sweating
- Palpitations
- Tremors
- Smooth, warm, flushed skin
- Fine, soft hair
- Exophthalmos
- Nausea and vomiting
- Oligomenorrhea or amenorrhea

DX: Thyroid function tests, imaging studies (ultrasound, radioactive thyroid scanning), needle aspiration
TX: Medication (thyroid replacement therapy, antibiotics [if indicated]), radiation therapy (if goiter exists), surgery
F/U: Referral to endocrinologist

Additional differential diagnosis: tumor

Other causes: drugs (lithium, sulfonamides, phenylbutazone, para-aminosalicylic acid) ▪ foods containing goitrogens (peanuts, cabbage, soybeans, strawberries, spinach, rutabagas, radishes)

Tinnitus

Tinnitus literally means ringing in the ears, although many other abnormal sounds fall under this term. For example, tinnitus may be described as the sound of escaping air, running water, or the inside of a seashell or as a sizzling, buzzing, or humming noise. Occasionally, it's described as a roaring or musical sound. This common symptom may be unilateral or bilateral and constant or intermittent. Although the brain can adjust to or suppress constant tinnitus, intermittent tinnitus may be so disturbing that some patients contemplate suicide as their only source of relief.

Tinnitus can be classified in several ways. Subjective tinnitus is heard only by the patient; objective tinnitus is also heard by the observer who places a stethoscope near the patient's affected ear. Tinnitus aurium refers to noise that the patient hears in his ears; tinnitus cerebri, to noise that he hears in his head.

Tinnitus is usually associated with neural injury within the auditory pathway, resulting in altered, spontaneous firing of sensory auditory neurons. Commonly resulting from ear disorders, tinnitus may also stem from cardiovascular and systemic disorders and from the effects of drugs. Nonpathologic causes of tinnitus include acute anxiety and presbycusis. (See *Common causes of tinnitus*.)

History and physical examination

Ask the patient to describe the sound he hears, including its onset, pattern, pitch, location, and intensity. Ask whether it's accompanied by other symptoms, such as vertigo, headache, or hearing loss. Next, take a health history, including a complete drug history.

Using an otoscope, inspect the patient's ears and examine the tympanic membrane. To check for hearing loss, perform the Weber's and Rinne tests. Also, auscultate for bruits in the neck. Then compress the jugular or carotid artery to see if this affects the tinnitus. Finally, examine the nasopharynx for masses that might cause eustachian tube dysfunction and tinnitus.

An expectant mother's use of ototoxic drugs during the third trimester of pregnancy can cause labyrinthine damage in the fetus, resulting in tinnitus.

Common causes of tinnitus

Tinnitus usually results from disorders that affect the external, middle, or inner ear. Below are some of its more common causes and their locations.

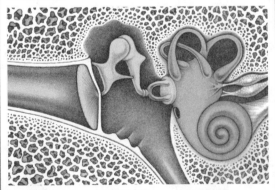

EXTERNAL EAR
- Ear canal obstruction by cerumen or a foreign body
- Otitis externa
- Tympanic membrane perforation

MIDDLE EAR
- Ossicle dislocation
- Otitis media
- Otosclerosis

INNER EAR
- Acoustic neuroma
- Atherosclerosis of the carotid artery
- Labyrinthitis
- Ménière's disease

TINNITUS

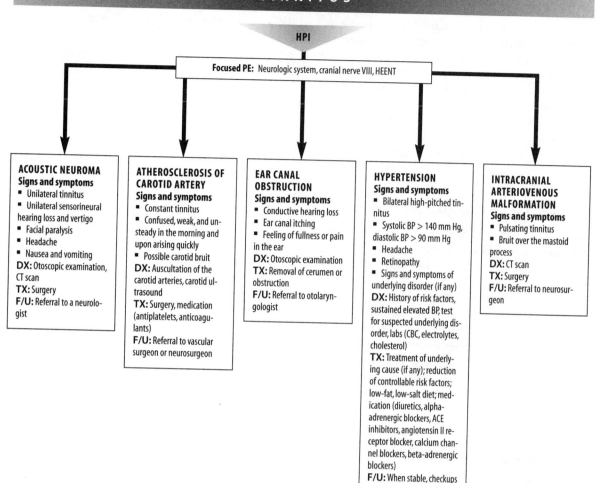

HPI

Focused PE: Neurologic system, cranial nerve VIII, HEENT

ACOUSTIC NEUROMA
Signs and symptoms
- Unilateral tinnitus
- Unilateral sensorineural hearing loss and vertigo
- Facial paralysis
- Headache
- Nausea and vomiting

DX: Otoscopic examination, CT scan
TX: Surgery
F/U: Referral to a neurologist

ATHEROSCLEROSIS OF CAROTID ARTERY
Signs and symptoms
- Constant tinnitus
- Confused, weak, and unsteady in the morning and upon arising quickly
- Possible carotid bruit

DX: Auscultation of the carotid arteries, carotid ultrasound
TX: Surgery, medication (antiplatelets, anticoagulants)
F/U: Referral to vascular surgeon or neurosurgeon

EAR CANAL OBSTRUCTION
Signs and symptoms
- Conductive hearing loss
- Ear canal itching
- Feeling of fullness or pain in the ear

DX: Otoscopic examination
TX: Removal of cerumen or obstruction
F/U: Referral to otolaryngologist

HYPERTENSION
Signs and symptoms
- Bilateral high-pitched tinnitus
- Systolic BP > 140 mm Hg, diastolic BP > 90 mm Hg
- Headache
- Retinopathy
- Signs and symptoms of underlying disorder (if any)

DX: History of risk factors, sustained elevated BP, test for suspected underlying disorder, labs (CBC, electrolytes, cholesterol)
TX: Treatment of underlying cause (if any); reduction of controllable risk factors; low-fat, low-salt diet; medication (diuretics, alpha-adrenergic blockers, ACE inhibitors, angiotensin II receptor blocker, calcium channel blockers, beta-adrenergic blockers)
F/U: When stable, checkups every 3 to 6 months

INTRACRANIAL ARTERIOVENOUS MALFORMATION
Signs and symptoms
- Pulsating tinnitus
- Bruit over the mastoid process

DX: CT scan
TX: Surgery
F/U: Referral to neurosurgeon

Additional differential diagnoses: anemia ▪ cervical spondylosis ▪ glomus jugulare or tympanicum tumor ▪ labyrinthitis ▪ Ménière's disease ▪ ossicle dislocation ▪ otitis externa ▪ otitis media ▪ otosclerosis ▪ palatal myoclonus ▪ tympanic membrane perforation

---

Other causes: drugs ▪ alcohol ▪ loud noise

Tracheal deviation

Normally, the trachea is located at the midline of the neck — except at the bifurcation, where it shifts slightly toward the right. Visible deviation from its normal position signals an underlying condition that can compromise pulmonary function and possibly cause respiratory distress. A hallmark of life-threatening tension pneumothorax, tracheal deviation occurs in disorders that produce mediastinal shift due to asymmetrical thoracic volume or pressure. A nonlesional pneumothorax can produce tracheal deviation to the ipsilateral side. (See *Detecting slight tracheal deviation*.)

History and physical examination

Be alert for signs of respiratory distress (tachypnea, dyspnea, decreased or absent breath sounds, stridor, nasal flaring, accessory muscle use, asymmetrical chest expansion, restlessness, and anxiety). If possible, place the patient in semi-Fowler's position to aid respiratory excursion and improve oxygenation. Palpate for subcutaneous crepitation in the neck and chest, a sign of tension pneumothorax. If the patient doesn't display signs of distress, ask about a history of pulmonary or cardiac disorders, trauma, or infection. If he smokes, determine how much. Ask about associated symptoms, especially breathing difficulty, pain, and cough.

Detecting slight tracheal deviation

Although gross tracheal deviation is visible, detection of slight deviation requires palpation and perhaps even an X-ray. Try palpation first.

With the tip of your index finger, locate the patient's trachea by palpating between the sternocleidomastoid muscles. Then compare the trachea's position with an imaginary line drawn vertically through the suprasternal notch. Any deviation from midline is usually considered abnormal.

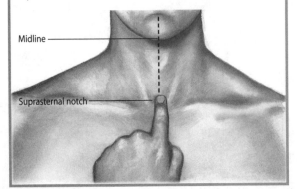

Midline

Suprasternal notch

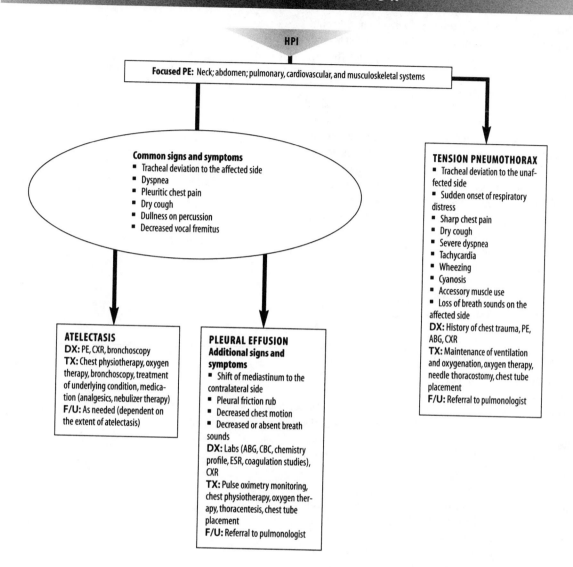

HPI

Focused PE: Neck; abdomen; pulmonary, cardiovascular, and musculoskeletal systems

Common signs and symptoms
- Tracheal deviation to the affected side
- Dyspnea
- Pleuritic chest pain
- Dry cough
- Dullness on percussion
- Decreased vocal fremitus

TENSION PNEUMOTHORAX
- Tracheal deviation to the unaffected side
- Sudden onset of respiratory distress
- Sharp chest pain
- Dry cough
- Severe dyspnea
- Tachycardia
- Wheezing
- Cyanosis
- Accessory muscle use
- Loss of breath sounds on the affected side

DX: History of chest trauma, PE, ABG, CXR

TX: Maintenance of ventilation and oxygenation, oxygen therapy, needle thoracostomy, chest tube placement

F/U: Referral to pulmonologist

ATELECTASIS

DX: PE, CXR, bronchoscopy

TX: Chest physiotherapy, oxygen therapy, bronchoscopy, treatment of underlying condition, medication (analgesics, nebulizer therapy)

F/U: As needed (dependent on the extent of atelectasis)

PLEURAL EFFUSION

Additional signs and symptoms
- Shift of mediastinum to the contralateral side
- Pleural friction rub
- Decreased chest motion
- Decreased or absent breath sounds

DX: Labs (ABG, CBC, chemistry profile, ESR, coagulation studies), CXR

TX: Pulse oximetry monitoring, chest physiotherapy, oxygen therapy, thoracentesis, chest tube placement

F/U: Referral to pulmonologist

Additional differential diagnoses: hiatal hernia ▪ kyphoscoliosis ▪ mediastinal tumor ▪ pulmonary fibrosis ▪ retrosternal thyroid ▪ thoracic aortic aneurysm

Tremors

The most common type of involuntary muscle movement, tremors are regular rhythmic oscillations that result from alternating contractions of opposing muscle groups. They're typical signs of extrapyramidal or cerebellar disorders and can also result from certain drugs.

Tremors can be characterized by their location, amplitude, and frequency. They're classified as resting, intention, or postural. *Resting tremors* occur when an extremity is at rest and subside with movement. They include the classic pill-rolling tremor of Parkinson's disease. Conversely, *intention tremors* occur only with movement and subside with rest. *Postural (or action) tremors* appear when an extremity or the trunk is actively held in a particular posture or position. A common type of postural tremor is called an *essential tremor*.

Tremorlike movements may also be elicited, such as asterixis — the characteristic flapping tremor seen in hepatic failure.

Stress or emotional upset tends to aggravate a tremor. Alcohol commonly diminishes postural tremors.

History and physical examination

Begin the patient history by asking the patient about the tremor's onset (sudden or gradual) and about its duration, progression, and any aggravating or alleviating factors. Does the tremor interfere with the patient's normal activities? Does he have other symptoms? Has he noticed any behavioral changes or memory loss (the patient's family or friends may provide more accurate information on this)?

Explore the patient's personal and family medical history for neurologic (especially seizures), endocrine, or metabolic disorders. Obtain a complete drug history, noting especially the use of phenothiazines. Also, ask about alcohol use.

Assess the patient's overall appearance and demeanor, noting mental status. Test range of motion and strength in all major muscle groups while observing for chorea, athetosis, dystonia, and other involuntary movements. Check deep tendon reflexes, and, if possible, observe the patient's gait.

PEDIATRIC POINTERS

- *A normal neonate may display coarse tremors with stiffening — an exaggerated hypocalcemic startle reflex — in response to noises and chills.*
- *Pediatric-specific causes of pathologic tremors include cerebral palsy, fetal alcohol syndrome, and maternal drug addiction.*

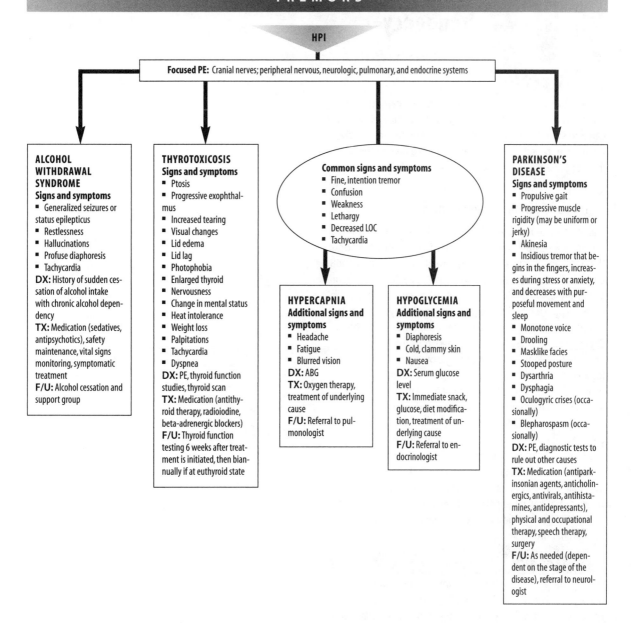

HPI

Focused PE: Cranial nerves; peripheral nervous, neurologic, pulmonary, and endocrine systems

ALCOHOL WITHDRAWAL SYNDROME
Signs and symptoms
- Generalized seizures or status epilepticus
- Restlessness
- Hallucinations
- Profuse diaphoresis
- Tachycardia

DX: History of sudden cessation of alcohol intake with chronic alcohol dependency
TX: Medication (sedatives, antipsychotics), safety maintenance, vital signs monitoring, symptomatic treatment
F/U: Alcohol cessation and support group

THYROTOXICOSIS
Signs and symptoms
- Ptosis
- Progressive exophthalmus
- Increased tearing
- Visual changes
- Lid edema
- Lid lag
- Photophobia
- Enlarged thyroid
- Nervousness
- Change in mental status
- Heat intolerance
- Weight loss
- Palpitations
- Tachycardia
- Dyspnea

DX: PE, thyroid function studies, thyroid scan
TX: Medication (antithyroid therapy, radioiodine, beta-adrenergic blockers)
F/U: Thyroid function testing 6 weeks after treatment is initiated, then biannually if at euthyroid state

Common signs and symptoms
- Fine, intention tremor
- Confusion
- Weakness
- Lethargy
- Decreased LOC
- Tachycardia

HYPERCAPNIA
Additional signs and symptoms
- Headache
- Fatigue
- Blurred vision

DX: ABG
TX: Oxygen therapy, treatment of underlying cause
F/U: Referral to pulmonologist

HYPOGLYCEMIA
Additional signs and symptoms
- Diaphoresis
- Cold, clammy skin
- Nausea

DX: Serum glucose level
TX: Immediate snack, glucose, diet modification, treatment of underlying cause
F/U: Referral to endocrinologist

PARKINSON'S DISEASE
Signs and symptoms
- Propulsive gait
- Progressive muscle rigidity (may be uniform or jerky)
- Akinesia
- Insidious tremor that begins in the fingers, increases during stress or anxiety, and decreases with purposeful movement and sleep
- Monotone voice
- Drooling
- Masklike facies
- Stooped posture
- Dysarthria
- Dysphagia
- Oculogyric crises (occasionally)
- Blepharospasm (occasionally)

DX: PE, diagnostic tests to rule out other causes
TX: Medication (antiparkinsonian agents, anticholinergics, antivirals, antihistamines, antidepressants), physical and occupational therapy, speech therapy, surgery
F/U: As needed (dependent on the stage of the disease), referral to neurologist

Additional differential diagnoses: alkalosis ▪ benign familial essential tumor ▪ cerebellar tumor ▪ general paresis ▪ kwashiorkor ▪ manganese toxicity ▪ multiple sclerosis ▪ porphyria ▪ thalamic syndrome ▪ Wernicke's disease ▪ West Nile encephalitis ▪ Wilson's disease

Other causes: herbal products (ephedra)

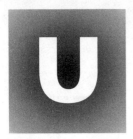

Urinary frequency

Urinary frequency refers to increased incidence of the urge to void. Usually resulting from decreased bladder capacity, frequency is a cardinal sign of urinary tract infection. However, it can also stem from other urologic disorders, neurologic dysfunction, or pressure on the bladder from a nearby tumor or from organ enlargement (as with pregnancy).

History and physical examination

Ask the patient how many times a day he voids. How does this compare with his previous pattern of voiding? Ask about the onset and duration of the abnormal frequency and about any associated urinary symptoms, such as dysuria, urinary urgency, urinary incontinence, hematuria, nocturia, or lower abdominal pain with urination. Also ask about any neurologic symptoms, such as muscle weakness, numbness, or tingling. Explore his medical history for urinary tract infection, other urologic problems or recent urologic procedures, and neurologic disorders. With a male patient, ask about a history of prostatic enlargement. If the patient is a female of childbearing age, ask whether she is or could be pregnant.

Obtain a clean-catch midstream sample for urinalysis and culture and sensitivity tests. Then palpate the patient's suprapubic area, abdomen, and flanks, noting any tenderness. Examine his urethral meatus for redness, discharge, or swelling. In a male patient, palpate the prostate gland for enlargement or abnormalities. If the patient's medical history reveals symptoms or a history of neurologic disorders, perform a neurologic examination.

PEDIATRIC POINTER

Urinary tract infection (UTI) is a common cause of urinary frequency in children, especially girls. Congenital anomalies that can cause UTI include a duplicated ureter, congenital bladder diverticulum, and an ectopic ureteral orifice.

ELDER CARE CUE

Men older than age 50 are prone to frequent non–sex-related UTIs. In postmenopausal women, decreased estrogen levels cause urinary frequency, urgency, and nocturia.

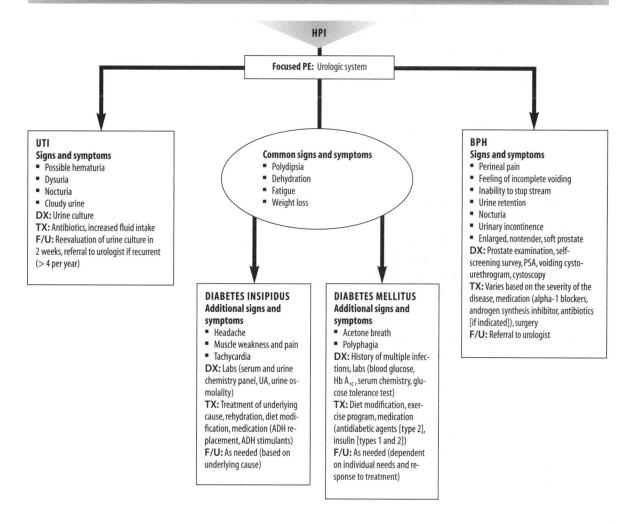

HPI

Focused PE: Urologic system

UTI
Signs and symptoms
- Possible hematuria
- Dysuria
- Nocturia
- Cloudy urine

DX: Urine culture
TX: Antibiotics, increased fluid intake
F/U: Reevaluation of urine culture in 2 weeks, referral to urologist if recurrent (> 4 per year)

Common signs and symptoms
- Polydipsia
- Dehydration
- Fatigue
- Weight loss

BPH
Signs and symptoms
- Perineal pain
- Feeling of incomplete voiding
- Inability to stop stream
- Urine retention
- Nocturia
- Urinary incontinence
- Enlarged, nontender, soft prostate

DX: Prostate examination, self-screening survey, PSA, voiding cysto-urethrogram, cystoscopy
TX: Varies based on the severity of the disease, medication (alpha-1 blockers, androgen synthesis inhibitor, antibiotics [if indicated]), surgery
F/U: Referral to urologist

DIABETES INSIPIDUS
Additional signs and symptoms
- Headache
- Muscle weakness and pain
- Tachycardia

DX: Labs (serum and urine chemistry panel, UA, urine osmolality)
TX: Treatment of underlying cause, rehydration, diet modification, medication (ADH replacement, ADH stimulants)
F/U: As needed (based on underlying cause)

DIABETES MELLITUS
Additional signs and symptoms
- Acetone breath
- Polyphagia

DX: History of multiple infections, labs (blood glucose, Hb A_{1c}, serum chemistry, glucose tolerance test)
TX: Diet modification, exercise program, medication (antidiabetic agents [type 2], insulin [types 1 and 2])
F/U: As needed (dependent on individual needs and response to treatment)

Additional differential diagnoses: multiple sclerosis ▪ rectal tumor ▪ Reiter's syndrome ▪ reproductive tract tumor ▪ spinal cord lesion

Other causes: radiation therapy ▪ diuretics

Urinary hesitancy

Urinary hesitancy — difficulty starting a urinary stream — can result from a urinary tract infection, a partial lower urinary tract obstruction, a neuromuscular disorder, or use of certain drugs. Occurring at all ages and in both sexes, it's most common in older men with prostatic enlargement. It also occurs in women with gravid uterine tumors in the reproductive system, such as uterine fibroids or ovarian, uterine, or vaginal carcinoma. Hesitancy usually arises gradually, commonly going unnoticed until urine retention causes bladder distention and discomfort.

History and physical examination

Ask the patient when he first noticed hesitancy and if he's ever had the problem before. Ask about other urinary problems, especially reduced force or interruption of the urinary stream. Ask if he's ever been treated for a prostate problem or urinary tract infection or obstruction. Obtain a drug history.

Inspect the patient's urethral meatus for inflammation, discharge, and any other abnormalities. Examine the anal sphincter and test sensation in the perineum. Obtain a clean-catch sample for urinalysis. In a male patient, the prostate gland requires palpation. A female patient requires a gynecologic examination.

PEDIATRIC POINTER

The most common cause of urinary obstruction in male infants is posterior strictures. Infants with this problem may have a less forceful urinary stream and may also present with fever due to urinary tract infection, failure to thrive, or a palpable bladder.

URINARY HESITANCY

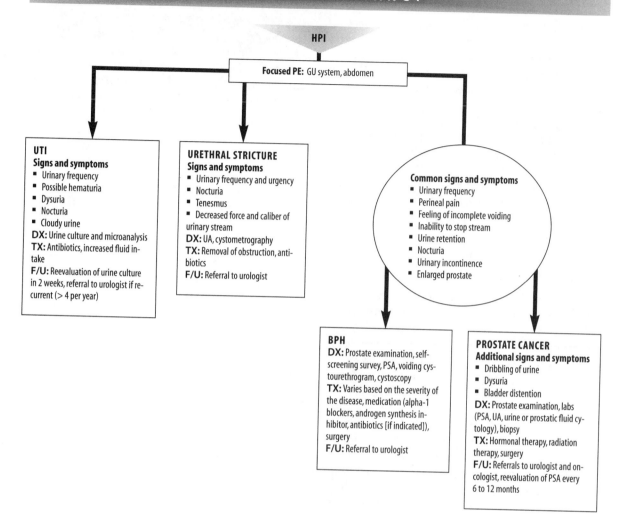

HPI

Focused PE: GU system, abdomen

UTI
Signs and symptoms
- Urinary frequency
- Possible hematuria
- Dysuria
- Nocturia
- Cloudy urine

DX: Urine culture and microanalysis
TX: Antibiotics, increased fluid intake
F/U: Reevaluation of urine culture in 2 weeks, referral to urologist if recurrent (> 4 per year)

URETHRAL STRICTURE
Signs and symptoms
- Urinary frequency and urgency
- Nocturia
- Tenesmus
- Decreased force and caliber of urinary stream

DX: UA, cystometrography
TX: Removal of obstruction, antibiotics
F/U: Referral to urologist

Common signs and symptoms
- Urinary frequency
- Perineal pain
- Feeling of incomplete voiding
- Inability to stop stream
- Urine retention
- Nocturia
- Urinary incontinence
- Enlarged prostate

BPH
DX: Prostate examination, self-screening survey, PSA, voiding cystourethrogram, cystoscopy
TX: Varies based on the severity of the disease, medication (alpha-1 blockers, androgen synthesis inhibitor, antibiotics [if indicated]), surgery
F/U: Referral to urologist

PROSTATE CANCER
Additional signs and symptoms
- Dribbling of urine
- Dysuria
- Bladder distention

DX: Prostate examination, labs (PSA, UA, urine or prostatic fluid cytology), biopsy
TX: Hormonal therapy, radiation therapy, surgery
F/U: Referrals to urologist and oncologist, reevaluation of PSA every 6 to 12 months

Additional differential diagnosis: spinal cord lesion

Other causes: drugs (anticholinergics, TCAs, nasal decongestants, some cold remedies, general anesthesia)

Urinary incontinence

Urinary incontinence, the uncontrollable passage of urine, results from either bladder abnormalities, neurologic disorders, or aging. A common urologic sign, incontinence may be transient or permanent and may involve large volumes of urine or scant dribbling. It can be classified as stress, overflow, urge, or total incontinence. *Stress incontinence* refers to intermittent leakage resulting from a sudden physical strain, such as a cough, sneeze, or quick movement. *Overflow incontinence* is a dribble resulting from urine retention, which fills the bladder and prevents it from contracting with sufficient force to expel a urinary stream. *Urge incontinence* refers to the inability to suppress a sudden urge to urinate. *Total incontinence* is continuous leakage resulting from the bladder's inability to retain any urine.

History and physical examination

Ask the patient when he first noticed the incontinence and whether it began suddenly or gradually. Have him describe his typical urinary pattern: Does incontinence usually occur during the day or at night? Does he have any urinary control, or is he totally incontinent? If he sometimes urinates with control, ask him the usual times and amounts voided. Determine his normal fluid intake. Ask about other urinary problems, such as urinary hesitancy, frequency, and urgency, nocturia, and decreased force or interruption of the urinary stream. Also ask if he's ever sought treatment for incontinence or found a way to deal with it himself.

Obtain a medical history, especially noting urinary tract infection, prostate conditions, spinal injury or tumor, cerebrovascular accident, or surgery involving the bladder, prostate, or pelvic floor.

After completing the history, have the patient empty his bladder. Inspect the urethral meatus for obvious inflammation or anatomic defect. Have female patients bear down; note any urine leakage. Gently palpate the abdomen for bladder distention, which signals urine retention. Perform a complete neurologic assessment, noting motor and sensory function and obvious muscle atrophy.

- *A complete diagnostic evaluation usually is necessary to rule out organic disease.*

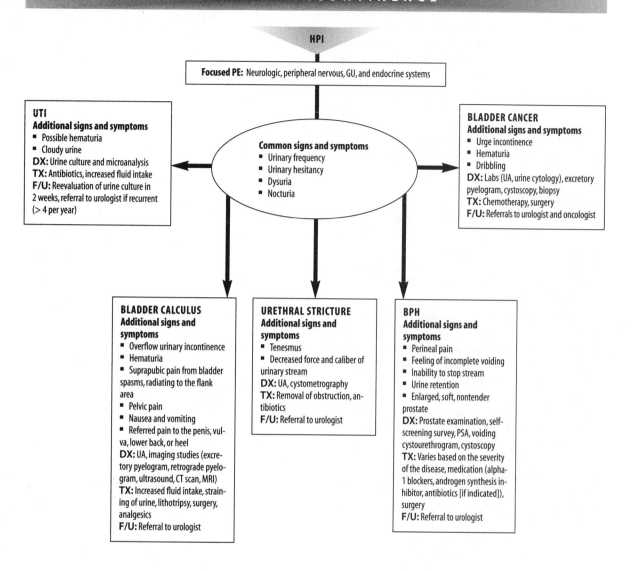

HPI

Focused PE: Neurologic, peripheral nervous, GU, and endocrine systems

Common signs and symptoms
- Urinary frequency
- Urinary hesitancy
- Dysuria
- Nocturia

UTI
Additional signs and symptoms
- Possible hematuria
- Cloudy urine

DX: Urine culture and microanalysis
TX: Antibiotics, increased fluid intake
F/U: Reevaluation of urine culture in 2 weeks, referral to urologist if recurrent (> 4 per year)

BLADDER CANCER
Additional signs and symptoms
- Urge incontinence
- Hematuria
- Dribbling

DX: Labs (UA, urine cytology), excretory pyelogram, cystoscopy, biopsy
TX: Chemotherapy, surgery
F/U: Referrals to urologist and oncologist

BLADDER CALCULUS
Additional signs and symptoms
- Overflow urinary incontinence
- Hematuria
- Suprapubic pain from bladder spasms, radiating to the flank area
- Pelvic pain
- Nausea and vomiting
- Referred pain to the penis, vulva, lower back, or heel

DX: UA, imaging studies (excretory pyelogram, retrograde pyelogram, ultrasound, CT scan, MRI)
TX: Increased fluid intake, straining of urine, lithotripsy, surgery, analgesics
F/U: Referral to urologist

URETHRAL STRICTURE
Additional signs and symptoms
- Tenesmus
- Decreased force and caliber of urinary stream

DX: UA, cystometrography
TX: Removal of obstruction, antibiotics
F/U: Referral to urologist

BPH
Additional signs and symptoms
- Perineal pain
- Feeling of incomplete voiding
- Inability to stop stream
- Urine retention
- Enlarged, soft, nontender prostate

DX: Prostate examination, self-screening survey, PSA, voiding cystourethrogram, cystoscopy
TX: Varies based on the severity of the disease, medication (alpha-1 blockers, androgen synthesis inhibitor, antibiotics [if indicated]), surgery
F/U: Referral to urologist

Additional differential diagnoses: Guillain-Barré syndrome ▪ multiple sclerosis ▪ spinal cord injury ▪ stroke

Other causes: surgery ▪ aging ▪ multiple pregnancies

Urinary urgency

Characterized by a sudden compelling urge to urinate, accompanied by bladder pain, urinary urgency is a classic symptom of urinary tract infection (UTI). As inflammation decreases bladder capacity, discomfort results from the accumulation of even small amounts of urine. Repeated, frequent voiding in an effort to alleviate this discomfort produces urine output of only a few milliliters at each voiding.

Urgency without bladder pain may point to an upper-motor-neuron lesion that has disrupted bladder control.

History and physical examination

Ask the patient about the onset of urinary urgency and whether he's ever experienced it before. Ask about other urologic symptoms, such as dysuria and cloudy urine. Also ask about neurologic symptoms such as paresthesia. Examine his medical history for recurrent or chronic UTIs or for surgery or procedures involving the urinary tract.

Obtain a clean-catch sample for urinalysis. Note urine character, color, and odor, and use a reagent strip to test for pH, glucose, and blood. Then palpate the suprapubic area and both flanks for tenderness. If the patient's history or symptoms suggest neurologic dysfunction, perform a neurologic examination.

PEDIATRIC POINTERS

- In young children, urinary urgency may appear as a change in toilet habits, such as a sudden onset of bed-wetting or daytime accidents in a toilet-trained child. Urgency may also result from urethral irritation caused by bubble bath salts.
- Girls may experience vaginal discharge and vulvar soreness or pruritus.

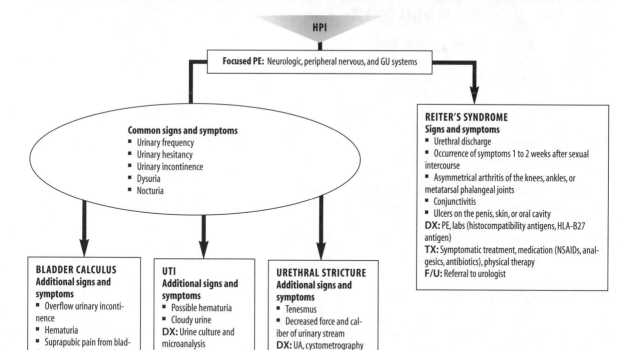

HPI

Focused PE: Neurologic, peripheral nervous, and GU systems

Common signs and symptoms
- Urinary frequency
- Urinary hesitancy
- Urinary incontinence
- Dysuria
- Nocturia

BLADDER CALCULUS
Additional signs and symptoms
- Overflow urinary incontinence
- Hematuria
- Suprapubic pain from bladder spasms, radiating to flank area
- Pelvic pain
- Referred pain to the penis, vulva, lower back, or heel

DX: UA, imaging studies (excretory pyelogram, retrograde pyelogram, ultrasound, CT scan, MRI)
TX: Increased fluid intake, straining of urine, lithotripsy, surgery, analgesics
F/U: Referral to urologist

UTI
Additional signs and symptoms
- Possible hematuria
- Cloudy urine

DX: Urine culture and microanalysis
TX: Antibiotics, increased fluid intake
F/U: Reevaluation of urine culture in 2 weeks, referral to urologist if recurrent (> 4 per year)

URETHRAL STRICTURE
Additional signs and symptoms
- Tenesmus
- Decreased force and caliber of urinary stream

DX: UA, cystometrography
TX: Removal of obstruction, antibiotics
F/U: Referral to urologist

REITER'S SYNDROME
Signs and symptoms
- Urethral discharge
- Occurrence of symptoms 1 to 2 weeks after sexual intercourse
- Asymmetrical arthritis of the knees, ankles, or metatarsal phalangeal joints
- Conjunctivitis
- Ulcers on the penis, skin, or oral cavity

DX: PE, labs (histocompatibility antigens, HLA-B27 antigen)
TX: Symptomatic treatment, medication (NSAIDs, analgesics, antibiotics), physical therapy
F/U: Referral to urologist

Additional differential diagnosis: ALS

Other cause: radiation therapy

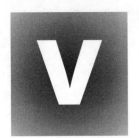

Vaginal bleeding (post-menopausal)

Postmenopausal vaginal bleeding — bleeding that occurs 6 or more months after menopause — is an important indicator of gynecologic cancer. But it can also result from infection, local pelvic disorders, estrogenic stimulation, atrophy of the endometrium, and physiologic thinning and drying of the vaginal mucous membranes. It usually occurs as slight, brown or red spotting developing either spontaneously or following coitus or douching, but it may also occur as oozing of fresh blood or as bright red hemorrhage. Many patients — especially those with a history of heavy menstrual flow — minimize the importance of this bleeding, delaying diagnosis.

History and physical examination

Determine the patient's current age and her age at menopause. Ask when she first noticed the abnormal bleeding. Then obtain a thorough obstetric and gynecologic history. When did she begin menstruating? Were her menses regular? If not, ask her to describe any menstrual irregularities. How old was she when she first had intercourse? How many sexual partners has she had? Has she had any children? Has she had fertility problems? If possible, obtain an obstetric and gynecologic history of the patient and the patient's mother, and ask about a family history of gynecologic cancer. Determine if the patient has any associated symptoms and if she's currently taking estrogen.

Observe the external genitalia, noting the character of any vaginal discharge and the appearance of the labia, vaginal rugae, and clitoris. Carefully inspect and palpate the patient's breasts for dimpling, color differences, and masses; also inspect and palpate the lymph nodes for nodules or enlargement. The patient should have pelvic and rectal examinations.

WOMEN'S HEALTH TIPS

- *Women can decrease their risk of getting vulvar cancer by practicing safer sex and by reducing controllable risk factors, such as hypertension, obesity, and diabetes.*
- *Eighty percent of postmenopausal vaginal bleeding is benign; endometrial atrophy is the predominant cause. Malignancy should be ruled out.*

HPI

Focused PE: Abdomen, GU system, pelvic examination

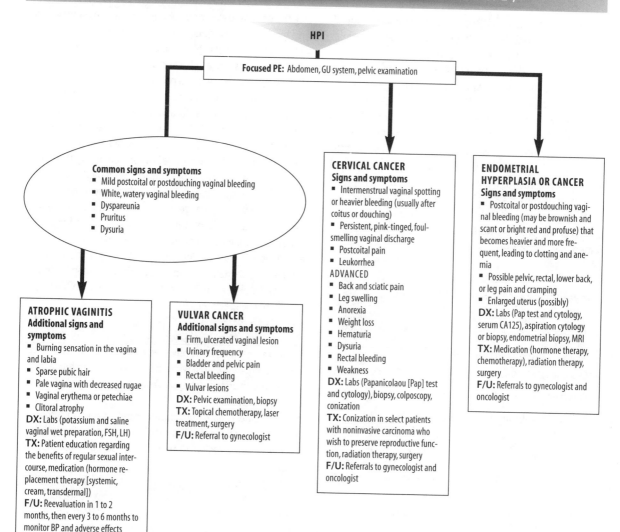

Common signs and symptoms
- Mild postcoital or postdouching vaginal bleeding
- White, watery vaginal bleeding
- Dyspareunia
- Pruritus
- Dysuria

ATROPHIC VAGINITIS
Additional signs and symptoms
- Burning sensation in the vagina and labia
- Sparse pubic hair
- Pale vagina with decreased rugae
- Vaginal erythema or petechiae
- Clitoral atrophy

DX: Labs (potassium and saline vaginal wet preparation, FSH, LH)
TX: Patient education regarding the benefits of regular sexual intercourse, medication (hormone replacement therapy [systemic, cream, transdermal])
F/U: Reevaluation in 1 to 2 months, then every 3 to 6 months to monitor BP and adverse effects

VULVAR CANCER
Additional signs and symptoms
- Firm, ulcerated vaginal lesion
- Urinary frequency
- Bladder and pelvic pain
- Rectal bleeding
- Vulvar lesions

DX: Pelvic examination, biopsy
TX: Topical chemotherapy, laser treatment, surgery
F/U: Referral to gynecologist

CERVICAL CANCER
Signs and symptoms
- Intermenstrual vaginal spotting or heavier bleeding (usually after coitus or douching)
- Persistent, pink-tinged, foul-smelling vaginal discharge
- Postcoital pain
- Leukorrhea
ADVANCED
- Back and sciatic pain
- Leg swelling
- Anorexia
- Weight loss
- Hematuria
- Dysuria
- Rectal bleeding
- Weakness

DX: Labs (Papanicolaou [Pap] test and cytology), biopsy, colposcopy, conization
TX: Conization in select patients with noninvasive carcinoma who wish to preserve reproductive function, radiation therapy, surgery
F/U: Referrals to gynecologist and oncologist

ENDOMETRIAL HYPERPLASIA OR CANCER
Signs and symptoms
- Postcoital or postdouching vaginal bleeding (may be brownish and scant or bright red and profuse) that becomes heavier and more frequent, leading to clotting and anemia
- Possible pelvic, rectal, lower back, or leg pain and cramping
- Enlarged uterus (possibly)

DX: Labs (Pap test and cytology, serum CA125), aspiration cytology or biopsy, endometrial biopsy, MRI
TX: Medication (hormone therapy, chemotherapy), radiation therapy, surgery
F/U: Referrals to gynecologist and oncologist

Additional differential diagnoses: cervical or endometrial polyps • ovarian tumors (feminizing)

Other cause: unopposed estrogen replacement therapy

Vaginal discharge

Common in women of childbearing age, physiologic vaginal discharge is mucoid, clear or white, nonbloody, and odorless. Produced by the cervical mucosa and, to a lesser degree, by the vulvar glands, this discharge may occasionally be scant or profuse due to estrogenic stimulation and changes during the patient's menstrual cycle. However, a marked increase in discharge or a change in discharge color, odor, or consistency can signal disease. The discharge may result from infection, sexually transmitted disease, reproductive tract disease, fistulas, and certain drugs. In addition, the prolonged presence of a foreign body, such as a tampon or diaphragm, in the patient's vagina can cause irritation and an inflammatory exudate, as can frequent douching, feminine hygiene products, contraceptive products, bubble baths, and colored or perfumed toilet papers.

Identifying causes of vaginal discharge

The color, consistency, amount, and odor of your patient's vaginal discharge provide important clues about the underlying disorder. For quick reference, use this chart to match common characteristics of vaginal discharge and their possible causes.

CHARACTERISTICS	POSSIBLE CAUSES
Thin, scant, watery white discharge	Atrophic vaginitis
White, curdlike, profuse discharge with yeasty, sweet odor	Candidiasis
Mucopurulent, foul-smelling discharge	Chancroid
Yellow, mucopurulent, odorless, or acrid discharge	*Chlamydia* infection
Scant, serosanguineous, or purulent discharge with foul odor	Endometritis
Thin, green or grayish white, foul-smelling discharge	*Gardnerella* vaginitis
Watery discharge	Genital herpes
Profuse, mucopurulent discharge, possibly foul-smelling	Genital warts
Yellow or green, foul-smelling discharge from the cervix or occasionally from Bartholin's or Skene's ducts	Gonorrhea
Chronic, watery, bloody, or purulent discharge, possibly foul-smelling	Gynecologic cancer
Frothy, greenish yellow, and profuse (or thin, white, and scant) foul-smelling discharge	Trichomoniasis

History and physical examination

Ask the patient to describe the onset, color, consistency, odor, and texture of her vaginal discharge. How does the discharge differ from her usual vaginal secretions? Is the onset related to her menstrual cycle? Also ask about associated symptoms, such as dysuria and perineal pruritus and burning. Does she have spotting after coitus or douching? Ask about recent changes in her sexual habits and hygiene practices. Is she or could she be pregnant? Next, ask if she has had vaginal discharge before or has ever been treated for a vaginal infection. What treatment did she receive? Did she complete the course of medication? Ask about her current use of medications, especially antibiotics, oral estrogens, and contraceptives.

Examine the external genitalia and note the character of the discharge. (See *Identifying causes of vaginal discharge.*) Observe vulvar and vaginal tissues for redness, edema, and excoriation. Palpate the inguinal lymph nodes to detect tenderness or enlargement, and palpate the abdomen for tenderness. A pelvic examination may be required. Obtain vaginal discharge specimens for testing.

PEDIATRIC POINTERS

- *Female neonates who have been exposed to maternal estrogens in utero may have a white mucous vaginal discharge for the 1st month after birth; a yellow mucous discharge indicates a pathologic condition.*
- *In the older child, a purulent, foul-smelling and, possibly, bloody vaginal discharge commonly results from a foreign object placed in the vagina. The possibility of sexual abuse should be considered.*

ELDER CARE CUE

The postmenopausal vaginal mucosa becomes thin due to decreased estrogen levels. Together with a rise in vaginal pH, this reduces resistance to infectious agents, increasing the incidence of vaginitis.

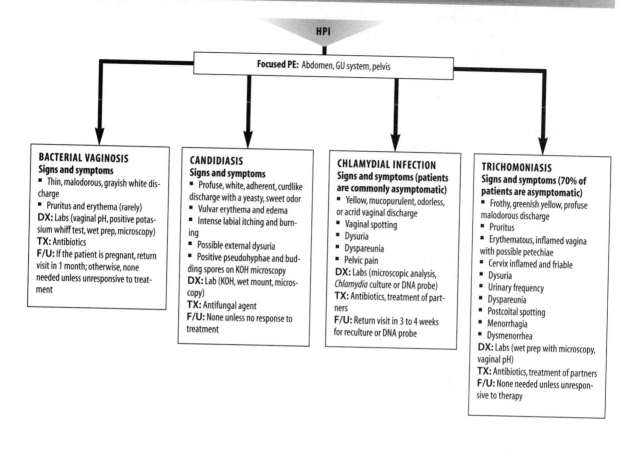

HPI

Focused PE: Abdomen, GU system, pelvis

BACTERIAL VAGINOSIS
Signs and symptoms
- Thin, malodorous, grayish white discharge
- Pruritus and erythema (rarely)

DX: Labs (vaginal pH, positive potassium whiff test, wet prep, microscopy)
TX: Antibiotics
F/U: If the patient is pregnant, return visit in 1 month; otherwise, none needed unless unresponsive to treatment

CANDIDIASIS
Signs and symptoms
- Profuse, white, adherent, curdlike discharge with a yeasty, sweet odor
- Vulvar erythema and edema
- Intense labial itching and burning
- Possible external dysuria
- Positive pseudohyphae and budding spores on KOH microscopy

DX: Lab (KOH, wet mount, microscopy)
TX: Antifungal agent
F/U: None unless no response to treatment

CHLAMYDIAL INFECTION
Signs and symptoms (patients are commonly asymptomatic)
- Yellow, mucopurulent, odorless, or acrid vaginal discharge
- Vaginal spotting
- Dysuria
- Dyspareunia
- Pelvic pain

DX: Labs (microscopic analysis, *Chlamydia* culture or DNA probe)
TX: Antibiotics, treatment of partners
F/U: Return visit in 3 to 4 weeks for reculture or DNA probe

TRICHOMONIASIS
Signs and symptoms (70% of patients are asymptomatic)
- Frothy, greenish yellow, profuse malodorous discharge
- Pruritus
- Erythematous, inflamed vagina with possible petechiae
- Cervix inflamed and friable
- Dysuria
- Urinary frequency
- Dyspareunia
- Postcoital spotting
- Menorrhagia
- Dysmenorrhea

DX: Labs (wet prep with microscopy, vaginal pH)
TX: Antibiotics, treatment of partners
F/U: None needed unless unresponsive to therapy

Additional differential diagnoses: atrophic vaginitis ▪ chancroid ▪ endometritis ▪ genital warts ▪ gonorrhea ▪ gynecologic cancer ▪ herpes simplex (genital)

Other causes: contraceptive creams and jellies ▪ drugs (such as oral contraceptives and antibiotics) ▪ radiation therapy

Vertigo

Vertigo is an illusion of movement in which the patient feels that he's revolving in space (subjective vertigo) or that his surroundings are revolving around him (objective vertigo). He may complain of a feeling of being pulled sideways, as though drawn by a magnet.

A common symptom, vertigo usually begins abruptly and may be temporary or permanent, mild or severe. It may worsen when the patient moves and often subsides when he lies down. Frequently, it's confused with dizziness — a sensation of imbalance and light-headedness that's nonspecific. However, unlike dizziness, vertigo is commonly accompanied by nausea, vomiting, nystagmus, and tinnitus or hearing loss. Although the patient's limb coordination is unaffected, vertiginous gait may occur.

Vertigo may result from neurologic or otologic disorders that affect the equilibratory apparatus (the vestibule, semicircular canals, eighth cranial nerve, vestibular nuclei in the brain stem and their temporal lobe connections, and eyes). However, this symptom may also result from alcohol intoxication, hyperventilation, postural changes (benign postural vertigo), and the effects of certain drugs, tests, and procedures.

History and physical examination

Ask your patient to describe the onset and duration of his vertigo, being careful to distinguish this symptom from dizziness. Does he feel that he's moving or that his surroundings are moving around him? How often do the attacks occur? Do they follow position changes, or are they unpredictable? Find out if the patient can walk during an attack, if he leans to one side, and if he's ever fallen. Ask if he experiences motion sickness and if he prefers one position during an attack. Obtain a recent drug history and note any evidence of alcohol abuse.

Perform a neurologic assessment, focusing particularly on eighth cranial nerve function. Observe the patient's gait and posture for abnormalities.

PEDIATRIC POINTER

Ear infection is a common cause of vertigo in children. Vestibular neuritis may also cause this symptom.

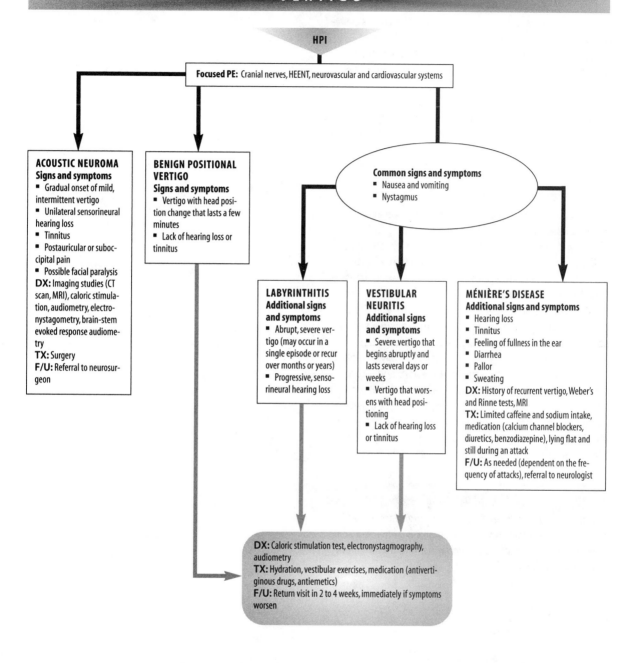

HPI

Focused PE: Cranial nerves, HEENT, neurovascular and cardiovascular systems

ACOUSTIC NEUROMA
Signs and symptoms
- Gradual onset of mild, intermittent vertigo
- Unilateral sensorineural hearing loss
- Tinnitus
- Postauricular or suboccipital pain
- Possible facial paralysis
DX: Imaging studies (CT scan, MRI), caloric stimulation, audiometry, electronystagometry, brain-stem evoked response audiometry
TX: Surgery
F/U: Referral to neurosurgeon

BENIGN POSITIONAL VERTIGO
Signs and symptoms
- Vertigo with head position change that lasts a few minutes
- Lack of hearing loss or tinnitus

Common signs and symptoms
- Nausea and vomiting
- Nystagmus

LABYRINTHITIS
Additional signs and symptoms
- Abrupt, severe vertigo (may occur in a single episode or recur over months or years)
- Progressive, sensorineural hearing loss

VESTIBULAR NEURITIS
Additional signs and symptoms
- Severe vertigo that begins abruptly and lasts several days or weeks
- Vertigo that worsens with head positioning
- Lack of hearing loss or tinnitus

MÉNIÈRE'S DISEASE
Additional signs and symptoms
- Hearing loss
- Tinnitus
- Feeling of fullness in the ear
- Diarrhea
- Pallor
- Sweating
DX: History of recurrent vertigo, Weber's and Rinne tests, MRI
TX: Limited caffeine and sodium intake, medication (calcium channel blockers, diuretics, benzodiazepine), lying flat and still during an attack
F/U: As needed (dependent on the frequency of attacks), referral to neurologist

DX: Caloric stimulation test, electronystagmography, audiometry
TX: Hydration, vestibular exercises, medication (antivertiginous drugs, antiemetics)
F/U: Return visit in 2 to 4 weeks, immediately if symptoms worsen

Additional differential diagnoses: brain stem ischemia ▪ head trauma ▪ herpes zoster ▪ multiple sclerosis ▪ posterior fossa tumor ▪ seizures

Other causes: caloric testing ▪ alcohol ▪ ear surgery ▪ high or toxic levels of salicylates ▪ aminoglycosides ▪ antibiotics ▪ quinine and oral contraceptives ▪ administration of overly warm or cold eardrops or irrigating solutions

Vesicular rash

A vesicular rash is a scattered or linear distribution of vesicles — sharply circumscribed lesions filled with clear, cloudy, or bloody fluid. The lesions, which are usually less than 0.5 cm in diameter, may occur singly or in groups. They sometimes occur with bullae — fluid-filled lesions larger than 0.5 cm in diameter.

A vesicular rash may be mild or severe and temporary or permanent. It can result from infection, inflammation, or allergic reactions.

History and physical examination

Ask your patient when the rash began, how it spread, and whether it has appeared before. Did other skin lesions precede eruption of the vesicles? Obtain a thorough drug history. If the patient has used any topical medication, what type did he use and when was it last applied? Also ask about associated signs and symptoms. Find out if he has a family history of skin disorders, and ask about immunizations, allergies, recent infections, insect bites, and exposure to allergens. Inquire about recent exposure to contagious viral infections.

Examine the patient's skin, noting if it's dry, oily, or moist. Observe the general distribution of the lesions and record their exact location. Note the color, shape, and size of the lesions, and check for crusts, scales, scars, macules, papules, or wheals. Palpate the vesicles or bullae to determine if they're flaccid or tense. Slide your finger across the skin to see if the outer layer of epidermis separates easily from the basal layer (Nikolsky's sign).

PEDIATRIC POINTER

Vesicular rashes in children are caused by staphylococcal infections (staphylococcal scalded skin syndrome is a life-threatening infection occurring in infants), varicella, hand-foot-and-mouth disease, and miliaria rubra.

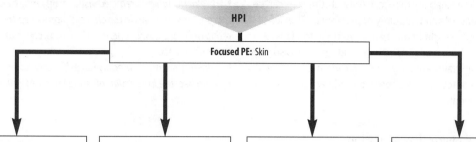

HPI

Focused PE: Skin

CONTACT DERMATITIS
Signs and symptoms
- Small vesicles on an erythematous base and edema that may ooze or scale
- Severe pruritus (possibly)

DX: Skin examination

TX: Medication (steroids [topical or systemic], antihistamine, antipruritic), cool tub baths with colloidal oatmeal, topical compresses of frozen (use for 15 to 20 minutes, three to four times per day), patient education on seeking immediate attention for SOB or chest tightness

F/U: None necessary if localized, 2 to 3 days if generalized

HERPES ZOSTER
Signs and symptoms
- Dermatomal pain, itching, and burning 4 to 5 days before eruption of vesicles
- Unilateral spread of vesicles on an erythematous base along dermatome
- Vesicles that dry and scab about 10 days after eruption
- Fever
- Headache
- Malaise
- Pruritus
- Paresthesia or hyperesthesia of involved area
- Involvement of thorax, extremities, and cranial nerves (possibly)

DX: Labs (Tzanck smear, viral antigen smear, viral culture, HIV testing)

TX: Cool compresses, medication (antivirals, NSAIDs, antidepressant, topical anesthetic)

F/U: Reevaluation in 7 to 10 days

SCABIES
Signs and symptoms
- Small, isolated serous vesicles on an erythematous base (may be at the end of a burrow)
- Burrows (gray or skin-colored ridges with a small, isolated red papule that contains the mite)
- Pustules and excoriations (possibly)
- Intense itching at night
- Rash commonly found on hands and finger webs but also occurring on the wrists, elbows, axillae, waistline, breasts, penis, and scrotum

DX: Microscopic identification of a mite or ova

TX: Medication (scabicide, antihistamine), treatment of all household members, laundering of all clothing and bedding in hot water and hot dryer cycle, cool bath with colloidal oatmeal, topical compresses wet with water kept in freezer (use for 15 to 20 minutes, three to four per day)

F/U: None unless treatment is ineffective

ERYTHEMA MULTIFORME
Signs and symptoms
- Sudden eruption of erythematous macules, papules, vesicles, and bullae
- Rash that appears on the hands, feet, arms, legs, face, and neck
- Vesiculobullous lesions that appear on mucous membranes and may rupture and ulcerate
- Thick yellow or white exudate
- Lymphadenopathy
- Pruritus

DX: Skin examination, positive Nikolsky's sign, biopsy

TX: Compresses, medication (antihistamines, analgesics, topical anesthetics)

F/U: As needed

Additional differential diagnoses: burns ▪ dermatitis herpetiformis ▪ dermatophytid ▪ herpes simplex ▪ insect bites ▪ pemphigoid (bullous) ▪ pemphigus ▪ pompholyx ▪ porphyria cutanea tarda ▪ tinea pedis ▪ toxic epidermal necrolysis

Vision loss

Vision loss — the inability to perceive visual stimuli — can be sudden or gradual and temporary or permanent. The deficit can range from a slight impairment of vision to total blindness. It results from ocular, neurologic, and systemic disorders as well as from trauma and reactions to certain drugs. The ultimate visual outcome may depend on early, accurate diagnosis and treatment.

History and physical examination

Sudden vision loss can signal an ocular emergency. Don't touch the eye if the patient has perforating or penetrating ocular trauma.

If the patient's vision loss occurred gradually, ask him if the vision loss affects one eye or both and all or only part of the visual field. Does the patient have corrective lenses or contacts? Is the visual loss transient or persistent? Did the visual loss occur abruptly or did it develop over hours, days, or weeks? What's the patient's age? Ask the patient if he has experienced photosensitivity, and ask him about the location, intensity, and duration of any eye pain. In addition, you should obtain an ocular history, including the date of the patient's last ocular examination and its outcome, as well as a family history of eye problems or systemic diseases that may lead to eye problems, such as hypertension; diabetes mellitus; thyroid, rheumatic, or vascular disease; infections; and cancer.

The first step in performing the eye examination is to assess visual acuity, with best available correction in each eye. Carefully inspect both eyes, noting edema, foreign bodies, drainage, or conjunctival or scleral redness. Observe whether lid closure is complete or incomplete, and check for ptosis. Using a flashlight, examine the cornea and iris for scars, irregularities, and foreign bodies. Observe the size, shape, and color of the pupils, and test the direct and consensual light and the effect of accommodation. Evaluate extraocular muscle function by testing the six cardinal fields of gaze.

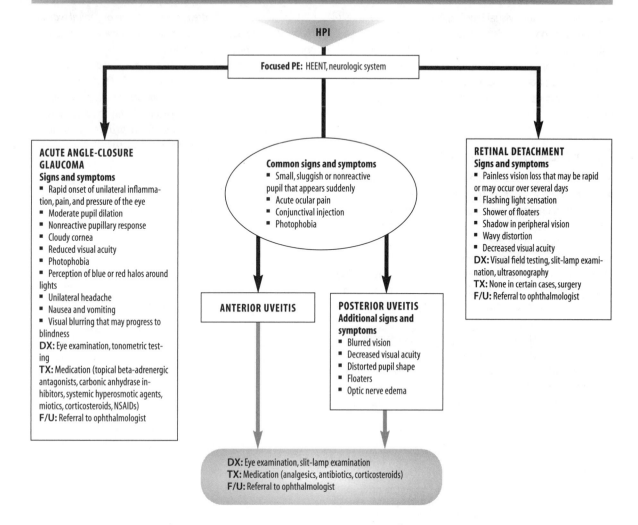

HPI

Focused PE: HEENT, neurologic system

ACUTE ANGLE-CLOSURE GLAUCOMA
Signs and symptoms
- Rapid onset of unilateral inflammation, pain, and pressure of the eye
- Moderate pupil dilation
- Nonreactive pupillary response
- Cloudy cornea
- Reduced visual acuity
- Photophobia
- Perception of blue or red halos around lights
- Unilateral headache
- Nausea and vomiting
- Visual blurring that may progress to blindness
DX: Eye examination, tonometric testing
TX: Medication (topical beta-adrenergic antagonists, carbonic anhydrase inhibitors, systemic hyperosmotic agents, miotics, corticosteroids, NSAIDs)
F/U: Referral to ophthalmologist

Common signs and symptoms
- Small, sluggish or nonreactive pupil that appears suddenly
- Acute ocular pain
- Conjunctival injection
- Photophobia

ANTERIOR UVEITIS

POSTERIOR UVEITIS
Additional signs and symptoms
- Blurred vision
- Decreased visual acuity
- Distorted pupil shape
- Floaters
- Optic nerve edema

RETINAL DETACHMENT
Signs and symptoms
- Painless vision loss that may be rapid or may occur over several days
- Flashing light sensation
- Shower of floaters
- Shadow in peripheral vision
- Wavy distortion
- Decreased visual acuity
DX: Visual field testing, slit-lamp examination, ultrasonography
TX: None in certain cases, surgery
F/U: Referral to ophthalmologist

DX: Eye examination, slit-lamp examination
TX: Medication (analgesics, antibiotics, corticosteroids)
F/U: Referral to ophthalmologist

Additional differential diagnoses: amaurosis fugax ▪ cataract ▪ concussion ▪ diabetic retinopathy ▪ endophthalmitis ▪ hereditary corneal dystrophies ▪ herpes zoster ▪ hyphema ▪ keratitis ▪ ocular trauma ▪ optic atrophy ▪ optic neuritis ▪ Paget's disease ▪ papilledema ▪ pituitary tumor ▪ retinal artery occlusion (central) ▪ retinal vein occlusion (central) ▪ senile macular degeneration ▪ Stevens-Johnson syndrome ▪ temporal arteritis ▪ trachoma ▪ vitreous hemorrhage

Other causes: chloroquine therapy ▪ phenylbutazone ▪ digitalis derivatives ▪ indomethacin ▪ ethambutol ▪ quinine ▪ methanol toxicity

Visual blurring

A common symptom, visual blurring refers to the loss of visual acuity with indistinct visual details. It may result from eye injury, neurologic and eye disorders, or disorders with vascular complications such as diabetes mellitus. Visual blurring may also result from mucus passing over the cornea, refractive errors, improperly fitted contact lenses, or the effects of drugs.

History and physical examination

If your patient has visual blurring accompanied by sudden, severe eye pain, a history of trauma, or sudden vision loss, order an ophthalmologic examination. If the patient has a penetrating or perforating eye injury, don't touch the eye.

If the patient isn't in distress, ask him how long he has had the visual blurring. Does it occur only at certain times? Ask about associated symptoms, such as pain or discharge. If visual blurring followed injury, obtain details of the accident, and ask if vision was impaired immediately after the injury. Obtain a medical and drug history.

Inspect the patient's eye, noting lid edema, drainage, or conjunctival or scleral redness. Also note an irregularly shaped iris, which may indicate previous trauma, and excessive blinking, which may indicate corneal damage. Assess for pupillary changes, and test visual acuity in both eyes. (See *Testing visual acuity.*)

- *Visual blurring in children may stem from congenital syphilis, congenital cataracts, refractive errors, eye injuries or infections, and increased intracranial pressure.*
- *Test vision in school-age children as you would in adults; test children aged 3 to 6 with the Snellen chart. Test toddlers with Allen cards, each illustrated with a familiar object, such as an animal. Ask the child to cover one eye and identify the objects as you flash them. Then ask him to identify them as you gradually back away. Record the maximum distance at which he can identify at least three pictures.*

Testing visual acuity

Use a Snellen letter chart to test visual acuity in the literate patient over age 6. Have the patient sit or stand 20′ (6.1 m) from the chart. Then, tell him to cover his left eye and read aloud the smallest line of letters that he can see. Record the fraction assigned to that line on the chart (the numerator indicates distance from the chart; the denominator indicates the distance at which a normal eye can read the chart). Normal vision is 20/20. Repeat the test with the patient's right eye covered.

If your patient can't read the largest letter from a distance of 20′, have him approach the chart until he can read it. Then, record the distance between him and the chart as the numerator of the fraction. For example, if he can see the top line of the chart at a distance of 3′ (1.9 m), record the test result as 3/200.

Use a Snellen symbol chart to test children ages 3 to 6 and illiterate patients. Follow the same procedure as for the Snellen letter chart but ask the patient to indicate the direction of the E's fingers as you point to each symbol.

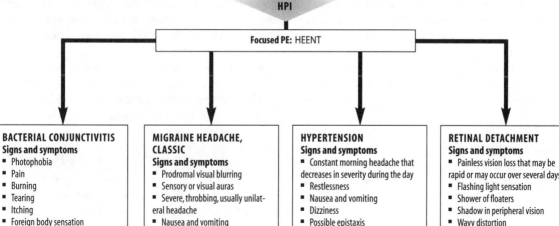

Focused PE: HEENT

BACTERIAL CONJUNCTIVITIS
Signs and symptoms
- Photophobia
- Pain
- Burning
- Tearing
- Itching
- Foreign body sensation
- Feeling of fullness around the eyes
- Erythema near the fornices
- Copious, mucopurulent, flaky drainage
- Matting of the eyelashes
- Edema of the eyelids

DX: Culture if chronic or recurrent condition
TX: Ophthalmic antibiotic
F/U: Reevaluation if there's no improvement in 24 to 48 hours or if the condition worsens, referral to ophthalmologist if recurrent

MIGRAINE HEADACHE, CLASSIC
Signs and symptoms
- Prodromal visual blurring
- Sensory or visual auras
- Severe, throbbing, usually unilateral headache
- Nausea and vomiting
- Photophobia
- Phonophobia
- Perspiration

DX: History
TX: Medication (NSAIDs, beta-adrenergic blockers, anticonvulsants, antidepressants, steroids, calcium channel blockers, ergots); headache diary; low-fat, high-complex carbohydrate diet
F/U: Referrals to ophthalmologist, neurologist, and headache center

HYPERTENSION
Signs and symptoms
- Constant morning headache that decreases in severity during the day
- Restlessness
- Nausea and vomiting
- Dizziness
- Possible epistaxis
- Fatigue
- Anxiety
- Peripheral edema

DX: Labs (CBC, BUN, creatinine, electrolytes, plasma renin, uric acid), renal ultrasound, 12-lead ECG
TX: Treatment of underlying condition for secondary hypertension, medication (beta-adrenergic blockers, ACE inhibitors, calcium channel blockers), BP diary
F/U: Return visit in 1 week, then every 4 weeks until hypertension is well controlled

RETINAL DETACHMENT
Signs and symptoms
- Painless vision loss that may be rapid or may occur over several days
- Flashing light sensation
- Shower of floaters
- Shadow in peripheral vision
- Wavy distortion
- Decreased visual acuity

DX: Visual field testing, slit-lamp examination, ultrasonography
TX: None in certain cases, surgery
F/U: Referral to ophthalmologist

Additional differential diagnoses: brain tumor ▪ cataract ▪ concussion ▪ conjunctivitis ▪ corneal abrasions ▪ corneal foreign bodies ▪ diabetic retinopathy ▪ dislocated lens ▪ eye tumor ▪ glaucoma ▪ hereditary corneal dystrophies ▪ hyphema ▪ iritis ▪ multiple sclerosis ▪ optic neuritis ▪ retinal vein occlusion (central) ▪ senile macular degeneration ▪ serous retinopathy (central) ▪ temporal arteritis ▪ uveitis (posterior) ▪ vitreous hemorrhage

Other causes: cycloplegics ▪ guanethidine ▪ reserpine ▪ clomiphene ▪ phenylbutazone ▪ thiazide diuretics ▪ antihistamines ▪ anticholinergics ▪ phenothiazines

Vomiting

Vomiting is the forceful expulsion of gastric contents through the mouth. Characteristically preceded by nausea, vomiting results from a coordinated sequence of abdominal muscle contractions and reverse esophageal peristalsis.

A common sign of GI disorders, vomiting also occurs with fluid and electrolyte imbalances; infections; and metabolic, endocrine, labyrinthine, central nervous system (CNS), and cardiac disorders. It can also result from drug therapy, surgery, and radiation.

Vomiting occurs normally during the 1st trimester of pregnancy, but its subsequent development may signal complications. It can also result from stress, anxiety, pain, alcohol intoxication, overeating, or ingestion of distasteful foods or liquids.

History and physical examination

Ask your patient to describe the onset, duration, and intensity of his vomiting. What started the vomiting? What does the vomitus look like? How often does vomiting occur? What makes it subside? If possible, collect, measure, and inspect the character of the vomitus. (See *Vomitus: Characteristics and causes.*) Explore any associated complaints, particularly nausea, abdominal pain, anorexia and weight loss, changes in bowel habits or stools, excessive belching or flatus, and bloating or fullness.

Obtain a medical history, noting GI, endocrine, and metabolic disorders; recent infections; and cancer, including chemotherapy or radiation therapy. Ask about current medication use and alcohol consumption. Inquire about recent diet history. If the patient is a female of childbearing age, ask if she is or could be pregnant. Ask which contraceptive method she's using.

Inspect the abdomen for distention, and auscultate for bowel sounds and bruits. Palpate for rigidity and tenderness, and test for rebound tenderness. Next, palpate and percuss the liver for enlargement. Assess other body systems as appropriate.

During the examination, keep in mind that projectile vomiting *unaccompanied* by nausea may indicate increased intracranial pressure, a life-threatening emergency. If this occurs in a patient with CNS injury, you should quickly check his vital signs. Be alert for widened pulse pressure or bradycardia.

PEDIATRIC POINTERS

- *In a neonate, pyloric obstruction may cause projectile vomiting, whereas Hirschsprung's disease may cause fecal vomiting.*
- *Intussusception may lead to vomiting of bile and fecal matter in an infant or toddler.*

ELDER CARE CUE

Although elderly patients can develop several of the disorders already mentioned, always rule out intestinal ischemia first — it's especially common in this age-group and has a high mortality rate.

Vomitus: Characteristics and causes

When you collect a sample of the patient's vomitus, observe it carefully for clues to the underlying disorder. Here's what this vomitus may indicate:

- *bile-stained (greenish) vomitus* — obstruction below the pylorus, as from a duodenal lesion
- *bloody vomitus* — upper GI bleeding, as from gastritis or peptic ulcer, if bright red; as from esophageal or gastric varices, if dark red
- *brown vomitus with a fecal odor*—intestinal obstruction or infarction
- *burning, bitter-tasting vomitus* — excessive hydrochloric acid in gastric contents
- *coffee-ground vomitus* — digested blood from slowly bleeding gastric or duodenal lesion
- *undigested food* — gastric outlet obstruction, as from gastric tumor or ulcer.

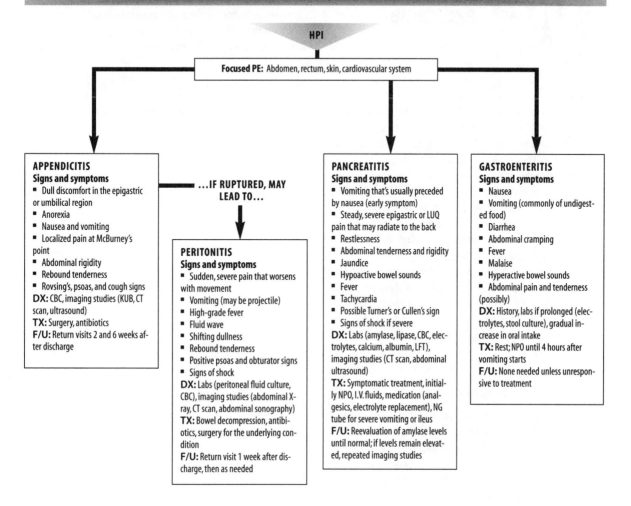

HPI

Focused PE: Abdomen, rectum, skin, cardiovascular system

APPENDICITIS
Signs and symptoms
- Dull discomfort in the epigastric or umbilical region
- Anorexia
- Nausea and vomiting
- Localized pain at McBurney's point
- Abdominal rigidity
- Rebound tenderness
- Rovsing's, psoas, and cough signs

DX: CBC, imaging studies (KUB, CT scan, ultrasound)
TX: Surgery, antibiotics
F/U: Return visits 2 and 6 weeks after discharge

...IF RUPTURED, MAY LEAD TO...

PERITONITIS
Signs and symptoms
- Sudden, severe pain that worsens with movement
- Vomiting (may be projectile)
- High-grade fever
- Fluid wave
- Shifting dullness
- Rebound tenderness
- Positive psoas and obturator signs
- Signs of shock

DX: Labs (peritoneal fluid culture, CBC), imaging studies (abdominal X-ray, CT scan, abdominal sonography)
TX: Bowel decompression, antibiotics, surgery for the underlying condition
F/U: Return visit 1 week after discharge, then as needed

PANCREATITIS
Signs and symptoms
- Vomiting that's usually preceded by nausea (early symptom)
- Steady, severe epigastric or LUQ pain that may radiate to the back
- Restlessness
- Abdominal tenderness and rigidity
- Jaundice
- Hypoactive bowel sounds
- Fever
- Tachycardia
- Possible Turner's or Cullen's sign
- Signs of shock if severe

DX: Labs (amylase, lipase, CBC, electrolytes, calcium, albumin, LFT), imaging studies (CT scan, abdominal ultrasound)
TX: Symptomatic treatment, initially NPO, I.V. fluids, medication (analgesics, electrolyte replacement), NG tube for severe vomiting or ileus
F/U: Reevaluation of amylase levels until normal; if levels remain elevated, repeated imaging studies

GASTROENTERITIS
Signs and symptoms
- Nausea
- Vomiting (commonly of undigested food)
- Diarrhea
- Abdominal cramping
- Fever
- Malaise
- Hyperactive bowel sounds
- Abdominal pain and tenderness (possibly)

DX: History, labs if prolonged (electrolytes, stool culture), gradual increase in oral intake
TX: Rest; NPO until 4 hours after vomiting starts
F/U: None needed unless unresponsive to treatment

Additional differential diagnoses: adrenal insufficiency ▪ bulimia ▪ cholecystitis (acute) ▪ cholelithiasis ▪ cirrhosis ▪ ectopic pregnancy ▪ electrolyte imbalances ▪ food poisoning ▪ gastric cancer ▪ gastritis ▪ heart failure ▪ hepatitis ▪ hyperemesis gravidarum ▪ increased ICP ▪ infection ▪ intestinal obstruction ▪ labyrinthitis ▪ mesenteric artery ischemia ▪ mesenteric venous thrombosis ▪ metabolic acidosis ▪ MI ▪ migraine headache ▪ motion sickness ▪ peptic ulcer ▪ preeclampsia ▪ renal and urologic disorders ▪ thyrotoxicosis ▪ ulcerative colitis

---

Other causes: drugs (such as antineoplastic agents, opiates, ferrous sulfate, levodopa, oral potassium, chloride replacement, estrogens, sulfasalazine, antibiotics, quinidine, anesthetic agents, and overdoses of digitalis and theophylline) ▪ radiation

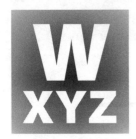

Weight gain, excessive

Weight gain occurs when ingested calories exceed body requirements for energy, causing increased adipose tissue storage. It can also occur when fluid retention causes edema. When weight gain results from overeating, emotional factors — most commonly anxiety, guilt, and depression — and social factors may be the primary causes.

Among elderly patients, weight gain often reflects a sustained food intake in the presence of the normal, progressive fall in basal metabolic rate. Among women, a progressive weight gain occurs with pregnancy, whereas a periodic weight gain usually occurs with menstruation. Weight gain also commonly occurs in menopause.

Weight gain, a primary symptom of many endocrine disorders, also occurs with conditions that limit activity, especially cardiovascular and pulmonary disorders. It can also result from drug therapy that increases appetite or causes fluid retention and from cardiovascular, hepatic, and renal disorders that cause edema.

History and physical examination

Determine your patient's previous patterns of weight gain and loss. Does he have a family history of obesity, thyroid disease, or diabetes mellitus? Assess his eating and activity patterns. Has his appetite increased? Does he exercise regularly or at all? Next, ask about associated symptoms. Has he experienced visual disturbances, hoarseness, paresthesia, or increased urination and thirst? Has he become impotent? If the patient is female, has she had menstrual irregularities or experienced weight gain during menstruation?

Form an impression of the patient's mental status. Is he anxious or depressed? Does he respond slowly? Is his memory poor? What medications is he currently using?

During your physical examination, measure skin-fold thickness to estimate fat reserves. Note fat distribution and the presence of localized or generalized edema and overall nutritional status. Inspect for other abnormalities, such as abnormal body hair distribution or hair loss and dry skin. Take and record the patient's vital signs.

 PEDIATRIC POINTERS

- *Weight gain in children can result from endocrine disorders such as hypercortisolism.*

- *Other causes include inactivity caused by Prader-Willi syndrome, Werdnig-Hoffmann disease, Down syndrome, late stages of muscular dystrophy, and severe cerebral palsy.*
- *Nonpathologic causes include poor eating habits, sedentary recreation, and emotional problems, especially among adolescents.*

 ELDER CARE CUE

Desired weights (associated with lowest mortality rates) increase with age.

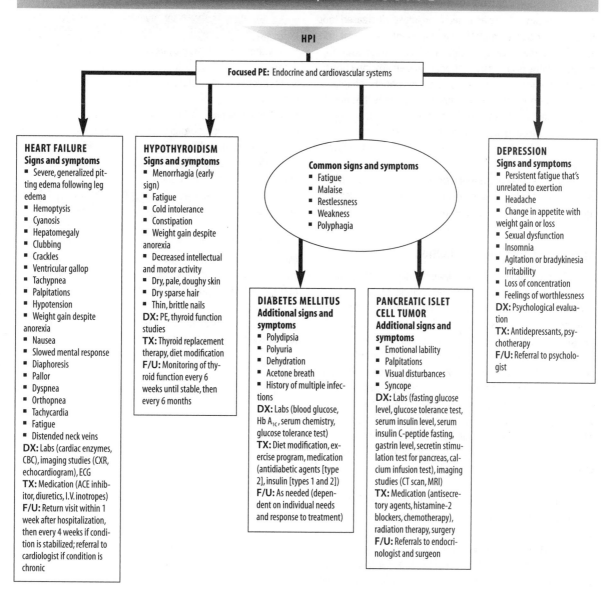

HPI

Focused PE: Endocrine and cardiovascular systems

HEART FAILURE
Signs and symptoms
- Severe, generalized pitting edema following leg edema
- Hemoptysis
- Cyanosis
- Hepatomegaly
- Clubbing
- Crackles
- Ventricular gallop
- Tachypnea
- Palpitations
- Hypotension
- Weight gain despite anorexia
- Nausea
- Slowed mental response
- Diaphoresis
- Pallor
- Dyspnea
- Orthopnea
- Tachycardia
- Fatigue
- Distended neck veins

DX: Labs (cardiac enzymes, CBC), imaging studies (CXR, echocardiogram), ECG
TX: Medication (ACE inhibitor, diuretics, I.V. inotropes)
F/U: Return visit within 1 week after hospitalization, then every 4 weeks if condition is stabilized; referral to cardiologist if condition is chronic

HYPOTHYROIDISM
Signs and symptoms
- Menorrhagia (early sign)
- Fatigue
- Cold intolerance
- Constipation
- Weight gain despite anorexia
- Decreased intellectual and motor activity
- Dry, pale, doughy skin
- Dry sparse hair
- Thin, brittle nails

DX: PE, thyroid function studies
TX: Thyroid replacement therapy, diet modification
F/U: Monitoring of thyroid function every 6 weeks until stable, then every 6 months

Common signs and symptoms
- Fatigue
- Malaise
- Restlessness
- Weakness
- Polyphagia

DIABETES MELLITUS
Additional signs and symptoms
- Polydipsia
- Polyuria
- Dehydration
- Acetone breath
- History of multiple infections

DX: Labs (blood glucose, Hb A$_{1c}$, serum chemistry, glucose tolerance test)
TX: Diet modification, exercise program, medication (antidiabetic agents [type 2], insulin [types 1 and 2])
F/U: As needed (dependent on individual needs and response to treatment)

PANCREATIC ISLET CELL TUMOR
Additional signs and symptoms
- Emotional lability
- Palpitations
- Visual disturbances
- Syncope

DX: Labs (fasting glucose level, glucose tolerance test, serum insulin level, serum insulin C-peptide fasting, gastrin level, secretin stimulation test for pancreas, calcium infusion test), imaging studies (CT scan, MRI)
TX: Medication (antisecretory agents, histamine-2 blockers, chemotherapy), radiation therapy, surgery
F/U: Referrals to endocrinologist and surgeon

DEPRESSION
Signs and symptoms
- Persistent fatigue that's unrelated to exertion
- Headache
- Change in appetite with weight gain or loss
- Sexual dysfunction
- Insomnia
- Agitation or bradykinesia
- Irritability
- Loss of concentration
- Feelings of worthlessness

DX: Psychological evaluation
TX: Antidepressants, psychotherapy
F/U: Referral to psychologist

Additional differential diagnoses: acromegaly ▪ hypercortisolism ▪ hyperinsulinism ▪ hypogonadism ▪ hypothalamic dysfunction ▪ nephrotic syndrome ▪ preeclampsia ▪ Sheehan's syndrome

---

Other causes: corticosteroids ▪ phenothiazines ▪ tricyclic antidepressants ▪ oral contraceptives ▪ cyproheptadine ▪ lithium

Weight loss, excessive

Weight loss can reflect decreased food intake, decreased food absorption, increased metabolic requirements, or a combination of the three. Its causes include endocrine, neoplastic, GI, and psychiatric disorders; nutritional deficiencies; infections; and neurologic lesions that cause paralysis and dysphagia. However, weight loss may accompany conditions that prevent sufficient food intake, such as painful oral lesions, ill-fitting dentures, and loss of teeth. It may be the metabolic sequela of poverty, fad diets, excessive exercise, and certain drugs.

Weight loss may occur as a late sign in such chronic diseases as heart failure and renal disease. In these diseases, however, it's the result of anorexia

History and physical examination

Begin with a thorough diet history because weight loss almost always is caused by inadequate caloric intake. If the patient hasn't been eating properly, try to determine why. Ask him about his previous weight and if the recent loss was intentional. Be alert to lifestyle or occupational changes that may be a source of anxiety or depression. For example, has he gotten separated or divorced? Has he recently changed jobs?

Inquire about recent changes in bowel habits, such as diarrhea or bulky, floating stools. Has the patient had nausea, vomiting, or abdominal pain, which may indicate a GI disorder? Has he had excessive thirst, excessive urination, or heat intolerance, which may signal an endocrine disorder? Take a careful drug history, noting especially any use of diet pills and laxatives.

Carefully check the patient's height and weight. Take his vital signs and note his general appearance: Is he well nourished? Do his clothes fit? Is muscle wasting evident? Ask about exact weight changes (with approximate dates).

Next, examine the patient's skin for turgor and abnormal pigmentation, especially around the joints. Does he have pallor or jaundice? Examine his mouth, including the condition of his teeth or dentures. Look for signs of infection or irritation on the roof of the mouth, and note any hyperpigmentation of the buccal mucosa. Also, check the patient's eyes for exophthalmos and his neck for swelling; evaluate his lungs for adventitious sounds. Inspect his abdomen for signs of wasting, and palpate for masses, tenderness, and an enlarged liver. Ask about any pain.

Conventional laboratory and radiologic investigations such as complete blood count, urinalysis, chest X-ray, and upper GI series usually reveal the cause. Almost all physical causes are clinically evident during the initial evaluation. Cancer, GI disorders, and depression are the most common pathologic causes.

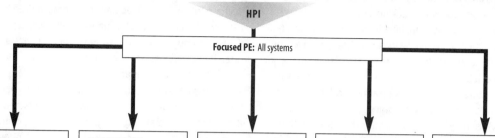

HPI

Focused PE: All systems

ADRENAL INSUFFICIENCY
Signs and symptoms
- Anorexia
- Weakness
- Fatigue
- Irritability
- Syncope
- Nausea and vomiting
- Abdominal pain
- Diarrhea or constipation
- Hyperpigmentation at the joints, beltline, palmar creases, lips, gums, tongue, and buccal mucosa
- Loss of axillary and pubic hair
- Amenorrhea

DX: Labs (CBC, BUN, creatinine, electrolytes, cortisol level, calcium, thyroid studies, adrenocorticotropic hormone stimulation test, 24-hour urinary cortisol level), imaging studies (CXR, CT scan), ECG

TX: Ventilation and circulation maintenance, medication (glucocorticoid and mineral corticoid hormone replacement therapy, electrolyte replacement), hydration, treatment of underlying condition

F/U: Referral to endocrinologist

MALIGNANCY
Signs and symptoms
- Fatigue
- Pain
- Nausea and vomiting
- Anorexia
- Abnormal bleeding
- Palpable mass (possibly)

DX: Labs (stool for occult blood, CBC with differential, UA, LFT, ESR), imaging studies (CXR, CT scan, mammogram)

TX: Varies based on the type of malignancy, diet modification, medication (analgesics, chemotherapy), radiation therapy, surgery

F/U: Referrals to oncologist and other specialist (based on type of malignancy)

DIABETES MELLITUS, TYPE 1
Signs and symptoms
- Polyphagia
- Polydipsia
- Polyuria
- Weakness
- Fatigue
- Blurred vision
- Listlessness
- Frequent infections
- Nocturnal enuresis in previously toilet-trained children
- Failure to grow

DX: Labs (serum glucose, Hb A_{1c}, postprandial serum C peptide, urine for ketones and protein)

TX: Diet modification, insulin therapy, blood glucose monitoring, teaching regarding managing hypoglycemia

F/U: Referrals to endocrinologist and diabetic counselor

ANOREXIA NERVOSA
Signs and symptoms
- Primary or secondary amenorrhea
- Emaciated appearance
- Compulsive behavior patterns
- Constipation
- Loss of scalp hair and lanugo on the face and arms
- Skeletal muscle atrophy
- Sleep disturbances

DX: Malnourished state, labs (electrolytes, CBC, renal studies, LFT, thyroid levels)

TX: Parenteral nutrition, psychological and nutritional counseling

F/U: Weekly return visits, then monthly visits if weight gain occurs; inpatient therapy if the condition doesn't improve

THYROTOXICOSIS
Signs and symptoms
- Ptosis
- Progressive exophthalmus
- Increased tearing
- Visual changes
- Lid edema
- Lid lag
- Photophobia
- Enlarged thyroid
- Nervousness
- Heat intolerance
- Tremors
- Palpitations
- Tachycardia
- Dyspnea

DX: PE, thyroid function studies, imaging studies (thyroid scan, ultrasound)

TX: Medication (antithyroid therapy, radioiodine, beta₂-adrenergic blockers)

F/U: Thyroid function testing 6 weeks after treatment is initiated, then biannually if at euthyroid state

Additional differential diagnoses: Crohn's disease ▪ cryptosporidiosis ▪ depression ▪ esophagitis ▪ gastroenteritis ▪ leukemia ▪ lymphoma ▪ pulmonary tuberculosis ▪ stomatitis ▪ thyrotoxicosis ▪ ulcerative colitis ▪ Whipple's disease

Other causes: amphetamines ▪ inappropriate dosages of thyroid preparations ▪ laxative abuse ▪ chemotherapeutic agents

Wheezing

Wheezing is an adventitious breath sound with a high-pitched, musical, squealing, creaking, or groaning quality. When wheezes (sibilant rhonchi) originate in the large airways, they can be heard by placing an unaided ear over the chest wall or at the mouth. When they originate in smaller airways, they can be heard by placing a stethoscope over the anterior or posterior chest. Unlike crackles and rhonchi, wheezes can't be cleared by coughing.

Usually, prolonged wheezing occurs during expiration when bronchi are shortened and narrowed. Causes of airway narrowing include bronchospasm; mucosal thickening or edema; partial obstruction from a tumor, a foreign body, or secretions; and extrinsic pressure, as in tension pneumothorax or goiter. With airway obstruction, wheezing occurs during inspiration.

History and physical examination

Examine the degree of the patient's respiratory distress. Is he responsive? Is he restless, confused, anxious, or afraid? Are his respirations abnormally fast, slow, shallow, or deep? Are they irregular? Can you hear wheezing through his mouth? Does he exhibit increased use of accessory muscles; increased chest wall motion; intercostal, suprasternal, or supraclavicular retractions; stridor; or nasal flaring? Take his other vital signs, noting hypotension or hypertension and an irregular, weak, rapid, or slow pulse. Institute emergency measures, if appropriate.

If the patient isn't in respiratory distress, obtain a history. What provokes his wheezing? Does he have asthma or allergies? Does he smoke or have a history of pulmonary, cardiac, or circulatory disorders? Does he have cancer? Ask about recent surgery, illness, or trauma or changes in appetite, weight, exercise tolerance, or sleep patterns. Obtain a drug history. Ask about exposure to toxic fumes or any respiratory irritants. If he has a cough, ask how it sounds, when it starts, and how often it occurs. Does he have paroxysms of coughing? Is his cough dry, sputum-producing, or bloody?

Ask the patient about chest pain. If he reports pain, determine its quality, onset, duration, intensity, and radiation. Does it increase with breathing, coughing, or certain positions?

Examine the patient's nose and mouth for congestion, drainage, or signs of infection, such as halitosis. If he produces sputum, obtain a sample for examination. Check for cyanosis, pallor, clamminess, masses, tenderness, swelling, distended neck veins, and enlarged lymph nodes. Inspect his chest for abnormal configuration and asymmetrical motion, and determine if the trachea is midline.

Percuss for dullness or hyperresonance, and auscultate for crackles, rhonchi, or pleural friction rubs. Note absent or hypoactive breath sounds, abnormal heart sounds, gallops, or murmurs. Also note arrhythmias, bradycardia, or tachycardia. (See *Evaluating breath sounds*.)

Evaluating breath sounds

Diminished or absent breath sounds indicate some interference with airflow. If pus, fluid, or air fills the pleural space, breath sounds will be quieter than normal. If a foreign body or secretions obstruct a bronchus, breath sounds will be diminished or absent over distal lung tissue. Increased thickness of the chest wall, such as with a patient who is obese or extremely muscular, may cause breath sounds to be decreased or inaudible. Absent breath sounds typically indicate loss of ventilation power.

When air passes through narrowed airways or through moisture, or when the membranes lining the chest cavity become inflamed, adventitious breath sounds will be heard. These include crackles, rhonchi, wheezes, and pleural friction rubs. Usually, these sounds indicate pulmonary disease.

Follow the auscultation sequences shown here to assess the patient's breath sounds. Have the patient take full, deep breaths, and compare sound variations from one side to the other. Note the location, timing, and character of any abnormal breath sounds.

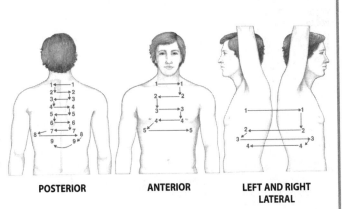

POSTERIOR   ANTERIOR   LEFT AND RIGHT LATERAL

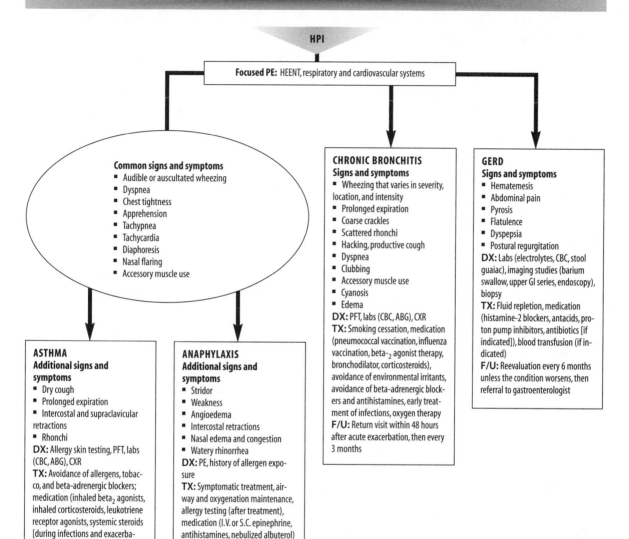

HPI

Focused PE: HEENT, respiratory and cardiovascular systems

Common signs and symptoms
- Audible or auscultated wheezing
- Dyspnea
- Chest tightness
- Apprehension
- Tachypnea
- Tachycardia
- Diaphoresis
- Nasal flaring
- Accessory muscle use

CHRONIC BRONCHITIS
Signs and symptoms
- Wheezing that varies in severity, location, and intensity
- Prolonged expiration
- Coarse crackles
- Scattered rhonchi
- Hacking, productive cough
- Dyspnea
- Clubbing
- Accessory muscle use
- Cyanosis
- Edema

DX: PFT, labs (CBC, ABG), CXR
TX: Smoking cessation, medication (pneumococcal vaccination, influenza vaccination, beta-$_2$ agonist therapy, bronchodilator, corticosteroids), avoidance of environmental irritants, avoidance of beta-adrenergic blockers and antihistamines, early treatment of infections, oxygen therapy
F/U: Return visit within 48 hours after acute exacerbation, then every 3 months

GERD
Signs and symptoms
- Hematemesis
- Abdominal pain
- Pyrosis
- Flatulence
- Dyspepsia
- Postural regurgitation

DX: Labs (electrolytes, CBC, stool guaiac), imaging studies (barium swallow, upper GI series, endoscopy), biopsy
TX: Fluid repletion, medication (histamine-2 blockers, antacids, proton pump inhibitors, antibiotics [if indicated]), blood transfusion (if indicated)
F/U: Reevaluation every 6 months unless the condition worsens, then referral to gastroenterologist

ASTHMA
Additional signs and symptoms
- Dry cough
- Prolonged expiration
- Intercostal and supraclavicular retractions
- Rhonchi

DX: Allergy skin testing, PFT, labs (CBC, ABG), CXR
TX: Avoidance of allergens, tobacco, and beta-adrenergic blockers; medication (inhaled beta$_2$ agonists, inhaled corticosteroids, leukotriene receptor agonists, systemic steroids [during infections and exacerbations]), peak expiratory flow monitoring
F/U: Reevaluation in 24 hours, then every 3 to 5 days, then every 1 to 3 months

ANAPHYLAXIS
Additional signs and symptoms
- Stridor
- Weakness
- Angioedema
- Intercostal retractions
- Nasal edema and congestion
- Watery rhinorrhea

DX: PE, history of allergen exposure
TX: Symptomatic treatment, airway and oxygenation maintenance, allergy testing (after treatment), medication (I.V. or S.C. epinephrine, antihistamines, nebulized albuterol)
F/U: Reevaluation within 24 hours

Additional differential diagnoses: aspiration of a foreign body ▪ aspiration pneumonitis ▪ bronchial adenoma ▪ bronchiectasis ▪ bronchogenic carcinoma ▪ chemical pneumonitis (acute) ▪ emphysema ▪ inhalation injury ▪ pneumothorax (tension) ▪ pulmonary coccidioidomycosis ▪ pulmonary edema ▪ pulmonary embolus ▪ pulmonary tuberculosis ▪ thyroid goiter ▪ tracheobronchitis ▪ Wegener's granulomatosis

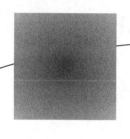

Appendices, selected references, and index

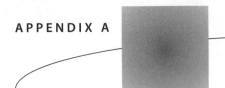

Normal laboratory test values

HEMATOLOGY

Activated partial thromboplastin time
21 to 35 seconds

Bleeding time
Duke: 1 to 3 minutes
Ivy: 3 to 6 minutes
Template: 3 to 6 minutes

Clot retraction
50% of size within 1 hour

Erythrocyte sedimentation rate
Males: 0 to 10 mm/hour
Females: 0 to 20 mm/hour

Fibrinogen, plasma
150 to 350 mg/dl

Fibrin split products
Screening assay: < 10 µg/ml
Quantitative assay: < 3 µg/ml

Hematocrit
Males: 42% to 54%
Females: 38% to 46%

Hemoglobin (Hb), total
Males: 14 to 18 g/dl
Females: 12 to 16 g/dl

Platelet aggregation
3 to 5 minutes

Platelet count
140,000 to 400,000/µl

Prothrombin consumption time
15 to 20 seconds

Prothrombin time
10 to 14 seconds

Red blood cell (RBC) count
Males: 4.5 to 6.2 million/µl venous blood
Females: 4.2 to 5.4 million/µl venous blood

Red cell indices
Mean corpuscular volume: 84 to 99 fl/cell
Mean corpuscular Hb: 26 to 32 pg/cell
Mean corpuscular Hb concentration: 30 to 36 g/dl

Reticulocyte count
0.5% to 2% of total RBC count

Sickle cell test
Negative

Thrombin time, plasma
10 to 15 seconds

White blood cell (WBC) count, blood
4,000 to 10,000/µl

WBC differential, blood
Basophils: 0.3% to 2%
Eosinophils: 0.3% to 7%
Lymphocytes: 16.2% to 43%
Monocytes: 0.6% to 9.6%
Neutrophils: 47.6% to 76.8%

Whole blood clotting time
5 to 15 minutes

Acid phosphatase
0.5 to 1.9 U/ml (based on assay method)

Alanine aminotransferase
Males: 10 to 35 U/L
Females: 9 to 24 U/L

Alkaline phosphatase, serum
Chemical inhibition method:
Males: 98 to 251 U/L
Females: 81 to 312 U/L

Amylase, serum
25 to 125 U/L

Arterial blood gases
Pao_2: 75 to 100 mm Hg
$Paco_2$: 35 to 45 mm Hg
pH: 7.35 to 7.45
Sao_2: 94% to 100%
HCO_3^-: 22 to 26 mEq/L

Aspartate aminotransferase
Males: 8 to 20 U/L
Females: 5 to 40 U/L

Bilirubin, serum
Direct: < 0.5 mg/dl
Indirect: ≤ 1.1 mg/dl

Blood urea nitrogen
8 to 20 mg/dl

Calcium, serum
Ionized: 4 to 5 mg/dl
Total: 8.9 to 10.1 mg/dl

Carbon dioxide, total, blood
22 to 34 mEq/L

Catecholamines, plasma
Supine: dopamine, 0 to 30 pg/ml; epinephrine, 0 to 110 pg/ml; norepinephrine, 70 to 750 pg/ml
Standing: dopamine, 0 to 30 pg/ml; epinephrine, 0 to 140 pg/ml; norepinephrine, 200 to 1,700 pg/ml

Chloride, serum
100 to 108 mEq/L

Cholesterol, total, serum
< 200 mg/dl (desirable)

C-reactive protein, serum
< 0.8 mg/dl

Creatine kinase (CK)
Total: males, 38 to 190 U/L; females, 10 to 150 U/L
CK-BB: None
CK-MB: < 6% of total CK
CK-MM: 90% to 100% of total CK

Creatinine, serum
Males: 0.8 to 1.2 mg/dl
Females: 0.6 to 0.9 mg/dl

Free thyroxine
0.8 to 3.3 ng/dl

Free triiodothyronine
0.2 to 0.6 ng/dl

Gamma-glutamyl transferase
Males: 6 to 38 U/L
Females: younger than age 45, 4 to 27 U/L; older than age 45, 6 to 37 U/L

Glucose, fasting, plasma
70 to 110 mg/dl

Glucose, plasma, oral tolerance
Peak at 160 to 180 mg/dl 30 to 60 minutes after challenge dose

Glucose, plasma, 2-hour postprandial
< 145 mg/dl

Iron, serum
Males: 70 to 150 µg/dl
Females: 80 to 150 µg/dl

Lactic acid, blood
0.93 to 1.65 mEq/L

Lactic dehydrogenase (LD)
Total: 35 to 378 U/L
LD1: 14% to 26% of total
LH2: 29% to 39% of total
LH3: 20% to 26% of total
LH4: 8% to 16% of total
LH5: 6% to 16% of total

Lipase
< 300 U/L

Lipoproteins, serum
High-density lipoprotein cholesterol:
Males: 37 to 70 mg/dl;
Females: 40 to 85 mg/dl

Low-density lipoprotein cholesterol:
Patients without coronary artery disease (CAD): < 130 mg/dl (desirable)
Patients with CAD: < 100 mg/dl (desirable)

Magnesium, serum
1.5 to 2.5 mEq/L
Atomic absorption: 1.7 to 2.1 mg/dl

Phosphates, serum
1.8 to 2.6 mEq/L
Atomic absorption: 2.5 to 4.5 mg/dl

Potassium, serum
3.8 to 5.5 mEq/L

Protein, total, serum
6.6 to 7.9 g/dl
Albumin fraction: 3.3 to 4.5 g/dl
Globulin level: Alpha$_1$ globulin, 0.1 to 0.4 g/dl; alpha$_2$ globulin, 0.5 to 1 g/dl; beta globulin, 0.7 to 1.2 g/dl; gamma globulin, 0.5 to 1.6 g/dl

Sodium, serum
135 to 145 mEq/L

Thyroxine, total, serum
5 to 13.5 µg/dl

Triglycerides, serum
Males: 40 to 160 mg/dl
Females: 35 to 135 mg/dl

Troponin I
0 to 0.4 µg/ml

Uric acid, serum
Males: 4.3 to 8 mg/dl
Females: 2.3 to 6 mg/dl

URINE CHEMISTRY

Amylase
10 to 80 U/hour

Bilirubin
Negative

Calcium
Males: < 275 mg/24 hours
Females: < 250 mg/24 hours

Catecholamines
dopamine: 0 to 400 µl/24 hours
epinephrine: 0 to 20 µl/24 hours
norepinephrine: 0 to 80 µl/24 hours

Creatinine
Males: 800 to 2,000 mg/24 hours
Females: 600 to 1,800 mg/24 hours

Creatinine clearance
Males (age 20): 85 to 146 ml/minute/1.73 m^2
Females (age 20): 81 to 134 ml/minute/1.73 m^2

Glucose
Negative

17-Hydroxycorticosteroids
Males: 4.5 to 12 mg/24 hours
Females: 2.5 to 10 mg/24 hours

17-Ketogenic steroids
Males: 4 to 14 mg/24 hours
Females: 2 to 12 mg/24 hours

Ketones
Negative

17-Ketosteroids
Males: 6 to 21 mg/24 hours
Females: 4 to 17 mg/24 hours

Proteins
up to 150 mg/24 hours

Sodium
30 to 280 mEq/24 hours

URINE CHEMISTRY *(continued)*

Urea
Maximal clearance: 64 to 99 ml/minute

Uric acid
250 to 750 mg/24 hours

Urinalysis, routine
Color: Straw to dark yellow
Odor: Slightly aromatic
Appearance: Clear
Specific gravity: 1.005 to 1.035
pH: 4.5 to 8
Protein: None
Glucose: None
Epithelial cells: 0 to 5
Casts: None, except occasional hyaline casts
Crystals: Present
Yeast cells: None

Urine concentration
Specific gravity:
Concentrated: 1.025 to 1.030+
Dilute: 1.001 to 1.010

Urine osmolality
50 to 1,400 mOsm/kg water

Urobilinogen
Males: 0.3 to 2.1 Ehrlich U/2 hours
Females: 0.1 to 1.1 Ehrlich U/2 hours

Vanillylmandelic acid
0.7 to 6.8 mg/24 hours

MISCELLANEOUS

Cerebrospinal fluid
Pressure: 50 to 180 mm water

Enzyme-linked immunosorbent assay for human immunodeficiency virus infection
Negative

HIVAGEN test
Negative

Lupus erythematosus cell preparation
Negative

Occult blood, fecal
< 2.5 ml

Rheumatoid factor, serum
Negative

Urobilinogen, fecal
50 to 300 mg/24 hours

Venereal Disease Research Laboratory test, serum
Negative

Western blot assay
Negative

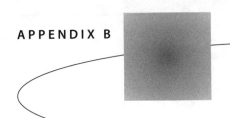

X-ray interpretation

When a radiologist assesses X-ray film, it's usually to find an answer to a particular problem or question. Examples include whether a chest tube or central line is positioned correctly, whether there's fluid in the lungs, and whether the bowel loops are distended.

Comparing an X-ray film with previous films is helpful, particularly when assessing progression of a clinical situation, such as pneumonia or pneumothorax. The patient's position when the film is taken should be noted. An anteroposterior (AP) versus a posteroanterior (PA) projection can change the apparent size of a structure because of its distance from the X-ray source. For example, the heart may appear enlarged in an AP projection because it was closer to the X-ray tube and farther from the film when exposed.

A decubitus film may be a more accurate projection for assessing fluid levels in the abdomen because the fluid is in a dependent position. Likewise, the quality and diagnostic usefulness of a portable film taken in a semi-upright position versus a full upright position are compromised because of fluid collecting in layers posteriorly and because the lungs aren't fully expanded. In many cases, the health care worker on the patient's unit decides whether the film is made in or out of the radiology department. Although it may be more convenient not to transport the patient, PA and lateral films taken in the radiology department ensure higher quality and greater diagnostic accuracy.

Differences in film quality, sharpness of detail, patient motion and positioning, and the lightness and darkness of structures can affect the diagnostic usefulness of an X-ray.

An X-ray should be considered a tool to aid the clinician in confirming a diagnosis or clinical finding. Wheezes or crackles in the lung bases heard on auscultation may be confirmed by the presence of fluid-filled, dense areas seen on a chest X-ray. In many cases, however, a standard X-ray can't give the clinician all the information needed to make a diagnosis. The clinician may then use another imaging modality to view anatomy or identify a pathologic process.

Normal chest X-ray

Bony and soft landmarks in this normal chest and upper abdomen X-ray stand out in this posteroanterior view.

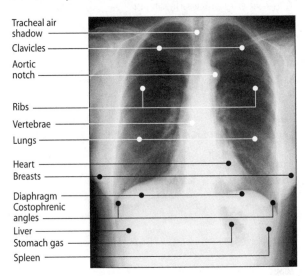

Tracheal air shadow
Clavicles
Aortic notch
Ribs
Vertebrae
Lungs
Heart
Breasts
Diaphragm
Costophrenic angles
Liver
Stomach gas
Spleen

Foreign object in lung

The child in these X-rays has inhaled an object, which has lodged in the left bronchus. The AP chest X-ray taken during inspiration appears normal. An X-ray taken during expiration shows the effect of the foreign object. Trapped air has hyperinflated the left lung ➤. The mediastinum has shifted right ➤ and, compared to the inspiratory X-ray, the dark air-filled area on the left has become more lucent.

INSPIRATION

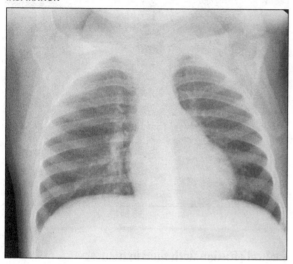

EXPIRATION

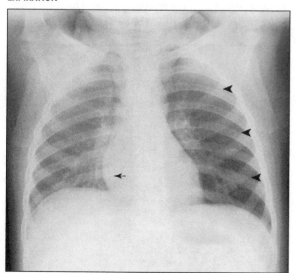

Heart valve replacement

This lateral chest X-ray taken after surgery to replace a defective heart valve shows the new valve in place ➤. It also shows a pleural effusion ➡.

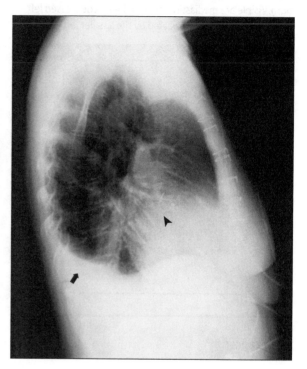

Lobar pneumonia

Typical signs of lobar pneumonia that involves the left lower lobe ➡ are apparent in this chest X-ray. Borders of the heart shadow and the left hemidiaphragm are hidden (silhouette sign). Visible are mediastinal shift to the left, depressed left hilum, and atelectasis (indicated by the smaller left lung) ➤.

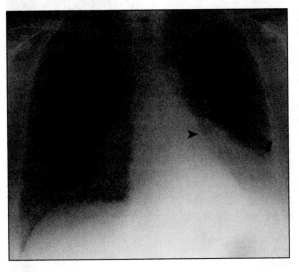

Pleural effusion

This PA chest X-ray of a patient with heart failure reveals pleural effusion. The right costophrenic angle is blunted by pleural fluid, and the upper border of the pleural fluid ▷ is concave.

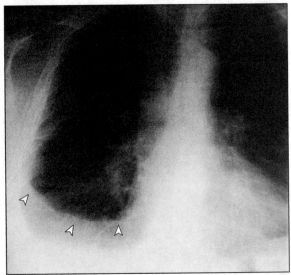

Lung cancer

In this chest X-ray, bronchogenic lung cancer shows up as a large mass ➡ with central cavitation ➤ in the right hilar area. Opacity of the right lower lobe indicates atelectasis caused by the tumor.

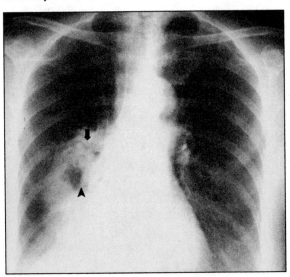

Pleural effusion with fluid in fissures

This lateral chest X-ray clearly demonstrates pleural fluid in the lung fissures ▷. These fissures, the spaces between the lung lobes, have been widened by the fluid.

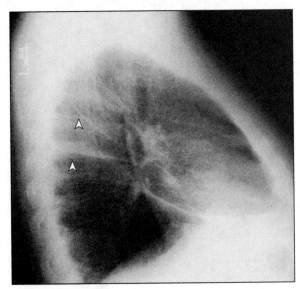

Pneumothorax with subcutaneous emphysema

This PA chest X-ray shows a pneumothorax as well as subcutaneous and mediastinal emphysema ⇢. Because the chest tube ⇨ has migrated outside the pleural space, the pneumothorax ▷ is larger than it was originally.

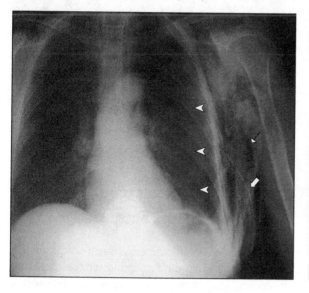

Rib fractures

This AP chest X-ray of a trauma patient shows lateral fractures of the fifth → and sixth ➡ ribs on the left side. Displacement and associated fractures of the left clavicle ➤ and left scapula ➤ have created separation at the fracture sites.

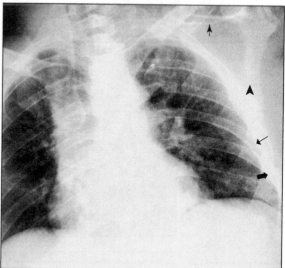

Pulmonary changes with asthma

The effects of asthma are apparent in this PA chest X-ray. The lungs ➤ are hyperinflated, the heart ▷ small, and the diaphragm ⇨ depressed.

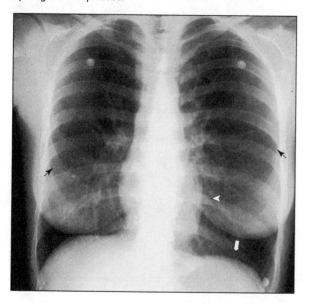

Bone tumor

A well-defined, eccentric, bubbly expansile tumor ▷ in the distal femoral diaphysis is clear in this plain X-ray.

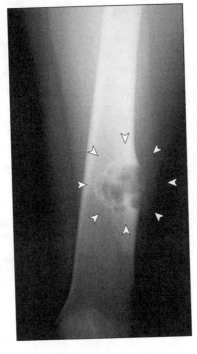

Osteoarthritis of the knee

This plain X-ray of a right knee shows narrowing of the medial joint space ➤ and mild osteophyte formation ▷.

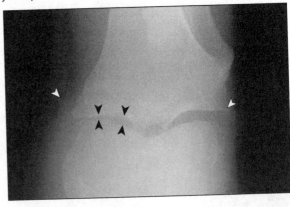

Leg fractures

This AP X-ray of the left leg and ankle shows the results of trauma. Visible are an oblique, comminuted fracture of the tibia ➤ and lateral displacement of distal parts as well as a comminuted avulsion-type fracture of the medial malleolus ➡.

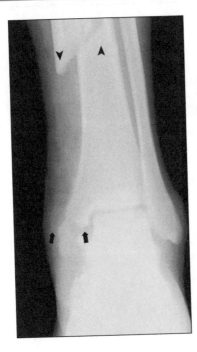

Rheumatoid arthritis of the hand

This plain X-ray of the left hand shows classic signs of advanced rheumatoid arthritis. Periarticular soft tissue swelling ➤ is evident as are many erosions involving the distal ulna, carpals, metacarpals, and phalanges ▷. Joint spaces are narrowed. In addition, periarticular osteoporosis encircles the metacarpal and phalangeal joints ✳.

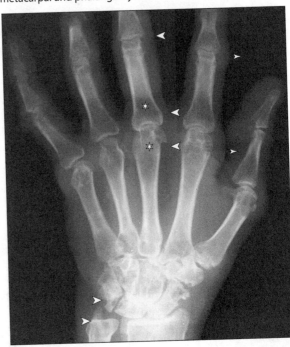

Rotator cuff tear and meniscal tear

The shoulder shown in this magnetic resonance imaging (MRI) scan (top right), clearly has a torn right rotator cuff ▷.

In the sagittal MRI image (bottom right), an oblique tear ➤ is evident in the posterior horn of the medial meniscus.

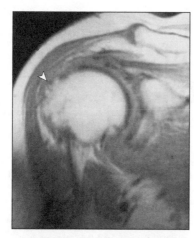

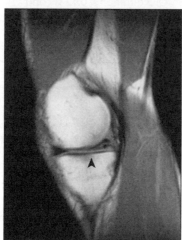

Small-bowel obstruction

In this plain abdominal X-ray, dilated, gas-filled bowel loops ▷ and a lack of colon gas indicate an obstruction of the small bowel.

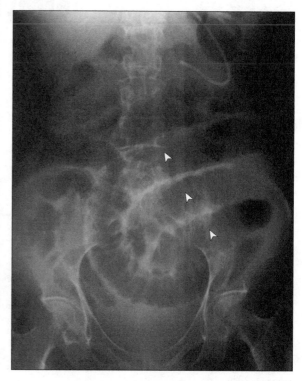

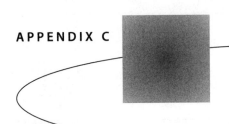

Types of cardiac arrhythmias

Use a standard electrocardiogram strip, if available, to compare normal cardiac rhythm configurations with the rhythm strips depicted here. (Note the various features, causes, and treatments of these common cardiac arrhythmias.) Characteristics of normal rhythm include :

- ventricular and atrial rates of 60 to 100 beats/minute
- regular and uniform QRS complexes and P waves
- PR interval of 0.12 to 0.20 second
- QRS duration < 0.12 second
- identical atrial and ventricular rates, with a constant PR interval.

ARRHYTHMIA AND FEATURES	CAUSES	TREATMENT
Sinus arrhythmia 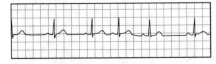 ▪ Irregular atrial and ventricular rhythms ▪ Normal P wave preceding each QRS complex	▪ Normal variation of normal sinus rhythm for athletes, children, and elderly people ▪ Also seen in digoxin toxicity and inferior wall myocardial infarction (MI)	▪ Atropine (0.5 to 1 mg I.V. push, repeated every 3 to 5 minutes to maximum of 2 mg) if rate decreases below 40 beats/minute and patient is symptomatic (for example, has hypotension)
Sinus tachycardia 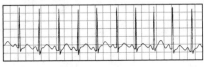 ▪ Atrial and ventricular rates regular ▪ Rate > 100 beats/minute; rarely, > 160 beats/minute ▪ Normal P wave preceding each QRS complex	▪ Normal physiologic response to fever, exercise, anxiety, pain, dehydration; may also accompany shock, left-sided heart failure, cardiac tamponade, hyperthyroidism, anemia, hypovolemia, pulmonary embolism, anterior wall MI ▪ May also occur with atropine, epinephrine, isoproterenol, quinidine, caffeine, alcohol, and nicotine use	▪ Correction of underlying cause
Sinus bradycardia 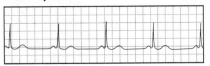 ▪ Regular atrial and ventricular rates ▪ Rate < 60 beats/minute ▪ Normal P wave preceding each QRS complex	▪ Normal in a well-conditioned heart, as in an athlete ▪ Increased intracranial pressure; increased vagal tone due to straining during defecation, vomiting, intubation, mechanical ventilation; sick sinus syndrome; hypothyroidism; inferior wall MI ▪ May also occur with anticholinesterase, beta-adrenergic blocker, digoxin, or morphine use	▪ For low cardiac output, dizziness, weakness, altered level of consciousness, or low blood pressure: atropine (0.5 to 1 mg I.V. push, repeated every 3 to 5 minutes to maximum of 2 mg) ▪ Temporary or permanent pacemaker ▪ Dopamine (5 to 20 mg/kg/minute) ▪ Epinephrine (2 to 10 mg/minute)

ARRHYTHMIA AND FEATURES	CAUSES	TREATMENT

Sinoatrial (SA) arrest or block *(sinus arrest)*

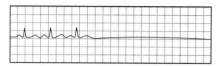

- Atrial and ventricular rhythms normal except for missing complex
- Normal P wave preceding each QRS complex
- Pause not equal to a multiple of the previous sinus rhythm

Causes:
- Acute infection
- Coronary artery disease (CAD), degenerative heart disease, acute inferior wall MI
- Vagal stimulation, Valsalva's maneuver, carotid sinus massage
- Digoxin, quinidine, or salicylate toxicity
- Pesticide poisoning
- Pharyngeal irritation caused by endotracheal intubation
- Sick sinus syndrome

Treatment:
- I.V. atropine (0.5 to 1 mg I.V. push, repeated every 3 to 5 minutes to maximum of 2 mg)
- Temporary or permanent pacemaker for repeated episodes

Wandering atrial pacemaker

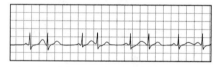

- Atrial and ventricular rates that vary slightly
- Irregular PR interval
- P waves irregular with changing configuration, indicating that they aren't all from SA node or single atrial focus; may appear after QRS complexes
- QRS complexes uniform in shape but irregular in rhythm

Causes:
- Rheumatic carditis due to inflammation involving the SA node
- Digoxin toxicity
- Sick sinus syndrome

Treatment:
- None necessary if patient is asymptomatic
- Treatment of underlying cause if patient is symptomatic

Premature atrial contraction *(PAC)*

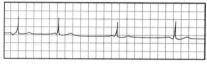

- Premature, abnormal-looking P waves that differ in configuration from normal P waves
- QRS complexes after P waves, except in very early or blocked PACs
- P wave often buried in the preceding T wave or identified in the preceding T wave

Causes:
- Coronary or valvular heart disease, atrial ischemia, coronary atherosclerosis, heart failure, acute respiratory failure, chronic obstructive pulmonary disease (COPD), electrolyte imbalance, and hypoxia
- Digoxin toxicity; use of aminophylline, beta-adrenergic blockers, or caffeine
- Anxiety

Treatment:
- None (usually)
- Treatment of underlying cause

Paroxysmal atrial tachycardia *(paroxysmal supraventricular tachycardia)*

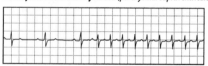

- Atrial and ventricular rates regular
- Heart rate > 160 beats/minute; rarely exceeds 250 beats/minute
- P waves regular but aberrant; difficult to differentiate from preceding T wave
- P wave preceding each QRS complex
- Sudden onset and termination of arrhythmia

Causes:
- Intrinsic abnormality of AV conduction system
- Physical or psychological stress, hypoxia, hypokalemia, cardiomyopathy, congenital heart disease, MI, valvular disease, Wolff-Parkinson-White syndrome, cor pulmonale, hyperthyroidism, systemic hypertension
- Digoxin toxicity; use of caffeine, marijuana, or central nervous system stimulants

Treatment:
- If patient is unstable, immediate cardioversion
- If patient is stable, vagal stimulation, Valsalva's maneuver, carotid sinus massage
- Adenosine (6 mg) by rapid I.V. bolus injection to rapidly convert arrhythmia
- If cardiac function is preserved: advanced cardiac life support (ACLS) treatment priority — calcium channel blocker, digoxin, and cardioversion; then possibly procainamide, amiodarone, or sotolol
- If ejection fraction is < 40% or the patient is in heart failure: ACLS treatment order — digoxin, amiodarone, and then diltiazem

ARRHYTHMIA AND FEATURES	CAUSES	TREATMENT

Atrial flutter

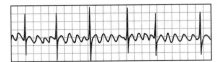

- Atrial rhythm regular rate; 250 to 400 beats/minute
- Ventricular rate variable, depending on degree of atrioventricular (AV) block (usually 60 to 100 beats/minute)
- Sawtooth P-wave configuration possible (F waves)
- QRS complexes uniform in shape but often irregular in rate

- Heart failure, tricuspid or mitral valve disease, pulmonary embolism, cor pulmonale, inferior wall MI, carditis
- Digoxin toxicity

- If patient is unstable with a ventricular rate > 150 beats/minute, immediate cardioversion
- If atrial flutter lasts > 48 hours and heart function is normal: calcium channel blocker or beta-adrenergic blocker to control rate
- If atrial flutter lasts < 48 hours and heart function is normal: amiodarone, ibutilide, flecainide, propafenone, or procainamide to convert rhythm
- If atrial flutter lasts > 48 hours and heart function is impaired: digoxin, diltiazem, or amiodarone, if appropriate
- Possibly synchronized cardioversion and anticoagulation therapy

Atrial fibrillation (AF)

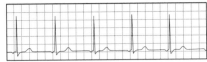

- Atrial rhythm grossly irregular; rate > 400 beats/minute
- Ventricular rate grossly irregular
- QRS complexes of uniform configuration and duration
- PR interval indiscernible
- No P waves, or P waves that appear as erratic, irregular, baseline fibrillary waves

- Heart failure, COPD, thyrotoxicosis, constrictive pericarditis, ischemic heart disease, sepsis, pulmonary embolus, rheumatic heart disease, hypertension, mitral stenosis, atrial irritation, complication of coronary bypass or valve replacement surgery

- If AF lasts > 48 hours and heart function is normal: calcium channel blocker or beta-adrenergic blocker to control rate
- If AF lasts < 48 hours and heart function is normal: amiodarone, ibutilide, flecainide, propafenone, or procainamide to convert rhythm
- In AF lasts > 48 hours and heart function is impaired: digoxin, diltiazem, or amiodarone
- Possibly elective cardioversion for rapid ventricular rate and anticoagulation therapy
- Treatment of underlying cause

Junctional rhythm

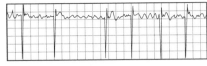

- Atrial and ventricular rates regular
- Atrial rate 40 to 60 beats/minute
- Ventricular rate usually 40 to 60 beats/minute (60 to 100 beats/minute is accelerated junctional rhythm)
- P waves preceding, hidden within (absent), or after QRS complex; usually inverted if visible
- PR interval (when present) < 0.12 second
- QRS complex configuration and duration normal, except in aberrant conduction

- Inferior wall MI or ischemia, hypoxia, vagal stimulation, sick sinus syndrome
- Acute rheumatic fever
- Valve surgery
- Digoxin toxicity

- Atropine (0.5 to 1 mg I.V. push, repeated every 3 to 5 minutes to maximum of 2 mg) for symptomatic slow rate
- Pacemaker insertion if patient is refractory to drugs
- Discontinuation of digoxin, if appropriate

Junctional contractions (junctional premature beats)

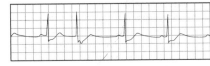

- Atrial and ventricular rhythms irregular
- P waves inverted; may precede, be hidden within, or follow QRS complexes
- PR interval < 0.12 second if P wave precedes QRS complex
- QRS complex configuration and duration normal

- MI or ischemia
- Digoxin toxicity and excessive caffeine or amphetamine use

- Correction of underlying cause
- None (usually)

ARRHYTHMIA AND FEATURES	CAUSES	TREATMENT

First-degree AV block

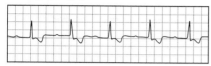

- Atrial and ventricular rhythms regular
- PR interval > 0.20 second
- P wave preceding each QRS complex
- QRS complex normal

- May be seen in a healthy person
- Inferior wall myocardial ischemia or MI, hypo-thyroidism, hypokalemia, hyperkalemia
- Digoxin toxicity; use of quinidine, procainamide, or propranolol

- Cautious use of digoxin
- Correction of underlying cause
- Possibly atropine (0.5 to 1 mg I.V. push, repeated every 3 to 5 minutes to maximum of 2 mg) if PR interval exceeds 0.26 second or bradycardia develops

Second-degree AV block *Mobitz I (Wenckebach)*

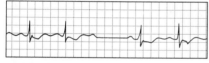

- Atrial rhythm regular
- Ventricular rhythm irregular
- Atrial rate exceeds ventricular rate
- PR interval progressively, but only slightly, longer with each cycle until QRS complex disappears (dropped beat); PR interval shorter after dropped beat

- Inferior wall MI, cardiac surgery, acute rheumatic fever, and vagal stimulation
- Digoxin toxicity; use of propranolol, quinidine, or procainamide

- Treatment of underlying cause
- Atropine (0.5 to 1 mg I.V. push, repeated every 3 to 5 minutes to maximum of 2 mg) or temporary pacemaker for symptomatic bradycardia
- Discontinuation of digoxin, if appropriate

Second-degree AV block *Mobitz II*

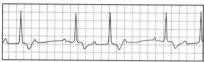

- Atrial rate regular
- Ventricular rhythm regular or irregular, with varying degree of block
- P-P interval constant
- QRS complexes periodically absent

- Severe CAD, anterior wall MI, acute myocarditis
- Digoxin toxicity

- Atropine (0.5 to 1 mg I.V. push repeated every 3 to 5 minutes to a maximum of 2 mg) for symptomatic bradycardia
- Temporary or permanent pacemaker
- Discontinuation of digoxin, if appropriate

Third-degree AV block *(complete heart block)*

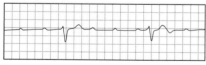

- Atrial rate regular
- Ventricular rate slow and regular
- No relation between P waves and QRS complexes
- No constant PR interval
- QRS interval normal (nodal pacemaker) or wide and bizarre (ventricular pacemaker)

- Inferior or anterior wall MI, congenital abnor-mality, rheumatic fever, hypoxia, postoperative complication of mitral valve replacement, Lev's disease (fibrosis and calcification that spreads from cardiac structures to the conductive tissue), Lenègre's disease (conductive tissue fibrosis)
- Digoxin toxicity

- Atropine (0.5 to 1 mg I.V. push repeated every 3 to 5 minutes to a maximum of 2 mg) for symptomatic bradycardia
- Temporary or permanent pacemaker
- Discontinuation of digoxin, if appropriate

ARRHYTHMIA AND FEATURES	CAUSES	TREATMENT

Junctional tachycardia

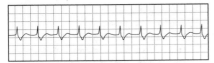

- Atrial rate > 100 beats/minute; however, P wave may be absent, hidden in QRS complex, or preceding T wave
- Ventricular rate > 100 beats/minute
- P wave inverted
- QRS complex configuration and duration normal
- Onset of rhythm often sudden, occurring in bursts

- Myocarditis, cardiomyopathy, inferior wall MI or ischemia, acute rheumatic fever, complication of valve replacement surgery
- Digoxin toxicity

- If patient is stable, vagal stimulation
- Adenosine (6 mg) by rapid I.V. bolus injection to convert arrhythmia
- If heart function is preserved: ACLS guidelines for amiodarone, calcium channel blocker, or beta-adrenergic blocker
- If ejection fraction is < 40% or the patient is in heart failure: ACLS guidelines for amiodarone

Premature ventricular contraction (PVC)

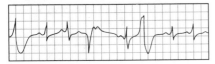

- Atrial rate regular
- Ventricular rate irregular
- QRS complex premature, usually followed by a complete compensatory pause
- QRS complex wide and distorted, usually > 0.14 second
- Premature QRS complexes occurring singly, in pairs, or in threes; alternating with normal beats; focus from one or more sites
- Ominous when clustered, multifocal, and with R wave on T pattern

- Heart failure; old or acute myocardial ischemia, MI, or contusion; myocardial irritation by ventricular catheter, such as a pacemaker; hypercapnia; hypokalemia, hypocalcemia
- Drug toxicity (cardiac glycosides, aminophylline, tricyclic antidepressants, beta-adrenergic blockers [isoproterenol or dopamine])
- Caffeine, tobacco, or alcohol use
- Psychological stress, anxiety, pain, exercise

- If symptomatic, lidocaine (1 to 1.5 mg/kg I.V. bolus, followed by continuous infusion 1 to 4 mg/minute), or procainamide (50 to 100 mg slow I.V. push up to 500 mg, followed by continuous infusion of 1 to 6 mg/minute)
- Treatment of underlying cause
- Discontinuation of drug causing toxicity
- Potassium chloride (40 mg rider) I.V. if PVC induced by hypokalemia

Ventricular tachycardia

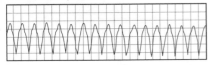

- Ventricular rate 140 to 220 beats/minute, regular or irregular
- QRS complexes wide, bizarre, and independent of P waves
- P waves not discernible
- May start and stop suddenly

- Myocardial ischemia, MI, or aneurysm; CAD; rheumatic heart disease; mitral valve prolapse; heart failure; cardiomyopathy; ventricular catheters; hypokalemia; hypercalcemia; pulmonary embolism
- Digoxin, procainamide, epinephrine, or quinidine toxicity
- Anxiety

- Cardioversion at any time to convert the rhythm
- If rhythm is monomorphic VT with normal heart function: procainamide or sotalol, amiodarone, and lidocaine
- If rhythm is monomorphic VT with impaired heart function: amiodarone or lidocaine; then synchronized cardioversion to convert rhythm
- If rhythm is polymorphic VT with normal baseline QT interval: treatment of ischemia, correction of electrolytes and, if appropriate, beta-adrenergic blocker, lidocaine, amiodarone, procainamide, or sotalol
- If rhythm is polymorphic VT with prolonged baseline QT interval (suggesting torsades de pointes): correction of electrolytes and magnesium, overdrive pacing, isoproterenol, phenytoin, or lidocaine
- Cardiopulmonary resuscitation (CPR), following ACLS protocol, if pulses are absent

ARRHYTHMIA AND FEATURES	CAUSES	TREATMENT

Ventricular fibrillation

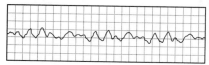

- Ventricular rhythm rapid and chaotic
- QRS complexes wide and irregular; no visible P waves

- Myocardial ischemia, MI, R-on-T phenomenon, untreated ventricular tachycardia, hypokalemia, hyperkalemia, hypercalcemia, alkalosis, electric shock, hypothermia
- Digoxin, epinephrine, or quinidine toxicity

- CPR, following ACLS protocol
- Defibrillation X 3 shocks
- Epinephrine or vasopressin followed by defibrillation
- Possibly antiarrhythmics (amiodarone, lidocaine, magnesium, or procainamide) and then defibrillation
- Possibly buffers
- Treatment of underlying cause

Asystole

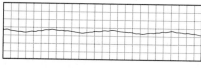

- No atrial or ventricular rate or rhythm
- No discernible P waves, QRS complexes, or T waves

- Myocardial ischemia, MI, aortic valve disease, heart failure, hypoxemia, hypokalemia, severe acidosis, electric shock, ventricular arrhythmias, AV block, pulmonary embolism, heart rupture, cardiac tamponade, hyperkalemia, electromechanical dissociation
- Cocaine overdose

- CPR, following ACLS protocol
- Transcutaneous pacemaker
- Treatment of underlying cause
- Epinephrine (1 mg I.V. push repeated every 3 to 5 minutes)
- Atropine (1 mg I.V. repeated every 3 to 5 minutes to a maximum of 0.04 mg/kg)

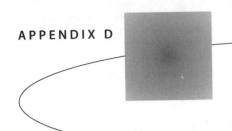

Resources for professionals, patients, and caregivers

General health care Web sites

- *www.healthfinder.gov* — from the U.S. government; searchable database with links to Web sites, support groups, government agencies, and not-for-profit organizations that provide health care information for patients
- *www.healthweb.org/* — from a group of librarians and information professionals at academic medical centers in the midwestern United States; offers searchable database of evaluated Web sites for patients and health care professionals
- *www.medmatrix.org/reg/login.asp* — includes journal articles, abstracts, reviews, conference highlights, and links to other major sources for health care professionals
- *www.mwsearch.com* — named Medical World Search, this site searches thousands of selected medical sites

Organizations

- American Academy of Family Physicians — includes "Family Medicine Online," offering handouts and other resources to patients and health care professionals, plus links to other sites: *www.aafp.com*
- Joint Commission on Accreditation of Healthcare Organizations (JCAHO): *www.jcaho.org*

Government agencies

- Agency for Healthcare Research and Quality (AHRQ)/National Guideline Clearinghouse: *www.ahcpr.gov;* TDD, 888-586-6340, hearing impaired only
- Centers for Medicare & Medicaid Services (formerly HCFA): *www.hcfa.gov*

- Centers for Disease Control and Prevention — check under "Topics A to Z": *www.cdc.gov*
- U.S. Department of Health & Human Services (DHHS): *www.dhhs.gov*
- Food and Drug Administration: *www.fda.gov*
- National Center for Complementary and Alternative Medicine: *www.nccam.nih.gov*
- Specialized Information Services/U.S. Government Resources (online listing of government bureaus with links to their sites): *www.sis.nlm.nih.gov/tehwwg.cfm*

Links to Spanish-language sites

- Agency for Healthcare Research and Quality (AHRQ): *www.ahcpr.gov* (click on Información en español)
- CANCERCare, Inc.: *www.cancercare.org* (click on Información en español)
- CancerNet: *www.cancernet.nci.nih.gov/sp_menu.htm*
- Healthfinder: *www.healthfinder.gov* (click on español)
- Immunization Action Coalition, Screening Questionnaire for Adult Immunization: *www.immunize.org* (click on Spanish)

Condition-specific sites

Aging
- Administration on Aging: *www.aoa.dhhs.gov*
- American Society on Aging (ASA): *www.asaging.org*
- National Institute on Aging: *www.nih.gov/nia;* 800-222-2225; TTY, 800-222-4225

AIDS/HIV/STDs
- CDC National Prevention Information Network: *www.cdcnpin.org*

- HIV/AIDS Treatment Information Service (ATIS); *www.sis.nlm.nih.gov/aids/aidstrea.html* or *www.hivatis.org;* 800-TRIALS-A (874-2572); 800-448-0440 (Spanish available); TTY, 888-430-3739
- *JAMA* Women's Health Sexually Transmitted Disease Information Center: *www.amaassn.org/special/std/std.htm*
- National AIDS Hotline (24 hours): 800-342-AIDS; Spanish, 800-344-SIDA; TTY, 800-243-7889
- Office of AIDS Research (OAR): *www.sis.nlm.nih.gov/aids/oar.html*

Allergies and Asthma
- Allergy & Asthma Disease Management Center: *www.aaaai.org/aadmc*
- Allergy & Asthma Network — Mothers of Asthmatics, Inc.: *www.aanma.org;* 800-878-4403
- Allergy, Asthma & Immunology Online: *www.allergy.mcg.edu*
- American Academy of Allergy Asthma & Immunology: *www.aaaai.org;* 800-822-2762
- Global Initiative For Asthma: *www.ginasthma.com*
- Joint Council of Allergy, Asthma and Immunology: *www.jcaai.org*
- National Asthma Education and Prevention Program: *www.nhlbi.nih.gov/nhlbi/othcomp/opec/naepp/naeppage.htm*
- National Institute of Allergy and Infectious Diseases: *www.niaid.nih.gov*

Alzheimer's disease
- Agency for Healthcare Research and Quality (AHRQ) Early Alzheimer's Disease/Clinical Practice Guideline/Patient and Family Guide: *www.ahcpr.gov/clinic/alzcons.htm*
- AHRQ's Recognition and Assessment Guideline: *www.ahcpr.gov/clinic/alzover.htm*
- Alzheimer Europe: *www.alzheimer-europe.org*
- Alzheimer's Association: *www.alz.org;* 800-272-3900
- Alzheimer's Disease Education & Referral (ADEAR) Center: *www.alzheimers.org;* 800-438-4380
- AlzWell Caregiver Page: *www.alzwell.com*

Arthritis
- American Autoimmune Related Diseases Association, Inc. (AARDA): *www.aarda.org/*
- American College of Rheumatology: *www.rheumatology.org*
- Arthritis Foundation: *www.arthritis.org;* 800-283-7800

- National Institute of Arthritis and Musculoskeletal and Skin Diseases: *www.nih.gov/niams*

Attention deficit disorder/hyperactivity
- National Attention Deficit Disorder Association (ADDA): *www.add.org*

Cancer
- American Cancer Society (ACS): *www.cancer.org;* 800-ACS-2345
- CANCERCare, Inc.: *www.cancercare.org;* 800-813-HOPE
- CANCERLit Topic Searches (National Cancer Institute): *www.cnetdb.nci.nih.gov/cancerlit.shtml*
- CancerNet (National Cancer Institute): *www.cancernet.nci.nih.gov*
- Cancer News on the Net: *www.cancernews.com*
- Cancer Trials — National Cancer Institute: *cancertrials.nci.nih.gov*
- National Breast Cancer Awareness Month: *www.nbcam.org*
- National Cancer Institute, International Cancer Information Center: 800-4-CANCER or 800-422-6237
- National Center for Chronic Disease Prevention and Health Promotion: *www.cdc.gov/nccdphp/cancer.htm*
- National Comprehensive Cancer Network: *www.nccn.org*
- Susan G. Komen Breast Cancer Foundation: 800-462-9273
- Y-Me National Breast Cancer Organization: *www.y-me.org;* 800-221-2141; 800-986-9505 (Español)

Cardiac
- American Heart Association: *www.americanheart.org;* 800-242-8721
- Mayo Health Oasis Heart Resource Center: *www.mayohealth.org*
- National Heart, Lung, and Blood Institute: *www.nhlbi.nih.gov*
- National Stroke Association; 800-STROKES

Diabetes
- American Association of Diabetes Educators (AADE): *www.aadenet.org;* 800-338-3633
- American Diabetes Association: *www.diabetes.org*
- Diabetes self-care equipment for the visually impaired: Palco Labs, Inc.: *www.palcolabs.com;* 800-346-4488,
- Joslin Diabetes Center: *www.joslin.harvard.edu/wlist.html*

- National Institute of Diabetes & Digestive & Kidney Diseases: *www.niddk.nih.gov*

Disabilities
- University of Virginia: General Resources About Disabilities: *www.curry.edschool.virginia.edu/go/cise/ose/resources/general.html*; Assistive Technology Resources, *www.curry.edschool.virginia.edu/go/cise/ose/resources/asst_tech.html*

Elder abuse
- National Center for Crime Victims: *www.nvc.org*
- National Center on Elder Abuse (NCEA): *www.elderabusecenter.org*

Gastrointestinal
- American Liver Foundation: 800-GO LIVER (465-4837)
- National Institute of Diabetes & Digestive & Kidney Diseases: *www.niddk.nih.gov*; 301-654-3810
- National Kidney Foundation: *www.kidney.org*; national office, 800-622-9010

Musculoskeletal
- American College of Foot and Ankle Surgeons: 888-843-3338
- Amputee Coalition of America: *www.amputee-coalition.org*; 888-AMP-KNOW (267-5669)
- National Association of the Physically Handicapped, Inc.: *www.naph.net*
- National Institutes of Health, Osteoporosis and Related Bone Diseases National Resource Center: 800-624-BONE
- National Osteoporosis Foundation: *www.nof.org*

Neurology
- ALS Association, National Office: *www.alsa.org*; information and referral service, 800-782-4747; all others, 818-880-9007
- ALS Association of Massachusetts: 800-258-3323
- American Brain Tumor Association: *www.abta.org*; 800-886-2282
- Association of Late-Deafened Adults, Inc., 10310 Main St., #274, Fairfax, VA 22030; TTY, 404-289-1596; fax, 404-284-6862
- EAR Foundation/Meniere's Network, American Academy of Otolaryngology, One Prince St., Alexandria, VA 22314; 703-836-4444

- National Association of the Deaf: *NADinfo@nad.org*
- National Federation of the Blind: *www.nfb.org*; 1800 Johnson Street, Baltimore, MD 21230; 410-659-9314
- National Institute of Neurological Disorders and Stroke (NINDS): *www.ninds.nih.gov*
- National Institute on Deafness and Other Communication Disorders (NIDCD): *www.nidcd.nih.gov*

Pediatrics
- CFUSA-Cystic Fibrosis USA: *www.cfusa.org*
- Children with Diabetes: *www.childrenwithdiabetes.com*
- Cystic Fibrosis Foundation: *www.cff.org*; 800-FIGHT CF, (344-4823)
- Cystic Fibrosis Mutation Data Base: *www.genet.sickkids.on.ca/cftr*
- Down's Heart Group: *www.downs-heart.downsnet.org*
- Emory University Sickle Cell Information Center (24 hours): *www.emory.edu* (enter "sickle cell" in the search box); 404-616-3572
- Families of S.M.A. (Spinal Muscular Atrophy): *www.fsma.org*; 800-886-1762
- Growth Charts for Children with Down Syndrome: *www.growthcharts.com*
- Internet Resources for Special Children (IRSC): *www.irsc.org*
- National Down Syndrome Society: *www.ndss.org*
- National Institute of Child Health & Human Development (NICHD): *www.nichd.nih.gov*
- NPAN, the National Pediatric AIDS Network: *www.npan.org*
- Spina Bifida Association of America: *www.sbaa.org*; 800-621-3141
- United Cerebral Palsy UCPnet: *www.ucpnatl@ucpa.org*; 800-872-5827

Psychiatry
- American Psychological Association: *www.apa.org*; 800-374-3120
- National Alliance for the Mentally Ill: *www.nami.org*; 800-950-NAMI (950-6264)
- National Depressive and Manic-Depressive Association: *www.ndmda.org*; 800-826-3632
- National Mental Health Association: *www.nmha.org*; 800-969-6642

Respiratory
- American Association for Respiratory Care: *www.aarc.org*

- American Heart Association: 800-242-8721 (smoking cessation information)
- American Lung Association: *www.lungusa.org;* 800-LUNG-USA (local affiliates answer)
- National Emphysema Foundation: *www.emphysemafoundation.org*

Skin
- National Pressure Ulcer Advisory Panel (NPUAP) (information on the PUSH tool and monitoring ulcers): *www.npuap.org*
- Wound Care Information Network — information for patients and professionals, including support groups: *www.medicaledu.com*
- Wound Care Institute, Inc. — newsletter, free products for financial hardships: *www.woundcare.org;* 305-919-9192
- Wound, Ostomy and Continence Nurses Society: *www.wocn.org;* 888-224-WOCN

Substance abuse
- Al-Anon & Alateen: *www.al-anon.alateen.org;* 888-4AL-ANON (425-2666) (Spanish and French language options)
- Alcoholics Anonymous: *www.alcoholics-anonymous.org* (Spanish and French language options)
- Narcotics Anonymous World Services: *www.wsoinc.com*
- National Centers for Disease Control and Prevention, National Center for Chronic Disease Prevention: *www.cdc.gov/tobacco*
- National Council on Alcoholism and Drug Dependence: 800-NCA-CALL (622-2255)
- National Institute on Alcohol Abuse and Alcoholism: *www.niaaa.nih.gov;* 301-443-3860
- Substance Abuse & Mental Health Services Administration: *www.samhsa.gov*

Women's health
- American College of Cardiology: *www.acc.org*
- American Heart Association: *www.women.americanheart.org*
- American Medical Women's Association:*www.amwadoc.org*
- *JAMA* Women's Health Information Center: *www.ama-assn.org/special/womh/womh.htm*
- Johns Hopkins Intelihealth: *www.intelihealth.com/specials/htWomen.htm*

- Office on Women's Health/U.S. Department of Health & Human Services: *www.4women.gov/owh*
- Womens' Health Initiative (WHI): *www.nhlbi.nih.gov/whi*

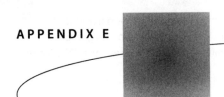

Commonly used medical abbreviations

Here is a list of commonly used medical abbreviations. You may find this list helpful when you're using the flowcharts in this book.

AAA	abdominal aortic aneurysm		AROM	active range of motion; artificial rupture of membranes
ABC	airway, breathing, and circulation		ASA	acetylsalicylic acid (aspirin)
ABG	arterial blood gas		ASD	atrial septal defect
ACE	angiotensin-converting enzyme		AV	atrioventricular
ACLS	advanced cardiac life support		AVM	arteriovenous malformation
ACTH	adrenocorticotropic hormone		BBB	bundle-branch block
ADH	antidiuretic hormone		BCP	birth control pill
ADLs	activities of daily living		BE	barium enema
AED	automated external defibrillator		b.i.d.	two times per day
AFB	acid fast bacilli		BKA	below-knee amputation
AFIB	atrial fibrillation		BM	bowel movement
AIDS	acquired immunodeficiency syndrome		BMR	basal metabolic rate
AKA	above-knee amputation		BP	blood pressure
ALL	acute lymphocytic leukemia		BPH	benign prostatic hyperplasia
ALS	amyotrophic lateral sclerosis		BSA	body surface area
AMA	against medical advice		BUN	blood urea nitrogen
ANA	antinuclear antibody		BW	birth weight
AP	anteroposterior; apical pulse		C	centigrade; Celsius
ARDS	adult respiratory distress syndrome		Ca	calcium
ARF	acute renal failure; acute respiratory failure		CABG	coronary artery bypass graft

CAD	coronary artery disease		DNA	deoxyribonucleic acid
CAPD	continuous ambulatory peritoneal dialysis		DNR	do not resuscitate
CAVH	continuous arteriovenous hemofiltration		DOA	date of admission; dead on arrival
CBC	complete blood count		DOB	date of birth
CC	chief complaint		DPT	diphtheria, pertussis, and tetanus
CCU	coronary care unit		*DSM-IV*	*Diagnostic and Statistical Manual of Mental Disorders,* 4th ed.
CDC	Centers for Disease Control and Prevention		DTR	deep tendon reflex
CEA	carcinoembryonic antigen		DVT	deep vein thrombosis
CF	cystic fibrosis		D5W	dextrose 5% in water
CK	creatine kinase		DX	diagnosis
CMV	cytomegalovirus		ECF	extended care facility; extracellular fluid
CNS	central nervous system		ECG	electrocardiogram
COPD	chronic obstructive pulmonary disease		ECMO	extracorporeal membrane oxygenator
CP	cerebral palsy		ECT	electroconvulsive therapy
CPAP	continuous positive airway pressure		ED	emergency department
CPP	cerebral perfusion pressure		EDC	estimated date of confinement
CPR	cardiopulmonary resuscitation		EDD	estimated date of delivery
C&S	culture and sensitivity		EEG	electroencephalogram
CSF	cerebrospinal fluid		EENT	eyes, ears, nose, and throat
CT	computed tomography		EF	ejection fraction
CV	cardiovascular		ELISA	enzyme-linked immunosorbent assay
CVP	central venous pressure		EMG	electromyogram
CXR	chest X-ray		EMS	emergency medical services
DC	direct current		ENT	ear, nose, and throat
DHEA	dehydroepiandrosterone		EOM	extraocular movements
DIC	disseminated intravascular coagulation		ER	emergency room; expiratory reserve
DJD	degenerative joint disease		ERCP	endoscopic retrograde cholangiopancreatography
DKA	diabetic ketoacidosis		ERV	expiratory reserve volume
DM	diabetes mellitus		ESR	erythrocyte sedimentation rate

ETOH	ethanol (ethyl alcohol)
F	Fahrenheit
FBS	fasting blood sugar
FDA	Food and Drug Administration
FEF	forced expiratory flow
FEV	forced expiratory volume
FFP	fresh frozen plasma
FH	family history
FHR	fetal heart rate
FRC	functional residual capacity
FSH	follicle-stimulating hormone
FSP	fibin split products
F/U	follow-up
FUO	fever of unknown origin
FVC	forced vital capacity
G	gravida
g	gram
GB	gallbladder
GBS	gallbladder series
GERD	gastroesophageal reflux disease
GFR	glomerular filtration rate
GI	gastrointestinal
GP	general practitioner
gr	grain
gtt	drops
GU	genitourinary
GVHD	graft-versus-host disease
GYN	gynecology
Hb	hemoglobin

HBIG	hepatitis B immunoglobulin
HBsAg	hepatitis B surface antigen
HCG	human chorionic gonadotropin
HCT	hematocrit
HEENT	head, ears, eyes, nose and throat
Hg	mercury
H/H	hemoglobin and hematocrit
HHA	home health aide
HHNS	hyperosmolar hyperglycemic nonketotic syndrome
HIV	human immunodeficiency virus
HLA	human leukocyte antigen
HMO	health maintenance organization
H_2O	water
H_2O_2	hydrogen peroxide
HOB	head of bed
HPI	history of present illness
h.s.	hour of sleep
HSV	herpes simplex virus
IABP	intra-aortic balloon pump
ICD	implantable cardioverter defibrillator
ICP	intracranial pressure
ICU	intensive care unit
I&D	incision and drainage
I.M.	intramuscular
I&O	intake and output
IOP	intraocular pressure
IPPB	intermittent positive-pressure breathing
IU	international unit
IUD	intrauterine device

I.V.	intravenous		Mg	magnesium
IVP	intravenous pyelography		mg	milligram
JVD	jugular venous distention		MI	myocardial infarction
K	potassium		MIBG	meta-iodobenzylguanidine
KCl	potassium chloride		ml	milliliter
kg	kilogram		MRA	magnetic resonance angiography
KUB	kidneys, ureters, and bladder (X-ray)		MRI	magnetic resonance imaging
KVO	keep vein open		MS	multiple sclerosis; mitral stenosis
L	left, liter		Na	sodium
LDH	lactate dehydrogenase		N/A	not applicable
LDL	low-density lipoprotein		NaCl	sodium chloride
LE	lower extremity		NAD	no acute distress
LFT	liver function tests		NAS	no added salt
LH	luteinizing hormone		NG	nasogastric
LLL	left lower lobe		NICU	neonatal intensive care unit
LLQ	left lower quadrant		NKA	no known allergies
LMP	last menstrual period		NMR	nuclear magnetic resonance
LOC	level of consciousness		NPO	nothing by mouth
LP	lumbar puncture		NSAID	nonsteroidal anti-inflammatory drug
LUE	left upper extremity		NSR	normal sinus rhythm
LUL	left upper lobe		NWB	non-weight bearing
LUQ	left upper quadrant		OB	obstetrics
LVEDP	left ventricular end-diastolic pressure		o.d.	daily
LVH	left ventricular hypertrophy		OOB	out of bed
MAO	monoamine oxidase		OPV	oral polio vaccine
MAP	mean arterial pressure		OR	operating room
mcg	microgram		ORIF	open reduction internal fixation
MCL	midclavicular line		OT	occupational therapy
mEq	milliequivalent		OTC	over the counter

P	pulse		RAI	radioactive iodine
PAT	paroxysmal atrial tachycardia		RAP	right atrial pressure
PAWP	pulmonary artery wedge pressure		RBBB	right bundle-branch block
PCA	patient-controlled analgesia		RBC	red blood cell
PCI	percutaneous coronary intervention		REM	rapid eye movement
PDA	patent ductus arteriosus		Rh	Rhesus factor
PE	physical examination		RICE	rest, ice, compression, elevation
PERRLA	pupils equal, round, react to light and accommodation		RLE	right lower extremity
PET	positron-emission tomography		RLL	right lower lobe
PFT	pulmonary function tests		RLQ	right lower quadrant
PICC	peripherally inserted central catheter		RML	right middle lobe
PID	pelvic inflammatory disease		ROM	range of motion
PIH	pregnancy-induced hypertension		RR	respiratory rate
PKU	phenylketonuria		R/T	related to
PMI	point of maximal impulse		RUL	right upper lobe
PMS	premenstrual syndrome		RUQ	right upper quadrant
P.O.	by mouth		Rx	prescription, treatment, or therapy
PRBC	packed red blood cells		SBE	self-breast examination
p.r.n.	as needed		S.C.	subcutaneous
PROM	passive range of motion		SG	specific gravity
PSA	prostate-specific antigen		SIDS	sudden infant death syndrome
PT	prothrombin time		S.L.	sublingual
PTCA	percutaneous transluminal coronary angioplasty		SLE	systemic lupus erythematosus
PTT	partial thromboplastin time		SNF	skilled nursing facility
PVC	premature ventricular contraction		SOB	shortness of breath
PVD	peripheral vascular disease		SSE	soapsuds enema
q.h.	every hour		SSRI	selective-serotonin reuptake inhibitors
q.o.d.	every other day		STD	sexually transmitted disease
RA	right atrium; right arm; renal artery		STS	serologic test for syphilis

SVD	spontaneous vaginal delivery
T_3	triiodothyronine
T_4	thyroxine
TAH	total abdominal hysterectomy
TB	tuberculosis
Tc	technetium
TCA	tricyclic antidepressants
TEE	transesophageal echocardiogram
TENS	transcutaneous electrical nerve stimulation
TIA	transient ischemic attack
TIBC	total iron-binding capacity
t.i.d.	three times per day
TMJ	temporomandibular joint
T.O.	telephone order
TPN	total parenteral nutrition
TPR	temperature, pulse, and respirations
TSH	thyroid stimulating hormone
TUR	transurethral resection
TURP	transurethral resection of the prostate
TX	treatment
U	unit
UA	urinalysis
UE	upper extremity
URI	upper respiratory infection
USP	*United States Pharmacopeia*
UTI	urinary tract infection
UV	ultraviolet
VAD	vascular access device; ventricular assist device
VC	vital capacity

VD	venereal disease
VDRL	Venereal Disease Research Laboratory (test)
VF	ventricular fibrillation
VO	verbal order
$\dot{V}/\dot{Q}$	ventilation-perfusion
VSD	ventricular septal defect
VT	ventricular tachycardia
V_T	tidal volume
WBC	white blood cell
WNL	within normal limits
WPW	Wolff-Parkinson-White (syndrome)

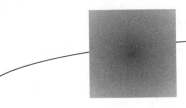

Selected references

Abeloff, M., et al. Clinical Oncology. New York: Churchill-Livingstone, Inc., 1999

American Heart Association. *Guidelines for Cardiopulmonary Resuscitation and Emergency Cardiovascular Care.* Dallas: 2000.

Apple, S., and Lindsay, J. *Principles & Practice of Interventional Cardiology.* Baltimore: Lippincott Williams & Wilkins, 2000.

Aronson, B.S. "Update on Acute Pancreatitis," *Med-Surg Nursing* 8(1):9-16, February 1999.

Association of Women's Health, Obstetric, and Neonatal Nurses, Mandeville, L.K., and Troiano, N.H., eds. *AWHONN's High Risk and Critical Care Intrapartum Nursing,* 2nd ed. Philadelphia: Lippincott Williams & Wilkins, 1999.

Auscultation Skills: Breath and Heart Sounds. Springhouse, Pa.: Springhouse Corporation, 1999.

Bartlett, J.G. *2002 Pocket Book of Infectious Disease Therapy,* 11th ed. Baltimore: Lippincott Williams & Wilkins, 2002.

Bartlett, J.G. *Management of Respiratory Tract Infections,* 3rd ed. Baltimore: Lippincott Williams & Wilkins, 2001.

Beattie, S. "Cut the Risks for Cardiac Cath Patients," *RN* 62(1):50-55, January 1999.

Beers, M., et al. *Merck Manual Diagnosis and Therapy.* Whitehouse Station, N.J.: Merck and Co., Inc., 1999.

Bickley, L.S., and Hoekelman, R.A. Bates' Guide to Physical Examination and History Taking, 7th ed. Philadelphia: Lippincott Williams & Wilkins, 1999.

Blank-Reid, C., and Reid, P. "Taking the Tension out of Traumatic Pneumothoraxes," *Nursing99* 29(4):41-46, April 1999.

Bullock, B.L., and Henze, R.L. *Focus on Pathophysiology.* Philadelphia: Lippincott Williams & Wilkins, 2000.

Bunevicius, R., et al. "Effects of Thyroxine as Compared with Thyroxine Plus Triiodothyronine in Patients with Hypothyroidism," *New England Journal of Medicine* 340(6):424-29, February 1999.

Burroughs, A., and Leifer, G. *Maternity Nursing: An Introductory Text,* 8th ed. Philadelphia: W.B. Saunders Co., 2001.

Busse, W., et al. "Pathology of Severe Asthma." *Journal of Allergy and Clinical Immunology* 106(6):1033-42 December 2000.

Chernecky, C.C., and Berger, B.J. *Laboratory Tests and Diagnostic Procedures,* 3rd ed. Philadelphia: W.B. Saunders Co., 2001.

Christensen, B.L., and Kockrow, E.O. *Foundations of Nursing,* 3rd ed. St. Louis: Mosby–Year Book, Inc., 1999.

Copel, L.C. *Nurse's Clinical Guide: Psychiatric and Mental Health Care.* 2nd ed. Springhouse, Pa.: Springhouse Corp., 2000.

Critical Care Nursing Made Incredibly Easy (CD-ROM). Springhouse, Pa.: Springhouse Corp., 2001.

Darovic, G.O., and Franklin, C.M. *Handbook of Hemodynamic Monitoring.* Philadelphia: W.B. Saunders Co., 1999.

DeVita, V., et al. *Cancer: Principle and Practice of Oncology.* Philadelphia: Lippincott Williams & Wilkins. 2000

Diagnostic and Statistical Manual of Mental Disorders, 4th ed. Washington, D.C.: American Psychiatric Association, 1994.

Diagnostics: An A-to-Z Nursing Guide to Laboratory Tests & Diagnostic Procedures. Springhouse, Pa.: Springhouse Corp., 2001.

Diepenbrock, N.H. *Quick Reference to Critical Care.* Philadelphia: Lippincott Williams & Wilkins, 1999.

Dillon, J.J. "Continuous Renal Replacement Therapy or Hemodialysis for Acute Renal Failure?" *International Journal of Artificial Organs* 22(3):125-27, March 1999.

Diseases, 3rd ed. Springhouse, Pa.: Springhouse Corp., 2001.

Dolan, B., and Holt, L. *Accident and Emergency Care: Theory into Practice.* Philadelphia: W.B. Saunders Co., 1999.

Dudek, S.G. *Nutrition Handbook for Nursing Practice,* 4th ed. Philadelphia: Lippincott Williams & Wilkins, 2001.

ECG Cards, 3rd ed. Springhouse, Pa.: Springhouse Corp., 2000.

ECG Interpretation Made Incredibly Easy, 2nd ed. Springhouse, Pa.: Springhouse Corp., 2001.

Elkin, M.K., et al. *Nursing Interventions and Clinical Skills,* 2nd ed. St. Louis: Mosby–Year Book, Inc., 2000.

Falk, K.M. "Cancer Treatment" in *Principles and Practices for the Acute Care NP.* Stanford, Conn.: Appleton & Lange, 1999.

Fitzpatrick, T.B., et al. *Color Atlas and Synopsis of Clinical Dermatology: Common and Serious Diseases,* 4th ed. New York: McGraw-Hill Book Co., 2001.

Fleischer, A.B., Jr. *20 Common Problems in Dermatology.* New York: McGraw-Hill Book Co., 2000.

Fluids and Electrolytes Made Incredibly Easy, 2nd ed. Springhouse, Pa.: Springhouse Corp., 2001.

Fraunfelder, F.T., and Roy, F.H. *Current Ocular Therapy,* 5th ed. Philadelphia: W.B. Saunders Co., 2000.

Goldman, L., and Bennett, J.C. *Cecil Textbook of Medicine*, 21st ed. Philadelphia: W.B. Saunders Co., 2000.

Greinenko, A. "Rapid Screening for Disordered Eating in College-Aged Females in the Primary Care Setting," *Journal of Adolescent Health* 26(5):338-42, 2000.

Grenvik, A., et al. *Textbook of Critical Care,* 4th ed. Philadelphia: W.B. Saunders Co., 2000

Handbook of Geriatric Nursing Care. Springhouse, Pa.: Springhouse Corp., 1999.

Harwood-Nuss, A.L. *The Clinical Practice of Emergency Medicine,* 3rd ed. Philadelphia: Lippincott Williams & Wilkins, 2000.

Heitz, U.E., et al. *Pocket Guide to Fluid, Electrolyte, and Acid-Base Balance,* 4th ed. St. Louis: Mosby–Year Book, Inc., 2000.

Humes, H. "Limiting Acute Renal Failure," *Hospital Practice* 34(1):31-38,41-42,47-48, January 1999.

Humes, H.D., et al. *Kelley's Textbook of Internal Medicine,* 4th ed. Philadelphia: Lippincott Williams & Wilkins, 2000.

Ignatavicius, D.D., et al., eds. *Medical-Surgical Nursing Across the Health Care Continuum,* 3rd ed., Philadelphia: W.B. Saunders Co., 1999.

Isaacs, A. *Lippincott's Review Series: Mental Health and Psychiatric Nursing.* Philadelphia: Lippincott Williams & Wilkins, 2000.

Isselbacher, K.J., et al., eds. *Harrison's Principles of Internal Medicine,* 15th ed. New York: McGraw-Hill Book Co., 2001.

Katz, D.L. *Nutrition in Clinical Practice.* Philadelphia: Lippincott Williams & Wilkins, 2001.

Kern, M.J. *The Cardiac Catheterization Handbook,* 3rd ed. St. Louis: Mosby–Year Book, Inc., 1999.

Ketner, K. "Identifying the Adolescent at Risk" in *Summary of 23rd Annual California Coalition of Nurse Practitioners Educational Conference.* 2000.

Kingsley, R.E. *Concise Text of Neuroscience,* 2nd ed. Philadelphia: Lippincott Williams & Wilkins, 1999.

Kirsner, J.B., ed. *Inflammatory Bowel Disease,* 5th ed. Philadelphia: W.B. Saunders Co., 2000.

Kluth, D.C., and Rees, A.J. "New Approaches to Modify Glomerular Inflammation," *Journal of Nephrology* 12(2):66-75, 1999.

Kooperman, W. *Arthritis and Allied Conditions: A Textbook of Rheumatology,* 14th ed. Philadelphia: Lippincott Williams & Wilkins, 2000.

Lahita, R., et al. *Textbook of Autoimmune Diseases.* Philadelphia: Lippincott Williams & Wilkins, 2000.

Lamkin, J.C. *Massachusetts Eye & Ear Infirmary Review Manual for Ophthalmology,* 2nd ed. Philadelphia: Lippincott Williams & Wilkins, 1999.

Lanken, P.N. *The Intensive Care Unit Manual.* Philadelphia: W.B. Saunders Co., 2001.

Lee, K.J. *Essential Otolaryngology: Head and Neck Surgery,* 7th ed. Stamford, Conn.: Appleton & Lange, 1999.

Leifer, G. *Thompson's Introduction to Maternity and Pediatric Nursing,* 3rd ed. Philadelphia: W.B. Saunders Co., 1999.

Lewis, A.M. "Gastrointestinal Emergency!" *Nursing99* 29(4):52-54, April 1999.

Lewis, S.M., et al., ed. *Medical-Surgical Nursing: Assessment and Management of Clinical Problems,* 5th ed. St. Louis: Mosby–Year Book, 2000.

Lowdermilk, D.L., et al. *Maternity Nursing,* 5th ed. St. Louis: Mosby–Year Book, Inc., 1999.

Maas, M., et al. *Nursing Care of Older Adults: Diagnoses, Outcomes, and Interventions.* St. Louis: Mosby–Year Book, Inc., 2000.

Mahan, L.K., and Escott-Stump, S. *Krause's Food, Nutrition, and Diet Therapy,* 10th ed. Philadelphia: W.B. Saunders Co., 2000.

Mauch, P., et al. *Hodgkin's Disease.* Philadelphia: Lippincott Williams & Wilkins. 1999.

Melson, K.A., et al. *Maternal-Infant Care Planning,* 3rd ed. Springhouse, Pa.: Springhouse Corp., 1999.

Miracle, V.A., and Sims, J.M. "Making Sense of the 12-Lead ECG," *Nursing99* 29(7):34-39, July 1999.

Novak, J.C., and Broom, B.L. *Ingalls and Salerno's Maternal and Child Health Nursing,* 9th ed. St. Louis: Mosby–Year Book, Inc., 1999.

Nursing Procedures, 3rd ed. Springhouse, Pa.: Springhouse Corp., 2000.

Oman, K.S., et al. *Emergency Nursing Secrets.* Philadelphia: Lippincott Williams & Wilkins, 2000.

Pillitteri, A. *Maternal and Child Health Nursing: Care of the Childbearing and Childrearing Family,* 3rd ed. Philadelphia: Lippincott Williams & Wilkins, 1999.

Pomerantz, J. "Managed Care and Suicide Prevention," *Drug Benefit Trends* 12(6):5-6, June 2000.

Rakel, R.E., ed. *Conn's Current Therapy, 2001.* Philadelphia: W.B. Saunders Co., 2001.

Rhee, D.J., and Pyfer, M.F. *The Wills Eye Manual: Office and Emergency Room Diagnosis and Treatment of Eye Disease,* 3rd ed. Philadelphia: Lippincott Williams & Wilkins, 1999.

Savage, L.S., and Canody C. "Life with a Left Ventricular Assist Device: The Patient's Perspective," *American Journal of Critical Care* 8(5):340-43, September 1999.

Shortall, S.P., and Perkins L.A. "Interpreting the Ins and Outs of Pulmonary Function Tests," *Nursing99* 29(12):41-46, December 1999.

Simon, R.P., et al. *Clinical Neurology,* 4th ed. Stamford, Conn.: Appleton & Lange, 1999.

Singleton, J.K., et al. *Primary Care.* Philadelphia: Lippincott Williams & Wilkins, 1999.

Smeltzer, S., and Bare, B. *Brunner & Suddarth's Textbook of Medical-Surgical Nursing*, 9th ed. Philadelphia: Lippincott Williams & Wilkins, 2000.

Smith, R., et al. "American Cancer Society Guidelines for Early Detection of Cancer" *CA-A Journal for Clinicians* 50: 34-49, 2000.

Stone, D.R., and Gorbach, L.S. *Atlas of Infectious Diseases*. Philadelphia: W.B. Saunders Co., 2000.

Thiedke, C., and Rosenfeld, J.A. *Women's Health (American Academy of Family Physicians)*. Philadelphia: Lippincott Williams & Wilkins, 2000.

Tierney, L.M., et al. *Current Medical Diagnosis and Treatment 2002,* New York: McGraw-Hill Book Co., 2001.

Tintinalli, J., ed. *Emergency Medicine: A Comprehensive Study Guide,* 5th ed. New York: McGraw-Hill Book Co., 2000.

Townsend, M.C. *Psychiatric Mental Health Nursing: Concepts of Care*, 3rd ed. Philadelphia: F.A. Davis Co., 1999.

Turjanica, M.A. "Anatomy of a Code: How Do You Feel at the Start of a Code Blue?" *Nursing Management* 30(11):44-49, November 1999.

Vaughan, D., et al. *General Ophthalmology,* 15th ed. Stamford, Conn.: Appleton & Lange, 1999.

White, G., and Cox, N. *Diseases of the Skin: A Color Atlas and Text.* St. Louis: Mosby–Year Book, Inc., 2000.

Zerbe, K.J. *Women's Mental Health in Primary Care.* Philadelphia: W.B. Saunders Co., 1999.

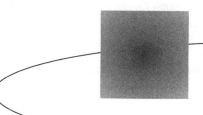

Index

i refers to an illustration; t refers to a table

i refers to an illustration; t refers to a table

i refers to an illustration; t refers to a table

Brain abscess
  apraxia and, 35i
  complex partial seizures and, 363i
  decorticate posture and, 113i
  headache and, 193i
  level of consciousness decrease and, 237i
  simple partial seizures and, 365i
  spastic gait and, 179i
Brain lesion, muscle flaccidity and, 257i
Brain neoplasms, anosmia and, 25i. *See also* Brain tumor.
Brain stem glioma, gag reflex abnormalities and, 175i. *See also* Brain stem tumor, absent doll's eye and.
Brain stem infarction
  absent corneal reflex and, 99i
  absent doll's eye sign and, 127i
  decerebrate posture and, 111i
Brain stem injury, absent corneal reflex and, 99i
Brain stem involvement
  analgesia and, 21i
  apnea and, 33i
Brain stem stroke, dysarthria and, 131i
Brain stem tumor, absent doll's eye sign and, 127i. *See also* Brain stem glioma, gag reflex abnormalities and.
Brain tumor. *See also* Brain neoplasms, anosmia and.
  aphasia and, 31i
  apraxia and, 35i
  athetosis and, 45i
  Babinski's reflex and, 47i
  confusion and, 93i
  decorticate posture and, 113i
  diplopia and, 123i
  headache and, 193i
  level of consciousness decrease and, 237i
  nystagmus and, 281i
  ocular deviation and, 283i
  simple partial seizures and, 365i
  spastic gait and, 179i
Breast abscess
  breast nodule and, 67i
  breast pain and, 69i
  nipple discharge and, 275i
  peau d'orange and, 305i
Breast cancer
  breast nodule and, 67i
  breast ulcer and, 71i
  nipple discharge and, 275i
  peau d'orange and, 305i
Breast cyst, breast pain and, 69i
Breast nodule, 66, 67i
Breast pain, 68, 69i
Breast trauma, breast ulcer and, 71i

Breast ulcer, 70, 71i
Breath, abnormal, 72, 73i
Breath sounds, evaluating, 416i
Bronchiectasis, hemoptysis and, 205i
Bronchitis
  asterixis and, 41i
  barrel chest and, 51i
  clubbing and, 91i
  cough and, 103i
  hemoptysis and, 205i
  rhonchi and, 355i
  wheezing and, 417i
Brudzinski's sign, 74, 75i
  testing for, 74i
Bruits, 76, 77i
Buerger's disease, cyanosis and, 109i
Bulimia, polyphagia and, 315i
Burns, erythema and, 155i
Bursitis, arm pain and, 38i
Butterfly rash, 78, 79i
  recognizing, 78i

C

Cancer, anorexia and, 23i. *See also specific type.*
Candida albicans infection, breast ulcer and, 71i
Candidiasis, vaginal discharge and, 401i
Carbon monoxide poisoning, propulsive gait and, 178i
Cardiac arrhythmia
  bounding pulse and, 327i
  bradycardia and, 63i
  dizziness and, 125i
  palpitations and, 297i
  syncope and, 375i
  tachycardia and, 377i
  types of, 430-435i
Cardiac tamponade
  abnormal pulse pressure and, 329i
  jugular vein distention and, 231i
  pulsus paradoxus and, 333i
Cardinal fields of gaze, 122i
Cardiogenic shock
  anxiety and, 29i
  blood pressure decrease and, 55i
  clammy skin and, 367i
Cardiomyopathy. *See also* Hypertrophic cardiomyopathy.
  atrial gallop and, 181i
  bradycardia and, 63i
  murmurs and, 253i
  ventricular gallop and, 181i
Carotid artery aneurysm
  hemianopia and, 203i
  mydriasis and, 263i

i refers to an illustration; t refers to a table

i refers to an illustration; t refers to a table

i refers to an illustration; t refers to a table

i refers to an illustration; t refers to a table

i refers to an illustration; t refers to a table

i refers to an illustration; t refers to a table

i refers to an illustration; t refers to a table

Mesenteric artery occlusion
  absent bowel sounds and, 59i
  hypoactive bowel sounds and, 61i
MI. *See* Myocardial infarction.
Migraine headache
  light flashes and, 239i
  paresthesia and, 303i
  scotoma and, 359i
  visual blurring and, 409i
Miosis, 248, 249i
Mitral insufficiency
  atrial gallop and, 181i
  murmurs and, 253i
  ventricular gallop and, 181i
Mitral prolapse, palpitations and, 297i
Mitral regurgitation. *See* Mitral insufficiency.
Mitral stenosis, palpitations and, 297i
Mobitz I, 433i
Mobitz II, 433i
Mononucleosis, throat pain and, 381i
Mouth lesions, 250, 250i, 251i
Multiple sclerosis
  footdrop and, 173i
  muscle atrophy and, 255i
  muscle spasms and, 259i
  muscle weakness and, 261i
  ocular deviation and, 283i
  paresthesia and, 303i
  Romberg's sign and, 357i
  spastic gait and, 179i
  spasticity and, 259i
Murmurs, 252, 253i
  identifying, 252i
Muscle atrophy, 254, 255i
Muscle cramps, 258, 259i
Muscle flaccidity, 256, 257i
Muscle hypertonicity, 258, 259i
Muscle spasms, 258, 259i
Muscle strain, chest pain and, 85i
Muscle strength, testing, 260
Muscle weakness, 260, 261i
Myasthenia gravis
  dysarthria and, 131i
  dysphagia and, 139i
  gag reflex abnormalities and, 175i
  masklike facies and, 243i
Mydriasis, 262, 263i
Myocardial infarction
  anxiety and, 29i
  atrial gallop and, 181i
  blood pressure decrease and, 55i

Myocardial infarction *(continued)*
  bradycardia and, 63i
  chest pain and, 83i
  diaphoresis and, 119i
  jaw pain and, 229i
  ventricular gallop and, 181i
Myoclonus, 264, 265i
Myotonic dystrophy, ptosis and, 323i
Myringitis, otorrhea and, 293i
Myxedema, generalized edema and, 150i

N

Nasal flaring, 266, 267i
  respiratory distress in infants and, 266i
Nasal neoplasms, anosmia and, 25i
Nasal obstruction, 268, 269i
Nasal polyps
  anosmia and, 25i
  nasal obstruction and, 269i
Nasal speculum, how to use, 352i
Nausea, 270, 271i
Neck pain, 272, 273i
  applying a Philadelphia collar for, 272i
Necrotizing ulcerative gingivitis, gum bleeding and, 185i
Neoplasms
  anosmia and, 25i
  fever and, 169i
Neuromuscular failure, apnea and, 33i
Nipple discharge, 274, 275i
  eliciting, 275i
Nocturia, 276, 277i
Non-Hodgkin's lymphoma, purpura and, 339i
Nuchal rigidity, 278, 279i
  testing for, 278i
Nummular dermatitis, scaly skin and, 369i
Nystagmus, 280, 281i
  classifying, 280i

O

Occipital lobe lesion, hemianopia and, 203i
Ocular deviation, 282, 283i
  cranial nerve damage and, 282t
Oculomotor nerve palsy
  mydriasis and, 263i
  nonreactive pupils and, 335i
Oligomenorrhea, 284, 285i
Oliguria, 286, 287i
Ophthalmic migraine, diplopia and, 123i
Ophthalmoplegic migraine, ocular deviation and, 283i
Opisthotonos, 288, 289i
  as sign of meningeal irritation, 288i

i refers to an illustration; t refers to a table

i refers to an illustration; t refers to a table

i refers to an illustration; t refers to a table

Pulse pressure, abnormal, 328, 329i
Pulsus bisferiens, 330, 331i
Pulsus paradoxus, 332, 333i
Pupillary light reflexes, innervation of, 334i
Pupils
    grading size of, 262l
    nonreactive, 334, 335i
    sluggish, 336, 337i
Purpura, 338, 339i
    identifying lesions of, 338i
Pustular rash, 340, 341i
Pustule, identifying, 340i
PVC. *See* Premature ventricular contraction.
Pyelonephritis
    dysuria and, 145i
    oliguria and, 287i
    polyuria and, 317i
Pyrosis, 342, 343i

R

Raynaud's disease, cyanosis and, 109i
Raynaud's phenomenon, pallor and, 295i
Rectal cancer, rectal pain and, 345i
Rectal pain, 344, 345i
Reflux esophagitis
    dysphagia and, 139i
    pyrosis and, 343i
Regurgitation, mechanism and cause of, 342
Reiter's syndrome
    dysuria and, 145i
    urinary urgency and, 397i
Renal artery occlusion, anuria and, 27i
Renal artery stenosis, bruits and, 77i
Renal calculi
    abdominal pain and, 7i
    flank pain and, 171i
    hematuria and, 201i
Renal cancer
    flank pain and, 171i
    hematuria and, 201i
Renal disease, end-stage, abnormal breath and, 73i
Renal failure, acute
    generalized edema and, 150i
    major causes of, 26i
Renal failure, chronic, agitation and, 13i
Renal failure, end-stage
    bradypnea and, 65i
    Cheyne-Stokes respirations and, 87i
Renovascular stenosis, blood pressure increase and, 57i

Respirations
    abnormal, 346, 347i, 348i, 349i
    Cheyne-Stokes, 86
Respiratory distress, nasal flaring and, 266i
Respiratory distress syndrome
    grunting respirations and, 347i
    retractions and, 351i
Respiratory failure, end-stage, bradypnea and, 65i
Respiratory insufficiency, severe, asterixis and, 41i
Retinal detachment
    light flashes and, 239i
    vision loss and, 407i
    visual blurring and, 409i
Retractions, 350, 351i
    observing, 350i
Retropharyngeal abscess, drooling and, 129i
Rheumatoid arthritis, 428i
    mottled skin and, 368i
    nuchal rigidity and, 279i
Rhinitis, anosmia and, 25i
Rhinorrhea, 352, 353i
Rhonchi, 354, 355i
Rib fracture, 427i
Right ventricular infarct, pulsus paradoxus and, 333i
Romberg's sign, 356, 357i
Rosacea
    butterfly rash and, 79i
    papular rash and, 299i
    pustular rash and, 341i
Rotator cuff tear
    arm pain and, 37i
    and meniscal tear, 429i
Ruptured esophagus, subcutaneous crepitation and, 107i
Ruptured major bronchus, subcutaneous crepitation and, 107i
Ruptured trachea, subcutaneous crepitation and, 107i

S

Scabies, vesicular rash and, 405i
Scleritis, exophthalmos and, 157i
Scotoma, 358, 359i
Scrotal swelling, 360, 361i
Scurvy. *See* Vitamin C deficiency.
Sebaceous cyst, infected, breast pain and, 69i
Seborrheic dermatitis
    alopecia and, 15i
    erythema and, 155i
    scaly skin and, 369i
Second-degree atrioventricular block, 433i
Seizure disorder, myoclonus and, 265i
Seizures, 362, 363i, 364i, 365i
    amnesia and, 19i

i refers to an illustration; t refers to a table

i refers to an illustration; t refers to a table

i refers to an illustration; t refers to a table

i refers to an illustration; t refers to a table